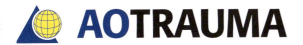

Klaus Dresing | Peter Trafton
Jos Engelen (Cast Technician)

Casts, Splints, and Support Bandages—Nonoperative Treatment and Perioperative Protection

WO 170 DRE

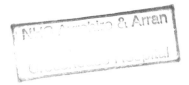

WO 170 DRE

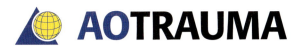

Klaus Dresing | Peter Trafton
Jos Engelen (Cast Technician)

Casts, Splints, and Support Bandages—Nonoperative Treatment and Perioperative Protection

Includes 2497 illustrations and images and 55 videos

Library of Congress Cataloging-in-Publication Data will be available from the publisher.

Copyright © 2014 by AO Foundation, Switzerland, Clavadelerstrasse 8, CH-7270 Davos Platz
Distribution by Georg Thieme Verlag, Rüdigerstrasse 14, DE-70469 Stuttgart and Thieme New York, 333 Seventh Avenue, US-New York, NY 10001

Layout: nougat GmbH, CH-4056 Basel
Illustration: AO Education Institute

ISBN: 9783131753410
e-ISBN: 9783131753519

Foreword

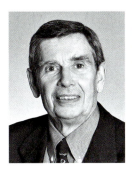

Thomas P Rüedi, MD, FACS
Founding Member AO Foundation
Consultant AOTrauma Education
Schellenbergstr. 20, Im Brisig
7304 Maienfeld
Switzerland

Finally, after many attempts and with great anticipation, AOTrauma has provided a publication specifically on non-operative fracture treatment. This book *Casts, Splints, and Support Bandages—Nonoperative Treatment and Perioperative Protection* is an indication that "AO" does not stand for "Always Operate" but rather for a comprehensive approach to the various treatment options for musculoskeletal injuries.

The two editors, from Germany and the US, together with 20 authors from around the world, have produced a book that covers all the major issues on the topic in a very didactic and self-explanatory way.

After an introduction to the basic principles of casting, the guidelines and indications of nonoperative fracture management are discussed critically based on the AO classification. There are indepth chapters about the treatment of fractures in the upper and lower extremities, while the chapters on injuries of the ligaments, and as a result of overload, are well chosen. Other important aspects discussed include pediatric fractures, a main domain of nonoperative treatment, as well as the management of spine injuries. Finally, the techniques of cast, splint, and bandage application are illustrated step-by-step for locations throughout the upper and lower extremities, as well as the spine, using different fixation materials.

The authors are to be congratulated for the very detailed presentation of the various techniques by two masters in casting, which is most helpful especially for all those that have not had the chance to learn the special "art of casting" with its many important tricks and hints.

If applied correctly by an expert, nonoperative treatment can be superior and preferable to poorly attempted surgery in many types of fractures, especially so in developing countries where the risk of infection after surgery is still very high and much more problematic than a minor malalignment or even a nonunion.

This book should find its place on the shelf of every casting room, at the disposal of residents and technicians, and for surgeons requiring up to date knowledge on the latest casting techniques.

Thomas P Rüedi

Acknowledgements

Casts, Splints, and Support Bandages — Nonoperative Treatment and Perioperative Protection would not have been possible without the dedicated assistance and support of a wonderfully diverse group of people. From the education design, development and filming of videos, medical and graphical illustrations, research and text development, editing and proof reading, typesetting, and final completion and print production, this book has indeed been a labor of love for which we would like to thank many people.

To begin, we would like to especially acknowledge the following:

- Urs Rüetschi, Director of the AO Education Institute, as well as the members of the AOTrauma Education Commission, for accepting and supporting the idea to develop this comprehensive text, and for providing extensive resources to do so
- The AO Education Institute Video Production Team, led by Robin Greene, for helping us to coordinate and film our extensive range of demonstration videos, and a very special thanks to Mike Laws for his countless hours spent in the editing suite, compiling and editing raw footage and turning it into clear and highly professional medical procedure demonstrations
- Our dedicated authors, who donated many hours researching and developing their chapters in their own rare spare time
- Prof Dr Thomas Rüedi, one of the founders of AO Foundation, who supported the idea for this book and kindly wrote his dedicatory foreword
- We especially thank our tireless and dedicated colleague Jos Engelen, not just for his expertise in cast and splint application, his starring role in the demonstration videos, and his thorough and precise editorial support in many of the chapters, but for his constant availability and friendship throughout every stage of this text

- Kathrin Lüssi from the AO Education Institute, and Cristina Lusti and Michael Gleeson, our hard working Project Coordinators, who provided invaluable administrative and editorial support to us throughout the life of the project
- Tom Wirth, Jecca Reichmuth, and Olivier Jallard for their exceptional work in designing and illustrating the book, as well as to the staff at AO Surgery Reference
- Our typesetters Nougat, our language editor Barbara Gernert, and our partner publisher Thieme Publishing for print production and distribution
- Carl Lau and Sue Klein for proof reading
- Our tremendous cast of video demonstration models, comprising Endre Varga Jr, Priska Inauen, Fabian Duttenhoefer, Sebastian Fäh, Kathrin Lüssi, and Cristina Lusti
- The AO Socioeconomic Committee, as steadfast supporters of nonoperative fracture management in the less-developed parts of the world
- 3M Germany, for providing synthetic casting materials for the video filming
- Lohmann & Rauscher, Germany, for providing plaster of Paris casting materials for the video filming
- Berger Medical Products, for the use of images of cast instruments
- Andreas Wuffli from the University Hospital Zürich, for providing us with cast tables and equipment for the video filming
- And finally to our own partners and families, without whose unquestioning support we could never have been able to bring together this important medical text.

Our sincere thanks to each of you.

Klaus Dresing, Peter Trafton

Preface

Klaus

I remember being introduced to nonoperative fracture treatment during my residency in Düsseldorf, Germany. We treated almost 60% of fractures conservatively. I later pursued further training in a level-1 trauma center where nonoperative care was taught well, and practiced significantly. As residents there, each of us was assigned to teach a plaster course for medical students. Over time, we began to include synthetic cast material and innovative new techniques into our practice and teaching. As a faculty member at the University Medical Center in Göttingen, Germany, I have always included cast application as a part of my therapeutic armament. Our group has developed increasingly sophisticated techniques, using plaster of Paris, as well as synthetic materials in both rigid and semirigid forms. This familiarity with the use of various casting techniques, as a surgeon, and as a teacher, meant that I was well prepared, and greatly honored, to accept AOTrauma's invitation to undertake this exciting and worthwhile book and video project *Casts, Splints, and Support Bandages—Nonoperative Treatment and Perioperative Protection*.

And it was a happy coincidence that led to my collaboration with Peter Trafton. Several years ago, my wife Petra (a quilt maker) and I held a charity auction, "Quilts for Malawi", to support a children's hospital in Blantyre, Malawi, in southeast Africa. Through our independent AOTrauma activities, Peter and I began to meet regularly, and I soon learned that, incredibly, he had also visited Blantyre as a volunteer orthopedic surgeon. We shared our experiences in the developing world, where financial constraints limit the use of osteosynthesis. We agreed that the AO needed up-to-date teaching resources for immobilization techniques, as alternatives and as supplements to operative fracture treatment, as well as for other orthopedic conditions. Having found a kindred spirit, I was delighted when Peter accepted my invitation to join me as co-editor.

Peter

Like Klaus, my training in trauma and orthopedic surgery began early in the transition from nonoperative treatment to modern practice, with its far greater emphasis on the surgical stabilization of fractures. Operative fracture care is indeed successful when practiced effectively and safely, and worldwide, we have adopted countless new internal and external fixation techniques, to which the AO community has contributed so much. However, the unintended consequence is that educators and surgical trainees have devoted so much time, energy, and attention to developing operative skills that nonoperative techniques have been left to wither away. But they are still a crucial part of our patient care, in first-world trauma centers, as well as everywhere else where musculoskeletal injuries and other disorders are encountered and treated. I am grateful that my teachers helped me acquire this knowledge and skills, and that my role as an educator has helped me improve my understanding and clinical practice. As a resident, I was privileged to work with Vert Mooney at Rancho Los Amigos, and subsequently to develop collegial relationships with Augusto Sarmiento and Loren Latta, who have contributed so much to functional fracture bracing.

More recently, my involvement in volunteer activities in lower and middle income locations have brought me back to my less-operative roots. In such settings, I am especially grateful for what I learned as a young resident. It is particularly rewarding that the AO, such a strong force in the development of operative musculoskeletal care, has embraced this effort to help preserve and further nonoperative techniques as well. Without doubt, a complete surgeon should be equally skilled in both approaches.

Together

In our great AO family, many friends and colleagues are involved in nonoperative fracture care. We are delighted and grateful that so many have supported this book with excellent chapters. With their help, we offer you this effort to maintain expertise in nonoperative immobilization techniques, for future generations, and for the care of musculoskeletal and soft tissue conditions today.

Klaus Dresing, Peter Trafton

Contributors

Editors

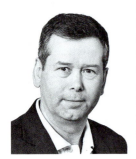

Klaus Dresing, Prof Dr med
Leitender Oberarzt
Klinik für Unfallchirurgie, Plastische und
Wiederherstellungschirurgie
Universitätsmedizin Göttingen
Georg-August-Universität
Robert-Koch-Strasse 40
37075 Göttingen
Germany

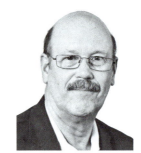

Peter G Trafton, Prof MD
The Warren Alpert Medical School of Brown
University
222 Richmond Street
Providence, RI 02903
USA

Cast technician

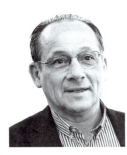

Jos Engelen
Cast Technician
aescoLOGIC AG
Alter Garten 60-62
51371 Leverkusen
Germany

Authors

Kamel Afifi, MD FMH
Consultant Orthopaedic and Hand Surgeon
Chairman of the Orthopaedic Department
Jordan Hospital and Medical Center
Queen Nour Street
Amman 11152
Jordan

E Walter Buchinger, em Prim Dr
(Former Chief Physician of the Trauma Unit Horn, Lower Austria)
Brentenmaisstr. 58
3012 Wolfsgraben
Austria

Matej Cimerman, Prof PhD MD
University Clinical Center Ljubljana
Department for Traumatology
Zaloska 7
1000 Ljubljana
Slovenia

Juan Manuel Concha Sandoval, MD
Orthopaedic Surgeon
Universidad del Cauca
Facultad de Medicina
Calle 5
Popayan
Colombia

Miles Francis T Dela Rosa, MD FPOA FPCS
Senior Consultant
Philippine Orthopaedic Center
Maria Clara Street
Quezon City
Philippines

Klaus Dresing, Prof Dr med
Leitender Oberarzt
Klinik für Unfallchirurgie, Plastische und Wiederherstellungschirurgie
Universitätsmedizin Göttingen
Georg-August-Universität
Robert-Koch-Strasse 40
37075 Göttingen
Germany

Clemens Dumont, PD Dr
Geschäftsführender Oberarzt
Klinik für Unfallchirurgie und Orthopädie
Abteilung für Unfallchirurgie, Plastische und Wiederherstellungschirurgie
Universitätsmedizin Göttingen
Georg-August Universität
Robert-Koch-Strasse 40
37075 Göttingen
Germany

Jos Engelen
Cast Technician
aescoLOGIC AG
Alter Garten 60-62
51371 Leverkusen
Germany

Florian Gebhard, Univ Prof Dr med
Director and Chair Department for Orthopaedic Trauma
Ulm University
Zentrum für Chirurgie
Klinik für Unfallchirurgie, Hand-, Plastische- und Wiederherstellungschirurgie
Albert-Einstein-Allee 23
89081 Ulm
Germany

Beate P Hanson, MD MPH
Director AO Clinical Investigation and Documentation
Stettbachstrasse 6
8600 Dübendorf
Switzerland

WJ Harrison, Prof MD
Consultant in Trauma and Orthopaedics
Countess of Chester NHS Foundation Trust
Liverpool road
Chester
United Kingdom

Richard Kdolsky, Prof Dr
Universitätsklinik für Unfallchirurgie
Medizinische Universität Wien
AKH, Währinger Gürtel 18–20
1090 Wien
Austria

Rami Mosheiff, Prof MD
Head of Orthopaedic Trauma Unit
Hadassah University Medical Center
Ein Kerem
PO Box 12000
91120 Jerusalem
Israel

Thomas Neubauer, Prim Dr
Waldviertelklinikum Horn
Unfallchirurgie
Spitalgasse 10
3580 Horn
Austria

Peter Richter, Dr med
Ulm University
Zentrum für Chirurgie
Klinik für Unfallchirurgie, Hand-, Plastische- und Wiederherstellungschirurgie
Albert-Einstein-Allee 23
89081 Ulm
Germany

Bastian Scheiderer, Dr med
Ulm University
Zentrum für Chirurgie
Klinik für Unfallchirurgie, Hand-, Plastische- und Wiederherstellungschirurgie
Albert-Einstein-Allee 23
89081 Ulm
Germany

Jan Philipp Schüttrumpf, Dr med
Assistenzarzt für Orthopädie und Unfallchirurgie
Klinik für Unfallchirurgie und Orthopädie
Abteilung für Unfallchirurgie, Plastische und Wiederherstellungschirurgie
Universitätsmedizin Göttingen
Georg-August Universität
Robert-Koch-Strasse 40
37075 Göttingen
Germany

Franz Seibert, Prim Ao Univ Prof Dr Mag
Medical Director
UKH-Graz, AUVA
Teaching Hospital of the Medical University Graz
Göstingerstrasse 24
8020 Graz
Austria

Peter G Trafton, Prof MD
The Warren Alpert Medical School of Brown University
222 Richmond Street
Providence, RI 02903
USA

Endre Varga, Prof MD
Professor of Trauma Surgery
Head of Department of Traumatology
President of Hungarian Trauma Society
University of Szeged
Albert Szentgyörgyi Clinical Center
Department of Traumatology
6725 Szeged, Semmelweis u.6.
Hungary

Abbreviations

AC	acromioclavicular		**Mpa**	megapascals of pressure
ACL	anterior cruciate ligament		**MRI**	magnetic resonance imaging
AP	anterior/posterior		**MT**	muscle tendon injury/muscle and tendon lesions
ATFL	anterior talofibular ligament		**MTP**	metatarsophalangeal
CFL	calcaneofibular ligament		**NCV**	nerve conduction velocity
COA	center of angulation		**NCS**	nerve conduction study
CRP	c-reactive protein		**NIBP**	noninvasive blood pressure monitor
CT	computed tomography		**Nm**	Newton meters
DIP	distal interphalangeal		**NSAIDs**	nonsteroidal antiinflammatory drugs
DRUJ	distal radioulnar joint		**NV**	neurovascular injury/nerve and vessel injuries
DVT	deep vein thrombosis		**OR**	operating room
EBM	evidence-based medicine		**ORIF**	open reduction and internal fixation
EBO	evidence-based orthopedics		**PACS**	picture archiving and communication system
ECG	electrocardiogram		**PCL**	posterior cruciate ligament
ED	emergency department		**PE**	pulmonary embolism
EN	European norm		**PET**	positron emission tomography
ESIN	elastic stable intramedullary nailing		**PIP**	proximal interphalangeal
ESR	erythrocyte sedimentation rate		**POP**	plaster of Paris
FDP	flexor digitorum profundus		**PP**	proximal phalanx
FDS	flexor digitorum superficialis		**PTB**	patella tendon bearing
Gpa	gigapascals of pressure		**PTFL**	posterior talofibular ligament
GH	glenohumeral		**RCTs**	randomized controlled trials
IC	integument closed (closed skin lesion)		**RICE**	rest, ice, compression, elevation
IDDM	insulin-dependent diabetes mellitus		**ROM**	range of motion
IMN	intramedullary nailing		**RPS**	regional pain syndrome
INR	international normalized ratio		**SLAP**	superior labrum anterior and posterior tear
IP	interphalangeal		**SpO2**	saturation of peripheral oxygen
IO	integument open (open skin lesions)		**TMT**	tarsometatarsal
IPC	intermittent pneumatic compression		**UCL**	ulnar collateral ligament
LCL	lateral collateral ligament		**UFH**	unfractionated heparin
LMWH	low-molecular-weight heparin		**VTE**	venous thromboembolism prophylaxis
MCL	medial collateral ligament		**WBC**	white blood cell count
MCP	metacarpophalangeal			

Table of contents

Table of contents

PRINCIPLES

Principles of Casting

Principles

1 Introduction

Klaus Dresing, Peter Trafton

Authors   Klaus Dresing, Peter Trafton

1 Introduction

1 Background

Over the past several decades, and particularly since the founding of the AO Foundation in 1958, the operative treatment of fractured bones has developed and expanded rapidly. As the arts and sciences of open reduction and internal fixation have flourished, the earlier techniques and skills of external immobilization have left the repertoire of trauma and orthopedic surgeons. Older surgeons, nearing retirement, often remark that today's trainees, as well as most colleagues trained in the last 30 years, are quite unfamiliar with the application and appropriate use of casts, splints, and support bandages. One might easily assume that operative fixation has replaced the use of such techniques, particularly for the treatment of unstable and displaced fractures. But is it really correct to conclude that external immobilization is no longer a necessary part of the surgeon's skill set, or that it can be delegated to other members of the medical care team—nurses, technologists, or orthotists? The authors and editors of this book strongly believe that the answer is "no".

Although early active motion is a valid goal for rehabilitation, postoperative external immobilization is often still desirable for the protection of healing tissues, to prevent contractures, and to assist with functional rehabilitation. Children, whose fractures heal rapidly and who are far less likely to develop permanently stiff joints after immobilization, are still usually treated with casts, even after open reduction. Finally, as Charles Court-Brown and his colleagues recently reported from their Edinburgh trauma centers (highly regarded for surgical experience and expertise), the nonoperative management of fractures continues to predominate. Nonoperative techniques were found to have been used for three quarters of the fractures they had treated—two thirds of the adults, and more than 90% of the children [1].

In other medical care settings, particularly in developing healthcare systems, the resources for operative fracture care can be quite limited, and nonoperative techniques must be relied upon even more. Valid outcome measurements are the basis for determining optimal management for a given fracture in a particular setting. Also necessary is consideration of all relevant patient characteristics as well as the resources and experience of the treating team. Patient-based outcome measures are the gold standard for evaluation of treatment results. As such assessment techniques are increasingly used, they occasionally reveal that the results of nonoperative care are at least as good as those achieved with operations, often to the surprise of surgeons and patients that have come to believe that surgery is required for good outcomes.

It is widely recognized that both technical skill and appropriate equipment are important for operative treatment. We believe that the same is true for external immobilization used for musculoskeletal disorders.

The work of Lorenz Böhler, including his *The Treatment of Fractures*, which was updated and expanded over many decades and translated into eight languages, clearly showed how important and effective plaster cast immobilization is in the treatment of bone fractures [2]. Major contributions to the understanding and use of external immobilization were provided by many others, including Jean Lucas-Campionniere and George Perkins. Particularly notable is John Charnley, whose work *The Closed Treatment of Common Fractures* [3] remains a valuable textbook today 64 years after its initial publication. Augusto Sarmiento, a Colombian working in the USA, with his engineer colleague Loren Latta, advanced the use of functional casts and braces, as well as the understanding of the mechanics of external immobilization.

Supportive immobilization is an essential component of primary care for unstable and painful skeletal injuries. In addition to nonoperative treatment, it is often used perioperatively in both trauma treatment and reconstructive surgery, as well as for the care of wounds or infections. Thus, knowledge of materials and techniques for casts, splints, and support bandages remains important in today's trauma and orthopedic surgery.

Furthermore, the prescription and application of these devices must remain the surgeon's responsibility. A poorly planned or poorly applied cast may not provide the needed immobilization. It can also result in complications with potential permanent harm stemming from pressure sores, nerve palsies, contractures, or compartment syndrome. Even when the actual application of a cast or other supporting bandage is delegated, the surgeon must be able to plan appropriately and to evaluate the applied device, to recognize when it is satisfactory, and when it must be revised.

Time and innovation have brought changes to materials and techniques for external immobilization. Today, mineral plaster of Paris casts and splints have been partly replaced by casts, splints, and orthoses made of synthetic material. These are typically lighter, more comfortable, and accommodate improved function. Rigidity can be chosen for an optimal balance between support and functional use. Increased durability, water resistance, and in some cases, the ability to be removed by the patient or family, are also available options.

Casts, Splints, and Support Bandages—Nonoperative Treatment and Perioperative Protection has been created as a comprehensive reference for the immobilization of an extensive range of musculoskeletal disorders. It is intended for surgeons, as well as other members of the treating team, particularly nurses and orthopedic technologists, and students preparing for these professions. It provides an extensive overview of the history, principles, methods, and techniques for applying a plaster or synthetic cast, for nonoperative care as well as perioperatively.

2 Contents and structure

The book comprises three sections:
• Principles of casting
• Guidelines for nonoperative treatment and perioperative protection
• Techniques of casts, splints, and support bandages.

2.1 Principles of casting

The first section, Principles of casting, presents basic information about external immobilization. Chapters 2 and 6 chart the progress from early plaster casts to today's variety of materials for such dressings: modern plaster of Paris, rigid synthetics, and also more compliant synthetics for semirigid casts, so-called soft casts. Chapter 3 explores the key principles of casting, including the principles of bone healing, types of splints and casts, reduction and stabilization, and responding to bone malalignment with cast wedging. Chapter 4 discusses thromboembolic risks related to injuries and immobilization, and reviews prophylaxis. Chapter 5 provides a detailed overview of the resources, equipment, lighting and electrical supply, and staffing needed to run a safe and well stocked modern day cast room. Logistical and economic issues are reviewed in chapter 7, recognizing technical issues and the differences between more and less-developed healthcare systems. Finally, chapter 8 considers evidence-based outcomes from nonoperative treatment, demonstrating its importance for the care of appropriately selected injuries.

2.2 Guidelines

The second section, Guidelines, comprises chapters that explore specific nonoperative treatment for fractures, ligament, nerve, and soft-tissue injuries, overload injuries, and infections, in the upper and lower extremities and the spine, and in pediatric patients. A comprehensive approach is presented to help the reader understand the indications and plan appropriate immobilization for optimal patient benefit.

Authors   Klaus Dresing, Peter Trafton

2.3   Techniques

Finally, the third section called Techniques provides step-by-step descriptions of 55 individual casting, splinting, orthotic, and bandaging techniques, presented in two ways. In the printed book, the demonstrations comprise still photographs and illustrations with explanatory text. However, the reader can also review each of the 55 immobilization demonstrations in high-quality video, by using the access code on the inside cover of the book and visiting the Thieme Media Center website.

The book does not present a single comprehensive view of primarily nonoperative fracture treatment, in the manner of Lorenz Böhler. Our world-wide group of authors, members of AOTrauma, have all contributed their individual viewpoints, based on personal experience and practices. While each is an expert in surgical trauma care, they all recognize the importance of nonoperative immobilization as a primary treatment, and as an adjunct to surgery. An often-repeated joke is that "AO stands for Always Operate" but this text presents a more eclectic vision of trauma care. All five geographic regions of AOTrauma are represented among the authors. It was a great honor that each of the authors immediately accepted the editors' invitation to contribute from their great experience in nonoperative and operative trauma surgery. The result is this new AOTrauma book, which presents a vitally important, but currently poorly documented, part of our care for injured patients.

The editors and authors are aware that some indications or presented techniques may be unfamiliar, and that alternative care regimens and techniques are abundant. We have not attempted to present or discuss the wide variety of available orthoses, either mass produced or custom-made by an orthotist, as to do so would have exceeded the book's scope. We chose instead to illustrate the principles of immobilization and support with techniques that use materials available in the typical surgical cast room. Indeed, we hope that what we have selected will provide valuable guidance for effective practice and further advancement of trauma care. We are confident that this AOTrauma book *Casts, Splints, and Support Bandages—Nonoperative Treatment and Perioperative Protection* will help improve patient care around the world.

3   References

1. **Court-Brown CM, Aitken S, Hamilton TW, et al**. Nonoperative fracture treatment in the modern era. *J Trauma.* 2010 Sep; 69(3):699–707.
2. **Böhler L**. *The Treatment of Fractures.* 4th ed English. Baltimore: William Wood and Company; 1936.
    Alternatively: **Böhler L**. *Die Technik der Knochenbruchbehandlung.* 13th ed. Vienna: Verlag Wilhem Maudrich; 1996. German.
3. **Charnley J**. *The Closed Treatment of Common Fractures.* 4th ed. United Kingdom. Cambridge University Press; 2010.

PRINCIPLES

2 History of casting—from the beginning to the present day

Walter E Buchinger

Author   Walter E Buchinger

2   History of casting—from the beginning to the present day

1   Introduction

From our earliest existence, humans have found innumerable ways to injure the bones and supporting structures of our fragile skeletal system. Yet, over time, we have also slowly developed a greater understanding of the workings of the human body. Today, highly trained surgeons and other medical professionals use incredible skill, operative and nonoperative techniques, and state of art instruments to repair even the most damaged bones and extremities. So, before we explore the underlying principles of modern casting, it is important to first outline the critical moments and historical figures that helped bring the knowledge of casting to where it is today.

2   First findings

In the analysis of prehistoric skeletons and well-preserved Egyptian mummies, it was discovered that, even in ancient times, some kind of treatment for fractures by means of splinting and dressing was performed. In the *Edwin Smith Papyrus*, an ancient Egyptian scroll known as the world's "oldest surgical textbook" (dating back to the 17th century BC), there are specific references to fracture treatment [1, 2]. Even today, in some parts of Asia, South America, and Africa, "bonesetters" provide treatment based on ancient magic spells and ointments in conjunction with splints made from cardboard or plywood (bamboo poles in China) for the purpose of fracture immobilization [3].

3   Pre-Christian era

In ancient Greece, numerous wars took place among the Greek city states, and other groups, during the second pre-Christian millennium. Additionally, though glorified today as a means of peaceful competition, the ancient Olympic Games included extremely brutal fighting and wrestling events (**Fig 2-1**). Victory meant great prestige to the fighter as well as to his region of origin, but the resulting injuries to the loser (or winner) created a need for suitable "treatment centers". Thus, a large number of medical schools were founded.

The most famous name of this era is, no doubt, Hippocrates (460–370 BC). The *Hippocratic Corpus*, published in several volumes, lists exact instructions pertaining to the treatment of fractures [4]. It includes detailed information on fracture treatment, and describes how bandages were stiffened by applying a mixture of wax and resin, on top of which splints from wood or iron were placed. It also provides fixation times for the most common types of fracture, and describes a kind of external fixator for the treatment of lower-leg fractures composed of rings placed on the knee and ankle joints, and connected by rods (**Fig 2-2**) [5, 6]. It is unclear how much of the complete work can be attributed to Hippocrates himself due to different dates of publications and varying quality of the text—sometimes the text even contradicts itself. Nevertheless, his theories provided great insight into early medicine and fracture treatment.

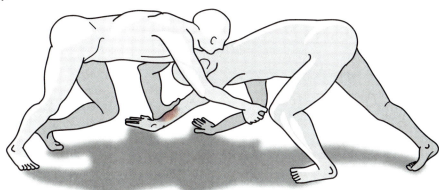

Fig 2-1   Through Olympic wrestling bouts and hand to hand combat, the ancient Greeks learned that the full weight of an opponent, or a direct blow to an unprotected limb, could easily cause sprain or fracture.

Following the foundation of Alexander the Great's empire, the center of medical science moved from the Greek motherland to the capital Alexandria, newly established in 331 BC, with its famous library that, among its 700,000 scrolls, also contained the Hippocratic Corpus.

The conquest by Augustus and the incorporation of Egypt as a Roman protectorate introduced Greek sciences, and thus medicine, to the Roman Empire. For a long time, Alexandria, as the second largest city of the Roman Empire, remained its cultural and intellectual center and Greek doctors, usually trained in Alexandria, were highly sought specialists.

4   Roman era

In regards to the treatment of injuries in early medicine, one name remains outstanding, Galen of Pergamon, who was renowned for treating gladiators (**Fig 2-3**). He lived and worked in Rome in the 2nd century AD. In his work *De Ossibus ad Tirones*, which freely translates into "About bones for beginners", he described and refined the methods listed in the Hippocratic Corpus [8].

5   Rise of Arabic knowledge

With the expansion of the Arabic/Islamic world in the second half of the first millenium AD, a new empire emerged, extending from the Himalayas to the Pyrenees. Based on Greek and Roman principles, the Arabic medical practitioners developed new insights, and the art of medical healing experienced major improvements. Rhazes Athuriscus (865–925) (**Fig 2-4**), for example, recommended the use of cloth saturated with lime or plaster, which held the limb firm, as was found to be effective for the fixation of bone fractures.

6   Middle Ages

Once the Greek and Roman empires had been destroyed, the practice and study of medicine in Europe was limited to religious monasteries. Since the church disapproved of all pagan rituals and practices (and this included the highly developed Arabic medicine), medical progress in Europe stagnated. Recognition of the value of Arabic medicine (as well as its Greek and Roman origins) moved only slowly. One of the last clerical doctors was Guy de Chauliac (Chaulhiaco) (1300–1368), who in his works *Chirurgia Magna* described in great detail immobilizing bandaging techniques (listing materials such as wood, leather, iron, and horn, already mentioned in Arabic and Greek texts) and also recommended the use of steady traction (extension) over a cylinder in order to avoid bone shortening [9].

7   The 13th–16th centuries

From the 13th century, the career opportunities of clerical doctors were severely reduced by a church reformation. It has been argued that one of the triggers for this crack down on the practice of medicine was that some practitioners were applying medicine for their own benefit rather than the patient's well-being. The field of modern surgery shares a somewhat similar history.

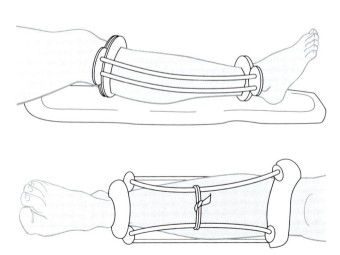

Fig 2-2   Wooden splint fracture fixation by Hippocrates [7].

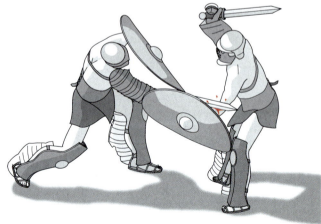

Fig 2-3   Galen of Pergamon explored ways to treat bone fractures following gladiatorial contests with swords, clubs, and even spiked iron balls.

Author   Walter E Buchinger

Initially, moderately complex surgery was practiced by barber surgeons and "quack" doctors—when in fact the word surgery in its translation from Greek means craftsman or "working with one's hands". At other times, it was taught on an academic level. Despite this, the era for critical scrutiny and questioning of traditional thinking had begun. As an example, in the 16th century, Andreas Vesalius (1514–1564) was able to correct large parts of Galen's teachings through findings he gathered from human autopsies.

Eventually, surgery began to be well-practiced by some of these craftsmen, as demonstrated by the barber surgeon Ambroise Paré, who received little if any university training. He worked at a time when injuries caused by firearms were considered to be poisonous and had to be cauterized by heated iron or scalding hot oil. During the French campaigns of the 16th century (when oil had become scarce), Paré realized that a mixture of essence of rose, egg yolk, and turpentine showed better results [10]. In peace times, he focused on the primary description of fractures of the femoral neck, among other activities.

8   The 17th–18th centuries

During the 17th and 18th centuries, numerous textbooks on trauma surgery were published. Their authors, Duverney, Petit, Larrey, Heister, Schultes, Desault, Malgaigne (also without university training), Pott, Jones, Smith, were all well-known and are still recognized today. Statistical reworking and follow-up examinations were introduced, and conclusions regarding diagnosis and therapy were drawn from autopsy results.

In 1792, Jean Dominique Larrey (Napoleon's personal physician and later, surgeon-in-chief for the entire Napoleonic Army) (**Fig 2-5**) invented the albumen dressing, which took two days to completely dry. However, because of this delay (and its thick padding) it provided enough elasticity to allow room for the initial swelling that usually occurs after fracture injuries. This particular dressing could be left on until the fracture had healed and, unlike Hippocrates' version, did not require frequent changing, which at the time was high in cost and material. However, even though the new dressing was superior in terms of stiffness to the previous splints made from wood, leather, etc, the longer drying time and high demand on raw materials were still considered a disadvantage. For each lower-leg fracture, 50–70 eggs were needed. It is likely that this high demand would have posed a significant challenge for the supply officers in the Napoleonic army, even though stringent pressure was imposed on the rural population of any occupied territories [11].

At that time, plaster was also already used in the form of the plaster mold, in which the extremity in question was placed in a case, and plaster was then molded around it until 2/3 of the respective limb was covered. The potential disadvantages of this method included heat damage, skin maceration, and, just as with Larrey's dressing, an obligatory lengthy bed rest. Most likely, the procedure for taking off the cast with hammer and chisel would not have contributed much to a trustful relationship between doctor and patient [8].

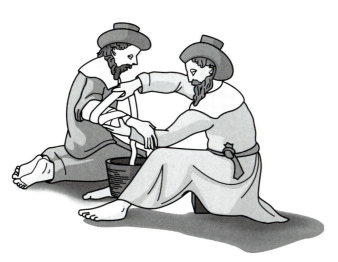

Fig 2-4   Rhazes Athuriscus used cloth saturated with lime or plaster for the fixation of bone fractures.

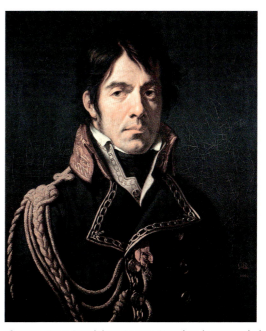

Fig 2-5   Jean Dominique Larrey—Napoleon's personal physician. (Painting by Anne-Louis Girodet De Roussy-Trioson (1804) © RMN-Grand Palais (Musée du Louvre). Thierry Le Mage)

9   The 19th–20th centuries

The 19th century first brought an innovation impetus for immobilizing dressings, followed by advances in general surgery. Stability of the Larrey dressing was increased in the first half of the century by the Belgian general practitioner LJ Seutin (1793–1862) as he used glue made from flour to impregnate the dressing. Splitting the cast was obligatory, as well as fenestration in the case of open fractures. After reduction of the swelling, the bandaging was closed or adapted by cutting out parts as needed. For the first time, this kind of treatment could even be accomplished on an out-patient basis [12].

In the second half of the 19th century, Antonius Mathijsen (1805–1878) (**Fig 2-6**), a Dutch navy surgeon, optimized fracture treatment by introducing cotton soaked with plaster of Paris [13]. He is generally considered to be the inventor of the plaster cast, however, at the same time, Russian surgeon Nikolai Pirogoff (1810–1881) described the same kind of technique, which he used during the Crimean war [14].

Around the same time, a number of new inventions completely changed the surgical routine. Knowledge of pain management and anesthesia were transferred from America to Europe, the importance of antisepsis (Semmelweis, Lister, Friedrich) became evident, and the invention of x-ray technology enabled the premortem analysis of fractures. At that time, only 10% of all injured patients with open fractures kept their limbs; 50% died, and 40% had to endure amputation (**Fig 2-7**). Moreover, the mortality rate of primary amputations was about 75% [15].

Inappropriate application of the now stiff dressing initially led to a number of complications, such as decubitus, circu-

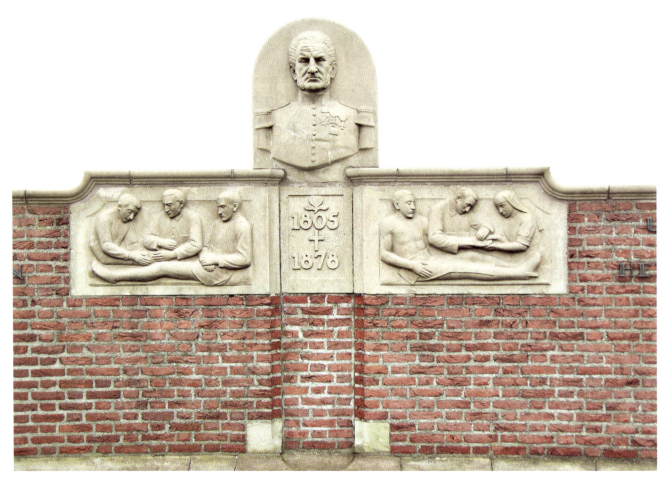

Fig 2-6   Antonius Mathijsen, who is generally considered as the inventor of the plaster cast. Monument at his birthplace, Budel, in The Netherlands.

Author   Walter E Buchinger

latory disturbance, contractures, and necrosis. Lack of experience regarding the duration of fixation and weight bearing as well as the importance of exercising the immobilized extremity—extreme rest was recommended—resulted in nonunion, muscular atrophy, and/or joint stiffness.

Slim plaster without the heavy padding allowed better assessment of the position of the axis. The technique of including the neighboring joints within the fixation, which had been practiced since the 18th century, proved to be useful in avoiding malrotation. However, it was not suitable to avoid shortening in the case of lower-extremity fractures. The earlier methods applied for extension treatment were unsuitable, as traction was attached directly to the skin via loops or bandages, which resulted in lesions of the skin, the perineum, or axilla caused by the necessary counterstrain.

In later years, Percival Pott pointed out that relaxation of the leg muscles by bending hip and knee joints might result in a distinct decrease of the required weight, needed to avoid bone shortening. This was well employed by Robert Chessher, who introduced a double-inclined frame. FH Hamilton came up with a simple solution for the problem of the counterstrain—he elevated the foot end of the bed [16]. Problems were finally solved by attaching traction devices directly to the bone. In the German-speaking countries, the term "Steinmann Nagel" (Steinmann Pin), coined by the Swiss surgeon Fritz Steinmann, is well known [17]. Since penetrating the cortex with a nail might cause fissures, in 1927 Martin Kirschner suggested drilling in a wire instead, a method which has become wide-spread [18].

As always, it took a while before experience with new techniques overcame initial failures (hypercorrection due to too much weight, resulting in problems with soft tissues and nonunion, inappropriate extension times, etc).

9.1   Nonoperative treatment and the Great War

One name closely connected with perfecting nonoperative techniques is Lorenz Böhler (1885–1973) (**Fig 2-8**). While working in a military hospital about 30 km from the river Isonzo, during World War I, he gained a lot of experience using immobilizing dressings and traction, applied either alone or in combination. Furthermore, he meticulously kept medical records and documented results and presented them to the board of the compensating insurance body in Austria after the war. It was discovered that the compensation paid by the Arbeiterunfallversicherung (AUVA) for worker's compensation after an industrial accident was much larger than for a comparable war injury that had been treated according to Böhler's principles. This made his techniques quite convincing.

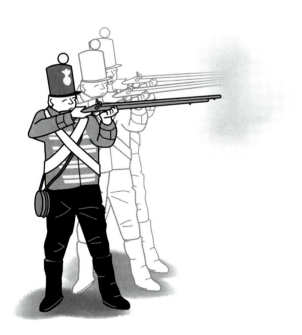
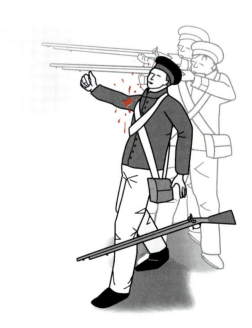

Fig 2-7   Throughout history, much medical knowledge was acquired on the battlefield. Until the discoveries made by wartime surgeons such as Larrey, Mathijsen, and Pirogoff, open fractures from gunshot wounds or shrapnel were regularly treated with amputation.

In 1925, the first trauma hospital of the AUVA was founded, with a total capacity of 52 beds. Within one year, Böhler was able to prove that the amount saved on compensation exceeded the running costs. Over the years, the thin script written for his students evolved into a four-volume reference book called *The Treatment of Fractures*, which had been published, with multiple editions, in German and eight other languages (including Chinese) by 1970. Every maneuver in fracture reduction and immobilization was described in great detail, including timeframes for immobilization as well as the consequences of not adhering to the given guidelines [19].

The successful "Böhler's school" was based on three pillars:
- Standardized guidelines for nonoperative techniques, which had to be strictly adhered to
- Strict organization, and
- The possibility to treat and observe patients from day 1 until full recuperation and their return to work.

"Fracture reduction, immobilization, training" were his guiding principles. Traction had to be checked twice a day and plaster dressings were only allowed without padding as this ensured that the reduced fractures were kept in the correct position. This of course was only possible by constant and organized observation and follow-up treatment. If needed, in case of pain or swelling, immediate action such as fenestration, splitting, or reapplication of the dressing had to be carried out. All immobilized patients had to participate in special programs of physical therapy and, thus, muscular atrophy and joint stiffening (the so-called "cast disease") could be avoided. Though Böhler, as well as his successors,

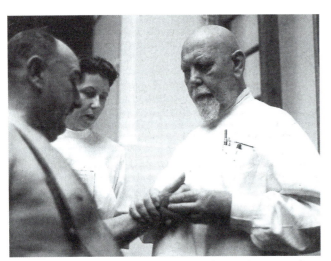

Fig 2-8 Lorenz Böhler, author of the four-volume reference work Techniques of Fracture Treatment during a critical review of a treatment outcome.

published an extremely large number of treated cases (more than even in cumulative studies today) with excellent follow-up results, these reports were astonishingly still under discussion by recent authors.

With the introduction of anesthesia and asepsis, the number of serious efforts for treating bone fractures surgically increased (Berard, Lambotte, Lane, Hansmann, Hey Groves, and others). However, surgical insufficiencies of the techniques applied at that time could now be demonstrated exactly by radiology, which had become generally available. Thus, many surgeons initially disapproved of osteosynthesis or regarded it as an 'ultima ratio' salvage procedure.

9.2 Müller and the AO Working Group

The break-through finally came with systematic research in metallurgy, biomechanics, and bone healing under conditions of osteosynthesis. This was initiated by the Swiss ME Müller (1918–2009), who, in conjunction with notable surgeons and a manufacturer of surgical instruments, founded the "working group on questions related to osteosynthesis" (Arbeitsgemeinschaft für Osteosynthese), now the AO Foundation, in 1958.

A new era of fracture treatment began and times started to change as nonoperative treatment measures subsided gradually. However, there was no mutual understanding among followers of the nonoperative treatment and those of the surgical treatment philosophy. Perhaps this was due to the fact that experience with nonoperative techniques outside Böhler's sphere of influence was not well established. In the 1950's, the amount of compensation the Swiss insurance company (SUVA) paid for femoral fractures was four times higher than that paid in Austria, the amount for lower-leg fractures was 10 times higher [6].

But eventually, even the most fervent advocates of nonoperative techniques had to accept that osteosynthesis provided an essential advantage compared with nonoperative treatment, even if the achieved results with both methods were comparable, because the patient's comfort improved. Nonoperative methods soon lost popularity and became an outside option; today, only a limited number of emergency departments actually know how to apply these methods. This seems to be an unfortunate development because:
- There are patients whose general condition or pattern of injury do not allow surgical intervention; insufficient knowledge of nonoperative methods will result in unsatisfactory results, which are usually attributed to the method rather than to the incorrectly applied technique—due to its not being common anymore

Author Walter E Buchinger

- There are countries in which, due to infrastructural deficiencies, knowledge transfer of nonoperative techniques rather than surgical techniques is more advantageous
- There are current operative techniques that surely would benefit from knowledge of fracture-reduction maneuvers of the nonoperative "old school", as can be demonstrated, eg, for the minimally invasive plate-osteosynthesis technique.

9.3 Plastics, synthetic, and closed functional fracture treatment

During the 1950s, casts made from plastic first made their appearance. In the beginning, their handling was quite complicated, some requiring very high temperatures or UV lights for hardening. They were also not as comfortable to wear as those with the water proof, lightweight fiberglass or polyester materials used today.

In the 1970s, other types of synthetic cast materials were introduced to fracture care. At first, fiberglass textile fabrics impregnated with a light-activated resin were used. The stability of the cast was induced by exposure to ultra-violet light. In the late 1970s, water-activated synthetic cast material was used for the first time. Today, knitted fabrics of polyester, fiberglass, and fiberglass-free polymer materials are in use, which are impregnated with polyurethane or resins of polyurethane. Water exposure accelerates the polymerization and the hardening process. Corresponding to the material composition, the results vary from rigid to semirigid casts.

In 1981, Sarmiento and Latta introduced "closed functional fracture treatment". This method involves a brace covering only the broken bone, thus preventing lateral giving-way of the surrounding soft-tissue and, at the same time, it functions as a pulley tension belt that also spreads the pressure over the entire fractured area [20]. Compared to Böhler's method, axis distortion and shortening are more frequent, therefore, application in various body regions (eg, in the case of lower-leg fractures) should be handled with caution. Additionally, it is necessary to check and adjust the brace frequently according to the amount of swelling of the soft-tissue.

The last extensive description of nonoperative fracture treatment was done by one of Böhler's students, H Jahna (1920–2003). In 1985, together with H Wittich, he published *Conservative Methods in Bone Fracture Treatment* [21]. Even today, his work is considered highly meticulous and exemplary in terms of reduction techniques and use of materials. It also includes a large chapter on how to produce immobi-

lizing dressings on one's own. Unfortunately, what is missing is a critical review of certain methods mentioned only for the sake of completeness. Some methods were already regarded as outdated by the authors. Exactly this was picked up by critics of the book; the baseline study and standardizing of nonoperative treatment options intended by authors was not fully appreciated everywhere.

In 1916, Hey Groves pointed out that a traumatologist/orthopedic surgeon should be able to carry out nonoperative treatment just as skillfully as if it was a surgical procedure [22]. It would be wonderful to finally achieve this demand in a field of expertise nearly 100 years after it was first developed.

10 Summary

- The unique properties of plaster have been known since ancient times, yet the earliest forms of casts and splints comprised such materials as wood, leather, wax, or eggs
- Hippocrates of Greece developed a set of instructions for fracture treatment, and further knowledge was developed during Roman, and later, Arabic periods
- In the 1800s, wartime surgeons such as Larrey, Mathijsen, and Pirogoff used plaster casts to treat open wound fractures, which dramatically improved the chances of survival for both limb and patient
- From his experiences in the First World War, Böhler published a 4-volume set on fracture treatment; he is considered a founding father of modern casting
- More recently, plastics and lighter synthetic materials were developed for casting, and the Sarmiento technique of functional treatment was introduced, using braces, which allows the limb some movement to reduce muscle breakdown during immobilization.

11 References

1. **Jäger K**. [Contributions to prehistoric surgery (Paleosurgery)]. *Dtsch Zschr Chir.* 1909; 102:109–140. German.
2. **Meyerhof M**. [About Papyrus Edwin Smith—the world's oldest surgery book]. *Dtsch Zschr Chir.* 1931; 231:645–690. German.
3. **Nwachukwu BU, Okwesili IC, Harris MB, et al**. Traditional bonesetters and contemporary orthopaedic fracture care in a developing nation: historical aspects, contemporary status and future directions. *Open Orthop J.* 2011 Jan; 5:20–26.
4. **Adams F.** The Hippocratic Corpus (translation). *The Internet Classics Archive;* 1994–2009. http://classics.mit.edu/Browse/browse-Hippocrates.html. [Accessed Nov 2012].
5. **Sigerist HE**. [*The Beginnings of Medicine: from Primitive and Archaic Medicine until the Golden Age in Greece*]. Zürich: Europa-Verlag. 1963. German.
6. **Povacz F**. [*The History of Trauma Surgery*]. 2nd ed. Berlin Heidlberg New York: Springer Verlag; 2007. German.
7. **Bick EM.** *Sourcebook of Orthopaedics.* 2nd ed. Baltimore: The Williams & Wilkins Company; 1948.
8. **Kullmann W, Althoff J, Asper M (eds)**. [*Categories of Scientific Literature in the Ancient World*]. Tübingen: Gunter Narr Verlag; 1998. German.
9. **de Chaulhiaco G**. Inventarium Sive Chirurgia Magna. McVaugh MR, Ogden MS (eds). *Studies in Ancient Medicine.* Vol 1. Leiden, New York: EJ Brill; 1997.
10. **Hamby WB**. *Ambroise Paré (1510–1590) Surgeon of the Renaissance.* St Louis: WH Green; 1967.
11. **Horndasch M**. [*Napoleon's Surgeon: The Life of Jean Dominique Larrey*]. 2nd ed. Bonn: Karl Glöckner Verlag; 1949. German.
12. **Seutin LJ**. [Essay on the method of non-removability-removability of a cast]. *Mémoire de l'Académie Royale de Médicine.* 1st ed. Brussels; 1835. French.
13. **Mathijsen A**. [*Gypsum Dressing*]. Crefeld: Kühler Verlag; 1857. German.
14. **Pirogoff N**. [*Basic Principles of General Military Surgery*]. 1st ed. Leipzig: Vogel Verlag; 1864. German.
15. **Malgaigne GB**. [*Treatment of Fractures and Luxations*]. Paris: Bailliere; 1847. French.
16. **Hamilton FH**. *A Practical Treatise on Fractures and Dislocations.* 1st ed. Philadelphia: Blanchard and Lea; 1860.
17. **Steinmann F (ed)**. [Nail extension of bone fractures]. *New German Surgery.* Vol 1. 1st ed. Stuttgart: Enke Verlag; 1912. German.
18. **Kirschner M**. [Improvement of wire extensions (Kirschner-wire)]. *Arch klin Chir.* 1927; 148:651–657. German.
19. **Böhler L**. [*The Treatment of Fractures*]. 1st ed. Wien: Wilhelm Maudrich; 1929. German.
20. **Sarmiento A, Latta HH**. *Closed Functional Treatment of Fractures.* 1st ed. Berlin Heidelberg New York: Springer-Verlag; 1981.
21. **Jahna H, Wittich H**. [*Conservative Methods in Bone Fracture Treatment*]. 1st ed. Wien, München, Baltimore: Urban & Schwarzenberg; 1985. German.
22. **Hey Groves EW**. *On Modern Methods of Treating Fractures.* 1st ed. Bristol: John Wright & Sons Ltd; 1916.

3 Principles of casting

Klaus Dresing, Franz Seibert, Jos Engelen

Authors   Klaus Dresing, Franz Seibert, Jos Engelen

3   Principles of casting

1   Introduction   Klaus Dresing, Franz Seibert, Jos Engelen

A fracture not only causes the loss of stability of the bone, the extremity itself also loses its physiological stability while the surrounding soft tissues are more or less compromised. As a nonoperative (ie, noninvasive) technique of fracture treatment, casting helps to keep the fracture in the reduced position by stabilizing the fracture fragments from outside and by "immobilizing" the fracture during the healing process of the bone. However, casting with reduction and immobilization of a fracture is a challenging task for every trauma surgeon. In recent decades, a lot of nonoperative fracture care knowledge has been lost due to an increased preference for operative fracture care, yet the old principles, which are still applicable and approved, should be remembered and accepted.

Although the old principles of casting have proven to be (and still are) effective, problems can still occur, such as the stiffening of joints or the occasional tremendous loss of muscle. Initially, physicians began to follow Lucas-Championnière, who was not only the first to highlight these problems but also the first to start teaching that with only a little immobilization, and a lot of functional therapy and massage, the fracture would heal quite well [1]. Later, an even more effective process was developed by Lorenz Böhler, whose technique was based on the principle of immobilizing the bone fragments and adjacent joints in a functional position, and for only as long as necessary, for a good clinical outcome. His method of fracture treatment was thought to achieve the best results, and he was also the author of several important books and numerous publications on nonoperative fracture treatment [2, 3].

This chapter therefore explores the fundamental principles of casting as developed over time by the leaders in the field, and provides an overview of other important principles including the basics of bone healing, functional treatment, cast wedging, and patient information.

2   Principles of bone healing   Klaus Dresing

In bone healing, there is a difference between "direct" and "indirect" healing. While indirect bone healing is the usual way of healing during nonoperative fracture care in a cast or splint, direct bone healing normally needs absolute stability (eg, rigid fixation with lag screws or compression plate, so as to prevent interfragmentary motion).

2.1   Direct bone healing

In direct (or primary) bone healing, the fracture gap is very small (ie, less than 0.5 mm). Osteons, the channels and blood vessels of which cortical bone is comprised, cross from one side of the fracture to the other. The cortical bone from both fracture sides reconnects by the end of the process. Direct bone healing occurs under conditions of absolute fracture stability by direct osteonal remodeling without callus formation.

The osteons (known as Haversian systems) run longitudinally along the cortex, and are bound to each other by cement lines. Osteons are formed around a central vessel, with surrounding layers called lamellae, which are orientated into a helical fashion, each twisting in the opposite direction to its neighbor. On the bone's surface is the periosteum, with an outer fibrous layer, and an inner cambium layer, which contains progenitor cells that replace old and injured cells (**Fig 3-1**).

During the process of healing, the bone is remodeled. There is a constant state of turnover as old bone is removed and new bone is continually laid down. Cells called osteoclasts remove bone, while osteoblasts lay down new bone. The balance between bone removal and bone deposit is determined by the biomechanical loads on the skeleton and the metabolic need to mobilize, or store, calcium ions (Ca++) (**Fig 3-2**).

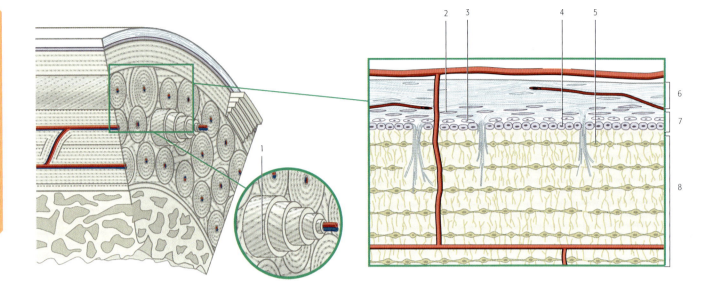

Fig 3-1 Schematic cut-through of cortical bone. Each helical orientated osteon (Haversian system) twists in the opposite direction to its neighbor (middle). The bone's surface is covered by the periosteum, including its inner cambium layer, which contains a variety of progenitor cells (right).

1   Helical lamellae
2   Osteoprogenitors
3   Preosteoblasts
4   Osteoblasts
5   Osteocytes
6   Periosteum
7   Cambium layer
8   Cortical bone

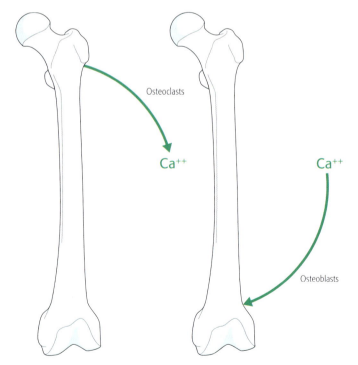

Fig 3-2 In normal bone there is continual turnover; old bone is removed by osteoclasts (Ca++ release) and new bone is laid down by osteoblasts (Ca++ intake).

Authors   Klaus Dresing, Franz Seibert, Jos Engelen

The remodeling phase starts with cutting cones crossing the cortical fracture zone from each direction. The advancing osteons, with osteoclastic cutting cones at their tips, become transformational units that remove woven (immature) bone (which has an irregular structure and orientation), followed by osteoblasts laying down cylinders of new lamellar bone (with highly organized and oriented structure) (**Fig 3-3**).

2.2   Indirect bone healing

Indirect (or secondary) bone healing, which occurs during nonoperative fracture treatment, involves callus formation around the fracture area. It is divided into three phases:

- Reactive phase
- Reparative phase
- Remodeling phase.

2.2.1   Reactive phase

2.2.1.1   Fracture and inflammation

Following the impact or cause of the fracture, soft-tissue damage, disruption of blood vessels, and separation of bony fragments can occur. A hematoma forms and the periosteum partly ruptures (**Fig 3-4**). Some bony fragments are without soft-tissue attachment, and with that, become devascularized and necrotic (**Fig 3-5**).

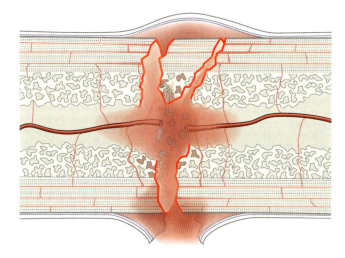

Fig 3-4   Hematoma formation and partial rupture of the periosteum.

Fig 3-3   Cutting cones create cylindrical bone formations. At the tip, osteoclasts remove old bone, followed by osteoblasts, which lay down new lamellar bone.

1   Central vessel
2   Osteocytes
3   Osteoblasts
4   Osteoclasts
5   Woven bone

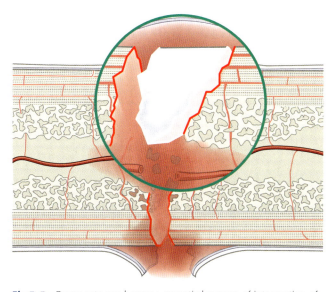

Fig 3-5   Fragments can become necrotic because of interruption of blood circulation.

Following this, the vessels dilate, causing a rise in local tissue temperature. Inflammation then occurs, because in the fracture hematoma a range of cells start to accumulate including macrophages, neutrophil granulocytes, mesenchyme stem cells, and cytokines, all of which help to remove and replace old and injured cells. From the periosteal cambium layer, progenitor cells are delivered to the fracture site (**Fig 3-6**). Osteoinductive growth factors stimulate the proliferation and differentiation of mesenchymal stem cells.

Osteoclasts remove necrotic bone parts, and the hematoma starts to become stabilized by fibrin fibers forming a hematoma callus (**Fig 3-7**).

2.2.1.2 Granulation

In this part of the reactive phase, chemical and mechanical factors stimulate callus formation and mineralization. New vessels invade the hematoma, and the hematoma is colonized by cells called fibroblasts, which derive from the periosteum. Granulation tissue develops in the fracture gap, consisting of collagen fibers, which are produced by the fibroblasts. These collagen fibers loosely link the bone fragments (**Fig 3-8**).

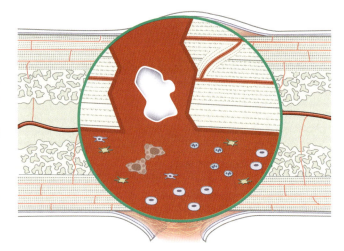

Fig 3-6   Delivery of progenitor cells from the periosteal cambium layer.

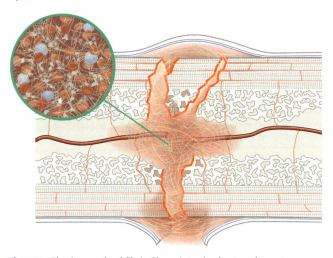

Fig 3-7   The ingrowth of fibrin fibers into the fracture hematoma starts to stabilize it (hematoma callus).

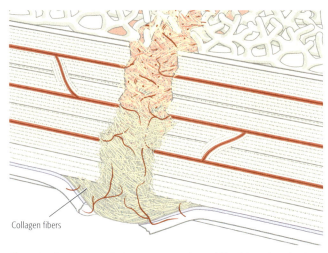

Collagen fibers

Fig 3-8   During granulation, new vessels and fibroblasts invade the hematoma. The fibroblasts produce collagen fibers, which loosely link the fragments together.

Authors   Klaus Dresing, Franz Seibert, Jos Engelen

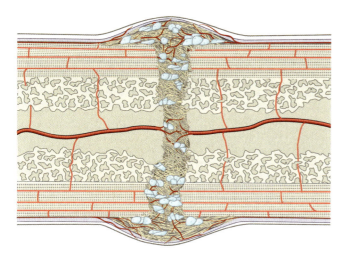

Fig 3-9   Granulation tissue gradually differentiates into fibrous tissue and fibrocartilage.

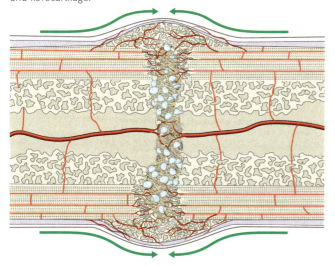

Fig 3-10   Callus cuff formation always starts at the periphery moving towards the fracture gap.

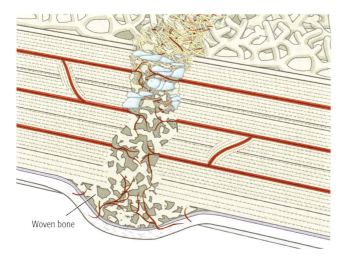

Woven bone

Fig 3-11   The cartilaginous callus is transformed into woven bone.

2.2.2   Reparative phase

2.2.2.1 Cartilage callus formation

In the reparative phase, the granulation tissue gradually differentiates into fibrous tissue and cartilage to form soft callus (**Fig 3-9**). Soft callus is an unorganized network of woven bone.

2.2.2.2 Lamellar bone deposition

In the next step, the cartilaginous tissue becomes calcified, transforming into hard callus. After soft-callus lining of the fracture ceases, the hard callus stage starts and lasts until the fragments are firmly united by new bone (3–4 months postinjury).

Endochondral ossification forms spindle-shaped bone cuffs, starting at the periphery and moving towards the center, further stiffening the healing tissue. The callus cuff is always thicker than the normal diameter of the bone, resulting in a longer lever arm, which is biomechanically more appropriate (**Fig 3-10**). Finally, the callus is converted into woven bone (**Fig 3-11**).

3

PRINCIPLES

2.2.3 Remodeling phase

In the final phase of indirect bone healing, bone remodeling occurs, either under traction (distractive strain) or compression (compressive strain). Cutting cones transform the woven bone into lamellar bone. The fracture healing process is completed with the remodeling of the medullary canal and removal of part of the external callus.

2.3 Factors influencing normal bone healing

Fracture healing greatly depends on the biological status of the bone fragments and on the local soft tissue, especially the periosteum. But fracture healing is also influenced by the amount and kind of movement.

2.3.1 Mobilization and movement

During the soft-callus phase, too much movement or excessive strain risks tearing the repairing tissue and can compromise callus formation, a potential cause of "delayed union" or "nonunion" (**Fig 3-12, Fig 3-13**). Yet, movement is necessary for bone healing because it increases muscle activity, stimulates vascularity (venous and arterial flow), stimulates callus maturation, and prevents thromboembolic complications (see topic 9 Functional treatment in this chapter and chapter 4 Thrombosis prophylaxis). But the mobilization and physiotherapy must be adapted to fit its stage of fracture healing (see **Table 3-1**). The problem in mobilizing a patient with a fractured extremity is to find the correct balance between too much and too little.

2.3.2 Delayed union and nonunion

After a bone fracture, normal bone healing will occur within 6–8 weeks, depending on the location and the type of fracture. In a period of 3–4 months, fractures normally heal over soft callus, and there is formation of hard callus. However, too much movement in the early phases of bone healing can result in delayed union or even nonunion. Other factors that can affect healing include soft-tissue injury with devascularization, the noncompliance of the patient, vascular diseases with insufficient perfusion of bone and soft tissue, and smoking.

When a fracture has not healed within the usual time frame (variously estimated but typically by 4 months), there is said to be a delayed union. If a fracture ceases radiographic progress toward union over a 3 month interval, and remains ununited after 6 months, there is nonunion (**Fig 3-13**).

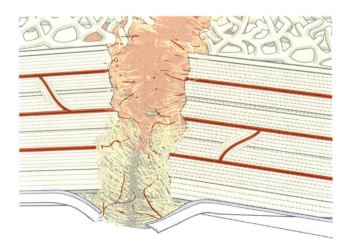

Fig 3-12   Too much strain during the healing process can rupture the granulation tissue; the collagen fibers break, and the process of bone healing is altered so much that delayed or nonunion results.

Authors   Klaus Dresing, Franz Seibert, Jos Engelen

Duration	Description	Symptomatology	Physiotherapy
Day 1–5	Hematoma callus: fracture hematoma with subsequent coagulation Fibrin fibers stabilize the hematoma	Unstable Mobile fragments	Lymphatic and venous decongestant measures
Day 5–10	Within the hematoma, a gelatinous structure forms Capillaries pervade the hematoma, and the hematoma is converted to immature granulation tissue (connective tissue), a gelatinous callus	Muscle pull and muscle tone narrow the fracture gap Fragments are unstable	Lymphatic and venous decongestant measures
Day 10–15	Osteoclasts break down dead and necrotic bone Fibroblasts, chondroblasts, and osteoblasts proliferate Osteoid matrix and chondroid matrix are formed (granulation callus)	Fracture is mobile	Isometric strengthening of the muscles Passive movement
Day 15–21	Osteoclasts break down dead and necrotic bone (the resorption fracture gap becomes wider) Formation of new bone A callus cuff is formed (stabilization) Callus and osteoid transformation to bony trabeculae (endochondral ossification)	Decrease in movement between the fragments Elastic fixation	Transformation from passive to active mobilization
Day 21–60	Volume of callus decreases (modeling) Restructuring of callus Reconstitution of medullary canal and medullary fat	Fracture is stable for exercises Bony consolidation in the x-ray	Progressive weight bearing

Table 3-1   Periods of fracture healing in humans in relation to symptomatology and physiotherapy.

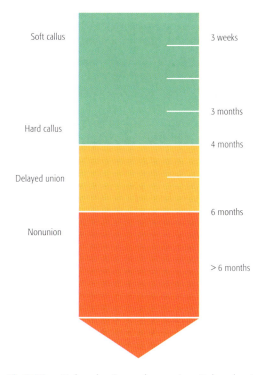

Fig 3-13a   Delayed union and nonunion. Delayed union occurs if the fracture has not healed after approximately 4 months. If the fracture has still not healed after 6 months or more, there is nonunion.

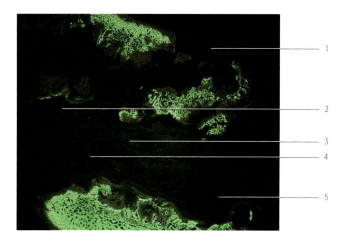

Fig 3-13b   An example of nonunion, as shown under fluorescent staining, showing connective tissue but no bone detection within the nonunion gap.

1   Proximal fragment
2   Fluorescent staining
3   Nonunion gap
4   No bone detection, but connective tissue
5   Distal fragment

3 Nonoperative fracture care   Franz Seibert

Each body region has its own criteria, but in general, there are a number of preconditions for the use of a plaster or synthetic cast in fracture treatment. One of the most important of these is that the soft-tissue envelope allows for the application of a cast; as opposed to the case of an infected wound needing daily change of dressing, or if the fracture was unstable and so an external fixator would be more suitable. Additionally, patients that need continued intubation and anesthesia over a longer period of time would particularly benefit from surgical fracture stabilization, as skin conditions cannot be checked daily beneath a plaster cast, and if unconscious, the patient cannot communicate the feeling of pain beneath the cast, eg, from pressure sores.

Nevertheless, there are a number of advantages that nonoperative fracture care has over operative treatment. Moreover, as society lives longer, the number of patients not suitable for surgery due to their medical and mental status continues to rise. And for those in poorer countries, an economic point of view also has to be taken into consideration when choosing treatment options. Therefore, any nonoperative treatment must be conducted as effectively as possible, keeping in mind that later on, the patient's status might not allow follow-up surgery. Providing that good results are achieved by reducing the fragments, the question of how to proceed, either nonoperatively or surgically, must be determined early on, together with the patient. Both patient and surgeon have to be aware of all the options for their further planning.

The principles of casting are governed by three important key points, the three Rs:
• Reduction
• Retention
• Rehabilitation.

Reduction: Fracture fragments must be reduced in order to restore contact with each other, ie, the distal fragment with the central fragment(s) and the proximal fragment, and recreate functionally acceptable limb alignment (ie, axis, rotation, and length).

Retention: Fracture fragments must be kept in the reduced position and immobilized until bone healing of the fracture is achieved.

Rehabilitation: Restoration of function with an early start to functional therapy; first, the free joints during cast immobilization, followed by functional therapy of the entire extremity after cast removal.

The primary goal of cast treatment after trauma is to achieve a painless and well-functioning extremity as early as possible, using the three Rs. Every step of treatment has to focus on this final goal and, in some cases, might need adaptation of therapeutic options or even changes in the treatment algorithm.

3.1 Advantages of nonoperative fracture care

The great advantages of nonoperative fracture treatment over operative treatment are:
• No need for surgical resources and logistics
• Normally, no danger of surgically-induced or implant-related infection or complications
• Reduced risk from general anesthesia
• No need for subsequent implant removal by surgery.

Additionally, there are circumstances that make some fractures more suitable for conservative therapy by plaster or synthetic casts than others. Yet, even knowing that every fracture can be treated nonoperatively, it is a question of acceptance of the expected result, especially in regard to the expectations of surgeon and patient concerning the radiological and, even more importantly, the clinical outcome.

Authors   Klaus Dresing, Franz Seibert, Jos Engelen

The decision must be based on:

- The form of the fracture (shaft, metaphyseal, intraarticular without step-off or impaction)
- The absence of displacement, especially after reduction
- The degree of malalignment
  - Limited axial (varus, valgus, antecurvation, or retrocurvation < 5°)
  - Rotational (internal, external rotation < 10°)
- Length discrepancy.

Physicians must remember the importance of overall anatomical alignment, as well as the fact that limb shortening is more acceptable for consolidation than a gap with no fracture fragment contact.

Moreover, it is important that patients whose fractures are treated without surgical reduction and fixation receive periodic reassessment by x-ray check of reduction, and clinical examination with continuous documentation of capillary refill (undisturbed blood flow), active and passive neurological integrity (no sensation deficit or loss of muscle activity), and painless intact skin conditions.

> Every immobilization using a cast should be followed by regular recheck of motor function, vascularization, and sensitivity, starting directly after the cast is applied.

3.2   Disadvantages of nonoperative fracture care

Some disadvantages of nonoperative fracture management with plaster or synthetic casts must also be addressed:

- Casts require intensive surveillance (at least once a week under normal circumstances), and a cooperative patient
- Full functional recovery can at times be delayed; also depending on the age of the patient
- There is the possibility of developing "fracture disease" with contracture, loss of muscle and/or bone (demineralization), accompanied by pain and swelling, which can lead to a disastrous loss of function, the so-called complex regional pain syndrome (reflex sympathetic dystrophy, with associated demineralization called Sudeck's atrophy).

We must remember that the father of conservative fracture treatment, Lorenz Böhler, stated in 1929 in his book *The Treatment of Fractures* that conservative (nonoperative) fracture treatment needs careful attention, exact technique, and able physicians [2].

4 Cast treatment for bruises, sprains and strains, infections, and nerve impairments

Klaus Dresing, Franz Seibert, Jos Engelen

Today, casts and splints are not only used for fracture treatment but also as a preliminary measure to prepare or condition soft tissues, and very often for patients not immediately fit enough for surgery. In addition, casts are often indicated as postoperative protection devices. After surgical intervention, the postoperative inflammation can be diminished by short-term cast immobilization. Additionally, protection by external immobilization is sometimes needed with noncompliant patients, or whenever the stabilized osteosynthesis is not adequate to allow weight bearing or exercise.

Severe bruises, and joint sprains and strains may require short-term cast immobilization in order to reduce pain and swelling. Ruptures of tendons and muscles can also be treated with immobilization, with functional bracing or casting (see chapter 11.1 Ligament and tendon injuries).

Cast immobilization or treatment by orthosis may be indicated to improve limb function in patients with nerve impairments, palsy or paresis, eg, palsy of the radial nerve or common peroneal nerve (see chapter 11.2 Nerve injuries).

Adjuvant immobilization in cases of infected limbs, arthritis, and aseptic swelling can support nonoperative treatment and reduce treatment time (see chapter 12 Indications for nonoperative treatment of infections).

Special dynamic casts (for example, a Quengel-hinge (extension-desubluxation) orthosis for the knee, or for the finger joints to regain flexion and extension in the PIP joint) could be indicated when restriction of movement or joint stiffness is observed after treatment.

5 Forms of splints, casts, and orthoses

Klaus Dresing, Jos Engelen

Casts can be distinguished according to the various materials involved in the immobilization:

- Plaster of Paris
- Synthetic materials
- Bandages
- Tapes

and by the specific techniques and applications used:

- Splints
- Casts
- Split casts
- Orthoses.

Casts are custom made for a patient using bandage-like materials that harden during application. Chapter 6 Properties of cast materials outlines the specific features of these materials. They can also be used to make splints. A great variety of prefabricateed and custom-made orthoses are also available for immobilization and for functional fracture treatment. This book presents fracture braces and other orthoses made from casting materials.

Both plaster of Paris (POP) and synthetic materials can be applied for primary, temporary, secondary, or definitive treatment of acute fractures, sprains, or strains. For immobilizing infected soft tissues and tendons, extremities, or joints, simple longitudinal splints can be used. Splints using a U-shaped slab technique (where the material is applied down one side of the limb and back up the other) or sugar-tong splints (Böhler U-POP casts) are used to immobilize the upper extremity, forearm, or injuries of the ankle joint.

Fig 3-14 shows examples of a splint (**a**), a cast (**b**), a split cast (**c**), and an orthosis (a custom-fabricated fracture brace) (**d**).

Authors   Klaus Dresing, Franz Seibert, Jos Engelen

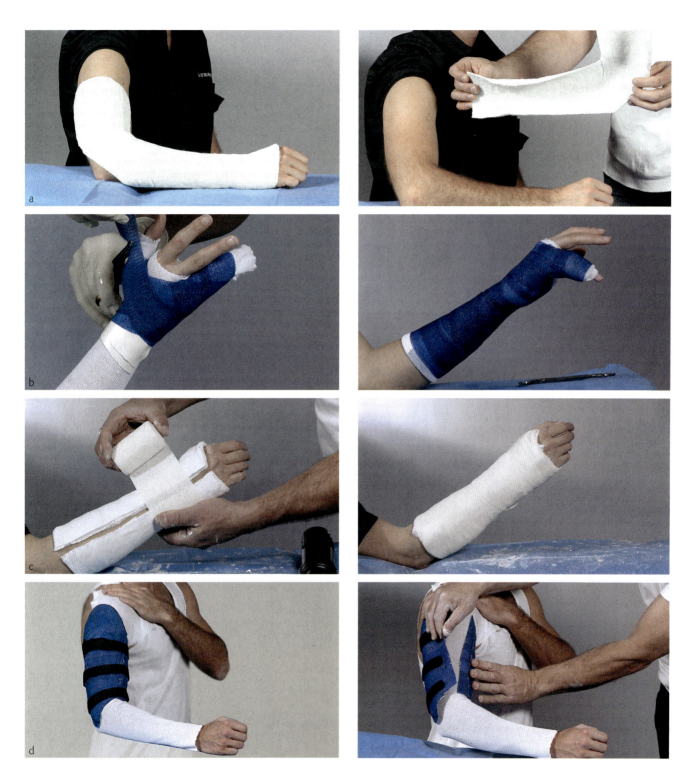

Fig 3-14a–d   The major forms of splints and casts.
a   An example of a splint.
b   An example of a fully circumferential cast.
c   An example of a split cast, which has been split and rewrapped with gauze bandage to allow for swelling.
d   An example of an orthosis (showing a fracture brace) where velcro straps permit easy removal and readjustment of tightness.

3

PRINCIPLES

5.1 Splints

If complete immobilization is not required, eg, in order just to decrease swelling or to protect against further soft-tissue damage, a noncircumferential "splint" made out of POP or synthetic material can be applied. During primary treatment of fractures and joint injuries in the emergency department, these types of noncircular casts are normally applied since acute and secondary swelling can occur in the course of treatment.

Another indication for the application of a splint is postoperative treatment or as protection after osteosynthesis in order to ensure that the cast does not conflict with postoperative swelling.

Before applying a splint, a tube bandage or stockinette is pulled over the extremity, and the appropriate amount of padding is applied. It is important to understand that excessive padding will compromise the immobilization effect of the splint as there will be too much space between the various layers of the cast and the skin. Lorenz Böhler preferred a nearly unpadded but well molded plaster. He only used padding to protect bony prominences.

When using plaster of Paris or synthetic material, the location of the injury and the strength of the patient determine how many layers of undercast padding should be used.

To increase stability, the splint should cover about two thirds of the circumference of the extremity. Another possibility is the use of small strips of splint material to reinforce its strength in areas where more stability is needed, eg, around joints.

When using POP, a splint for the upper extremity typically consists of 8–10 layers, and for the lower extremity 12–16 layers are needed. As the rigidity of synthetic material is greater, the number of layers needed for the upper extremity is only 6–8, and for the lower extremity 9–12 layers is sufficient.

5.2 Casts

A circumferential "cast" is used whenever a higher degree of immobilization is needed, or in secondary treatment. The stability of a fully circular cast is much higher than in a splint and it allows the patient to be more active. A cast allows weight bearing and walking, which is not possible with a splint or split cast.

To make the cast stable enough for weight bearing it might be necessary to combine the circular windings with additional strips or longuettes of splint material in order to reinforce those areas of the cast where it might break easily, especially in the vicinity of joints.

In a cast, the extremity is covered with a tube bandage (stockinette) and the required amount of padding is applied. The cast roll is then wrapped around the limb from distal to proximal. While winding, the cast material should overlap at least 50% in order to avoid weak spots (throughout this text this is referred to as the "half-overlapping technique"). In areas where the maximum load on the extremity occurs, more windings are necessary. For a cast, 8–10 layers of POP or 4–6 layers of synthetic are required in order to achieve enough stability for the upper extremity. For lower extremity casts, 12–14 layers of POP or 6–8 layers of synthetic cast material are recommended.

All circumferential casts applied for primary treatment (first cast after injury or surgical procedure) must be split completely and secured with an adhesive bandage. Otherwise, postoperative soft-tissue swelling will be limited by the cast resulting in compression of the soft tissues. This might cause a compartment syndrome. Moreover, since some cast materials and bandages can shrink as they dry, the physician/cast technician should not only split and loosen the cast, but also divide all underlying layers of padding after the cast material has set (hardened).

Authors   Klaus Dresing, Franz Seibert, Jos Engelen

5.3   Split casts

When a circumferential cast is applied to a fresh fracture, or postoperatively, it should be opened or split longitudinally to become a "split cast", to allow posttraumatic or postoperative swelling to occur without increasing tissue pressure (see topic 11 Cast splitting techniques and cast removal in chapter 14.1 Overview of cast, splint, orthosis, and bandage techniques). Without splitting the cast, complications can occur, such as impaired venous or arterial circulation, nerve irritation, or compartment syndrome, with potentially permanent injury to soft tissues, especially muscles and nerves.

The cast is split completely using scissors or a cast saw and widened with a cast spreader. Another technique is to remove a 1 cm strip in order to achieve more space. This gap is filled with padding and the split cast is then wrapped with an elastic bandage in order to prevent swelling along the gap.

5.4   Orthoses and removable casts

An "orthosis" is a removable external orthopedic device that prevents or controls the movement of the limbs, head, or spine. While casts are the domain of the surgeon and cast technician, orthoses are typically applied by other healthcare professionals, such as orthotists and occupational therapists, and the devices themselves are usually easy to remove and reapply, even by the patient. Examples of orthoses include the halo vest or cervical collars for the head and neck area, or strap-on braces for the arm or ankle. The main types of orthoses include:

• Commercially available prefabricated devices, with variation in their ability to be contoured to fit the patient
• Custom-fabricated devices made of leather, plastic, metal, and other components, with or without using a mold of the patient's limb
• Devices made from sheets of thermoplastic material specifically molded to the contours of the patient's limb
• Removable casts and splints made with synthetic casting materials, developed specifically for each patient.

There is great variation in the costs and access to the first three categories of orthosis around the world, and are beyond the scope of this book, but still may be worthy of consideration for certain therapeutic needs. However, orthoses made from casting materials are made to specifically meet the needs and shape of the patient, and the materials have a lower cost. And by incorporating other materials, their combined adjustability and removability represent a valuable advance in the development of cast technology.

Orthoses made from casting materials are often referred to as "fracture braces" and are particularly well suited for functional fracture treatment (functional exercises, ambulation with partial or full weight bearing, and use of the immobilized part for selected activities of daily living) (see chapters 15.5 Sarmiento humeral brace using synthetic, combicast technique; and 16.9 Sarmiento tibial brace using synthetic, combicast technique).

It is best to apply an orthosis after posttraumatic swelling has resolved. If a fracture brace is designed so that tightness of fit can be adjusted by the patient for optimal support, it becomes even more adaptable. Temporary fracture brace removal can also be helpful for some physical therapy treatments.

3

PRINCIPLES

Removable splints and casts can be secured in various ways. In addition to an over-wrapping bandage, straps with hook and loop fasteners (eg, velcro) permit easy application and removal, and the opportunity to increase brace tightness for functional activities.

Sometimes, a cast can be split twice (bivalved), usually 180° apart, making its removal and reapplication easy. But even with multiple wraps, stability is compromised because circumferential tightening is not possible. If the split in a cast is made so it overlaps adjustably, both fit and mechanical support can be optimized.

6 Pretreatment medical information and informed consent
Klaus Dresing

After complete examination of the patient and study of the type of fracture shown in the x-ray, the patient is informed about the intended treatment. Physicians should take into consideration that an informed patient is a more cooperative patient and thus the outcome will usually be better. The personal rights of the patient have to be respected at all times.

The surgeon needs to distinguish two situations:
- Emergency procedures
- Elective procedures.

In emergency cases, the informed consent is often only given orally. The surgeon has to confirm and document that the treatment and the special procedure (reduction, cast) are required immediately.

In nonemergency fracture treatment, the patient has to be informed about the risks and alternative treatment options prior to treatment. This requires a written informed consent. If the patient is not able to sign, eg, because of fracture or injury of the dominant hand, the oral informed consent is documented by the surgeon and, if possible, signed by a witness. In case of minor patients, written parental consent is always required.

In some countries (such as Germany), medical treatment without valid consent is legally regarded as an injury according to civil or criminal law, even if the outcome is successful [4]. Exemption from punishment requires authorization by the consent of the patient. Such "informed consent" includes documentation that the physician has informed the patient about their medical conditon and the relevant aspects of treatment [4].

In special clinical situations, it is difficult to obtain informed consent from the patient, either because the patient is unable to provide consent or because of a life-threatening situation that requires immediate intervention [5]. The informed consent document must specify the risks and consequences of the intervention [5].

Consent should be obtained prior to casting procedures whenever the patient is able to follow the explanations. The patient should be informed about alternative treatment procedures, and about the course and risks of treatment [6]. The informed consent should be understandable for patients of all ages. In case of minors, the legal guardian(s) have to be informed and they have to sign the form.

Authors   Klaus Dresing, Franz Seibert, Jos Engelen

The list of possible local risks after cast application comprises:
- Skin and soft-tissue alteration
- Bruising beneath the cast
- Pressure necrosis
- Allergic reaction to cast material
- Skin lesions, abrasions by cast saws
- Burn injuries
- Swelling
- Disturbed arterial or venous blood circulation
- Nerve irritation
- Pressure injury of a nerve (eg, peroneal, ulnar, and superficial (sensory) radial nerve)
- Muscle reduction/atrophy
- Compartment syndrome
- Redisplacement of the fracture
- Secondary redislocation of joints
- Displacement of the cast
- Breaking of the cast, especially when using POP
- Joint stiffness
- Muscular contractures
- Shoulder overload or overuse injuries from using crutches
- Pain in adjacent joints caused by abnormal posture.

The list of possible general risks after cast application comprises:
- Thrombosis and embolism of the immobilized limb
- Muscular atrophy
- Osteopenia
- Regional pain syndrome (RPS)
- Back pain after unilateral reduction of weight
- Back pain by relative limb lengthening of the casted lower extremity
- Shoulder-neck pain syndrome with an upper extremity cast.

Surgeons applying casts have to be informed and trained in the correct application of casts, otherwise their treatment might (in some countries) be classified as willful negligence. The professional, medical, and ethical diligence is violated if, under similar conditions, a prudent and trained healthcare provider would carry out treatment in a different manner or if the treatment published in literature differs completely.

The surgeon prescribing the cast must take final responsibility. Although surgeons may delegate the task to a resident or cast technician, the final liability for indication, information, informed consent, as well as problems with the cast lies with the surgeon.

Always remember that at the beginning of any nonoperative fracture treatment, patients and their relatives, parents, or those accompanying them, should first be informed about the risks of a cast, and advice should be given by the surgeon on how to respond in case of problems. When problems do arise with the cast, the patient is obliged to immediately return to the clinic.

3

PRINCIPLES

7   Reduction of bone fractures   Franz Seibert

As the first option in treating a fracture should always be nonoperative treatment, the fracture should be "reduced" as early and as accurately as possible. If the initial conservative trial has failed, operative fracture treatment then becomes the only option. All patients have the right to get the full attention and receive the best efforts of their surgeon in order to achieve a good result, even when receiving nonoperative treatment.

Prompt reduction of the fractured bone is very important whenever the skin is endangered due to inner pressure caused by displaced bone fragments. In special regions, eg, the distal tibia, the ankle joint, and above the knee—especially in the case of displacements with tension on the skin—immediate reduction in order to prevent subsequent skin problems or even necrosis is of utmost importance. The same is true if deformity impairs arterial blood flow, as may happen with a child's supracondylar humeral fracture, or a knee dislocation. A surgical incision through badly injured skin and subcutaneous tissue may break down after an early operation. Delaying the operation until the soft-tissue envelope has recovered helps to avoid such problems.

Open fracture wounds are less serious if caused by indirect trauma, typically a torsional injury resulting in a spiral fracture with sharp pointed ends. These can perforate the skin from inside out. Unless seriously contaminated (eg, from farm yard or industrial dirt), the risk of infection of such injuries is little more than that of closed injuries, assuming adequate wound toilette has been achieved without undue delay.

Open fracture wounds due to a force applied directly to the bone at the fracture site produce more damage to the surrounding skin and soft tissues (fracture zone), often with greater contamination from outside (eg, car against leg). Increased soft-tissue injury is associated with higher rates of infection and impaired fracture healing. Fractures due to direct trauma are usually transverse, short oblique, and/or comminuted. Adequate debridement, combined with the prompt release of any soft-tissue tension from swelling or deformity, are surgical measures intended to reduce the risks of infection and delayed fracture healing. A bone end trapped outside the skin, typically through a tight open wound, can be re-placed inside the soft-tissue envelope with an instrument, sterile gloved finger, or by enlarging the wound with a scalpel. This measure also serves to protect the partially traumatized skin from additional pressure by the bone and to prevent subsequent skin necrosis. Healing of bone is only possible with healthy and intact soft tissues surrounding the fracture zone. Otherwise, consolidation will at least be prolonged, and if worse comes to worst, infection can set in, which can even endanger the patient's life.

Reduction of a fracture is achieved by traction and reversing the fracture mechanism in order to bring the distal fragment back into place. To keep the patient free of pain, local or general anesthetics can be used. Traction can be done either by hand or by placing weight on an extremity in one step or continuously. Traction can only be removed after stabilization (hardening/setting of the plaster) and immobilization of the fractured bone(s) is achieved.

In a so-called Colles' fracture, in which the distal fragment of the radius is impacted, dorsally displaced, dorsally angulated, and supinated, the distal fragment needs first to be disimpacted by manipulative manual traction, increasing displacement, and then moved anteriorly over the proximal fragment followed by palmar flexion at the fracture. Then, releasing traction restores contact of the volar cortical surface at the fracture site, increasing stability, if dorsiflexion of the fracture is prevented. Finally, pronation is added to correct the typical supination malalignment, and increase stability. Simple traction alone almost never corrects the Colles' fracture's multiple deformities.

Because closed manipulation and cast or splint application can be insufficient to reduce some fractures, it is helpful to have additional aids. An assistant, or weights with slings, can improve countertraction. Sometimes, one or more percutaneously inserted pins or wires can help achieve reduction, or maintain traction, perhaps by being incorporated into the cast proximally or distally to the fractures. Sterile equipment and technique are of course essential. Fluoroscopy, with appropriate protective shielding, can also be helpful.

In some instances, it is possible to use preformed splints or bandages, but more often than not, standard cast materials, expertly applied, provide better fit, better padding, and thus optimal immobilization for a fresh fracture.

There are some commercially available knee braces that are useful to limit motion in special situations, eg, healing of

Authors   Klaus Dresing, Franz Seibert, Jos Engelen

the medial collateral ligament or after meniscus repair. They allow controlled joint movement that accelerates healing and improves orientation of collagen fibrils within the healing scar tissue. Tendon healing is known to be improved by a low traction force, but excessive tension can cause failure of a tendon repair. Thus, in some cases, it is helpful to use removable immobilizing splints or casts, which allow limited physical therapy, local wound control, and scar therapy.

Whenever immobilization is needed but compromised soft tissues are present, it is sometimes helpful to incorporate windows within the plaster (more information on cast windows is found in chapter 14.1 Overview of cast, splint, othosis, and bandage techniques). If the patient is allowed to bear weight and the cast has a window over the lateral ankle, this must be closed securely during walking to prevent severe local swelling ("window edema").

The main principle is to first keep the patient alive, and then to keep the limb alive as well. Accurate reduction of fractures provides the best possible foundation for good nonoperative treatment. The goal, full recovery of function, always has to be kept in mind.

8   Stabilization of fractures
Franz Seibert

Stabilization of fracture fragments or joints helps to reduce pain by avoiding motion. Pain relief is one of the most important prerequisites of healing. If patients feel pain, they will feel ill. If patients try to move, the fracture fragments will move as well, and thus cause pain and, as the antidromic contracture of the adjacent muscles tries to stabilize the fragments, even more pain will be caused and the malalignment could worsen. Under such conditions, it will be impossible to encourage patients to move or even to get out of bed. Moreover, there may be an increased loss of muscle and bone. Due to the reduced muscle function and the resulting reduced blood flow, swelling will not subside. Therefore, trophic changes will diminish the chance for good results and healing will take much longer or, under such circumstances, might not be achieved at all.

Stabilization of fracture fragments can either be achieved by external immobilization (casts or splints), or internally by plating and bridging or by an intramedullary rod, typically with proximal and distal locking bolts to maintain length and rotational alignment. Intraarticular fractures with gaps and/or depressed areas have to be reduced anatomically, sometimes augmented by bone substitutes or cancellous bone grafts, and fixed with absolute stability, usually using lag screws and butress plates. Early motion of articular fractures should be encouraged but significant load bearing should await radiographic signs of healing, and progress gradually, guided by absence of pain. Another option for fracture stabilization is the external fixator. This involves an external frame, connected with wires or pins to bone proximally and distally to a fracture. Such a frame can be attached to both ends of a fractured bone, or may cross a joint, in the case of an articular fracture, to avoid loading the articular surface of the injured joint. Depending upon their design and application, external fixators can permit weight bearing and/or joint motion, as chosen for a particular injury and patient.

For all fractures, it is important to provide enough stability to control pain, maintain fracture alignment, promote healing of bone and soft tissues, and permit mobilization of the patient. As soon as the fracture is stable enough, considering its pattern, location, means of therapeutic stabilization, and extent of healing, progressive functional use should be encouraged, within the patient's range of comfort.

PRINCIPLES

37

Immobilization of fractures with a POP cast may also need stabilization of the adjacent joint in order to minimize motion of the fracture fragments and reduce pain and swelling. If stabilization of the fragments is not adequate, each muscle contraction and motion at the ends of the fracture fragments will cause pain. Therefore, the fragments should have good contact as well as correct axial and rotational alignment. As there is swelling and hematoma in the first phase after the fracture, care must be taken that the cast is not too tight. Otherwise, pain will increase and pressure damage to the surrounding tissues might bring about disastrous results perhaps even leading to amputation. Therefore, primary immobilization cannot be done with a closed (circular) cast. Noncircumferential splints or split casts are the methods of choice. After swelling is reduced and the hematoma has been resorbed, a circular cast can be applied and more activity allowed. Early range of motion exercises for all mobile joints are encouraged in order to prevent stiffness. Elevation of the injured limb helps to control swelling, as does functional use, which also helps to avoid atrophy and joint stiffness, as well as to promote fracture healing.

Duration of stabilization should be as short as necessary, and the cast should extend only as far as needed. Normally, the "three-point stabilization technique" (see **Fig 3-16** in topic 10 of this chapter) will keep alignment, axis, and rotation within acceptable limits for the duration of immobilization and bony healing.

9 Functional treatment   Klaus Dresing

"Functional fracture treatment" is the early and progressive use of the injured limb during fracture healing, as opposed to enforced rest and restrictive immobilization. It typically includes use of casts or fracture braces that allow as much function as possible, while providing enough support to keep fracture site motion within the limits required for bone healing, as well as to preserve adequate fracture alignment. Examples include:

- Early mobilization and exercises within pain tolerance for patients with stable vertebral or pelvic fractures
- Slings and exercises for many proximal humerus fractures
- Fracture braces, range of motion and muscle isometrics for humeral shaft fractures
- Abbreviated forearm casts or braces for isolated ulnar fractures
- Weight bearing patella tendon bearing casts or braces for tibial shaft fractures.

With nonoperative fracture treatment, the physician must distinguish between immobilization and nonimmobilizing functional treatment, as cast-free functional treatment is a therapeutic option for some fracture indications. Functional treatment after surgery, especially intramedullary fracture fixation, is also an important postoperative tool.

9.1 Benefits of functional treatment
The complete immobilization of an extremity leads to cast-mediated bone mineral loss [7], as first described by Wolff in Berlin in 1892 [8]. This is associated not only with decreased physical activity due to limb fractures [9], but also measurably altered activity of the brain, as well as induced rapid reorganization of the sensorimotor system [10]. Fur-

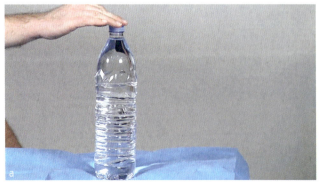
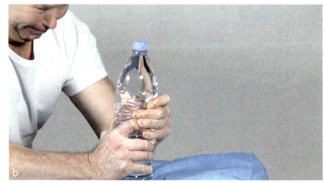

Fig 3-15a–d   Comparison of the stability of a tight-fitting cast using filled (**a, b**) and empty (**c, d**) plastic soda bottles as an example.

Authors   Klaus Dresing, Franz Seibert, Jos Engelen

thermore, these changes in the cortex are also associated with skill transfer from the injured to the uninjured extremity [11]. Trauma and the subsequent immobilization together induce alterations of the soft and hard tissues. Immobilization leads to progressive decrease in muscle mass, strength, and tension based on a decrease of muscle fiber diameter [10]. The collagen fibers develop cross-links, which are followed by lessened flexibility of tendons and ligaments. During immobilization, cartilage degeneration starts with proteoglycan decrease [10]. With immobilization, the normal feedback system between muscle spindle and skin and joint receptors is also influenced.

Partial immobilization, however, inhibits certain movements of joints and extremities but does not completely immobilize the joint. A second option is to keep extremities and joints from bearing loads but to preserve the functional activity of the musculoskeletal apparatus [12–16]. With partial immobilization, functional treatment is possible and thus the usual disadvantages of immobilization can be prevented or at least reduced.

After the first period of wound healing, no later than after the first postoperative or postinjury week, functional follow-up treatment should start. The amount of mobilization depends on fracture location, displacement, joint dislocation (if any), soft-tissue involvement, nonoperative versus operative fracture care, and the compliance of the patient.

The positive outcomes from functional immobilization result from:
• Mechanical effects
• Exteroceptive effects
• Sensomotor effects
• Psychological effects.

Mechanical effects:
The various cast and immobilization materials have different physical properties according to elasticity, bending force, and adhesive force. These support bandages and cast materials build a coherent system together with the underlying soft tissues and skin. Therefore, these tissues are exposed to the bending and compressive forces transmitted to and/or relayed by the cast material.

Exteroceptive effects:
The coherent system (cast and bandage material with underlying soft tissue and skin) stimulates mechanoreceptors resulting in an activation of muscles, tendons, and joint capsules.

Sensomotor effects:
Functional dressing and bandaging will result in functioning sensomotor pathways in muscles and joints.

Psychological effects:
A functional bandage or bracing can result in a feeling of safety, especially with anxious patients.

Sarmiento et al first described functional bracing in 1977 [13]. His brace consisted of anterior and posterior synthetic half-shells that were fixed together with velcro straps. The reduced fracture was kept in position through soft-tissue compression, and with decreasing swelling, the brace was tightened. The principle is comparable to the high stability of a filled plastic soda/water bottle (**Fig 3-15**).

Functional fracture treatment makes use of the biology of fracture and soft-tissue healing. The normal feedback of the body, including that initiated by pain, is helpful in functional treatment.

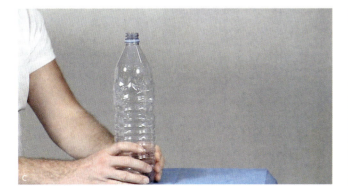

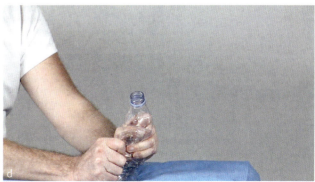

Functional treatment is normally an early mobilization therapeutic regime. The goal of functional treatment is that the extremity at the end of treatment recovers maximal possible function with:

- Improvement of joint function
- Prophylaxis of contractions
- Improved coordination
- Strengthening of muscles and function
- Possibility for endurance training
- Possibility for training of fine and gross motor skills.

9.2 Indications for functional treatment

Functional treatment is especially indicated in nonoperative fracture care of fractured long bones. Fractures of the clavicle or pediatric fractures of the tibia are further indications. Functional treatment is also indicated after various osteosyntheses of long bones, ie, metaphyseal and articular fractures.

At the final checkup of every cast, splint, or orthosis, the free movement of all joints that do not require immobilization must be possible.

Although there are numerous advantages of functional nonoperative fracture care, operative fracture treatment is preferred in many countries. The expenditure of time and personnel is nearly the same as for operative treatment. Fracture braces for functional treatment need individually adapted adjustments by a cast specialist/orthopedic technician. However, hospitals can earn more money by operative fracture treatment than with functional fracture care.

In developing countries, on the other hand, many patients obtain a favorable outcome from this low-cost nonoperative treatment option.

10 Biomechanics of casts

Franz Seibert, Klaus Dresing, Jos Engelen

Whenever an extremity is relaxed and not in motion it is in balance. Forces applied to this extremity will lead to movement and result in motion, which in turn will lead to a change in position. Mechanics is a science devoted to studying forces and the results of these forces. Biomechanics is the implementation of mechanical principles incorporated into the musculoskeletal system and also pertains to immobilized extremities in casts [17]. Physicians dealing with immobilization should understand these principles, as they are essential for the selection and application of a splint or cast.

In the case of fractures, there may be an imbalance between the forces on the extremity resulting in displacement of the different parts of the fractured bone. The cause of this displacement can come from the trauma itself, from direct force on the extremity, or from the leverage of the inserted muscles pulling on the fracture fragments instead of an intact bone [18].

In theory, a support (or a force) to counter these forces is needed to stabilize the broken bone or the unstable joint. The way to correct this imbalance also depends on the amount of force. For example, there is much more tension on the various fragments in a broken forearm than in a broken clavicle. Therefore, the need for stabilization or immobilization is much higher in a forearm fracture.

Using splints or casts means using an external force. Stabilizing only two points, distally and proximally of the fracture, will not be sufficient for control of angulation. A third point is needed in order to counteract the forces on the various fragments once the muscle pulls. The three-point fixation technique is necessary in order to stabilize or immobilize a fracture as this will achieve a new balance between the different fragments (**Fig 3-16**) [19].

As already mentioned, the necessary amount of counterforce depends on the amount of force applied to the extremity. In a forearm fracture, an above-elbow cast or splint has to be applied otherwise the resulting forces on the fragments would exceed the counterforce provided by the cast. On the other hand, a fracture in the ankle is so far from the proximal side of the tibia or fibula that a below-knee cast will suffice to counteract the forces exerted on the fragments. There is no need to accommodate the three-point principle, as the resulting forces are counteracted by means of the proximal tibia or fibula. One should always aim to leave as much movement as possible, and if there is no need to immobilize the proximal joint it should not be done. However, a proximal bandage

Authors   Klaus Dresing, Franz Seibert, Jos Engelen

that is too short or too loose will lose its stabilizing effect and will lead to more leverage, resulting in a loss of reduction or even a rotation of the fracture.

Another way to stabilize a fracture in a long bone is to apply a certain type of compression by means of the soft tissues (hydraulic effect) as published by Sarmiento on his brace techniques (for example, see **Fig 3-14d**). These techniques offer the possibility of leaving both joints of the fracture (distal and proximal) free. A stabilizing or immobilizing bandage will only stabilize or immobilize if the principles of mechanics and biomechanics have been applied properly. It must also be acknowledged that the design and application of casts for fracture treatment is an art, passed from teacher to student. Collected clinical experience informs us of indications and likely results, based upon fracture analysis and classification.

If needed, include joints in a functional manner so that contracture can be prevented. Extended casts, eg, upper-arm casts for forearm fractures, should only stay on for as short a time as necessary and be in a functional position (90° elbow flexion) in order to allow early motion after cast reduction. The same applies to long leg POP casts for a lower-leg fracture. As soon as possible, the cast should be exchanged for a Sarmiento-like patellar bearing cast in order to allow knee flexion by controlling alignment and axis of the lower-leg fractures.

In some special cases and fractures, a Steinman pin will need to be incorporated within the plaster (eg, Steinman pin in-serted in the calcaneus in a tibial pilon fracture). This will allow you to apply traction while keeping the fragments in the correct position at first. Special padding will allow correcting the axes during the first period of immobilization and formation of the first callus, which is still flexible enough to allow correction.

Sometimes, it is also helpful to incorporate elastic devices (elastic bands or springs) in immobilizing splints or casts in order to help avoid active motion in the direction needing protection. For example, after suture repair of flexor tendons, active flexion, which puts tension on tendons and sutures, has to be avoided during the first period after surgery. Therefore, flexion is achieved passively by springs or elastic bands while active extension/stretching of the fingers is encouraged in order to allow tendon gliding and to avoid adhesions and scaring around the tendons. Even the process of healing will be improved by better circulation and forming of a new fibrous channel after surgical opening of the flexor tendon sheath to permit tendon repair.

A special lesson can be learned from Sarmiento. He made use of the muscle pressure from the surrounding muscles to bring fracture fragments into place by distributing the pressure from the cast via muscle activity directly onto the bone in order to achieve good alignment. Sarmiento gained great experience and success by bracing fractures, which is still a common practice today with humeral shaft fractures, and isolated ulnar shaft fractures. He also reported good results for closed tibial shaft fractures, particularly those due to lower energy injuries, and characterized by lesser degrees of displacement and shortening. Today, the Sarmiento version of the below-knee cast is still used. It partly incorporates the femoral condyles, helping control rotation, and, through good contact and molding, improves fracture stability (see chapters 16.8 Sarmiento (patella tendon bearing) cast using plaster of Paris and 16.9 Sarmiento tibial brace using synthetic, combicast technique). With this method, the time needed for long leg plaster immobilization of a tibial fracture is reduced, and weight bearing ambulation is restored sooner, with less dependence on crutches, and faster overall rehabilitation.

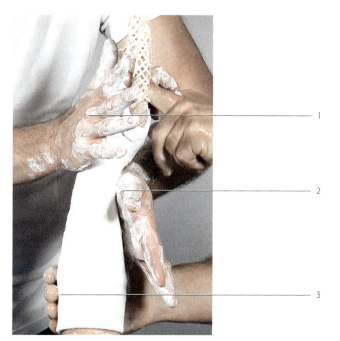

Fig 3-16   The three-point principle, using the example of a traction and reduction cast for the distal radius using POP. This fracture presented with typical dorsal displacement and angulation of the distal fragment.

1   Point one: dorsal molded rim.
2   Point two: palmar aspect, where the surgeon's palm is situated.
3   Point three: proximal shaft of the cast (where the four fingers are shown).

3

PRINCIPLES

11 Posttreatment patient information and cast check

Klaus Dresing

Before patients are allowed to leave the emergency department or doctor's surgery after application of a cast, the doctor must inform them about cast care, recognition of potential problems, and how to address them. This information should be discussed with the patient and any available caregivers, and presented in written form. It should always include telephone numbers and addresses for further advice, prompt assessment, and any necessary urgent care. A copy of the advice form, acknowledged by the patient, is placed in the medical record to confirm the discussion. However, documentation alone can be insufficient. Patients need to understand basic ideas about the complications of casts, cast care, and that their behavior is an essential contribution to their fracture care and recovery. In some cases, earlier follow up, or attention from visiting nurses may be wise.

11.1 Cast care information

Written instructions in the patient's language concerning fracture and cast care and safety are remembered better than information only given orally [20]. The inclusion of illustrations, pictures, and cartoons to aid the visual understanding of concepts is advantageous [20]. Such an instruction leaflet should be provided after cast application, with instructions regarding how and when to contact his/her caregivers. An example has been developed by AOTrauma and is included as an appendix in this book and as a downloadable document from the Thieme website. Other examples are also easily found on the internet.

The medical information provided to a patient should address the following potential problems and issues (a selection) [21].

Patient advice and information
The patient should be advised to:
• Avoid wearing jewelry on the affected limb because of the swelling of the soft tissues and the possibility of pinching or constriction, especially by rings on fingers
• Remove opaque nail varnish/polish and artificial finger nails on the affected extremity in order to allow examination of capillary refill.

The patient should be informed about the following.
Pain:
• Significantly increased or unresponsive pain may indicate serious problems and should be discussed promptly with the surgeon or his / her representative by telephone or in person.

Swelling:
• If the limb swells, the cast will become too tight and cause injury because of interference with normal blood flow
• There could be swelling of the fingers or toes; normal skin color turns to dark red, to blue, or white.

Itching (pruritus):
• Itching inside a cast is not unusual, however, nothing should be pushed into the cast to "scratch the itch"
• A vacuum cleaner or (strictly) cold hair dryer may be used to suck or blow air through the cast, which can relieve itching sensation.

Neural signs:
• Sensation caused by cast fixing pins
• Sensory deficits (numbness, loss of feeling)
• Weakness or inability to move fingers or toes
• Burning sensations
• "Pins and needles" sensation.

Vascular signs/symptoms:
• Information about signs (deep pain in the calf) and symptoms of deep venous thrombosis, which can lead to pulmonary embolism
• Skin irritation
• Blisters
• Rubbing
• Humidity, wetness beneath the cast as signs of developing blisters (bullae)
• Foreign item beneath the cast, especially in children.

Authors Klaus Dresing, Franz Seibert, Jos Engelen

Loosening of cast:
- After swelling has reduced, the cast may become loose and the loss of support can result in a loss of reduction and correct position of the fracture fragments
- Or in cases of noncompliance, the patient manipulates or loosens the cast.

Cast care/fracture care:
- Mobilization of neighboring joints
- Movement of fingers or toes
- Elevation of the affected limb on a pillow in order to have a better and faster reduction of swelling
- (Limited) weight bearing as advised by the surgeon, use of crutches
- Use of cast shoes for the lower extremity in order to protect the cast
- Protection against humidity/wetting
  - No wetting the cast or dipping in water, especially POP, because this can destroy the cast or disintegrate the cast layers
  - Keep the cast covered under rainy conditions
  - Bathing instructions
  - If the POP cast has become wet, a new one should be applied
  - Synthetic casts are normally resistant to humidity/dampness but the padding used is not
  - Only use hairdryers, with protection against heat
- Protection from heat
  - Keep a distance from fire and other heat sources, because the heat build-up can cause skin irritation and even burns beneath the cast
- Protection against external forces or impact
  - The cast can break or crack if it receives a localized impact, especially POP casts
- Driving is not permitted with a cast
- Risks involving flights with casts
  - Increased risk of thrombosis with leg casts
- How to contact the physician, and coverage for routine questions, follow-up appointments, and for emergencies.

11.2 Routine cast check

The day after the application of a primary cast, it is essential that the patient is evaluated by the surgeon or an appropriate team member. The following items should be checked:

- Swelling distal to the cast
- Excessive or focal pain
- Inadequate blood circulation
  - Capillary refill
  - Pulses if available
- Motor strength
- Sensation
- Compartment syndrome signs
  - Excessive pain
  - Tight swelling
  - Passive stretch tolerance
  - Reduced sensation and/or strength.

Any abnormalities must be documented and addressed appropriately. The patient's understanding of his/her injury and care plan, as well as ability to cope with the activities of daily living, should also be reviewed and addressed as needed.

Depending on the type of fracture and body region, an x-ray of potentially unstable fractures or dislocations should be repeated periodically and compared with the earlier studies, as indicated by the guidelines of relevant regional and national professional societies. By reviewing the x-rays, physicians are able to detect redisplacement or unsatisfactory alignment of fractures and recommend timely corrections.

3

PRINCIPLES

12　Cast wedging

Klaus Dresing

During nonoperative treatment of long bone fractures, deformities can occur at the fracture site. This could be the result of an unsatisfactory initial reduction, or a subsequent loss of alignment. Deformity must be considered in several planes and directions. While one form might predominate in any given case, deformity typically involves a combination of deviations from normal alignment. Deformities, usually described in terms of location of the distal fragment relative to the proximal, involve:

- Length, usually shortening but occasionally distraction along the longitudinal axis
- Rotation, internally or externally, around the long axis of the bone
- Transverse displacement, ie, shift of the distal segment's location across a plane perpendicular to the long axis of the proximal segment (medially, laterally, anteriorly, posteriorly, or some combination thereof)
- Angulation, between the axes of distal and proximal segments.

Angulation is usually identified and described with the aid of AP and lateral x-rays through the patient's cast. If angulation is evident on both of these 90° opposed views, this indicates that the plane of maximal angulation is between the radiographic planes, and that the true angle of axis deviation is greater than that observed on either x-ray. For such angulation to be understood and corrected, the surgeon must identify the plane of maximal angulation, measure the angle accurately, and make an equivalent correction oriented in the plane. Paley discusses this as an "oblique plane deformity" [22]. Orthopedic tradition has been to separate angular deformities into those observed on the AP x-rays, called varus or valgus, and those on the lateral x-rays, called antecurvation (or apex anterior) and retro or recurvation (apex posterior). Only when no deformity is evident on the 90° opposed view will such a deformity be completely corrected by manipulation in either coronal or sagittal plane. By correcting angulation in the true plane of deformity (eg, properly orienting the direction of cast wedging) the surgeon is able to achieve a straight bone.

Relatively small deformities can be well tolerated, and possibly even not noticed, without careful examination. More significant long bone deformities compromise functional outcome, may be associated with posttraumatic arthritis, and can be unsightly, with resulting patient distress. While deformities in an immature skeleton can improve, if they are in the plane of motion of an adjacent joint, and if sufficient limb growth remains, those in skeletally mature patients are permanent without surgical correction. One of

the significant tasks of nonoperative fracture treatment is to recognize and correct a significant deformity before healing progresses to the point that nonoperative realignment is not possible. Shortening, transverse plane displacement, and significant rotation are harder to correct without surgery. A healing fracture remains "bendable" longer with a larger time window for correcting angulation.

The following approach is suggested for avoiding excessive deformity.

Length:
Long bone fractures treated nonoperatively tend to heal, with the amount of overlapping observed on initial x-rays (without any applied traction). If this overlapping seems excessive, measures must be taken to restore and maintain length until it is stable (eg, skeletal traction, external fixation, or internal fixation).

Rotation:
A careful visual examination, with the uninjured limb held in a position symmetric to the one in the cast, can be very helpful, for example, in assessing tibial rotational alignment. Rotation is not easily assessed with AP and lateral x-rays, but mismatched diameter of the fracture ends, and various specific landmarks for each long bone, suggest malrotation. Significant malrotation should be identified as soon as possible after the initial definitive cast is applied. If it cannot be corrected by remanipulation, early surgical correction is advisable. Precise measurement of rotational alignment can be done with fluoroscopic positioning techniques and more precisely with CT scans.

Transverse displacement:
Transverse displacement is often produced by overlapping. By itself, it poses few problems, unless a gap between the bone ends suggests interposed soft tissues. Such a finding should suggest an increased risk of delayed union, and perhaps at least a relative indication for open reduction and internal fixation.

Angulation:
Small degrees of angulation are quite acceptable for many fractures treated nonoperatively. However, there is a tendency for slight angulation to increase with time, especially for fractures in a metadiaphyseal location where a cast might not offer good control of the shorter bone segment. Patients with presumably acceptable angulation must be watched closely in order to provide a timely correction should the angulation increase. Correction of angular deformity may not only be possible, but easier to maintain, if it is done through bendable callus 2 or 3 weeks after injury, with

Authors   Klaus Dresing, Franz Seibert, Jos Engelen

either manipulation during a cast change or with well-planned cast wedging.

Wedging is an elegant way to correct angular deformity. However, only fractures immobilized in full casts are suitable for this method. Cast wedging allows controlled correction without the need for recasting but can potentially cause nerve palsy or skin irritation. Böhler proposed wedging for angular deformities of less than 15–20° [2].

Normally, anesthesia during the cast wedging process is not recommended [2] as it increases the danger of harming the underlying skin and soft tissues. Cast wedging has been shown to correct angulation of < 5° for fractures with isolated varus, valgus, or apex anterior deformities with a 90% success rate [23].

12.1   Steps for cast wedging
The steps for conducting cast wedging are as follows:
- Analyze the bone-axis deviation by x-ray
- Plan the wedging procedure
  - On plain x-rays, by drawing the correction axes on transparent overlay paper
  - In picture archiving and communication systems (PACS), by using IT tools
- Determine the wedge with resulting lengthening or shortening
  - In the interface of the main fragments
  - Or more distally or proximally of the fracture zone
  - With one or more cuts
- Mark the anatomical axis, the deviation axis, and the proposed cuts into the cast with a permanent felt marker or with short drawing pins [24]
- Split the cast as planned
  - ¾ around the circumference of the cast
  - Or alternatively, ½ of the circumference of the cast, with an additional shorter cut on the opposite side to avoid limb length alterations
- Reduce the fracture and realign the axis
  - Closing-wedge cast technique
    - Cutting out a ¾ circumferential cast wedge
  - Opening-wedge cast technique
    - One cut ¾ circumferentially and interposition of a spacer (piece of wood or cork) in the cast gap
    - Filling the remaining cast gap with additional padding material in order to avoid gap edema
- Close the gap with POP or synthetic cast material applied circularly over the gap
- Conduct x-ray controls
- Provide relevant patient information.

12.2   Analysis of malalignment
To determine the malalignment of the anatomical axis after the trauma or treatment, a clinical evaluation of movement as well as an analysis of the axis in the x-ray is required. At the conclusion of a surgical fracture reduction and fixation, assessment of fracture alignment, including passive ranges of motion, is routine before the patient is awakened. In nonoperative fracture treatment, this clinical checkup is limited because often the neighboring joints are immobilized. Therefore, x-ray controls and analysis of the axis are required.

The process requires that you mark the axes of the two main fragments. Firstly, the anatomical axis is marked on the x-ray (as an example, the anterior/posterior (AP) anatomical axis of the tibia is shown in **Fig 3-17**). Secondly, the deviation axis is determined. The axes will not meet in one line, instead they will intersect. This intersection of the two lines is called the "center of angulation".

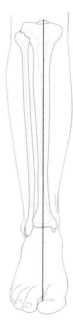

Fig 3-17   The anatomical axis of the tibia is defined as the line from the middle of the tibial plateau to the middle of the talus (AP view).

12.3 Valgus angulation

If a valgus (inward angled) deformation is diagnosed, the axes of the two main fragments are marked, and the angle between the axes (called the "deviation angle" or ∠ α) is measured (**Fig 3-18a**). This angle is then transferred to the fracture (fragments) planes (becoming the "correction angle" or ∠ α') (**Fig 3-18b**).

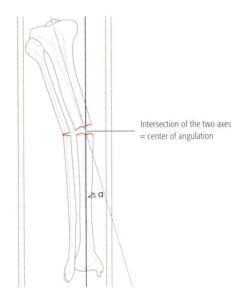

Intersection of the two axes
= center of angulation

a

12.3.1 Closing-wedge cast technique

To treat a valgus angulation using the closing-wedge cast technique, the cast is cut 2/3 of the way around the convex side of the main fracture line. The correction angle (∠ α') determines the length of wedge to be cut out of the cast (length a–b) as well as the two cutting planes (cut I and II) (**Fig 3-19a**). These cutting lines intersect at the "center of cutting" lateral to the fibula. The center of angulation (COA) is positioned close to the edge.

After removal of the wedge of cast (length a–b), the cast is closed medially and the anatomical axis is restored (**Fig 3-19b**). This must be followed with closing of the gap by applying POP or synthetic cast material over the gap, circularly around the cast.

When using the closing-wedge cast technique the leg will shorten when closing the wedge. Checkup with a new x-ray is mandatory.

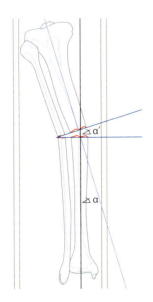

b

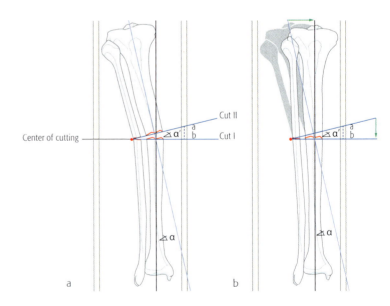

a   b

Fig 3-18a–b Valgus angulation in an AP (schematic) x-ray.
a The anatomical axis (black) and the deviation axis (blue) are marked. The angle between the anatomical and deviation axes is measured (the deviation angle ∠ α).
b The deviation angle is transferred to the medial aspect of the cast (becoming the correction angle ∠ α').

Fig 3-19a–b Closing-wedge cast technique.
a The correction angle (∠ α') determines the length to be cut out of the cast as well as the two cutting planes. These lines intersect in the center of cutting lateral to the fibula (red dot).
b Once the cast wedge is removed, the cast is closed medially (in the direction of the green arrows) and the anatomical axis is restored.

Authors   Klaus Dresing, Franz Seibert, Jos Engelen

12.3.2   Opening-wedge cast technique

To treat a valgus angulation using the opening-wedge cast technique, the cast is cut 2/3 of the way around the concave side. The correction angle ($\angle$ α′) determines the length the cast must be spread apart (length a–b) (**Fig 3-20a**).

A cast spreader is inserted into the newly created space. The cast is spread and a cork or wood spacer of length a–b is inserted. The anatomical axis is restored (**Fig 3-20b**). The remaining cast gap is filled with additional padding material in order to avoid gap edema, and the gap is closed and stabilized with POP or synthetic cast material applied over the gap circularly (**Fig 3-21**).

When using the opening-wedge cast technique the leg will lengthen when opening the wedge. Checkup with a new x-ray is mandatory.

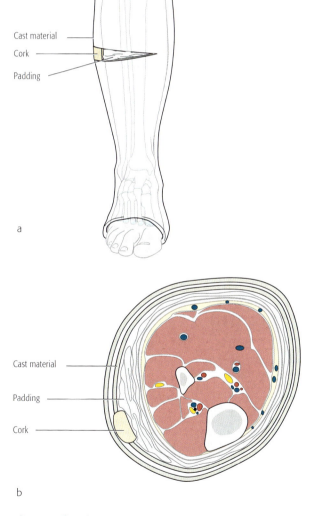

a

b

Fig 3-21a–b   Closing the gap.
a   The cast gap is filled with additional padding material in order to avoid gap edema.
b   The gap is closed and stabilized with POP or synthetic cast material applied over the gap circularly.

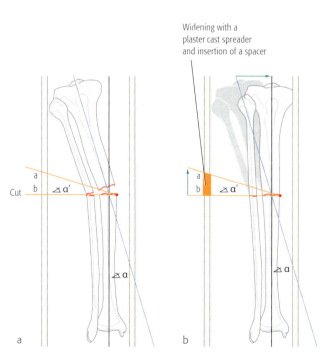

Fig 3-20a–b   Opening-wedge cast technique.
a   The cast is cut once on the concave side. The correction angle ($\angle$ α′) determines the distance the cast must be spread apart (length a–b).
b   The cast is spread and a spacer of length a–b (orange line) is inserted to restore the anatomical axis.

A comparison of the opening-wedge and closing-wedge cast techniques for correction of a valgus angulation is shown in **Fig 3-22**.

12.3.3 Cast wedging without length change of the limb

If no alteration of limb length is indicated, the center of the wedge is placed in the middle of the cast, the first cut is done on the convex side, and a supplementary short cut is done horizontally on the opposite side. When spreading the cast incision on the convex side with a plaster cast spreader, no lengthening or shortening will occur (**Fig 3-23**).

12.4 Varus angulation

If a varus (outward angled) deformation is diagnosed, the axes of the two main fragments are marked. The deviation angle between the axes is measured and transferred to the fracture (fragments) planes, becoming the correction angle (**Fig 3-24**).

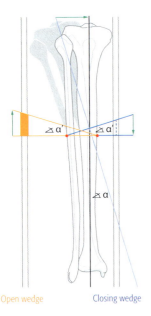

Open wedge   Closing wedge

Fig 3-22 Comparison of opening-wedge and closing-wedge cast techniques in valgus angulations. The intersection points of the angles are located medially and laterally.

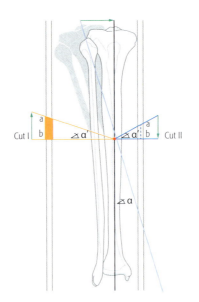

Fig 3-23 Cast wedging without lengthening or shortening of the limb. The deviation angle (∠ α) is transferred to the cutting area (∠ α') on the medial aspect of the cast.

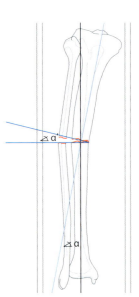

Fig 3-24 Varus angulation in an AP (schematic) x-ray. The anatomical and deviation axes are marked, the varus deviation angle is measured (∠ α), and the angle is then transferred to the cutting area on the lateral aspect of the cast (∠ α').

Authors   Klaus Dresing, Franz Seibert, Jos Engelen

12.4.1 Closing-wedge cast technique

To treat a varus angulation using the closing-wedge cast technique, the cast is cut on the concave side along the fracture line. The correction angle determines the length of wedge to cut out (length a–b) as well as the two cutting planes (**Fig 3-25a**).

After removal of the wedge, the cast is closed (**Fig 3-25b**). The leg will shorten when closing the wedge and a checkup with a new x-ray is mandatory.

12.4.2 Opening-wedge cast technique

To treat a varus angulation using the opening-wedge cast technique, the cast is cut on the convex side (**Fig 3.26a**). The cast is spread (length a–b) and a spacer is inserted (**Fig 3-26b**). The remaining cast gap is filled with additional padding material in order to avoid gap edema and the gap is closed and stabilized.

The bone will lengthen when opening the wedge and a checkup with a new x-ray is mandatory.

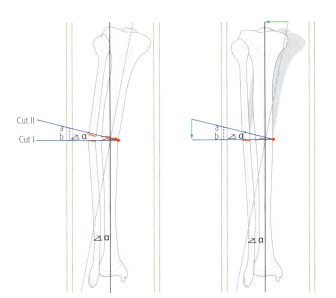

Fig 3-25a–b   The closing-wedge cast technique to treat a varus angulation.

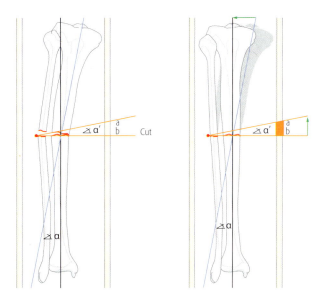

Fig 3-26a–b   The opening-wedge cast technique to treat a varus angulation.

3

PRINCIPLES

12.4.3 Cast wedging without length change of the limb

If no alteration of limb length is indicated, the center of the wedge is placed in the middle of the cast. The first cut is done on the concave side and a supplementary short cut is done horizontally on the opposite side. When spreading the cast incision on the concave side with a cast spreader, no lengthening or shortening will result (**Fig 3-27**).

12.5 Antecurvation angulation

An antecurvation (apex anterior) angulation occurs when there is a slight degree of forward curvature of a fractured diaphyseal bone. Again, two cast wedging methods are possible, ie, closing-wedge or opening-wedge cast technique.

The axes of the two main fragments are marked, and the angle between the axes is measured and transferred (see **Fig 3-28** and **Fig 3-29)**.

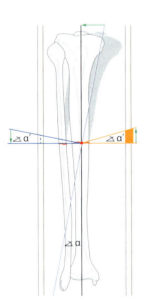

Fig 3-27   Cast-wedging without changing limb length.

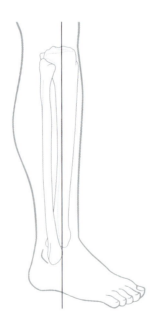

Fig 3-28   The anatomical axis of the lower limb marked in the lateral (schematic) x-ray view.

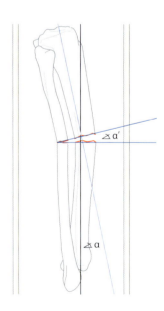

Fig 3-29   Antecurvation angulation. The anatomical and deviation axes are marked. The deviation angle (∡ α) determines the correction angle (∡ α').

Authors   Klaus Dresing, Franz Seibert, Jos Engelen

12.5.1 Closing-wedge cast technique

To treat an antecurvation angulation using the closing-wedge cast technique, the correction angle ($\measuredangle$ α') indicates the length of the wedge to be cut from the cast (length a–b) as well as the two cutting planes (cut I and II) (**Fig 3-30a**). These lines intersect dorsally at the center of cutting.

The wedge is cut out of the anterior aspect of the cast and the anatomical axis is restored by closing of the wedge (**Fig 3-30b**).

12.5.2 Opening-wedge cast technique

To treat an antecurvation angulation using the opening-wedge cast technique, a dorsal wedge is inserted and filled after the correction (**Fig 3-31**). A cast spreader is inserted within the dorsal cut and opened to the length a–b corresponding to the correction angle ($\measuredangle$ α'). The intersection line of the two planes is ventral to the tibia.

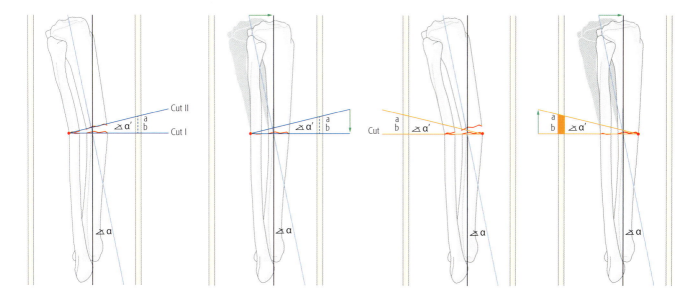

Fig 3-30a–b   The closing-wedge cast technique to treat an antecurvation angulation.

Fig 3-31a–b   The opening-wedge cast technique to treat an antecurvation angulation.

3

12.6 Retrocurvation angulation

Whenever a rare retrocurvation (apex posterior) angulation is observed, a correction with cast wedging may be indicated. The axes of the two main fragments are marked, and the angle between the axes is measured and transferred.

12.6.1 Closing-wedge cast technique

In the closing-wedge cast technique, a wedge on the dorsal aspect of the cast is cut out (**Fig 3-32**).

After analysis of the deviation, a wedge is cut out of the dorsal aspect of the cast (length a–b) corresponding to the correction angle ($\angle$ α'). The intersection line of the two planes is ventral to the tibia. The anatomical axis is restored by closing of the wedge.

12.6.2 Opening-wedge cast technique

In the opening-wedge cast technique, a wedge on the ventral aspect of the cast is removed (**Fig 3-33**).

After analysis of the deviation, an incision is cut on the ventral aspect of the cast and widened with a cast spreader (length a–b) corresponding to the correction angle ($\angle$ α'). The intersection line of the two planes is dorsal to the tibia. A spacer is inserted within the gap and the remaining gap is filled with padding and closed with POP or synthetic cast material.

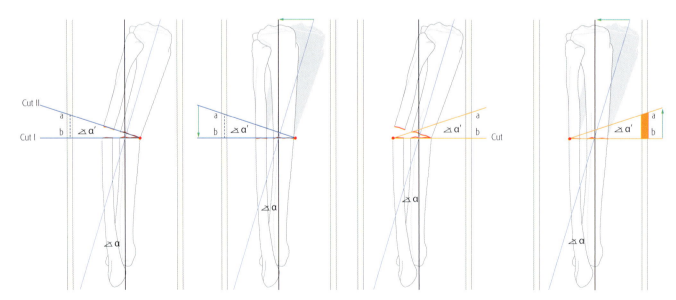

Fig 3-32a–b The closing-wedge cast technique to treat a retrocurvation angulation.

Fig 3-33a–b The opening-wedge cast technique to treat a retrocurvation angulation.

Authors   Klaus Dresing, Franz Seibert, Jos Engelen

13   Summary

- Fractures treated nonoperatively heal indirectly, through the reactive, reparative, and remodeling phases, with callus that becomes new woven bone
- Direct bone healing (osteonal remodeling) only occurs with absolutely stable surgical fixation
- Fractures that have not healed within the appropriate period of time are said to have delayed union, and by six months are experiencing nonunion
- Fractures can be treated nonoperatively using casting as it keeps the fracture in a reduced position by stabilizing the fracture fragments from the outside
- Nonoperative fracture care avoids many of the risks and financial costs that come with surgery, however, casting requires intensive surveillance, and cannot always be recommended
- Casting is effective not just to treat fractures, but also postsurgery, or to treat ligament, tendon and nerve damage, or infection
- The major types of casting techniques include: splints, when full immobilization is not required; fully circumferential casts; split casts, which allow for swelling; and removable orthoses and braces

- Splints and casts are typically made of two types of material: plaster of Paris known as POP; or rigid or semirigid synthetic
- Functional treatment, which encourages progressive protected use of a fractured limb, promotes recovery and fracture healing, while limiting disuse atrophy, weakness, and joint stiffness; it often involves the use of fracture braces designed to allow some joint motion and weight bearing
- Malalignment or fracture redisplacement can develop during nonoperative fracture treatment, and must be corrected if it is severe enough to compromise results
- Angulation of a fracture immobilized in a fully circumferential cast can be corrected by cast wedging, in which a section of cast is cut at a certain angle and removed, the deformity is straightened, and the cast is repaired
- Patients need to be fully informed about the various treatments being undertaken both before and after treatment; the patient's understanding of and level of compliance with directions can either support or delay the healing process.

14   References

Klaus Dresing, Franz Seibert, Jos Engelen

1. **Lucas-Championnière J**. The treatment of fractures by mobilization and massage (1908). *Hand Clin.* 1996 Feb; 12(1):167–171.
2. **Böhler L**. [*Treatment of Fractures*]. 1st ed. Wien: Wilhelm Maudrich; 1929. German.
3. **Böhler L**. *Verbandlehre für Schwestern, Helfer, Studenten und Ärzte.* Wien: Wilhelm Maudrich; 1943. German.
4. **Gropp W**. [Medical care as physical injury from the viewpoint of the law and jurisdiction]. *Z Arztl Fortbild Qualitatssich.* 1998 Oct; 92(8-9):536–542. German.
5. **Acea B**. [Informing the surgical patient. Reflections on the basic law of patient autonomy]. *Cir Esp.* 2005 Feb; 77(2):60–64. Spanish.
6. **Ludolph E, Hierholzer G**. [Conservative or operative fracture treatment — alternative information in relative indications]. *Unfallchirurgie.* 1986 Feb; 12(1):44–51. German.
7. **Ceroni D, Martin X, Delhumeau C, et al**. Decrease of physical activity level in adolescents with limb fractures: an accelerometry-based activity monitor study. *BMC Musculoskelet Disord.* 2011 May 4; 12:87.
8. **Wolff JD**. [*The Law of Transformation of the Bone/Das Gesetz der Transformation der Knochen*]. Berlin: August Hirschwald; 1892. German.
9. **Ceroni D, Martin X, Delhumeau C, et al**. Effects of cast-mediated immobilization on bone mineral mass at various sites in adolescents with lower-extremity fracture. *J Bone Joint Surg Am.* 2012 Feb 1; 94(3):208–216.
10. **Culav EM, Clark CH, Merrilees MJ**. Connective tissues: matrix composition and its relevance to physical therapy. *Phys Ther.* 1999 Mar; 79(3):308–319.
11. **Langer N, Hänggi J, Müller NA, et al**. Effects of limb immobilization on brain plasticity. *Neurology.* 2012 Jan 17; 78(3):182–188.
12. **Sarmiento A**. A functional below-the-knee brace for tibial fractures: a report on its use in one hundred and thirty-five cases (1970). *J Bone Joint Surg Am.* 2007 Sep; 89 Suppl 2 Pt.2:157–169.
13. **Sarmiento A, Kinman PB, Galvin EG, et al**. Functional bracing of fractures of the shaft of the humerus. *J Bone Joint Surg Am.* 1977 Jul; 59(5):596–601.
14. **Sarmiento A, Latta LL**. Fractures of the middle third of the tibia treated with a functional brace. *Clin Orthop Relat Res.* 2008 Dec; 466(12):3108–3115.
15. **Sarmiento A, Latta LL**. Functional treatment of closed segmental fractures of the tibia. *Acta Chir Orthop Traumatol Cech.* 2008 Oct; 75(5):325–331.
16. **Sarmiento A, Zagorski JB, Zych GA, et al**. Functional bracing for the treatment of fractures of the humeral diaphysis. *J Bone Joint Surg Am.* 2000 Apr; 82(4):478–486.
17. **Schuren J**. *Working with Soft Cast — a Manual on Semi-rigid Immobilisation.* 2nd ed. Borken: 3M Minnesota Mining & Manufacturing; 1994: 9–29.
18. **Schäpe T**. [*Immobilization Techniques: Theory and Practice*]. Reed Business information; 1993. Dutch.
19. **Charnley J**. *The Closed Treatment of Common Fractures.* 4th ed. United Kingdom. Cambridge University Press; 2010.
20. **Hossieny P, Carey Smith R, Yates P, et al**. Efficacy of patient information concerning casts applied post-fracture. *ANZ J Surg.* 2012; 82(3):151–155.
21. **Harp JH**. Complications from casting: pitfalls and pearls. *AAOS Bulletin.* 2005 Dec.
22. **Paley D**. *Principles of Deformity Correction.* Berlin: Springer Verlag; 2002.
23. **Wells L, Avery AL, Hosalkar HH, et al**. Cast wedging: a "forgotten" yet predictable method for correcting fracture deformity. *University of Pennsylvania Orthopaedic Journal (UPOJ).* 2010; 20:113–116.
24. **Holman L, Davies H, Scott JM**. Fracture localisation for cast wedging. *Ann R Coll Surg Eng.* 2009 Nov; 91(8):714.

15   Further reading

Klaus Dresing, Franz Seibert, Jos Engelen

AO Surgery Reference. Casting. Colton CL, Schatzker J, Trafton P (eds). AO Foundation. Available at http://www.aosurgery.org. [Accessed July 2011].

Rüedi TP, Buckly RE, Moran CG. *AO Principles of Fracture Management.* 2nd ed. Vol 1. Stuttgart: Thieme; 2007: 276–279

4 Thrombosis prophylaxis

Jan Philipp Schüttrumpf

4

PRINCIPLES

Author   Jan Philipp Schüttrumpf

4   Thrombosis prophylaxis

1   Introduction

Patients with reduced mobility, either due to a lower-extremity injury or surgery, are generally considered to carry an increased risk of incurring venous thromboembolic disease. Therefore, patients requiring immobilization due to a lower-extremity sprain, fracture, or tendon rupture, regardless of whether they are treated with or without surgery, should be considered for venous thromboembolism prophylaxis. Causation of venous thromboembolic disease (VTE) is still thought to be related to Virchow's triad of factors:

- Venous stasis
- Endothelial injury
- Hypercoagulability.

Prophylaxis attempts to modify one or more of these factors, primarily stasis and hypercoagulability.

The incidence of symptomatic deep vein thrombosis in the general public is 90–130 per 100,000 inhabitants [1, 2]. Several factors clearly increase the risk of VTE, notably older age, malignancy, prior VTE, family history of VTE, and obesity. The prevalence of VTE in the absence of prophylaxis is particularly significant in some categories of orthopedic and trauma patients, for example, 40–80% after multiple trauma and 40–60% after hip fracture or total hip/knee replacement [3, 4]. The frequency of VTE in immobilized patients (cast or splint) with isolated lower-extremity injuries or orthopedic surgery is less well established. There is some evidence that patients with more proximal lower-extremity injuries, at the knee or above, carry a higher risk [4]. Ettema et al estimated that, without any prophylaxis, approximately 17% of patients without obvious risk factors would develop VTE [5]. Healy reported a 6.3% rate of symptomatic VTE events in 208 unprophylaxed patients with Achilles tendon ruptures [6]. Available data, summarized in a review by the American College of Chest Physicians reports a risk of symptomatic deep vein thrombosis (DVT) of 24 per 1,000 and 3 per 1,000 for nonfatal pulmonary embolism (2.7% overall) among immobilized patients in the control groups of randomized trials of anticoagulation [4].

The decision for or against VTE prophylaxis as well as its specific form should best be based upon the rational assessment of risk for each individual patient. Unfortunately, experts have not yet come to agree on how to assess the risks of VTE, nor upon the validity of available assessment tools. Nevertheless, surgeons still have to consider both the risks of VTE and of potential preventive measures, along with the effectiveness of various prophylactic regimens, in order to offer a rational recommendation for VTE prophylaxis for each patient.

Tosetto et al identified prior history of superficial phlebitis, obesity, and smoking as significant risk factors for patients with surgery or trauma [7]. Family history or oral contraceptive use were less associated in these patients, however, the presence of two or more risk factors increased the risk of VTE. In this context, the presence of hypercoagulability [8] as well as the presence of malignancy [9] are also worth mentioning. In the absence of a reliable and universally accepted algorithm, it remains challenging for surgeons to choose the most appropriate prophylactic regimen for a given patient that has to be immobilized for lower-extremity injury or orthopedic surgery.

However, before specific recommendations for selected situations are presented, different options for VTE prophylaxis are reviewed according to two main categories:

- Nonpharmacological, and
- Pharmacological.

2   Nonpharmacological prophylaxis

Drug-free measures for thrombosis prophylaxis—physical therapy, movement, active ankle exercises (calf muscle pump), and pneumatic compression therapy—are discussed in this topic.

2.1   Physical therapy

While following appropriate care for their injuries, patients should be mobilized as early as possible in order to stimulate the cardiovascular system and thereby increase the blood flow within the muscles and soft tissues of the lower extremities. Supervised physical therapy for both injured and intact body regions should be part of this program. All patients should be encouraged to learn appropriate exercises and practice them on their own between formal therapy sessions. Prior to elective surgery, patients can even be trained in appropriate postoperative exercises.

2.2   Movement/calf muscle pump

Resuming "normal" physiological gait or movement may be the best and easiest form of VTE prophylaxis. All unharmed body regions must be part of the program, as stated above. As soon as possible after injury or elective surgery, the use of the muscle pump in the calf should begin, with active dorsal/plantar flexion of the ankle joint and toe flexion/extension.

2.3   Compression therapy (static and active)

The use of static compression stockings deserves routine consideration. One example includes thromboembolic deterrent stockings, which have a compression pressure rating of around 18 mmHg in the ankle region, and a decreasing pressure gradient from distal to proximal. It is essential that these stockings fit the patient correctly, per manufacturer's instructions, and that constricting wrinkles are avoided. Special contraindications, in addition to the need for a cast or splint, include peripheral arterial insufficiency, severe neuropathy, extensive edema, and local infection or otherwise compromised tissues. The effectiveness of such elastic stockings, alone or combined with pharmacologic prophylaxis, has been reported [10].

Intermittent pneumatic compression is a useful auxilliary device for immobilized patients. At certain time intervals, one to three air chamber systems are automatically inflated and deflated with a pressure of up to 45 mmHg. Devices exist for the entire lower extremity or for the foot alone. Some can even be used inside a cast or splint. Cardiac insufficiency, local inflammations, injuries, and severe hypertension are common contraindications. Although intermittent pneumatic compression (IPC) is not used frequently in clinical settings due to logistical problems and high costs, the literature does support its effectiveness both when used faithfully as directed [11] as well as, with additional benefits, when used together with antithrombotic medication [4].

3   Pharmacological prophylaxis

The administration of any medication to prevent VTE is an additional step, beyond the nonpharmacological measures discussed above, which should always be used in order to reduce the frequency of thromboembolic complications. It seems to be apparent that adding pharmacological prophylaxis to the mechanical methods, which are generally free of complications, would provide more effective VTE prevention. Nevertheless, confirmatory evidence of safety and effectiveness is still required. As yet, this is not generally available, especially for lower-extremity injuries.

Pharmacological prophylaxis is routinely advised by physicians and surgeons in many parts of the world whenever a patient needs to be immobilized for a lower-extremity injury. This seems quite appropriate for patients with an evidentially increased risk of VTE, particularly if multiple risk factors are present [12]. However, pharmacological prophylaxis is not universally recommended as demonstrated by the American College of Chest Physicians (ACCP) Antithrobotic Guidelines, published in February 2012: "We suggest no prophylaxis rather than pharmacologic thromboprophylaxis in patients with isolated lower-leg injuries requiring leg immobilization" [13]. This recommendation is based on a meta-analysis of more than 1,000 patients that showed slight, but nonsignificant reduction of symptomatic DVT and nonfatal pulmonary embolism (PE), with a slightly elevated risk of bleeding events when low-molecular-weight heparin prophylaxis was compared with "usual care".

The following drugs are widely used in the application of drug-based VTE prophylaxis.

3.1   Acetylsalicylic acid (aspirin)

The use of aspirin as a single chemoprophylactic agent for VTE is controversial, though not uncommon in some parts of the world. Many experts consider its effectiveness too low to justify recommendation [13–15]. However, the most recent ACCP guidelines [16], revised from prior editions, now include aspirin, even when used alone, among a list of several pharmacological options for VTE prophylaxis. An additional recommendation suggests that aspirin might be less effective than low-molecular-weight heparin (LMWH).

Author   Jan Philipp Schüttrumpf

3.2   Unfractionated and fractionated heparin

Unfractionated heparin has a half-life of two hours and is eliminated in equal portions via the liver and kidneys. Unfractionated heparin (UFH) is typically injected subcutaneously two or three times a day for VTE prophylaxis. Monitoring of the anticoagulant effect is unnecessary [14].

Low-molecular-weight heparins are chemically derived from UFH through depolymerization. A number of such agents are available, and they are pharmacologically distinct from one another [17]. Drug properties including dosages and administration schedules are not the same. Since LMWH patents are now expiring, lower cost generic versions will soon become available, along with pressure to select the lower cost agents. However, international and national organizations have emphasized that LMWHs are not equivalent. Shared characteristics of LMWHs include longer duration of activity than UFH, purely renal elimination, and varying immunogenic similarity, which, however, does not prevent them from occasionally causing allergic reactions or thrombocytopenia similar to UFH. Patients with acute or chronic renal impairment, as well as those that are elderly, obese, or very small, should be considered for different dosages or alternative antithrombotic agents.

Heparin-induced thrombocytopenia is a rare but serious complication of both UFH and LMWH. A past history of this condition is a contraindication to the use of heparins. As a general precaution, platelet counts should be obtained at the beginning of heparin administration, and monitored regularly. The drug should be stopped if the platelet count falls below 100,000/mm^3.

Another concern regarding anticoagulants, including LMWH, is the associated risk of epidural hematoma after spinal or epidural anesthesia, and in the case of spinal fracture. A similar concern is posed by recent head injuries.

Comparing the use of UFH and LMWH, the lower DVT rate and reduced bleeding complications after orthopedic surgery, as well as the ease of a single daily injection and the evidence supporting the therapeutic effectiveness of LMWH, might indicate an advantage for the use of LMWH [14, 18–19]. The data on nonoperatively treated patients is limited, but no significant difference between UFH and LMWH could be found regarding effectiveness and safety [20].

3.3   Coumarins

Warfarin (half-life 24 hours) and phenprocoumon (half-life 120 hours) are the most common vitamin-k antagonists of the coumarin type, which can be administered orally. Their delayed effect, required blood tests (International Normal-

ized Ratio) with individually adjusted dosages, and relatively high risk of bleeding complications results in fairly rare use as first-line VTE prophylaxis for patients with isolated lower-leg immobilization [14].

3.4   Other anticoagulants

A variety of other drugs (eg, fondaparinux, apixaban, dabigatran, rivaroxaban, and adjusted-dose vitamin-k antagonists) that interfere with coagulation are occasionally recommended for use in orthopedic patients [4], but little evidence is as yet available concerning their safety and effectiveness for patients with lower-extremity injuries and immobilization.

In summary, first-line pharmaceutical VTE prophylaxis should usually involve LMWH (or UFH). A coumarin might be considered as an alternative [21–22]. However, the contraindications, namely the risk of bleeding and potential heparin-induced thrombocytopenia, should not be forgotten.

4   Specific recommendations for upper- or lower-extremity injuries with immobilizing treatment in a cast or splint

This topic gives recommendations for thrombosis prophylaxis according to international guidelines and up-to-date literature.

4.1   Upper extremity

In general, immobilization of the upper extremity does not require antithrombotic drugs. But the patient's own movement (eg, of the fingers, physiotherapy) is advantageous to decrease swelling of the soft tissue.

However, in individual cases with multiple or very significant risk factors, the additional use of an anticoagulant might be indicated [14].

4.2   Lower extremity

Plaster cast immobilization of the lower extremity, especially of the knee and ankle joint, and the inability to bear weight, is regarded as a moderate risk for thrombosis [4].

Contrary to the upper extremity, the lower extremity requires certain measures when injured and stabilized and immobilzed in a cast. The most effective measures are a muscle pump, walking, and other movement of the muscles, which compress the veins during contraction of the muscle, then let them refill with venous blood during the swing phase. This contraction and refilling allows the flow of blood from periphery to central, ensuring no stasis of blood in the veins, and therefore, less danger of thrombosis. An active rolling movement of the foot initiates and maintains this process.

There is limited evidence regarding the risk of VTE and the effectiveness and safety of prophylactic anticoagulation for patients immobilized with casts for lower-extremity injuries or surgery. Only four international guidelines make recommendations in regard to VTE prophylaxis for such patients [12]. Two recent investigations have shown that prophylaxis with LMWH reduces the VTE rate during immobilization of the lower extremities. Ettema et al (2008) performed a meta-analysis (including 1,456 patients from six randomized studies) where the VTE rate was reduced from 17.1 to 9.6% without any increase in bleeding complications [5]. Testroote et al (2008) made a Cochrane review where the VTE rate in patients with an immobilizing plaster cast for a minimum period of one week due to any sort of leg injury varied from 4.3–40% without any prophylaxis. These rates were significantly lower when LMWH was given once daily [19]. The most recent ACCP guidelines, based upon Testroote's review and including another multicenter study, repeated the meta-analysis and concluded, as mentioned above, that there was insufficient evidence to establish the benefit of thromboprophylaxis in the enrolled patients. However, it is important to recognize that higher-risk patients were excluded from these studies.

Knowledge about risks and prevention of VTE in patients with lower extremity casts is still growing and, thus, guidelines are likely to evolve accordingly. Regional differences in practice are understandable and should be taken into consideration by practitioners. Based on present knowledge, it seems most appropriate to apply nonpharmacological prophylaxis to the extent permitted by the patient's injuries [14]. Patients judged to have elevated risk of VTE should be considered candidates for drug-based prophylaxis, with LMWH generally being the first choice. If used, such drugs should be continued until the cast or splint has been removed and partial weight bearing of > 20 kilograms and a range of motion in the upper ankle joint of > 20° has been achieved [23–24].

5 Summary

- Following lower-extremity injury or surgery, patients with reduced mobility carry an increased risk of venous thromboembolic disease
- Every patient should be mobilized as early as possible in accordance with the extent and pattern of the injury
- The aim is to achieve at least partial weight bearing of > 15–20 kilograms and a range of motion in the upper ankle joint of 20° (rolling motion in the lower ankle joint and activation of muscle pump in the calf); exclusion of weight bearing should be avoided, if possible
- Prophylaxis against venous thromboembolism consists of general nonpharmacological measures with additional drug-based prophylaxis, at least for patients with increased risk of VTE.

Author   Jan Philipp Schüttrumpf

6   References

1. **Naess IA, Christiansen SC, Romundstad P, et al**. Incidence and mortality of venous thrombosis: a population-based study. *J Thromb Haemost.* 2007 Apr; 5(4):692–699.

2. **White RH, Zhou H, Murin S, et al**. Effect of ethnicity and gender on the incidence of venous thromboembolism in a diverse population in California in 1996. *Thromb Haemost.* 2005 Feb; 93(2):298–305.

3. **Stein PD, Beemath A, Olson RE**. Trends in the incidence of pulmonary embolism and deep venous thrombosis in hospitalized patients. *Am J Cardiol.* 2005 Jun 15; 95(12):1525–1526.

4. **Falck-Ytter Y, Francis CW, Johanson NA, et al**. Prevention of VTE in orthopedic surgery patients: Antithrombotic Therapy and Prevention of Thrombosis, 9th ed: American College of Chest Physicians Evidence-Based Clinical Practice Guidelines. *Chest.* 2012 Feb; 141(2 Suppl):e278S–e325S.

5. **Ettema HB, Kollen BJ, Verheyen CC, et al**. Prevention of venous thromboembolism in patients with immobilization of the lower extremities: a meta-analysis of randomized controlled trials. *J Thromb Haemost.* 2008 Jul; 6(7):1093–1098.

6. **Healy B, Beasley R, Weatherall M**. Venous thromboembolism following prolonged cast immobilisation for injury to the tendo Achillis. *J Bone Joint Surg Br.* 2010 May; 92-B (5):646–650.

7. **Tosetto A, Frezzato M, Rodeghiero F**. Prevalence and risk factors of non-fatal venous thromboembolism in the active population of the VITA Project. *J Thromb Haemost.* 2003 Aug; 1(8):1724–1729.

8. **Wu O, Robertson L, Langhorne P, et al**. Oral contraceptives, hormone replacement therapy, thrombophilias and risk of venous thromboembolism: a systematic review. The Thrombosis: Risk and Economic Assessment of Thrombophilia Screening (TREATS) Study. *Thromb Haemost.* 2005 Jul; 94(1):17–25.

9. **Blom JW, Doggen CJ, Osanto S, et al**. Malignancies, prothrombotic mutations, and the risk of venous thrombosis. *JAMA.* 2005 Feb 9; 293(6):715–722.

10. **Amaragiri SV, Lees TA**. Elastic compression stockings for prevention of deep vein thrombosis. *Cochrane Database Syst Rev.* 2000; (3):CD001484.

11. **Urbankova J, Quiroz R, Kucher N, et al**. Intermittent pneumatic compression and deep vein thrombosis prevention. A meta-analysis in postoperative patients. *Thromb Haemost.* 2005 Dec; 94(6):1181–1185.

12. **Struijk-Mulder MC, Ettema HB, Verheyen CC, et al**. Comparing consensus guidelines on thromboprophylaxis in orthopedic surgery. *J Thromb Haemost.* 2010 Apr; 8(4):678–683.

13. **Huo MH, Spyropoulos AC**. The eighth American college of chest physicians guidelines on venous thromboembolism prevention: implications for hospital prophylaxis strategies. *J Thromb Thrombolysis.* 2011 Feb; 31(2):196–208.

14. **Encke A, Haas S, Sauerland S, et al**. [S3-Guideline: Prophylaxis of venous thromboembolism (VTE)]. *Vasa.* 2009; 38(S76):1–131. German.

15. **Antiplatelet Trialists' Collaboration**. Collaborative overview of randomised trials of antiplatelet therapy-III: Reduction in venous thrombosis and pulmonary embolism by antiplatelet prophylaxis among surgical and medical patients. *BMJ.* 1994 Jan 22; 308:235–246.

16. **American College of Chest Physicians Evidence-Based Clinical Practice Guidelines (ed)**. Antithrombotic Therapy and Prevention of Thrombosis. 9th ed. *Chest.* 141(2 Suppl). (Online articles only). [Accessed 2011].

17. **Merli GJ, Groce JB**. Pharmacological and clinical differences between low-molecular-weight heparins: implications for prescribing practice and therapeutic interchange. *P T.* 2010 Feb; 35(2):95–105.

18. **Koch A, Ziegler S, Breitschwerdt H, et al**. Low molecular weight heparin and unfractionated heparin in thrombosis prophylaxis: meta-analysis based on original patient data. *Thromb Res.* 2001 May 15; 102(4):295–309.

19. **Testroote M, Stigter W, de Visser DC, et al**. Low molecular weight heparin for prevention of venous thromboembolism in patients with lower leg immobilization. *Cochrane Database Syst Rev.* 2008 Oct 8;(4).

20. **Mismetti P, Laporte-Simitsidis S, Tardy B, et al**. Prevention of venous thromboembolism in internal medicine with unfractionated or low-molecular-weight heparins: a meta-analysis of randomised clinical trials. *Thromb Haemost.* 2000 Jan; 83(1):14–19.

21. **Freedman KB, Brookenthal KR, Fitzgerald RH Jr, et al**. A meta-analysis of thromboembolic prophylaxis following elective total hip arthroplasty. *J Bone Joint Surg Am.* 2000 Jul; 82-A(7):929–938.

22. **Roderick P, Ferris G, Wilson K, et al**. Towards evidence-based guidelines for the prevention of venous thromboembolism: systematic reviews of mechanical methods, oral anticoagulation, dextran and regional anaesthesia as thromboprophylaxis. *Health Technol Assess.* 2005 Dec; 9(49):1–78.

23. **Eisele R, Greger W, Weikert E, et al**. Ambulatory prevention of thrombosis in traumatology. *Unfallchirurg.* 2001 Mar; 104(3):240–245.

24. **Eisele R, Weickert E, Eren A, et al**. The effect of partial and full weight-bearing on venous return in the lower limb. *J Bone Joint Surg Br.* 2001 Sep; 83(7):1037–1040.

4

PRINCIPLES

PRINCIPLES

4

5 Logistics and resources in the cast room

Klaus Dresing, Jos Engelen

PRINCIPLES

5

Authors   Klaus Dresing, Jos Engelen

5   Logistics and resources in the cast room

1   Introduction

The modern cast room (or plaster room) is situated in proximity to the emergency or operating department. In some settings, the cast room may be closer to the operating room (OR) or the inpatient wards than to the emergency department (ED). Sometimes, there may even be several such rooms. Cast room equipment and supplies certainly vary according to local customs and resources.

Today, in many hospitals, the cast room is not used exclusively for the application of plaster or synthetic casts but also for the application of bandages and orthoses. Orthoses are often custom-made by a cast technician, or occasionally, by other staff. These technicians are trained to treat orthopedic or trauma patients by applying different kinds of immobilization or stabilization techniques.

In theory, a modern cast room is a well-equipped working place. While in the past, the cast room was used exclusively for the application of plaster of Paris casts, today, the room is used for many different types of treatment. Often, several synthetic materials are used in combination. This requires a safe and clean working space for both the technician as well as the patient (**Fig 5-1**).

The cast room should also be used to store relevant equipment, materials, and instruments. The equipment for closed reduction of displaced fractures or dislocations, under sedation or regional anesthesia, should also be made available.

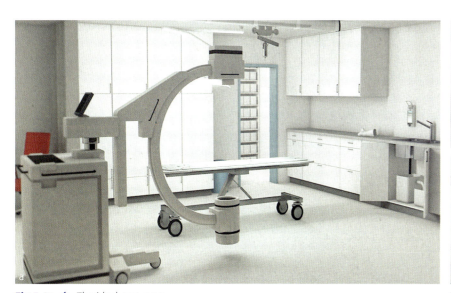
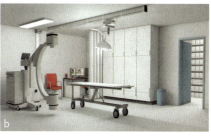
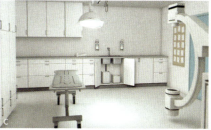
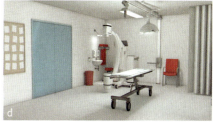

Fig 5-1a–d   The ideal cast room.

a   Cast room with (from left to right): mobile image intensifier (C-arm), ceiling-mounted traction (extension) system with mobile pulley, cast table, open storage room, shelves or cupboards for storage and daily use, working bank with plaster basin and installed plaster trap (seen through opened cupboard doors).

b   Space for documentation with PACS access and desk.

c   Ceiling-mounted examination lamp with enough space to position the C-arm.

d   Ceiling-mounted extension system and hygiene corner.

2 Cast room features and facilities

In any modern cast room, the following features and facilities are recommended and useful:

- Appliances for physiological monitoring during procedures
- Anesthesia facility
- Monitoring equipment (NIBP monitor, SpO_2 pulse oximeter, ECG)
- Resuscitation equipment is also necessary, with oxygen, suction, and ventilation aids, consistent with safety requirements for sedation and/or anesthesia
- Nitrous oxide delivery system or storage space for a portable nitrous oxide delivery system overhead service panel
- Energy and water supply
- Traction and reduction devices
- X-ray film viewer (two panels are preferable) or a digital imaging system (picture archiving computer system) station
- Space for documentation (conventional writing desk or computer)
- Plaster basin
- Sink and drain with a plaster trap
- Cast work bench
- Storage for bandages, and plaster and cast materials for daily usage
- Storage for other cast materials and crutches easily accessible from the cast room.

2.1 Cast room size

The space must be adequate, with an examination couch or equivalent, eg, a cast table that can be accessed from all sides. The room should be at least 20 m² but preferably closer to 35–40 m² in size, excluding storage areas for materials and crutches. The cast room should be large enough to roll a bed inside (see **Fig 5-1**).

2.2 Walls and floor

All surfaces should be washable. The edging strips between walls, ceiling, and floors should be curved in order to allow for better cleaning. The walls should be shielded in order to offer protection against radiation—this may be specified by national regulations—and preferably be treated with sprayed plastic skin or surfaced with epoxy resin paints. Although stainless steel surfaces are expensive, they allow excellent cleaning and are durable. Ceramic tiles are often porous and, therefore, do not allow effective cleaning. The floor surface should have a nonslip coating.

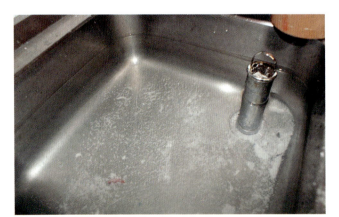

Fig 5-2a Plaster of Paris (POP) residue after dipping three slabs of POP splint (longuette). The drain is not closed completely, instead, a simple overflow system is used.

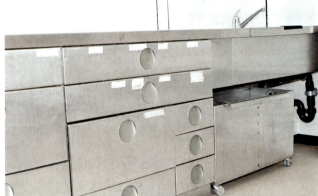

Fig 5-2b Cast bench with water basin (right) and a movable plaster trap beneath the basin.

Authors   Klaus Dresing, Jos Engelen

2.3   Energy and water supply, and waste disposal

The cast room should have appropriate electrical connections for an electric cast saw, anesthesia equipment, and other medical devices such as a light box on which to display the relevant x-rays.

A source of water is required, preferably clean tap water. The sink should have an overflow system in order to avoid inundations (**Fig 5-2a**). A floor drain is optional. A plaster trap (**Fig 5-2b**) is required for discarded plaster application water as the plaster residue will block normal drains.

A separate washbasin (**Fig 5-2c**) is necessary, with hot and cold water, for hand washing before and after patient contact as well as after applying a cast. Soap and disinfectant dispensers as well as a paper towel dispenser are thus required. If pneumatic devices are to be used, compressed air connectors are necessary.

A management system for used materials should be established, as some material residues can be recycled, and some can be reused. Some cast residues (waste) can be discarded with general hospital waste. National and international protocols for contaminated and/or potentially infectious medical waste disposal must be followed.

2.4   Cast room lighting

Wherever possible, access to natural daylight is ideal in the cast room from clerestory (high-set) windows, or access to light via glass corridor panels. The electric lighting should resemble daylight with a color temperature of approx. 5,500 Kelvin and an illumination corresponding to natural light (full spectrum light). Light bulbs or halogen bulbs are usually installed. In modern lighting technology, fluorescent tubes emitting natural light similar to daylight or full spectrum light are used. The color temperature corresponds to, eg, European norm (EN) 12,464 with 5,300–6,500 Kelvin, and the luminaire needs a capacity of 5,000–10,000 lux. In recent years, LED lamps have been introduced into lighting concepts in hospitals and cast rooms. The national guidelines of workplace lighting should be respected.

2.5   Surgical examination lamps

In order to examine wounds or skin problems, good light is needed. The examination light, eg, LEDs mounted on walls or the ceiling, can be focused and adjusted to illuminate the area of interest (**Fig 5-3**).

5

PRINCIPLES

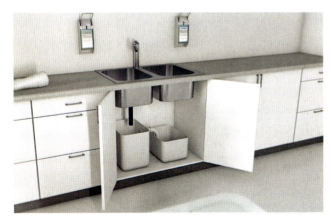

Fig 5-2c   Bench with separate wash basin.

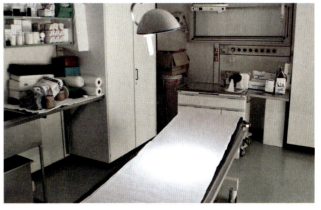

Fig 5-3   Ceiling-mounted examination light with focusable light beam. The image also shows a service unit (with sockets for oxygen, compressed air, electric supply, etc) mounted on the wall.

5

PRINCIPLES

2.6 Ventilation, air conditioning, and dust extraction

The cast room is not an aseptic operation theatre, however, adequate ventilation is required, preferably air conditioning. When using a cast saw, dust extraction via an extraction nozzle fixed directly to the oscillating cast saw blade is recommended. Surgical masks should be available in case of need.

2.7 Traction (extension) system

For the application of more elaborate casts, an extension table (eg, Cotrel or Hess) or a ceiling-mounted traction system is necessary to position and hold the patient or extremity in the right position (**Fig 5-4**). These systems are certainly required when pelvic POP casts or corsets for spine fractures are applied.

2.8 Storage room

A storage room is necessary for stocking the cast materials at room temperature, observing the required humidity levels, and ensuring security. If possible, the room should be directly accessible from the cast room.

2.9 Documentation, access to patient records, x-ray viewing station

The cast room must offer space for documentation and viewing of x-rays. At the very least, a conventional x-ray viewer (light box) should be available (**Fig 5-5**) as well as a desk or console for handwritten medical documentation.

In accordance with building requirements, access to the electronic hospital information system should be installed, which also means access to the picture archiving computer system (PACS) (**Fig 5-6**).

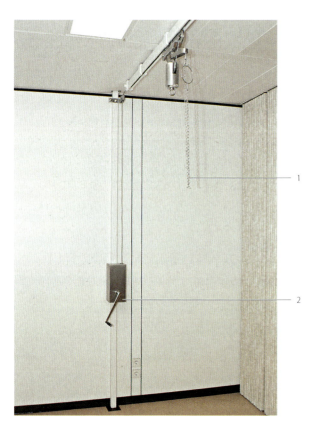

Fig 5-4 Traction (extension) system, eg, used for suspended finger traps to reduce distal radius fractures (see **Fig 9.1-10** in chapter 9.1 Fractures, dislocations, and subluxations of the upper extremity), with ceiling rail with crab.

1 By pulling the chain the crab can be moved and positioned over the patient.

2 Handle to release or tighten the chain.

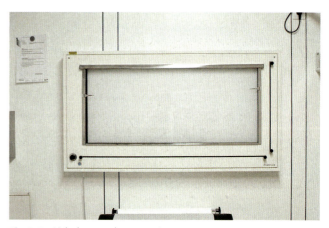

Fig 5-5 Light box, analog x-ray viewer.

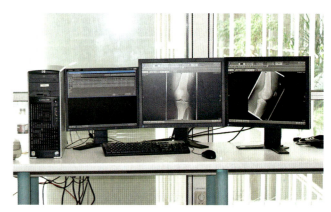

Fig 5-6 The PACS viewing station with three monitors, the left one for administration and medical documentation, the other two for image analysis and comparison.

Authors   Klaus Dresing, Jos Engelen

3   Cast room equipment

The following equipment within the cast room is useful and accepted:

- Storage space for bandages, plaster, and cast materials for daily usage
- Plaster and cast cart (trolley)
- Cast table
- Mobile image intensifier (C-arm) system for controlled fracture reduction
- Materials for reduction and stabilization.

3.1   Storage space for cast materials for daily usage

All materials and instruments needed in daily plaster or synthetic cast application should be easily accessible. The storage should be organized clearly and appropriately (**Fig 5-7**).

3.2   Plaster and cast cart (trolley)

For the cast trolley, it is preferable that a cart made of stainless steel is used, and which is both conveniently located and able to be moved into a comfortable working position. It also needs to be large enough to hold the required materials. Some trolleys accommodate a bucket or bowl for water (**Fig 5-8**).

3.3   Mobile cast table

Having access to an adequate cast table is important while applying a POP or synthetic cast (**Fig 5-9, Fig 5-10**). It supports the patient in the required position and offers enough space for the surgeon or technician to work in an appropriate manner. It should also be radiolucent, transportable, and easy to clean. If possible, the table should be adjustable in height.

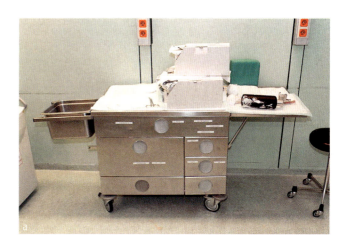

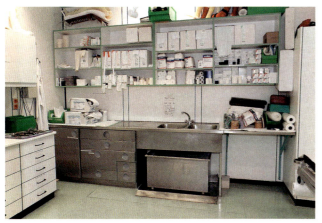

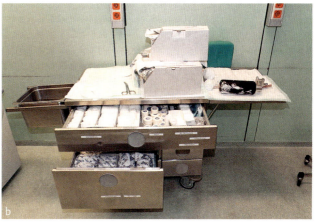

Fig 5-7   Equipped cast room at the University of Medicine in Göttingen, Germany. Materials for cast padding are stored above the cast work bank, POP splint (longuettes) on the left side of the cast work bench, and cushions for positioning extremities are on the right.

Fig 5-8a–b   Plaster and cast cart (trolley) for mobile use or in the cast room.
a   A mobile cast basin is mounted on the left.
b   Open drawers show a fully equipped cast trolley with cast and padding materials ready to use.

3.4   Image intensifier

A mobile x-ray/imaging apparatus or C-arm is recommended for the direct control of adequate reduction of fractures (**Fig 5-11**). Radiation safety measures are imperative, including staff training, protective shielding for patient and staff, and periodic radiation physics testing.

3.5   Stool for surgeon or cast technician

A stool with adjustable height is also required. This makes it more comfortable while working on the patient. In addition, it can be used when a limb needs to hang down off the table, eg, during application of a below-knee cast for a malleolar fracture. The surgeon can sit on the stool and rest the metatarsal heads on his knee in order to keep the ankle plantigrade while applying a molded below-knee cast.

3.6   Cushions and support for extremities

Positioning materials should also be available in proximity to the cast table (see **Fig 5-7**). Thigh supports are useful for the application of a long leg cast. Alternatively, a knee support is recommended (**Fig 5-12**).

A low footstool is a valuable aid for ambulatory patients transferring to the cast table. It also serves well as a lower seat, if such is required, for the cast technician or surgeon.

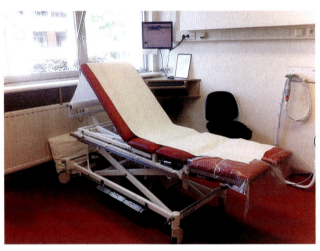

Fig 5-9   A movable cast table with hydraulic height-adjustable support plate, upholstered with foam covered by a washable fabric. At the top end, one third of the support plate is separately adjustable; a paper reservoir for single-use coverage of the support plate is fixed to the top end.

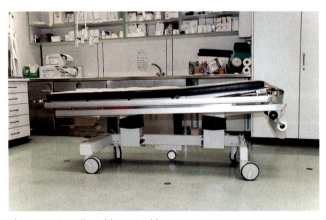

Fig 5-10   An adjustable cast table.

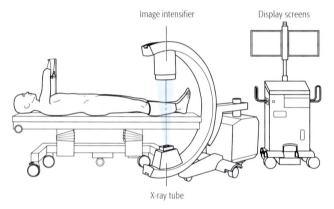

Fig 5-11   An image intensifier (C-arm) in position over the patient, with a trolley with double screen display.

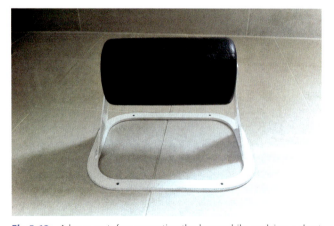

Fig 5-12   A knee rest, for supporting the knee while applying a short leg cast, or for supporting the leg while applying a long leg cast. The knee rest should be high enough to allow the knee to bend at about 45 degrees, and the padding should be covered in plastic vinyl sheeting, which is easily wiped clean after use.

Authors   Klaus Dresing, Jos Engelen

3.7   Instruments

Before starting the application of a cast, the surgeon or cast technician will prepare for the cast procedure. This includes making sure that all items needed are at hand because any interruption once the application of a cast has been started could result in problems. To interrupt the procedure, even for a short period, may result in a POP cast that is delaminated (layered or puff-pastry) and which, therefore, will be weakened. Thus, correct preparation is essential. In addition to the cast materials, padding, as well as the instruments needed for cutting or trimming the cast, should be readied.

Three major groups of instruments are in usage in the cast room (see **Fig 5-13** and **Table 5-1**):
- POP cutting shears and saws
- Plaster spreaders
- Scissors with a blunt protection end.

Cutting shears are used to split or remove a cast. An electric cast saw can be used instead. A cast knife or manual shears will only work to split wet POP casts. After splitting the cast, a spreader will help to widen the gap to allow the scissors to be introduced and to cut the padding and tube bandage (stockinette) completely.

An electric plaster saw is a wired or wireless oscillating saw for the removal or windowing of plaster or cast material. The saw can be used with a variety of saw blades, depending on the material to be cut or the opening to be made. Modern saws are often combined with a vacuum cleaner in order to avoid excessive dust. Electric cast cutters require blades to be replaced periodically. Spare blades and an appropriate wrench are necessary. For tips on the use of a cast saw see chapter 14.1 Overview of cast, splint, orthosis, and bandage techniques.

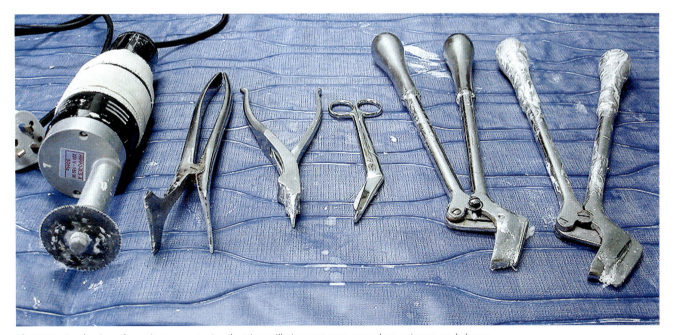

Fig 5-13   A selection of cast instruments. An electric oscillating cast saw, spreaders, scissors, and shears.

	Name	Function	Things to keep in mind
	Electric oscillating saw	For cutting the cast	• Electricity needed • Noisy • Frightening, especially for children
	Goniometer	To control the angle of the extremity	• Take care to ensure precise positioning
	Lister bandage scissors	For cutting padding and undercast materials, and to cut semirigid (soft) casts	• Ensure the blunt side of the scissors glide over the skin • Take caution with patients with skin problems
	Bruns scissors	Especially for POP	• Ensure the blunt side of the scissors glide over the skin • Take caution with patients with skin problems
	Universal scissors	For standard bandages	• Not appropriate for thick material • Becomes dull or blunt easily
	Stille plaster shears	To remove POP or synthetic casts	• Some strength needed • Difficulties in case of thick casts • Difficulties with sharp angles
	Plaster cast spreader	To spread or widen a bivalved plaster cast	• Ensure good positioning • Take care not to cut or scratch the skin
	Cast bender	To widen the cast at the borders To remove the POP casts of children	• Take care not to cut or scratch the skin
	Plaster saw	To handsaw POP casts	• Good when electricity is not available • Less frightening • More time consuming
	Plaster knife	To trim or cut (wet) POP casts	• The knife should be sharp • Care should be taken not to wound the patient • Technique: cut from bottom up and not from top down

Table 5-1   Selection of instruments needed for the application or removal of POP or synthetic casts.

Authors   Klaus Dresing, Jos Engelen

4   Maintenance

It is very important to use all instruments and devices in the appropriate manner. Maintenance with adequate cleaning, lubrication, and sharpening of tools will increase the lifetime of instruments and reduce costs. Somebody should take responsibility for the cast room. The tasks include cleaning and restocking inventory as well as the maintenance and ensuring the security of the equipment.

4.1   Cast technician

Each country has its own regulations in regard to who is allowed to apply and remove casts. The potential for harm is great, particularly in developing countries where patients may not be able to get help if complications arise. Only trained and licensed people should apply casts, and, while informally trained assistants can be helpful, they must be supervised and not left to apply or remove casts on their own.

The cast technician is a trained medical employee assisting or working under the supervision of a surgeon. The theoretical and practical training is focused on the anatomical and functional aspects of the musculoskeletal system. These paramedics have the required knowhow to deal with a variety of trauma or orthopedic related problems. They are familiar with the properties and application techniques of the different materials and are expert in preparing POP and synthetic splints and casts, braces, and other medical applications. These technicians are also responsible for trimming and removing the different types of casts and any traction (extension) systems.

4.2   Assistance during casting

Many casts can be applied more effectively with the help of a well-trained assistant. This assistant may be required to support a limb in a correct position, dip POP rolls into water, or even apply the plaster while the surgeon holds the limb in place. Adequate support for a fractured limb during casting reduces pain and allows a better cast to be applied.

5   Summary

- Typically situated in close proximity to the emergency or operating departments, the cast room is a clean area dedicated to the application of casts, support bandages, and other nonemergency treatments
- The cast room should have adequate size, storage, power supply, lighting, and ventilation
- The cast room should have the relevant equipment for daily application of casts and splints, including dedicated tables, light boxes or PACS for viewing x-rays, and a fully stocked cast trolley, as well as all relevant scissors, spreaders, and other cutting instruments
- An ideal situation is the employment of a dedicated cast technician to maintain the cast room and to provide skilled paramedic assistance.

PRINCIPLES

6   Properties of cast materials

Klaus Dresing, Jos Engelen

PRINCIPLES

6

76

Casts, Splints, and Support Bandages—Nonoperative Treatment and Perioperative Protection Klaus Dresing, Peter Trafton

Authors   Klaus Dresing, Jos Engelen

6   Properties of cast materials

1   Introduction

Plaster casts have been the standard rigid bandaging for posttraumatic or postoperative immobilization in trauma surgery and orthopedics for at least 150 years. However, over recent decades, synthetic alternatives with similar and/ or various differing properties have become increasingly available. The question for the physician is which material to use given a particular situation. This chapter therefore takes a closer look at the important properties, benefits, and disadvantages of each of the key cast materials.

2   Plaster of Paris

2.1   Discovery and term "plaster of Paris"

The earliest archeological evidence indicating the use of gypsum plaster dates back more than 9,000 years, with discoveries in Syria and Anatolia, Turkey. About 5,000 years ago, Egyptians began to produce a powder by heating gypsum in open-air fires. When mixed with water, this powder, a less hydrated form of gypsum, became a paste that hardened as it dried. The ancient Egyptians used this paste as grout in order to join stone blocks, like those of the Great Pyramid of Cheops. The Egyptians also applied plaster to the interior walls of the palaces and tombs of their pharaohs [1].

Powdered (dehydrated) gypsum came to be called "plaster of Paris" because the material was abundant and therefore widely used for building purposes by Parisians. In the 17th century, Paris had become the "capital of gypsum", and the King of France ordered that the wooden buildings of Paris be covered with plaster in order to protect them against spreading fires [1].

Initially, plaster of Paris (POP) was used by the construction industry, and was later adopted for treating unstable injuries, and for manufacturing. However, it was the Dutch army surgeon Antonius Mathijsen that was specifically given

credit for developing plaster bandages, during the Crimean War (1853–1856), as he developed a process for applying cotton bandages filled with dry, powdered POP, then wetting the bandages once the limb was appropriately positioned. He noted that as the bandages dried, they hardened, and surgeons could then shape them by hand while the plaster set. The ease and convenience of using these bandages led to their widespread adoption in preference to earlier types of splints [2] (see chapter 2 History of casting—from the beginning to the present day).

2.2   Properties

Plaster of Paris as used in casts or splints for fracture patients hardens due to a simple chemical reaction. However, it is possible to vary the features of the process (setting speed, strength, etc) according to different requirements.

2.3   Chemical and physical features

Gypsum is a soft sedimentary crystalline rock, plentiful where large bodies of water disappeared by evaporation in earlier geological eras. Chemically, it is calcium sulfate dihydrate ($CaSO_4 \cdot 2H_2O$). When heated at an appropriate temperature, gypsum gives off some of its water in the form of steam and turns into the dry white powder mentioned above (calcium sulfate hemihydrate), ie, POP. The reaction equation is $CaSO_4 \cdot 2H_2O + heat \rightarrow CaSO_4 \cdot \frac{1}{2}H_2O + 1\frac{1}{2}H_2O$. This process is called calcination. It occurs after naturally occurring gypsum has been crushed, surface-dried, and ground.

When the hemihydrate powder is subsequently mixed with water, an exothermic hydration reaction sets in leading back to the dihydrate state, ie, solid gypsum. While this reaction occurs, the material forms a paste, which expands slightly (about 1%) during setting [1]. Within minutes, the paste sets into a solid mass comprised of interlaced gypsum crystals, $CaSO_4 \cdot 2H_2O$. Additives can be used to vary the setting time. When potassium sulfate is utilized as an accelerator, or sodium borate as a retarder, the effect is a quicker or slower setting of the material.

6

PRINCIPLES

2.4   Qualities and types

Plaster is applied to a specially prepared fabric carrier that minimizes plaster loss from the dry fabric, and reduces its dustiness (**Fig 6-1**). Plaster of Paris bandages normally consist of a carrier fabric (cotton gauze or woven leno cloth) sprayed with hemihydrate plaster. The bandage is usually rolled on a round core for better handling and stability during the application process (**Fig 6-2**). Several roll widths are available to accommodate different body parts and sizes of patients. Before they are wet, plaster rolls can be cut into narrower widths with a sharp knife.

In addition to rolls, POP is also available as splints (also variously known as slabs or longuettes) which are individual strips of plaster-coated fabric of several different dimensions and package sizes (**Fig 6-3**). For convenience, splints (longuettes) are often packaged in folded groups of multiple layers. Slabs of splint (longuette) can also be formed from POP rolls, when they are unrolled to create a strip of the desired width, length, and number of layers. In some products, a zigzag-cut edge prevents fraying as well as cracking of the edges. Moisture resistant packaging protects the plaster bandages from undesired hardening in humid environments or during prolonged storage.

Additives added during the fabrication of plaster-fabric composites can be used to influence the properties of the plaster, eg, the time it takes the plaster to set (harden) [3].

> Since there are many varieties of plaster available worldwide, it is important that all users make themselves familiar with the products available in their hospital or clinic, particularly in regard to setting time and proper initial wetness.

The setting time is approximately 10–12 minutes when 20° C dipping water is used, and varies not only with the type of plaster but also with variations in water temperature. After moistening, most POP offers good to excellent conformability and modeling properties. Some preparations are very creamy, some are very durable. The plaster is easily molded, so it conforms closely to the body part to which it is being applied [4]. Shaping the plaster during setting is a technique that can be used in order to counteract deforming forces, to correct mobile deformity such as a pliable clubfoot, or a healing fracture before it completes consolidation, or to improve containment fit in order to stabilize an unstable fracture into anatomical alignment.

Appropriate padding must be placed between the skin and any immobilizing material. The importance of padding, an essential part of cast application, is discussed in more detail in this chapter in topic 5 Undercast materials.

Fig 6-1   Plaster of Paris is fixed on a specially prepared fabric carrier in order to minimize plaster loss during the dipping process and application.

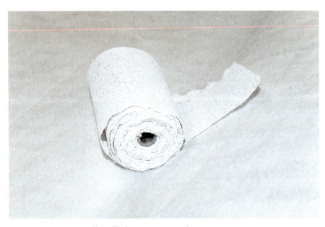

Fig 6-2   A POP roll, rolled onto a round core.

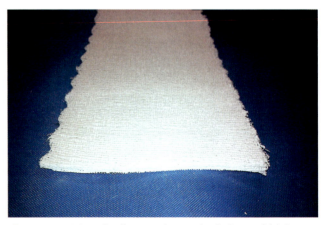

Fig 6-3 A   A POP splint (longuette) comprised of several fabric layers impregnated with POP.

Authors   Klaus Dresing, Jos Engelen

2.5   Application characteristics
2.5.1 Conformability and plasticity

The ability to loosen a circumferential cast is essential in order to relieve generalized tissue pressure, which occurs when a limb swells inside a noncompliant cast. This increasing pressure can cause compartment syndrome that results rapidly in potentially permanent loss of muscle and nerve function. Casts may also need to be altered to relieve focal pressure that might lead to a pressure sore or nerve injury. [5] So, it is desirable that the plaster is sufficiently pliable and plastically deformable in order to allow a circumferential cast to be spread apart along a single longitudinal cut, and thus loosened (often called "univalving", as opposed to "bivalving" with two cuts, which makes the cast removable but more unstable). Plaster of Paris is well-suited for this univalving technique, since a longitudinal saw cut can usually be spread enough to achieve the desired loosening.

2.5.2 Porosity and absorption

The porosity of plaster casts allows transmission of perspiration, which permits skin moisture to dry. However, plaster also absorbs liquids readily, as seen with wound drainage (**Fig 6-4**), or when the outside of a cast becomes wet. Absorb-

ing moisture weakens the plaster. Once the plaster cast becomes soaked, it softens and loses its rigidity. If this happens while it is still needed, the cast must be replaced.

2.5.3 Strength and stability

The final strength of the plaster cast material depends on its crystal structure. If the cast is manipulated while it is beginning to harden, or prevented from drying out, it will be weak because of impaired crystallization. Drying is delayed in cold or moist conditions and accelerated in a warm and dry environment.

The cast strength also depends on the layers of plaster (thickness) and the shape of the cast contoured around the injured extremity. As mentioned, excessive plaster increases weight, bulk, and heat production. But on the other hand, compliance of the trauma patient is also mandatory (**Fig 6-5**). It is important that a plaster cast does not become wet after drying, as the POP will literally dissolve.

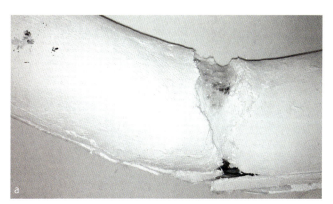

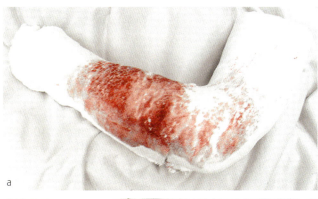

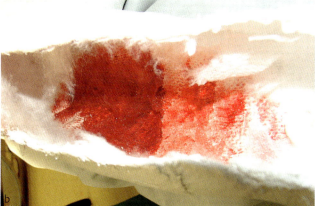

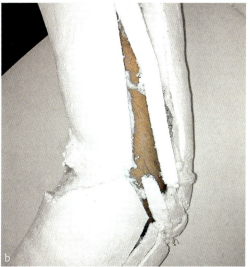

Fig 6-4a–b   Demonstration of moisture absorbance by a plaster cast.
a POP easily absorbs wound drainage and other liquids.
b Inner aspect of the POP cast: The hematoma has soaked the padding and POP cast.

Fig 6-5a–b   A POP cast can break if (**a**) not enough layers are applied, or (**b**) there is a conflict between the stability of the cast and the compliance of the patient.

It is thus important to add strength by proper casting techniques. For example, the molded longitudinal reinforcement ridges on the surface of a plaster cast or splint can double strength and stiffness with only a 20% increase in weight [6]. The caregiver must balance these factors in order to create a cast of optimal strength and weight, with minimal risk of thermal injury. Because it conforms so well to the underlying body contours, a properly molded POP cast or splint produces less friction (shear forces) on the skin surface than other cast materials. This provides an optimal environment for healing of wounds, including skin grafts [3].

Proper handling of the plaster is important and this starts with the dipping process. The water depth should be at least 20–30 cm, so that any roll used can be submerged vertically below the water surface. The column of water helps to press out the remaining air between the layers of plaster. The bandages rapidly become wet when placed into water in the correct manner (**Fig 6-6**). The immersion time is ap- proximately three seconds, or until air bubbles stop appearing, which indicates that the plaster is soaked completely.

The plaster must be uniformly wet. Dry spots decrease the quality and strength of the plaster. Dry layers cause delamination, producing so-called "puff pastry plaster" (**Fig 6-7**).

After dipping, the plaster roll or splint (longuette) must be squeezed just enough to remove excess water, and to distribute the remaining water uniformly. The latter is achieved by holding each end of the plaster roll while gently wringing or squeezing it as it is removed from the water after being soaked through. Sufficient water must remain in order to create a thick fluid plaster paste. The layers of plaster are smoothed together by manual longitudinal compression motions; the result is a homogenous cast or splint (**Fig 6-8**).

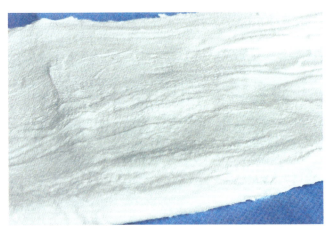

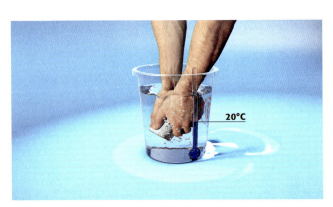

Fig 6-6   If dipped correctly into 20–30 cm water depth, air bubbles escape from the POP layers.

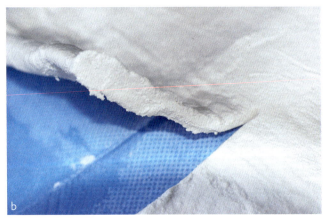

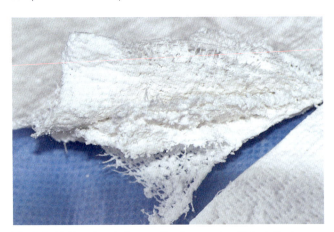

Fig 6-7   Puff pastry plaster resulting from an insufficient dipping process and delamination of the POP layers.

Fig 6-8a–b   Optimally prepared POP splint (longuette). It is a homogenous slab as the result of rubbing the moist paste of plaster into the fabric.
a View from above.
b Slab cut (view from the side). All layers form a homogenous composite.

Authors   Klaus Dresing, Jos Engelen

During application, it is important to rub the moist paste into the fabric in order to obtain a smooth, uniform composite in which the fabric threads are embedded (like reinforcing metal bars in structural concrete). Splints (longuettes) 4–12 layers thick should similarly be squeezed and rubbed to spread the plaster paste through the fabric before they are applied as reinforcement to a cast or as slab splints, held onto the surface of an extremity with a fabric roller bandage. Splints (longuettes) should be rubbed longitudinally, typically on a waterproof table top, so they adhere to each other and become a single composite. Several layers of padding can be added to the surface of a setting splint before it is placed on the patient. Using a circular application of POP, the layers of plaster should be molded similarly, after the wrapping. Rubbing the plaster while it is wet, during the early phase of setting, distributes the plaster uniformly through all fabric layers in order to produce a single composite that will not delaminate.

The strength of a POP cast measures between 5 and 10 megapascals of pressure (MPa), with a bending modulus of 2–3 gigapascals (GPa) [7]. Because of this relative stiffness, circumferential POP casts, applied to fresh injuries or postoperatively, should be split and spread apart at least along one side in order to accommodate swelling and to avoid excessive increase of interstitial fluid pressure. For the forearm, a dorsal split is more stable than others, and allows the cast to retain the reduction better [8].

Plaster of Paris is weaker in tension, but stronger in compression [9]. With low-tensile strength and normal loading, the material loses its rigidity over time [9]. Adding one or more longitudinal ridges to a POP cast or splint increases its strength and longevity [6].

2.6   Temperature sensitivity and heat formation

If a plaster bandage is immersed in cold water (< 15° C) the initial setting will be delayed and thus the working time lengthened. Conversely, if very rapid setting is required, soaking the bandage in warm water (> 25° C) accelerates the rate of reaction. However, water temperatures above 50° C will slow down setting and at 100° C no setting will occur at all.

The exothermic reaction during the hardening of POP may cause significant thermal burns [5, 10–13], especially if the dip water temperature is high. Using a normal water temperature of (18–20° C) is essential. Key elements that can cause burn injuries include cast thickness, dipping water temperature, and the use of pillows, especially with plastic covers, which prevents heat dissipation [12, 14, 15].

Because of the low strength-to-weight ratio of POP, thicker casts are often used. However, this produces more heat and increases the risk of burn injuries [5, 11].

The key factors that affect plaster cast application include:
- Water temperature used for dipping the plaster material
- Warmer water will accelerate setting time
- Colder water will slow down setting time
- Tepid water is recommended for plaster dipping
- Air temperature and humidity
- Plaster casts dry more rapidly when the cast is exposed to circulating, dry air.

Remember, a POP cast is not water resistant.

2.7   Working time

The plaster can only be worked for a period of 3–5 minutes, depending on water temperature and plaster brand. The initial setting time takes 10–12 minutes. The required time for complete setting, and if allowed first permissibility for weight bearing, is 24–48 hours depending on the thickness of the cast.

2.8   Removal of plaster of Paris casts

For removal and splitting of POP casts, cast saws are usually used. After complete hardening, POP casts are so hard and stiff that normal scissors or knives are useless. Special plaster scissors eg, Stille, can be used to open or remove the cast (see topic 3 in chapter 5 Logistics and resources in the cast room).

2.9   Possible problems/disadvantages

Potential disadvantages of plaster include the time required for hardening, the relatively heavier weight compared to lighter synthetic materials, the fact a POP cast can break easily and is affected by water and moisture, and the amount of heat that can be produced, particularly with warm dipping water and a thick plaster cast [16–20].

3   Synthetic cast materials

Synthetic cast materials typically consist of one layer of polyester knit, fiberglass fabric, polypropylene knit, or fiberglass free polymer (the latter also called thermoplastic). The important part of the material is the knitted fabric impregnated with a polyurethane resin, the prepolymer. The resin polymerizes and hardens after being exposed to humidity or water. As with plaster, uniform wetting is important, in this case, in order to achieve uniform polymerization. Gloves should be used during application because the resin adheres to skin and causes irritation.

3.1   Properties

Synthetic casts are often perceived as being more difficult to apply, and their moldability is less than plaster. However, they retain their strength even when wet [16] and they are lighter and interfere less with x-rays [19, 21, 22]. Synthetic casts harden rapidly, and soon achieve their final strength (**Fig 6-9**).

Modifications in the formula of the resin used can result in either a rigid (hard) or a semirigid (soft) cast. While light and durable, the hard cast technique nevertheless has some disadvantages. The materials are very rigid with hard and sharp edges and therefore an oscillating saw is usually needed for splitting and adjustment.

Semirigid (soft) casts provide significant stability by means of containment, comparable to a hydraulic cylinder. Their stability is often sufficient for maintaining alignment during functional use of the extremity, even including weight bearing. Sarmiento and others pointed out their benefits for early functional use both in fractures of the upper and lower extremities, and also demonstrated the effectiveness of such casts and braces for providing the necessary support [23–26].

The flexible, semirigid cylinder can adapt to the changing form of the musculature, leading to controlled compression and improved circulation [27]. Due to the hydrostatic principle of a semirigid tube, it is possible for the functional use of the

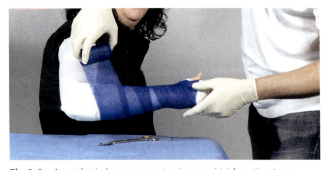

Fig 6-9   A synthetic long arm cast using semirigid casting tape.

injured limb to accelerate fracture healing [28]. While this perhaps is easier to achieve by a light, semirigid soft cast, this may also be accomplished by rigid casts. More important than the type of cast material is that the cast provides good support in a functional position and that the patient is appropriately taught and trained in functional use and exercises.

3.2   Qualities and types
3.2.1   Polyester

Synthetic cast material with a polyester fabric carrier is coated with polyurethane resin. Stability and flexibility of the cast can be adjusted individually by the number of layers applied. Fewer layers offer higher flexibility while more layers increase stability in order to provide increased immobilization if and where necessary. The cast is molded carefully to fit body contours. Depending on the number of layers used, cast scissors can be used to open the cast and adjust its size.

Polyester casting material interferes less with x-ray imaging than plaster does. The cast edges stay soft and flexible if the material is applied thinly near the edge. These casts can be used either as an initial or a subsequent application. Patients are often more comfortable and may be more compliant during rehabilitation. Yet another advantage is that this material produces less dust during cast removal.

3.2.2   Fiberglass–rigid and semirigid casts

Fiberglass fabric with water-activated polyurethane resin normally provides rigid, durable immobilization after a short setting time. Varying the amount or composition of resin can result in different levels of rigidity. Hardening can be activated by air humidity alone, but is more rapid after being dipped in water. The fiberglass material hardens quickly and can bear weight shortly after application [27].

Semirigid fiberglass material is easier to apply and to mold. Its setting time is approximately five minutes. The cast is ready for weight bearing after approximately 30 minutes. After hardening, soft casts are flexible, but lack elasticity. Semirigid casts are easy to reapply, to clean, and are ideal for treating trauma and in postoperative applications.

Gloves should be worn during application in order to protect the caregiver's skin from the polyurethane resin. But the edges of the finished semirigid cast are smooth and less abrasive than a rigid cast, which increases the patient's comfort. The layers consolidate well, offering improved strength without delamination.

Removal and adjustment of semirigid or soft casts can be done with cast scissors alone; there is no need for a saw.

Authors Klaus Dresing, Jos Engelen

However, rigid fiberglass casts require an oscillating cast saw for removal.

3.2.3 Thermoplastic

This variety of synthetic cast bandages consists of a flexible, knitted polyester fabric with a thermoplastic polyester coating. No resin is used. Thermoplastic cast material can be applied and molded without gloves. With thermoplastic moldable casting material, which is reversibly moldable, the self-adhesive characteristic is achieved by heating in a hot water bath or a steam heater. The thermoplastic polymer cast material starts to be moldable at or above the respective softening temperature. The material hardens again upon cooling. The material is water-resistant and permeable to air and water vapor. Its setting time is approximately five minutes; the cast is ready for weight bearing after approximately 20 minutes. Removal is possible with bandage or cast scissors.

3.2.4 Special synthetic materials and material combinations

3.2.4.1 Combicast applications

In the so-called "combicast" technique, rigid (hard cast) splint is integrated between two layers of semirigid (soft cast) material. This technique, also called "sandwich-technique", permits the connection of rigid splint with circular wraps of semirigid material, making the entire construction stable [27, 29]. Such immobilization can be applied by molding it using the three-point fixation technique as described by Charnley [30] (see topic 10 in chapter 3 Principles of casting). Providing flexibility in some portions of the combicast may permit more muscle function than is possible with a completely rigid cylindrical cast [27, 29].

3.2.4.2 Padded synthetic casting material

These prepadded splints can be applied directly to the patient's skin and secured with a fabric roller bandage. The rigid cast material knit is impregnated with polyurethane resin in order to form the moldable core of the splint. Multiple layers of a knitted fiberglass (or occasionally polyester) fabric are integrated between two layers of padding felt (eg, 100% polypropylene) on the side of skin contact or a film/padding cover on the outer side. The outer side is typically covered with a nonwoven, water-permeable fabric. When wet, this moistens the entire splint, ensuring rapid and uniform activation of the resin. The material can be handled without using gloves. Its setting time is approximately 3–5 minutes and the splint can withstand significant forces after approximately 20 minutes. Such casting material is available in several widths, in a thin, flattened moisture-proof aluminum foil tube. It is available in precut sizes as well as in a roll of several meters length. The desired length (with its wrapper)

is cut off with scissors. The cut end of the foil wrapper on the rest of the roll must then be clamped closed in order to avoid air moisture causing the remaining material to harden.

3.2.4.3 Precut unpadded fiberglass splints

These are available as strips of fiberglass or polyester fabric impregnated with polyurethane resin, individually sealed in aluminum foil. They are useful for applying splints over separate padding or for reinforcement of circular rigid or semirigid casts.

3.3 Temperature sensitivity and heat formation

Synthetic casting materials produce less heat during polymerization than is produced during the setting of POP casts. Additionally, because of their greater strength, less material is needed for a cast.

> The key factors that affect synthetic cast application include:
> - Temperature of water used for dipping the synthetic casting material
> - Warmer water accelerates setting time
> - Colder water slows setting time
> - Tepid water is recommended for synthetic materials.

3.4 Working time

There are two different ways to apply synthetic cast material. Normally the material is dipped into tepid water (around 18–20° C) and then applied to the limb. The working time using this technique is about 2–4 minutes and the initial setting time takes about 6–8 minutes.

Another way of applying synthetic cast material is the dry application method where the material is first applied to the limb and then moistened by spraying water on it or by wrapping it with a wet bandage. This technique gives the cast technician more working time and is advised for difficult applications. The working time using this technique is about 5–7 minutes and the initial setting time is 8–10 minutes.

The complete setting time and, if permitted, weight bearing is approximately 30 minutes in both application techniques.

3.5 Removal of synthetic casts

Semirigid casting material is simply removed with cast scissors. However, a cast saw is required for rigid synthetic casts.

> Using synthetic cast materials (fiberglass, polyester, and polypropylene) has advantages and disadvantages. Users must become familiar with the properties and optimal application techniques of the materials available in their practice.

4 Plaster of Paris versus synthetic cast materials

Synthetic materials, which are known to be lighter, stronger, and less prone to emit offensive odors, are often preferred by patients, especially for lower extremity immobilization [31]. But there are a wide range of factors to be considered when comparing POP versus synthetic materials. In brief, these include:

- Greater material costs of synthetic
- Shorter working time for the application of synthetic
- Less frequent need for recasting with synthetic
- Less abrasive and smoother edges in semirigid synthetic casting
- Heavier weight of POP
- Time required for complete setting with POP
- The amount of heat that can be produced in POP, particularly with warm dipping water or a thick plaster cast.

4.1 Hybrid casts

It is possible to create a best of both worlds hybrid cast by beginning with a thinner layer of POP in order to take advantage of its easy application and excellent molding properties. Once this layer is sufficiently set, it is reinforced with an outer layer of rigid synthetic material for extra strength and durability but less weight than if only plaster was used. Limiting the amount of synthetic cast material may be more cost effective as well. An oscillating saw is required for removal of such casts, especially for the outer layer of synthetic.

4.2 Cast removal

A major advantage of semirigid casts is that they can be split, adjusted, or removed with cast scissors instead of a cast saw. Particularly when treating children, the use of oscillating saws to split, cut, or remove the plaster or hard cast bandage constitutes a major problem. A recent case report ascribed death of a young child with cardiomyopathy to anxiety associated with the use of an electric cast saw [32]. The authors also noted tachycardia during cast removal in other patients and its amelioration when hearing protection was provided, particularly for patients younger than 13 years of age [32–34]. But while semirigid material can be removed with scissor cuts, a saw is usually needed for removal of plaster casts and always for rigid synthetic casts. An additional major concern is the possible carcinogenic risk for healthcare professionals with frequent exposure to sawdust from synthetic casts [35].

4.3 Weight of casts

As mentioned previously, synthetic cast materials are lighter than plaster. However, a prospective study recently demonstrated that the difference in weight was only significant for lower extremity casts [31].

4.4 Biomechanics

Mechanically, plaster bandages have a higher elastic modulus and substantially lower ultimate yield strength than synthetic materials [16, 17, 19, 36]. Pressure increases in the soft-tissue compartments after injury and surgery [37]. A study comparing more semirigid casts in patients with stable, nondisplaced fractures (distal radius, scaphoid, and fifth metatarsal or ankle) demonstrated that patients preferred these to closed circumferential plaster casts that were more rigid throughout [38].

4.5 Recommendations

Recognizing that, overall, plaster is stiffer but synthetic cast material is more durable, the authors offer the following clinical recommendations:

- In the acute phase, directly posttrauma or postoperatively, use plaster for immobilization
- In the secondary phase, use synthetic casts [16, 19, 29, 39, 40]
- Inexperienced caregivers must always exercise great caution [41].

Significant morbidity can result from use of a rigid circumferential cast for immobilizing an extremity at risk of swelling. In order to minimize the risks of harm from compartment syndrome, pressure sores, and/or complex regional pain syndrome, a circumferential cast should be split to the last layer of noncompliant material and then spread apart far enough to loosen it when immobilizing a fresh injury [41]. Alternatively, instead of a circumferential cast, a well-padded, rigid splint can be applied with compliant bandages. Optimizing comfort, function, and safety in the initial cast depends on a multitude of factors [42].

4.6 Semirigid casts

Semirigid below-knee walking casts provide greater immobilization at the ankle while allowing more forefoot movement. They are easier to walk in. Semirigid casting has measurable advantages when compared to rigid synthetic casts, and represents a further development in the nonoperative management of fractures and soft-tissue injuries [43]. Casts can be constructed with a greater degree of function, so that controlled motion and stabilization can be provided within the same cast [44].

Polyester casts with fewer layers are not as flexible as soft cast (fiberglass) material, but have nearly the same characteristics.

Authors   Klaus Dresing, Jos Engelen

4.7   Semirigid casts for acute injuries—primary definitive care

A semirigid cast should be split similarly to rigid casts whenever it is applied for an acute injury. Since a higher skin surface pressure has been measured under synthetic casts, and the unsplit cast cannot adapt to swelling, some authors advise against these materials for acute injuries [19, 45, 46]. Research by Kunze and Haberer showed that the expansion behavior of polyester and polypropylene is initially better, while POP shows no expansion at all [21], unless it is split. Typically, the synthetic materials spring back [21]. After the cast is applied, a clear pressure increase can occur under conventional plaster bandages and synthetic casts. In an experimental study, Davids was able to show that significant pressure increase occured under rigid fiberglass casts if wrapping is carried out with the standard technique [40]. The pressure increase is greater than under a plaster bandage [40]. When using the stretch-relax technique (see topic 10 Bandaging techniques in chapter 14.1 Overview of cast, splint, orthosis, and bandage techniques) and simulated swelling, the pressure values are significantly below the values measured inside a POP cast [40]. Other authors suggest that the characteristics of POP and fiberglass should best be combined [47, 48].

Semirigid casting has the best compliance and rate-dependency characteristics, accommodating significantly more volume of fluid compared to POP or rigid fiberglass material [49]. The use of semirigid material may thus be safer than other materials as far as response to swelling (volume expansion) is concerned [49].

Primary definitive care (where treatment involves the application of only one cast) with semirigid casting material provides adequate support for selected lower extremity indications [29]. The primary definitive cast technique with polyester materials has been practiced for some time [50]. As with the plaster technique, the primary definitive soft cast bandage should also be split completely. It is wrapped with an elastic bandage or held together with velcro straps. An advantage of the soft cast technique for acute injuries is that the split cast can be adjusted to fit more closely as the swelling subsides or muscles atrophy. A longitudinal strip of cast material is removed by cutting with scissors and the cast is "snugged" by wrapping with a bandage.

A Cochrane analysis found that there is good evidence for the beneficial effect of ankle supports in the form of semirigid orthosis or Aircast braces in order to prevent ankle sprains during high-risk sporting activities [51].

In a comparison of rigid and semirigid material, the following was found for grade III lateral collateral ligament sprains of the ankle:

- The semirigid cast group had a better range of motion and could walk better at the 2-week checkup, but these differences diminished at 6 weeks
- With the semirigid cast group, patient satisfaction was higher, need for a support for walking was less, and return to work was earlier.

Considering also its reduced cost of application, semirigid casting material is an excellent choice for the initial short-term immobilization for the functional treatment of acute ankle ligament injuries [52]. In the postoperative and conservative care of ligament injuries to the ankle joint, semirigid immobilization has been recommended for many years [53]. The semirigid cast technique allows more functional plantar flexion/dorsiflexion than other ankle casts [54]. Such greater mobility of the ankle within its normal range of motion appears to lead to improved results when ankle sprains are treated with semirigid casts or orthoses [55].

5   Undercast materials

In addition to the structural material used to build the cast, two kinds of undercast materials are typically needed:
- Tube bandages
- Cast padding.

5.1   Tube bandages
5.1.1   Stockinette tube bandages
Tubular fabric bandages, often called stockinette, are pulled over the skin in order to protect it from the cast material and padding. Both natural and synthetic textiles are available. Cotton is skin-friendly, and may also be mixed with rayon or small amounts of elastic fiber.

5.1.2   Tubular elastic bandages
Integrating elastane (spandex) into the fabric results in highly compliant bandages that can be applied without creases. This prevents slipping and conforms well to the contour of the body. The properties of the padding remain unimpaired over the entire period of wear. High permeability in regard to water vapor and air, as well as a low absorption volume, increase the wearer's comfort. Normally, the knitted material is smoother on the outer side, therefore, the outer side should be next to the skin, ie, the smoother and softer side will lie directly on top of the patient's skin. In the final step of applying a tubular elastic bandage, try to pull it in the direction of hair growth (ie, down, rather

than up the leg) in order to avoid leaving the skin hairs under tension.

5.1.3 Natural terry-cloth stockinette
More cushioning than a single layer of standard tube bandage can be obtained by using material with a terry-cloth weave. These terry-cloth stockinettes are ideal for the focused rigidity casting technique as well as for primary definitive treatment.

5.1.4 Synthetic tube bandage
These fabrics, knitted in tubes, are suitable for use with synthetic or POP casting materials. Some of the stockinettes have breathable properties, and some are water-repellent.

5.2 Cast padding
Orthopedic padding is used under a plaster or synthetic cast for protection of the skin, soft tissues, bony prominences, and superficial nerves, and protects them from pressure, ulceration, and abrasion while wearing the cast as well as during cast removal. Padding also helps protect the skin from thermal injury during cast hardening. Gently compressed undercast padding can help prevent edema.

Cast padding is available in many varieties. The most common cast paddings are rolled thin cotton (or viscose), which is readily stretched or torn by hand, and synthetic padding such as polyester. Sheet wadding (the batting/padding made for quilts) or other thick, compressible fiber sheets have also been used extensively. Conformable rolls are easiest to apply. Felt pads can be added in order to protect pressure points, and some synthetic materials are waterproof [5]. Generally, the authors recommend synthetic cast padding.

Poorly applied padding can produce sores, and too much padding results in an ill-fitting cast, poorer immobilization, and possibly impaired healing. Excessive padding thickness has been associated with secondary fracture displacement [56]. In cases with redisplacement, the plaster molding (cast index) and padding (padding index) were found to be significantly greater [57].

A sufficient layer of padding significantly protects the skin during cast removal, when the blade of the oscillating cast saw grows hot, and can protect against mechanical injuries (lacerations or abrasions) [58]. Clearly, the skillful application of padding is as essential as plaster molding in the production of a safe and effective therapeutic cast (**Fig 6-10**).

5.2.1 Cotton padding
Cotton padding is soft on the skin but is not very moldable and may result in lumps and/or ruptures of the material. It

is also not waterproof. The required sizes can be cut out of bigger packages. However, in some countries, the choice between cotton and synthetic padding is severely limited, with synthetic padding material either not available at all or restricted to special applications and treatments.

5.2.2 Synthetic padding
Unlike cotton padding, synthetic padding often comes in the form of nonabsorbent (yet highly breathable) material that wicks moisture away from the skin and reduces the risk of skin maceration. Some synthetic padding materials are even designed to be completely water resistant, in which case, if a synthetic cast is also used, patients can shower or swim while wearing casts with this padding, although air drying, perhaps with a cool hairdryer, is advised.

5.2.2.1 Polyester
The most commonly used synthetic cast padding is bandage made of low or nonabsorbent crinkled polyester fibers. Polyester padding facilitates application by requiring only a little tension on the fabric as it is rolled onto the limb, with some gentle smoothing with the other hand. The cushioning effect is maintained even under pressure and when moist. It stays permeable to air and perspiration. The material has a temperature-compensating effect and is easy to handle. During application it can easily be torn by hand as needed. Sterilization by autoclaving at 121° C is possible. The material is radiolucent.

5.2.2.2 Polyacrylate
This material is used for partial padding at the edges of the cast or weight-bearing zones. Individually cut shapes are used to protect exposed support zones when applying trunk or pelvis/leg casts. Polyacrylate padding mostly uses an adhesive backing, allowing the padding to be applied in strips. It involves a finely-porous foam, which provides good air permeability and high skin tolerance.

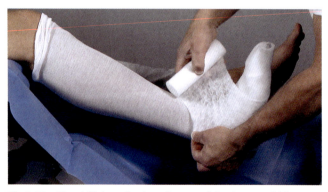

Fig 6-10 The skillful application of cast padding is essential in the production of a safe and effective therapeutic cast.

Authors   Klaus Dresing, Jos Engelen

5.2.2.3 Polyurethane (adhesive foam padding)

A bandage with an open-pored (open-cell) surface made out of polyurethane foam (**Fig 6-11**) provides additional protection to the skin, and is particularly suited for use on bony prominences. Foam padding should be used with an adhesive backing on one side, as this will adhere to the tube bandage (stockinette), holding it in place and avoiding movement inside the cast. It is typically air and moisture permeable and resistant to perspiration.

Polyurethane has been found to be highly effective in preventing pressure sores [59].

Closed-cell foam padding exists, and is occasionally used as a sports protection, but is not recommended in casting as it may contain rubber latex, which can cause allergic reactions.

5.2.2.4 Felt

Needle-felt padding, both with or without an adhesive backing, is an orthopedic felt used for additional patient comfort in splinting and casting techniques. This felt may be combined with foam for additional protection and cushioning.

5.2.2.5 Elastic foam tape

Adhesive elastic foam tape provides soft edges for casts and splints, or protection for bony prominences (**Fig 6-12**). It is particularly useful for the edging of removable casts and orthoses. The central high-stretch section makes it easy to fold over cast edges. It should be as thin as possible to avoid reducing stability.

5.2.2.6 Waterproof padding

A special knit structure lets water quickly drain from the cast (30–60 minutes). Most of the liquid runs out of the cast, the rest evaporates through the cast heated by body temperature. Water-permeable liners allow transpiration to escape from the cast. Especially in children, these liners may prevent skin irritation [60].

5.2.3 Padding anchorage

All padding material should be anchored in some way in order to avoid shifting under the cast. Extra pads can also be placed so they are in contact with the cast material to which they are likely to adhere.

5.2.3.1 Crepe paper

Crepe paper bandages are made of wood-free, fine crepe paper, used as a barrier between the dry padding and the wet POP. They are highly extensible, and easy to apply and to tear off; often the end of the bandage is slightly fastened with latex adhesive. They are slightly water resistant. Such materials may prove constricting if the cast is adjusted after its application (eg, cast wedging).

5.2.3.2 Synthetic roller bandages

Polyurethane bandages are often used instead of crepe paper. They are breathable and slip resistant.

5.2.3.3 Tapes, clips, and other fixing materials

During the process of making the cast, or to hold the padding or cast in place, a variety of fixation materials may be required. For example, gauze and elastic bandages are used to wrap and hold an opened (split) cast in place. Wrapped bandages are often secured by using surgical tape, adhesive tape, elastic clips, or safety pins (see chapter 18 Support bandages). And hook (scratchy) and loop (smooth) strips of velcro allow a splint or orthosis to be temporarily removed and reapplied later (eg, for bathing or physiotherapy).

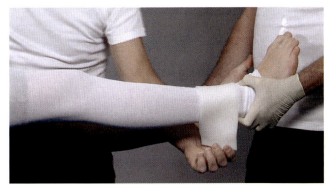

Fig 6-11   Open-poured adhesive foam padding provides additional protection to the skin and bony prominences.

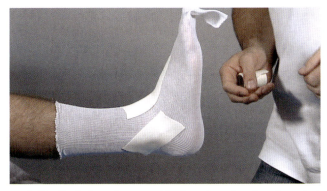

Fig 6-12   Elastic foam tape, used for the edges of casts or to protect bony prominences.

6 Summary

- Plaster of Paris is the gold standard for acute non-operative trauma care, especially when reduction is required; it is available world wide
- Synthetic cast material is more comfortable, lighter in weight, and more stable than POP, but is more expensive
- After hardening, semirigid (soft) synthetic material is flexible, but lacks elasticity
- Unlike rigid synthetics, semirigid materials do not need a cast saw for removal
- Physicians / cast technicians should ensure they are fully aware of the application working time, setting time (before hardening), and heat generation caused by both POP and synthetic casting materials, as incorrect application can lower the cast's effectiveness or cause potential harm
- Under each cast, tube bandages (stockinette) and padding are applied to protect the skin and soft tissues
- There are a wide range of other similarities and differences between plaster of Paris and synthetic casting materials; see **Table 6-1** for a comparison summary.

Item	Plaster of Paris (POP)	Rigid synthetic material	Semirigid synthetic material
Water resistance	–	+++	+++
Perspiration transfer	+	++	++
Skin irritation during application	+	++	++
Removal tools	Oscillating cast saw	Oscillating cast saw	Scissors
Gloves necessary	–	+++	+++
Exothermic reaction during application	++	+	–
Weight	+++	+	+
Radiolucency	–	++	++
Fast hardening speed	+	++	++
Immediate weight bearing	–	++	++
Conformability	+++	+	+
Bulkiness	++	–	–
Stability	+	+++	++
Resistance against tension	–	++	+
Resistance against compression	++	+++	+
Acute fracture care	+++	+	++
Maintains reduction	+++	+	+
Offers support and functional stabilization	+	++	+++
Thickness	+++	–	–
Molding properties	+++	+	+
Strength-to-weight ratio	Low	High	Medium-high (semirigid combicast)
Allows for a primary definitive cast	+	+	+++

Legend for Table 6-1.
- – Nil or not applicable
- + Slightly applicable
- ++ Moderately applicable
- +++ Strongly applicable

Table 6-1 Summary of cast material properties.

Authors   Klaus Dresing, Jos Engelen

7   References

1. **Sampson DH (ed)**. *Gypsum: Properties, Production and Applications (Chemical Engineering Methods and Technology)*. 1st ed. Hauppauge: Nova Science Pub Inc; 2011.

2. **Povacs F**. *[History of Trauma Surgery]*. 2nd ed. Heidelberg: Springer Medizin Verlag; 2007. German.

3. **Colditz JC**. Plaster of Paris: the forgotten hand splinting material. *J Hand Ther*. 2002 Apr-Jun; 15(2):144–157.

4. **Gurevitz S, Tjtium Y, Halperin C, et al**. Correlation between experience in plaster-cast application and weight of plaster of Paris. *Eur J Orthop Surg Traumatol*. 2004; 14(2):72–74.

5. **Halanski M, Noonan KJ**. Cast and splint immobilization: complications. *J Am Acad Orthop Surg*. 2008 Jan; 16(1):30–40.

6. **Stewart T, Cheong W, Barr V, et al**. Strong and light plaster casts? *Injury*. 2009 Aug; 40(8):890–893.

7. **Wytch R, Ross N, Wardlaw D**. Glass fibre versus non-glass fibre splinting bandages. *Injury*. 1992; 23(2):101–106.

8. **Nielsen DM, Ricketts DM**. Where to split plaster casts. *Injury*. 2005 May; 36(5):588–589.

9. **Schmidt VE, Somerset JH, Porter RE**. Mechanical properties of orthopedic plaster bandages. *J Biomech*. 1973 Mar; 6(2):173–185.

10. **Gannaway JK, Hunter JR**. Thermal effects of casting materials. *Clin Orthop Relat Res*. 1983 Dec; (181):191–195.

11. **Halanski MA, Halanski AD, Oza A, et al**. Thermal injury with contemporary cast-application techniques and methods to circumvent morbidity. *J Bone Joint Surg Am*. 2007 Nov; 89(11):2369–2377.

12. **Lavalette R, Pope MH, Dickstein H**. Setting temperatures of plaster casts. The influence of technical variables. *J Bone Joint Surg Am*. 1982 Jul; 64(6):907–911.

13. **Pope MH, Callahan G, Lavalette R**. Setting temperatures of synthetic casts. *J Bone Joint Surg Am*. 1985 Feb; 67(2):262–264.

14. **Ahmed SS, Carmichael KD**. Plaster and synthetic cast temperatures in a clinical setting: an in vivo study. *Orthopedics*. 2011 Jan; 34(2):99.

15. **Unal S, Aksoy A, Yilmaz C, et al**. Third-degree burn after plaster of Paris brace. *Plast Reconstr Surg*. 2004 Nov; 114(6):1686–1687.

16. **Berman AT, Parks BG**. A comparison of the mechanical properties of fiberglass cast materials and their clinical relevance. *J Orthop Trauma*. 1990; 4(1):85–92.

17. **Callahan DJ, Daddario N, Williams S, et al**. Three experimental designs testing orthopedic casting material strength. *Orthopedics*. 1986 May; 9(5):673–675.

18. **Callahan DJ, Harris BJ**. Short history of plaster-of-Paris cast immobilization. *Minn Med*. 1986 Apr; 69(4):195–196.

19. **Wehbé MA**. Plaster uses and misuses. *Clin Orthop Relat Res*. 1982 Jul; (167):242–249.

20. **Younger AS, Curran P, McQueen MM**. Backslabs and plaster casts: which will best accommodate increasing intracompartmental pressures? *Injury*. 1990 May; 21(3):179–181.

21. **Kunze K, Haberer KH**. [Comparative studies of synthetic and nonsynthetic cast dressings]. *Unfallchirurg*. 1994 Jun; 97(6):325–331. German.

22. **Mihalko WM, Beaudoin AJ, Krause WR**. Mechanical properties and material characteristics of orthopaedic casting material. *J Orthop Trauma*. 1989; 3(1):57–63.

23. **Martinez A, Sarmiento A, Latta LL**. Closed fractures of the proximal tibia treated with a functional brace. *Clin Orthop Relat Res*. 2003 Dec; (417):293–302.

24. **Sarmiento A, Zagorski JB, Zych GA, et al**. Functional bracing for the treatment of fractures of the humeral diaphysis. *J Bone Joint Surg Am*. 2000 Apr; 82(4):478–486.

25. **Sarmiento A, Latta LL**. 450 closed fractures of the distal third of the tibia treated with a functional brace. *Clin Orthop Relat Res*. 2004 Nov; (428):261–271.

26. **Stewart HD, Innes AR, Burke FD**. Functional cast-bracing for Colles' fractures. A comparison between cast-bracing and conventional plaster casts. *J Bone Joint Surg Br*. 1984 Nov; 66(5):749–753.

27. **Schuren J**. *Working with Soft Cast—a Manual on Semi-rigid Immobilisation*. 2nd ed. Borken, Germany: 3M Minnesota Mining & Manufacturing; 1994:9–29.

28. **Challis MJ, Welsh MK, Jull GA, et al**. Effect of cyclic pneumatic soft tissue compression on simulated distal radius fractures. *Clin Orthop Relat Res*. 2005 Apr; (433):183–188.

29. **Schleikis A**. [*Gypsum and Synthetic Cast. Conventional Fixation and Functional Stabilization*]. 2nd ed. Darmstadt: Steinkopff Verlag; 2006. German.

30. **Charnley J**. *The Closed Treatment of Common Fractures*. 4th ed. United Kingdom. Cambridge University Press; 2010.

31. **Kowalski KL, Pitcher JD Jr, Bickley B**. Evaluation of fiberglass versus plaster of Paris for immobilization of fractures of the arm and leg. *Mil Med*. 2002 Aug; 167(8):657–661.

32. **Katz K, Fogelman R, Attias J, et al**. Anxiety reaction in children during removal of their plaster cast with a saw. *J Bone Joint Surg Br*. 2001 Apr; 83(3):388–390.

33. **Carmichael KD, Westmoreland J**. Effectiveness of ear protection in reducing anxiety during cast removal in children. *Am J Orthop (Belle Mead NJ)*. 2005 Jan; 34(1):43–46.

34. **Wiggins CE, Brown KD**. Hearing protection and cast saw noise. *J South Orthop Assoc*. 1996 Spring; 5(1):14.

35. **Gallagher RP, Bajdik CD, Fincham S, et al**. Chemical exposures, medical history, and risk of squamous and basal cell carcinoma of the skin. *Cancer Epidemiol Biomarkers Prev*. 1996 Jun; 5(6):419–424.

36. **Callahan DJ, Carney DJ, Daddario N, et al**. A comparative study of synthetic cast material strength. *Orthopedics*. 1986 May; 9(5):679–681.

37. **Dresing K, Peterson T, Schmit-Neuerburg KP**. Compartment pressure in the carpal tunnel in distal fractures of the radius. A prospective study. *Arch Orthop Trauma Surg*. 1994; 113(5):285–289.

38. **Cohen AP, Shaw DL**. Focused rigidity casting: a prospective randomised study. *J R Coll Surg Edinb*. 2001 Oct; 46(5):265–270.

39. **Bowker P, Powell ES**. A clinical evaluation of plaster-of-Paris and eight synthetic fracture splinting materials. *Injury*. 1992; 23(1):13–20.

40. **Davids JR, Frick SL, Skewes E, et al**. Skin surface pressure beneath an above-the-knee cast: plaster casts compared with fiberglass casts. *J Bone Joint Surg Am*. 1997 Apr; 79(4):565–569.

41. **Böhler L**. [*The Treatment of Fractures*]. Vol 1 and 2. 11th ed. Wien: Wilhelm Maudrich; 1943. German.

42. **Spain D**. Casting acute fractures. Part 1—Commonly asked questions. *Aust Fam Physician*. 2000 Sep; 29(9):853–856.

43. **White R, Schuren J, Konn DR**. Semirigid vs rigid glass fibre casting: a biomechanical assessment. *Clin Biomech (Bristol, Avon)*. 2003 Jan; 18(1):19–27.

44. **White R, Schuren J, Wardlaw D, et al**. Biomechanical assessment of gait in below-knee walking casts. *Prosthet Orthot Int*. 1999 Aug; 23(2):142–151.

6

PRINCIPLES

45. **Kozin SH, Wood MB**. Early soft-tissue complications after fractures of the distal part of the radius. *J Bone Joint Surg Am*. 1993 Jan; 75(1):144–153.

46. **Marson BM, Keenan MA**. Skin surface pressures under short leg casts. *J Orthop Trauma*. 1993; 7(3):275–278.

47. **Philbin TM, Gittins ME**. Hybrid casts: a comparison of different casting materials. *J Am Osteopath Assoc*. 1999 Jun; 99(6):311–312.

48. **Charles MN, Yen D**. Properties of a hybrid plaster-fibreglass cast. *Can J Surg*. 2000 Oct; 43(5):365–367.

49. **Deshpande SV**. An experimental study of pressure-volume dynamics of casting materials. *Injury*. 2005 Sep; 36(9):1067–1074.

50. **Schleikis A**. [Fracture fixation with polyester. Primary care with polyester in selected forms of fractures]. *Pflege Z*. 1994; 47(12):664–665. German.

51. **Handoll HH, Rowe BH, Quinn KM, et al**. Interventions for preventing ankle ligament injuries. *Cochrane Database Syst Rev*. 2001; (3):CD000018.

52. **Avci S, Sayli U**. Comparison of the results of short-term rigid and semi-rigid cast immobilization for the treatment of grade 3 inversion injuries of the ankle. *Injury*. 1998 Oct; 29(8):581–584.

53. **Neugebauer H, Fasching G, Wallenböck E**. [Experiences with using the soft cast in injuries of the fibular ligament of the upper ankle joint]. *Unfallchirurg*. 1995 Sep; 98(9):489–492. German.

54. **Nishikawa T, Kurosaka M, Mizuno K, et al**. Protection and performance effects of ankle bracing. *Int Orthop*. 2000; 24(5):285–288.

55. **Losch A, Meybohm P, Schmalz T, et al**. [Functional results of dynamic gait analysis after 1 year of hobby-athletes with a surgically treated ankle fracture]. *Sportverletz Sportschaden*. 2002 Sep; 16(3):101–107. German.

56. **Singh S, Bhatia M, Housden P**. Cast and padding indices used for clinical decision making in forearm fractures in children. *Acta Orthop*. 2008 Jun; 79(3):386–389.

57. **Bhatia M, Housden PH**. Redisplacement of paediatric forearm fractures: role of plaster moulding and padding. *Injury*. 2006 Mar; 37(3):259–268.

58. **Shuler FD, Grisafi FN**. Cast-saw burns: evaluation of skin, cast, and blade temperatures generated during cast removal. *J Bone Joint Surg Am*. 2008 Dec; 90(12):2626–2630.

59. **Forni C, Loro L, Tremosini M, et al**. Use of polyurethane foam inside plaster casts to prevent the onset of heel sores in the population at risk: a controlled clinical study. *J Clinical Nursing*. 2011 March; 20(5):675–680.

60. **Kruse RW, Fracchia M, Boos M, et al**. Goretex fabric as a cast underliner in children. *J Pediatr Orthop*. 1991 Nov–Dec; 11(6):786–787.

7 Socioeconomic considerations

Klaus Dresing, Jim Harrison

7

PRINCIPLES

91

Authors Klaus Dresing, Jim Harrison

7 Socioeconomic considerations

1 Introduction

Plaster of Paris cast material is available in most medical facilities, worldwide. Synthetic materials may be harder to find, especially in less developed countries. The market for cast materials is not stable. As described in chapter 6 Properties of cast materials, there is a wide range of synthetic cast bandages, with a variety of properties and purposes. They are often described by use of their brand names, without which the exact product may be difficult to identify. Plaster of Paris (POP), similarly, is sold under a variety of brand names. Availability is regional. Preparations are not identical, and users readily distinguish differences and exhibit preferences [1]. While the widths of plaster bandages are more or less standard in either centimeters (eg, 5, 7.5, 10, 15, and 20 cm) or inches (eg, in US & sometimes in Canada: 2, 3, 4, 5, 6, and 8 inches), lengths of POP bandage rolls vary, so that equivalence cannot be presumed. It appears that materials for synthetic casts are at least as variable as those for POP. Brand names change occasionally, and producers and distributors come and go. Producers may work locally as well as for larger markets. Recently, several new producers of cast materials have opened for business in India and China. It seems likely that prices, availability, handling qualities, and other properties will continue to change for the foreseeable future.

2 Availability and distribution

The availability of cast supplies for the professional user depends largely upon the local distribution system. The specific brands of plaster, synthetic cast materials, cast padding, tubular bandages, and other supplies will almost definitely be determined by the distributors in a given region. Most manufacturers use distributors instead of selling and delivering directly to purchasers, who might be individual practitioners, small medical supply merchants, clinics, hospitals, purchasing cooperatives, regional healthcare systems, or governmental units, ranging up to a ministry of health or national government.

The costs of cast materials are not consistent, even in a single country. Prices paid for medical supplies are affected by the local distribution system, including delivery and storage, quantity purchased, and individually negotiated contracts between suppliers and purchasers. In some settings, quality control of supplies during shipping, warehouse storage, delivery, and on-site storage is an important issue. While poorly packaged POP, with potential to become unusable during storage, may have a lower purchase price, it could prove significantly more expensive per treatment. Furthermore, expenses are generated by suppliers' efforts to preserve freshness and quality. Product shelf-life may be a particularly significant issue in tropical environments. Practitioners must work closely with purchasing agents in order to obtain optimal value in relation to purchase price.

3 Prices and costs

While local "list prices" for cast supplies can be obtained from the internet or other sources, the actual cost to the purchaser as well as charges to the patients vary widely, and are sometimes not even closely related or are difficult to obtain. Medical costs and charges generally form a complex relationship. Depending upon the practice setting (hospital, clinic, surgeon's office, etc) and the local arrangements for healthcare delivery and its reimbursement, different costs will be quoted for materials, labor, and facility use. A single charge could be set for a given type of cast, with or without a separate allowance for materials. Taking all these issues into consideration, it is easy to understand how difficult it is to compare the costs of casts from one site of care to another.

Nonetheless, the practitioner must choose the most appropriate cast material for each patient from what is available. In addition to the practitioner's preference (eg, handling characteristics), the cost and comparative effectiveness must also be considered.

3.1 Direct and indirect costs

In assessing costs of materials, it is important to be aware of regional differences, as these might be helpful in negotiations for better prices. It is also important to consider all costs involved, both direct and indirect. Direct costs not only include the supplies that are used but also costs related to human resources, including training, time required for the entire service, and the necessary infrastructure to maintain and stock an adequate facility. Indirect costs include time and other costs for patients and their supporters. For example, if a particular choice of cast needs to be replaced more often during the treatment process, both direct and indirect costs of care will increase. Thus, in the long run, a more expensive cast material requiring fewer changes or revisions may turn out to be less expensive, particularly when the overall costs are considered instead of material costs alone. In 1997, Downing et al found that the cost to the hospital for treating diaphyseal tibia fractures in the UK was lower when using plaster casts than with intramedullary nails, but that the overall cost to the community was essentially the same [2]. However, a sophisticated analysis is needed in order to compute such costs. In a study of treatments for scaphoid fractures, Vinnars et al demonstrated that, when return to work was taken into consideration, the indirect costs were lower in nonmanual workers since they had shorter periods of disability [3].

Few comprehensive analyses of the costs of casts for extremities have been published. Those available are limited in extent and rarely up-to-date. They may not reflect current pricing, available materials, and clinical practice. No publication could be identified that addresses the personnel costs (time, labor, training, etc) of cast application.

3.2 Casting techniques

Several observations have been made regarding the cost of casts. It is clearly necessary to consider the total cost of cast treatment for the typical treatment duration. For example, a 2002 study in the USA reported the material cost for a POP short arm cast (elbow to finger) as $12.90 versus $15.40 for a similar cast made using fiberglass [4]. However, less expensive cast material, typically POP, can be less durable and require replacement more frequently [5, 6]. Therefore, a cast that can be adjusted instead of needing to be replaced might be more cost-effective.

A recent study from Göttingen, Germany, compared two different casting techniques for upper- and lower-extremity indications [7]. The first technique (ie, conventional) involved initial use of a POP cast, routinely followed by a change to a rigid synthetic cast. The second technique (ie, primary definitive) starts out with a semirigid synthetic cast, reinforced with additional rigid splint longuettes. This initial cast was split after being applied and secured with an elastic bandage or velcro tape. Instead of replacing this primary definitive cast, it was simply tightened once swelling resolved, removing some of the material along the split, if necessary. The time required, personnel costs (but not the physician's), and the cost of materials were compared. The second (ie primary definitive) technique was found to be less expensive by up to 30% [7]. Furthermore, primary definitive semirigid casts are more comfortable for patients, require less padding, and are even applicable for some indications involving the hand and fingers [6].

The amount of material used to apply a given cast can vary significantly based not only upon the material chosen but upon the technique of cast application, the size of the patient, and local customs. Typically, more layers of POP are required to obtain a cast of desired strength and durability compared with fiberglass-based synthetic. Use of a composite cast, in which the initial layers of cast material are POP but the outside is a stronger synthetic, result in greater strength and lower overall material cost. Use of splint ribs on convex surfaces, instead of additional circumferential layers of a cast bandage roll, increases strength and durability without adding as much material, thus reducing cost and weight [8].

3.3 International AO survey

Internationally, comparative price information for cast materials is not readily available. Therefore, in September 2011, a survey among AO surgeons from various parts of the world was carried out specifically for this publication. Information on personnel costs was not requested. The survey specifically addressed the cost of materials but not specific brands, types of synthetic cast materials, actual sizes of specified rolls, or the amount of material used per typical cast. Although relevance to the reader's situation will vary, the results are presented in order to provide an example of the variability of the costs of materials.

PRINCIPLES

7

Authors   Klaus Dresing, Jim Harrison

Table 7-1 presents the results of the global survey of AO-Trauma surgeons. The cost analysis is based on the information supplied by 77 AOTrauma members, with prices converted from their original currency to Euros (€). Unfortunately, no information was obtained for North America.

Material	Dimensions	Costs (average) currency (€)
Plaster of Paris roll	10 cm x 3 m	1.05
Plaster of Paris splint	15 cm x 20 m	1.78
Padding	1 roll	0.81
Synthetic casting tape	7.5 cm x 3.6 m	6.93
Synthetic splint	7.5 cm x 30 cm	8.06

Table 7-1   Average costs of casting materials (survey of 77 AO Trauma members).

Additionally, Table 7-2 presents the results of a global survey on casting materials among the same 77 AOTrauma surgeons, according to their geographic region, again with the exception of North America. Prices were again converted from the individual currencies into Euros (€).

While there is variation between the sizes and specifications of the materials, the tables nevertheless indicate that the costs for the same item can vary considerably from region to region.

A spreadsheet has been developed so that the reader can do their own local or regional calculation of the estimated costs of a cast procedure. This is available on the Thieme Media Center website.

Material	Dimensions	Middle East	Latin America	Asia-Pacific	Europe	Africa
Plaster of Paris roll	10 cm x 3 m	0.91 €	2.04 €	1.03 €	0.91 €	0.90 €
Plaster of Paris splint	15 cm x 20 m	1.30 €	2.46 €	1.56 €	1.67 €	1.38 €
Padding	1 roll	0.81 €	0.89 €	0.81 €	0.55 €	1.28 €
Synthetic casting tape	7.5 cm x 3.6 m	4.87 €	27.73 €	7.59 €	7.38 €	4.95 €
Synthetic splint	7.5 cm x 30 cm	4.60 €	14.51 €	7.83 €	8.06 €	12.62 €

Table 7-2   Comparison of material costs by region (survey of 77 AO Trauma members).

7

PRINCIPLES

4   Summary

- Casting materials and services comprise a range of direct and indirect costs that vary greatly around the world
- The cost of materials used is affected by a wide range of factors, such as types of suppliers, material quality and storage, even to the individual technique of the caregiver
- The cost of an individual POP cast is typically lower than that using synthetic cast material, however, the latter is more durable and does not need to be replaced as often
- When the expense of cast room personnel is taken into consideration, the overall costs of synthetic casts is often less because each cast lasts longer and, moreover, it is possible to use a semirigid synthetic cast for the initial immobilization, which can then be adjusted, rather than replaced, for a proper fit after the early swelling has resolved (primary definitive technique).

5   References

1. **Creswell T, Flowers M, Barton L, et al**. Staff opinions on casting material brands: a prospective study. *Injury*. 2008 Dec; 39(12):1467–1473.
2. **Downing ND, Griffin DR, Davis TR**. A comparison of the relative costs of cast treatment and intramedullary nailing for tibial diaphyseal fractures in the UK. *Injury*. 1997 Jun–Jul; 28(5–6):373–375.
3. **Vinnars B, Ekenstam FA, Gerdin B**. Comparison of direct and indirect costs of internal fixation and cast treatment in acute scaphoid fractures: a randomized trial involving 52 patients. *Acta Orthop*. 2007 Oct; 78(5):672–679.
4. **Kowalski KL, Pitcher JD Jr, Bickley B**. Evaluation of fiberglass versus plaster of Paris for immobilization of fractures of the arm and leg. *Mil Med*. 2002 Aug; 167(8):657–661.
5. **Marshall PD, Dibble AK, Walters TH, et al**. When should a synthetic casting material be used in preference to plaster-of-Paris? A cost analysis and guidance for casting departments. *Injury*. 1992; 23(8):542–544.
6. **Schleikis A**. [*Plaster and Synthetic Casts: Conventional Fixation and Functional Stabilization*]. 2nd ed. Darmstadt: Steinkopff Verlag; 2006. German.
7. **Dresing K, Schleikis A, Stürmer KM**. [Primary definitive cast therapy on the upper and lower extremities. Indications and cost analysis]. *Chirurg*. 2009 Mar; 80(3):223–230. German.
8. **Theopold C, Bush JA, Wilson SW, et al**. Optimal plaster conformation derived using a custom-made jig to obtain maximum strength of protective plaster of Paris for hand surgery. *J Trauma*. 2007 Nov; 63(5):1074–1078.

8 Outcomes after nonoperative fracture treatment—what information can be gained from evidence-based medicine?

Beate Hanson, Klaus Dresing

8

PRINCIPLES

PRINCIPLES

8

Authors   Beate Hanson, Klaus Dresing

8   Outcomes after nonoperative fracture treatment—what information can be gained from evidence-based medicine?

1   Introduction

The ability to assess and utilize evidence effectively in decision making is an important skill for physicians. To this end, physicians need clear recommendations on how to identify and apply the best available evidence to specific clinical scenarios. This chapter presents a brief description of what evidence is and why it is needed. The second section will include a discussion on how evidence can be incorporated within nonoperative fracture-related scenarios.

2   What is evidence and why is it needed in fracture care?

The balanced application of the evidence in clinical decision making is the central point of practicing evidence-based orthopedics, and involves, according to evidence-based medical principles, a combination of the surgeon's clinical expertise and judgment, the patient's perceptions and social values, and the best available research evidence.

Evidence-based orthopedics (EBO) involves careful attention to the design, statistical analysis, and critical appraisal of clinical research. The delineation between "outcomes" research and "evidence-based medicine" (EBM) is vague. Since the term evidence-based medicine was coined, orthopedic surgeons and researchers have adopted their own style of critical appraisal, often coined as "evidence-based orthopedics". They use a clear delineation of relevant clinical questions, a thorough search of the literature relating to the questions, a critical appraisal of available evidence and its applicability to the clinical situation, and finally, the balanced application of the conclusions to the clinical problem [1, 2]. Gaining momentum from the global EBM movement, the concepts and ideas attributed to and labeled collectively as EBO have become a part of daily clinical routine. Surgeons hear more and more about evidence-based guidelines, evidence-based care paths, and evidence-based questions and solutions. The controversy has shifted from whether to implement the new concepts to how to do so sensibly and efficiently, while avoiding potential problems associated with a number of misconceptions about what EBO is and what it is not. The EBO-related concepts of hierarchy of evidence, meta-analyses, confidence intervals, and study design have become so widespread that health care providers willing to use and comprehend today's medical literature have no choice but to become familiar with the principles and methodologies of EBO [3].

Given the increasing burden from to the rising number of publications, surgeons must be able to distinguish higher-quality studies from lower-quality studies in order to ensure informed clinical practice. In orthopedic literature, various classes of studies exist, including studies of therapy, prognosis, diagnosis, and economic analysis. These different classes of studies all have their individual hierarchies of evidence. Given that the majority of orthopedic literature consists of therapeutic studies, focus on the levels of evidence for a surgical therapy is typically the norm. Therapeutic studies are those investigating the effect of a treatment or intervention. These studies, which best minimize bias and are more likely to yield an accurate estimate of the truth (randomized controlled trials (RCTs)), are referred to as level-I studies (**Table 8-1**).

Level of evidence	Study design
I	Systematic review of homogenous RCTs RCT with narrow confidence intervals (high quality)
II	Systematic review of homogenous cohort studies Low-quality RCT (> 80% follow-up, lack of blinding, etc) and individual cohort study
III	Systematic review of homogenous case-control studies Individual case-control study
IV	Case series Poor quality cohort study or case-control study
V	Expert opinion

Table 8-1   Oxford levels of evidence [4].

With an understanding of the quality and level of evidence, investigators and physicians can apply it to their clinical practice using the EBM model. Evidence-based medicine was defined in 1996 by Sackett et al as "the conscientious, explicit, and judicious use of current best evidence in making decisions about the care of the individual patient" [5]. This model mainly focuses on using research evidence along with clinical expertise in order to make decisions based on individualized patient cases. At the time of its inception, the concept of EBM presented a profound paradigm shift in that, on its own, clinical experience was no longer sufficient. Clinical experience is gained by years of work as a clinician, education, and acquired skills [6] but now, this new paradigm suggests that experience alone is insufficient for medical decision making. Sackett et al state that "good doctors use both individual clinical expertise and the best available external evidence, and neither alone is enough" [5]. This paradigm shift certainly paved the way for the use of medical literature to effectively guide medical practice [7, 8].

Evidence-based medicine now requires physicians to learn new skills including efficient literature searches and the application of formal rules of evidence in evaluating the clinical literature [7–11]. Yet, even if the evidence is clear, individual situations vary in regard to benefits and risks, thus, the final decision should always be influenced by the values, preferences, and expectations of both clinician and patient as well as the availability and costs of the treatment [6, 10].

For example, consider the treatment of distal radius fractures. Even though they are the most frequently encountered extremity fracture, correct treatment is still controversial and debated within the literature. A search for the best available evidence produces several Cochrane reviews discussing the main therapeutic choices for distal radius fractures. One review covers conservative treatment and includes 37 randomized and quasi-randomized controlled clinical trials with 4,215 patients [12]. The included studies were of poor quality and heterogeneous and, therefore, meta-analytic statistics were not performed. The authors conclude that there is insufficient evidence from randomized controlled trials to determine the most appropriate conservative treatment in adults [12]. The other Cochrane reviews for treatment of distal radius fractures also only showed insufficient evidence [13].

In a continued search, physicians will come across a guideline and evidence report by the American Academy of Orthopaedic Surgeons [14]. Upon taking a closer look, this document only includes a summary of recommendations specifically limited to acute distal radius fractures. All

recommendations were made using "systematic evidence-based processes designed to combat bias, enhance transparency, and promote reproducibility" [14]. The strength of these recommendations is based on the amount and type of evidence supporting that statement. An example: "We suggest operative fixation for fractures with postreduction radius shortening > 3 mm, dorsal tilt > 10°, or intraarticular displacement or step-off > 2 mm as opposed to cast fixation." The strength of recommendation: moderate [14].

If the clinical outcomes and complication rates of operative versus nonoperative fracture care are compared across varying fracture types, according to the established search strategies of EBM, not many studies are available.

3   Incorporating evidence within nonoperative fracture care

Nonoperative fracture care avoids complications that can potentially follow surgery, eg, infection, hardware irritation of nerve structures, or soft-tissue irritation caused by prominent implants [15]. However, redisplacement and malunion are not uncommon after nonoperative fracture care [16] (see **Table 8-2**).

Item	Osteosynthesis	Nonoperative fracture care
Infection	Possible	Rarely
Hardware irritation	Possible	Not possible
Redisplacement	Rarely	Possible
Malunion	Possible	Possible
Stability	Immediate	Late
Return to activities of daily life	Earlier	Later
Return to work	Earlier	Later
Outpatient treatment	Less	More
Resources (OR, etc)	More	Less
In children	Less	More
In adults	More	Less

Table 8-2   Comparison of nonoperative and operative fracture treatment—a selection.

Since all included studies are of high quality, ie, evidence analogous to level-I RCTs, the result indicates that nonoperative fracture treatment carries less risk of complications [14]. The operative fracture treatment shows better clinical outcomes, but demonstrates an increased risk of complications [14, 17]. The difference in clinical outcome shows no statistical significance [17], and there is only a trend with 73.7% excellent and good results for the operative treatment

Authors   Beate Hanson, Klaus Dresing

group compared to 68.1% in the nonoperative group [14]. The pooled relative risk for complications showed a 23% risk reduction for complications in the nonoperative group [14].

Particularly in those parts of the world where resources and medical services are limited, conservative fracture treatment is still the treatment of choice. Well trained surgeons and cast technicians can provide good and comprehensive non-operative fracture treatment in these regions. Competent conservative fracture care always shows better results compared with inadequate operative fracture treatment.

4   Summary

- While there are demands placed on surgeons to be familiar with a wide range of evidence-based research, and to develop their own skills in literature searches, only the highest quality literature ensures informed clinical practice
- Evidence-based medicine (EBM) focuses on using both research evidence and clinical expertise in order to make the best decisions for patients
- Individual situations can vary, so regardless of the evidence, the final decision can be influenced by values, patient and clinician expectations, the experience level of the surgeon, and even costs of treatment
- In parts of the world where resources and services are limited, nonoperative fracture treatment is the most common, and can provide good results.

5   References

1. **Hoppe DJ, Bhandari M**. Evidence-based orthopaedics: a brief history. *Indian J Orthop.* 2008 Apr; 42(2):104–110.

2. **Petrisor B, Bhandari M**. The hierarchy of evidence: levels of evidence and grades of recommendation. *Indian J Orthop.* 2007 Jan; 41(1):11–15.

3. **Helfet DL, Hanson BP**. How to read the orthopedic literature. *Am J Orthop.* 2005 Sep; 34(9):418–419.

4. **Oxford Centre for Evidence-Based Medicine**. Levels of Evidence. 2009 March. Available from: http://www.cebm.net/. [Accessed August 2009].

5. **Sackett DL, Rosenberg WM, Gray JA, et al**. Evidence based medicine: what it is and what it isn't. *BMJ.* 1996 Jan 13; 312(7023):71–72.

6. **Bhandari M, Joensson A (eds)**. *Clinical Research for Surgeons.* New York: Georg Thieme Verlag; 2009: 20–27.

7. **Collins J**. Evidence-based medicine. *J Am Coll Radiol.* 2007 Aug; 4(8):551–554.

8. **Evidence-Based Medicine Working Group**. Evidence-based medicine. A new approach to teaching the practice of medicine. *JAMA.* 1992 Nov 4; 268(17):2420–2425.

9. **Dijkman BG, Kooistra BW, Pemberton J, et al**. Can orthopedic trials change practice? *Acta Orthop.* 2010 Feb; 81(1):122–125.

10. **Croft P, Malmivaara A, van Tulder M**. The pros and cons of evidence-based medicine. *Spine.* 2011 Aug 1; 36(17):E1121–E1125.

11. **Hanson BP, Bhandari M, Audigé L, et al**. The need for education in evidence-based orthopedics: an international survey of AO course participants. *Acta Orthop Scand.* 2004 Jun; 75(3):328–333.

12. **Petrisor BA, Bhandari M**. Principles of teaching evidence-based medicine. *Injury.* 2006 Apr; 37(4):335–339.

13. **Handoll HH, Madhok R**. Conservative interventions for treating distal radius fractures in adults. Cochrane Database Syst Rev. 2003; (2):CD000314.

14. **American Academy of Orthopaedic Surgeons**. The treatment of distal radius fractures. Guideline and evidence report 2009. Available from: www.aaos.org/research/guidelines/drfguideline.pdf. [Accessed 2012].

15. **Hanson BP, Dresing K**. Operative versus nonoperative treatment of fractures: a systematic analysis of the literature. Forthcoming 2014.

16. **Sanders DW, Tieszer C, Corbett B**. Operative versus nonoperative treatment of unstable lateral malleolar fractures: a randomized multicenter trial. *J Orthop Trauma.* 2012 Mar; 26(3):129–134.

17. **Földhazy Z, Ahrengart L**. External fixation versus closed treatment of displaced distal radial fractures in elderly patients: a randomized controlled trial. *Current Orthopaedic Practice.* 2010; 21(3):288–295.

PRINCIPLES

8

GUIDELINES

Guidelines for nonoperative treatment
and perioperative protection

Guidelines

9.1 Fractures, dislocations, and subluxations of the upper extremity

Richard Kdolsky, Clemens Dumont

Authors   Richard Kdolsky, Clemens Dumont

9.1 Fractures, dislocations, and subluxations of the upper extremity

1 Introduction
Richard Kdolsky, Clemens Dumont

In injuries of the upper extremity, nonoperative treatment should always be considered as a possible treatment option. Most metaphyseal and diaphyseal fractures, as well as intraarticular fractures with little to no displacement, and most dislocations can be treated nonoperatively with good or at least acceptable results. Yet, as operative treatment is steadily improving and the needs and wishes of patients are mounting, a lot of new operative options are constantly being established.

Despite this, the knowledge and skills regarding nonoperative treatment are still a prerequisite for every surgeon in order to be able to advise the patient correctly. The fair presentation of an alternative treatment option is crucial in times when medical treatment has to withstand legal review (see topic 6 in chapter 3 Principles of casting). This chapter therefore explores upper extremity injuries and presents effective nonoperative treatment options.

2 Clavicle, scapula, and shoulder
Richard Kdolsky

2.1 Diagnostics
The following sequence is recommended: history, physical examination, imaging, and reevaluation after analyzing the x-rays and other images.

2.1.1 History
History includes review of the injury (eg, direct or indirect trauma; high or low energy), and of any concomitant diseases.

2.1.2 Physical examination
Follow the sequence of inspection, palpation, and range of motion. Focus on:
- Wounds
- Excoriations
- Sore skin before perforation
- Swelling
- Range of motion (ROM) of elbow, wrist, and fingers
- Sensory innervation
- Perfusion.

2.1.3 Imaging
Standardized x-rays should be performed in at least two planes:
- Clavicle: PA and axial, both ends of the clavicle must be seen
- AC joint: AP and AP with loading compared with the noninjured side
- Scapula: AP and tangential
- Shoulder: AP and axial, and if necessary, outlet view (Morrison, Bigliani).

Computed tomography is used for the detailed evaluation of joint fracture dislocations, or for further information in unclear x-rays.

Magnetic resonance imaging is also highly valuable in shoulder joint dislocations and rotator-cuff injuries.

2.1.4 Reevaluation

Includes the findings of history, physical examination, imaging, concomitant injuries, and evaluation of the patient (age/profession/diseases). The treatment options can then be defined and presented to the patient.

2.2 Clavicle

In diaphyseal fractures of the clavicle, no definitive recommendation can be given on whether operative or nonoperative treatment is best [1]. Up to now, the majority of these fractures have been treated nonoperatively. Usually, a relevant shortening of the broken clavicle will be treated by surgical fixation with plates or intramedullary nails in addition to classic indications for surgery, ie, perforation or danger of perforation by displaced bone fragments [2]. In patients with concomitant ipsilateral fractures of the ribs, operative stable fixation of the clavicle is performed to facilitate ventilation. For nonoperative treatment, use a neck or shoulder sling or preferably a Gilchrist bandage (**Fig 9.1-1**) (see chapter 18.3 Gilchrist bandage).

A clavicle bandage (**Fig 9.1-2**) (see chapter 18.2 Clavicle bandage) is another option, however, the surgeon should keep in mind that due to the danger of circulatory disorders and skin injuries, problems can occur [3]. Nondisplaced lateral fractures of the clavicle are treated nonoperatively with a Gilchrist bandage. Displaced fractures of the lateral clavicle are seen as an indication for surgical treatment. However, it must be pointed out that in a long-term study with 15 years of results from 110 lateral clavicle fractures treated strictly nonoperatively, excellent results were shown [4].

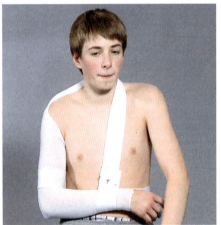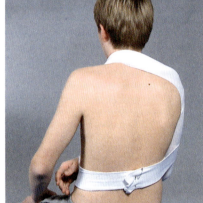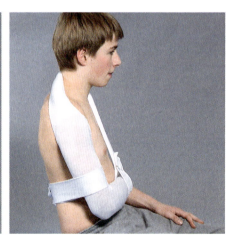

Fig 9.1-1   Example of a Gilchrist bandage.

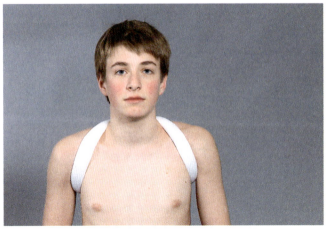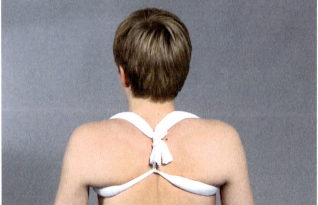

Fig 9.1-2   Clavicle bandage in an adolescent.

Authors   Richard Kdolsky, Clemens Dumont

2.3   Acromioclavicular dislocations

Rockwood grades I-III acromioclavicular dislocations (see chapter 11.1 Ligament and tendon injuries) can be treated nonoperatively using a simple sling or Gilchrist bandage (see chapter 18.3 Gilchrist bandage) until pain ceases. A clavicle bandage can also be very useful (see chapter 18.2 Clavicle bandage). Movement therapy is established and most patients are able to resume their work and sports activities after 2 to 4 weeks. In patients with persisting pain without elevation of the lateral clavicle, an arthroscopic resection of the AC joint can be successful. However, if pain persists and the lateral clavicle stays elevated, a lateral resection of the clavicle could be performed.

In Europe, for example, an operative approach is commonly favored in active patients with Rockwood II and III injuries. Special attention is necessary for manual workers, especially when heavy overhead work is to be performed.

2.4   Scapula

Fractures of the scapular body are treated nonoperatively with a sling or Gilchrist bandage (see chapter 18.3 Gilchrist bandage) until pain ceases. Only displaced fractures of the glenoid still present an indication for operative reconstruction. In floating-shoulder injuries, the indication for operative treatment depends on the extent of medial impaction of the glenoid fossa and the expected loss in range of motion, unless anatomical reconstruction is performed [5].

2.5   Shoulder dislocations

Dislocations of the shoulder are initially reduced and treated by a sling or a Gilchrist bandage (see chapter 18.3 Gilchrist bandage). In younger patients, the extent of the injury is assessed by magnetic resonance imaging (MRI). Especially in young men, operative treatment is recommended in most cases, in accordance with the expected outcome. In elderly patients, nonoperative treatment is performed using a Gilchrist bandage until pain ceases (ie, a maximum of 4 weeks). Physiotherapy is standard after removal of the bandage.

2.6   Rotator-cuff injuries

Most partial ruptures of the rotator-cuff can be treated nonoperatively. The prerequisite is an accurate clinical examination and evaluation of the injury by MRI, which is clear-cut in complete ruptures but less so for partial tears. Intensive physical therapy and regular clinical checkups are required in order to detect failure of the therapy early on and to change to operative treatment if necessary. In complete ruptures of the rotator-cuff, operative treatment is preferred depending on the patient's demands (work, sports, self-reliance in the elderly).

2.7   Indications for nonoperative treatment

An overview of the various fracture types for the clavicle, scapula, and shoulder, as well as their treatment options, is presented in **Table 9.1-1**.

Fracture pattern	Nonoperative treatment	Operative treatment
Scapular body	Slightly displaced	Widely displaced fractures of scapular body
Fractures of the scapular processes	Nondisplaced	Displaced fractures of the coracoid or acromion (take note of an os acromiale)
Fractures of the scapular neck	< 2 cm medial displacement	> 2 cm medial displacement
Fractures of glenoid rim (Bankart's fracture)	No dislocation	Instability and dislocation of the glenoid rim
Fractures of the glenoid fossa	Dislocation < 2 mm	Dislocation > 2 mm
Scapula fractures and ipsilateral clavicle fractures (floating shoulder)	Displacement < 5 mm	Displacement > 5 mm
Clavicle fractures (diaphyseal)	Displacement without skin and soft-tissue irritation	Open clavicle fractures Imminent skin or pleura perforation Injuries of the neurovascular bundle
Acromioclavicular joint injuries	Minor dislocation, type Rockwood grade I–III	Dislocation of acromioclavicular joint types Rockwood grade IV–VI
Lateral clavicle fractures	Nondisplaced	Displaced
Clavicle fractures with ipsilateral rib fractures	Not indicated	Operative stable fixation of the clavicle

Table 9.1-1   Overview of the fracture types and treatment options for the clavicle, scapula, and shoulder.

9.1

The individual steps for physical therapy of the shoulder are demonstrated in **Fig 9.1-3**.

2.8 Postoperative protection of the shoulder

As postoperative protection, a Gilchrist bandage (see chapter 18.3 Gilchrist bandage) can be applied for 4 weeks following repair of shoulder instability. Another advisable option is the use of an abduction brace for 6 weeks following rotator-cuff repair. Nevertheless, physiotherapy should start immediately after surgery.

Fig 9.1-3a–e Physical therapy after a shoulder injury.
a Gilchrist bandage. Used as passive support.
b Passive physical therapy.
c Hanging, passive. Can include a range of pendulum exercises (eg, straight-arm movement across the chest and to the side, or up and back beside the body).
d Hanging with weight. Oscillation, clockwise and anticlockwise.
e Active physical therapy of the shoulder.

3 Humerus

Richard Kdolsky

3.1 Diagnostics

For the humerus, diagnostics follows the sequence of history, physical examination, imaging, and reevaluation after analyzing the images and x-rays.

3.1.1 History

Includes review of the injury (eg, direct or indirect trauma; high or low energy), and concomitant diseases.

3.1.2 Physical examination

Follow the sequence of inspection, palpation, and ROM. Focus on:

- Wounds
- Excoriations
- Sore skin before perforation
- Swelling
- ROM of wrist and fingers (radial nerve)
- Sensory innervation (radial nerve)
- Perfusion.

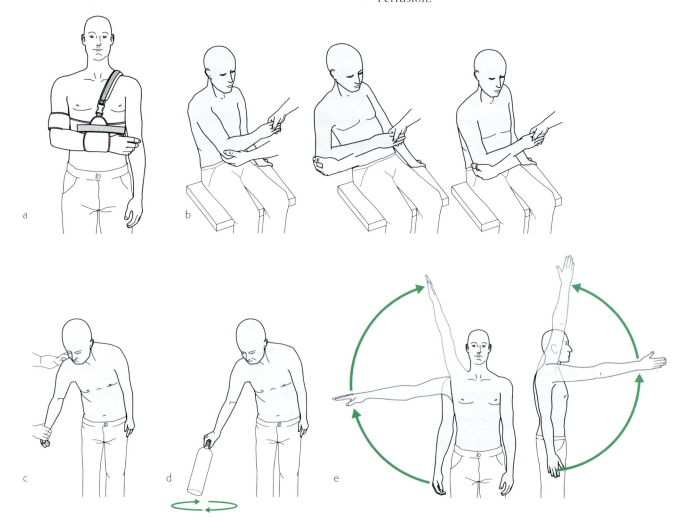

a   b   c   d   e

Authors   Richard Kdolsky, Clemens Dumont

3.1.3 Imaging
Conduct x-rays with the following aspects:
- Shoulder: AP and axial
- Humerus: PA with shoulder and elbow in two planes
- Elbow: volo-dorsal and humerus with elbow laterally.

Computer tomography (CT) can be used for the detailed evaluation of joint fracture dislocations.

3.1.4 Reevaluation
Reevaluation includes the findings of history, physical examination, imaging, concomitant injuries, and evaluation of the patient (age/profession/diseases). The treatment options can then be defined and presented to the patient.

3.2   Proximal humeral fractures
Most proximal humeral fractures will heal without surgery. Mainly proximal humeral fractures that are nondisplaced or only minimally displaced are indicated for nonoperative treatment. The therapeutic principle is to immobilize the upper arm by securing it to the chest until the patient is largely free of pain. Then physical therapy needs to be initiated, at first passive and subsequently active therapy and isometric strengthening exercises.

Fractures of the proximal humerus can be treated nonoperatively with a sling, a sling with swath (**Fig 9.1-4a**), a shoulder immobilizer (**Fig 9.1-4b**), or a Gilchrist bandage for 3 weeks (**Fig 9.1-4c**) (see chapter 18.3 Gilchrist bandage).

The swath is an additional support in order to restrict shoulder motion and is wrapped around the humerus and the chest.

In addition, a collar and cuff bandage (see chapter 18.1 Collar and cuff bandage) can also be indicated even though the weight of the arm is not supported significantly. By interposition of a padding roll at the axilla, bone alignment can be influenced when tightening the bandage. All bandages can be worn outside the patient's clothing.

The bandage is changed weekly and the fracture is checked by x-rays. The duration of application should be limited to 2–3 weeks.

Operative treatment is recommended for younger patients with severe fracture displacement. Although reconstruction in patients over 55 years of age with displaced three-fragment fractures is common, there is no evidence that operative treatment yields better results than nonoperative treatment. On the contrary, it was demonstrated that the complication rate is significantly higher following surgery by comparable functional outcome [6–8] (see the comparative graph at **Fig 9.1-5**).

3.3   Indications for nonoperative treatment— proximal humerus
An overview of the various types of proximal humeral fractures and the options for treatment are presented in **Table 9.1-2**.

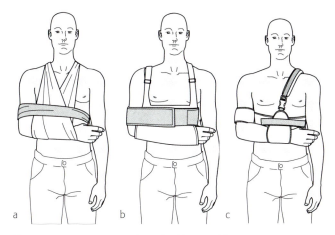

Fig 9.1-4a–c   Treatment of proximal humeral fractures.
a Sling with swath.
b Shoulder immobilizer.
c Gilchrist bandage.
Essentially, these or similar devices provide support for the shoulder joint.

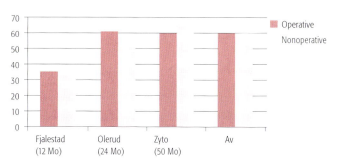

Fig 9.1-5   The graph shows the average Constant score at follow-up (prospective, randomized studies on three-part fractures using open reduction internal fixation vs nonoperative treatment) in patients > 55 years.

AO/OTA classification	Type of fracture	Fracture pattern	Nonoperative treatment	Operative treatment
11-A1		Tuberosity: 11-A1.1	Nondisplaced	Recommended treatment
		Displaced greater tuberosity fragment: 11-A1.2 and 11-A1.3	Not indicated	Recommended treatment
11-A2		Impacted metaphyseal: 11-A2.2 varus impacted	Indicated	High angulation – recommended treatment
11-A3		Nonimpacted metaphyseal: surgical neck fractures	Indicated	Possible
		With displacement	Only when there are severe underlying diseases	Recommended to avoid impingement
11-B1		Without metaphyseal impaction	Only when there are severe underlying diseases	Recommended to avoid impingement
11-B2		With glenohumeral dislocation	Only when there are severe underlying diseases	Recommended treatment
11-B3		With glenohumeral dislocation and displacement	Only when there are severe underlying diseases	Recommended treatment

Authors   Richard Kdolsky, Clemens Dumont

AO/OTA classification	Type of fracture	Fracture pattern	Nonoperative treatment	Operative treatment
11-C1		With slight displacement	Not indicated	Recommended treatment
11-C2		Impacted with marked displacement	Not indicated	Recommended treatment
11-C3		With dislocation	Not indicated	Recommended treatment

Table 9.1-2   Overview of proximal humeral fracture types and their treatment options.

3.4   Diaphyseal humeral fractures

Diaphyseal fractures of the humerus can be treated nonoperatively [9, 10]. The treatment starts with a Desault's bandage (binding the elbow to the patient's side), a Gilchrist bandage, or a Velpeau bandage (**Fig 9.1-6**), or a cast, such as a U-shape splint (**Fig 9.1-7**) for 2 weeks and subsequent change to a Sarmiento brace (see chapter 15.5 Sarmiento humeral brace using synthetic) (**Fig 9.1-8**) for another 4–6 weeks.

Patients are advised to actively move their shoulder and elbow within the brace. Shortening of the fracture and contact of fragments are prerequisites for this treatment. The focus is on the restoration of axis and rotation in contrast to the humerus, which will tolerate rotational misalignment of up to 30° without any functional deficits.

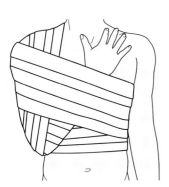

Fig 9.1-6   Velpeau bandage.

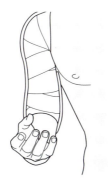

Fig 9.1-7   U-shape splint.

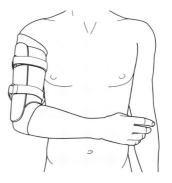

Fig 9.1-8   Sarmiento humeral brace.

3.5 Indications for nonoperative treatment—diaphysis

Long, spiral fractures in the middle of the diaphysis are ideally treated nonoperatively. However, the more transverse and the more proximal or distal the fracture occurs, the higher the rate of nonunion resulting from nonoperative treatment (see **Table 9.1-3**). After application of the cast, nerve function has to be reevaluated in order not to overlook secondary palsy of the radial nerve due to compression between the fragments. In that case, an absolute indication for prompt operative compression of the radial nerve and stabilization is constituted. The first checkup by x-ray is performed after 2 weeks.

In elderly patients, operative treatment is an option in order to prevent pulmonary complications due to restrictions of the thoracic mechanics of the cast.

AO/OTA classification	Type of fracture	Fracture pattern	Nonoperative treatment	Operative treatment
12-A1	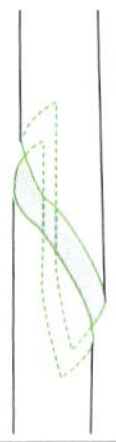	Simple spiral		(Applies for all fracture types) Major displacement of tuberosities (> 5 mm), shaft fragments (> 20 mm), or head angulation (> 45°) Floating shoulder Floating elbow Bilateral fracture of humeral shaft Vascular injury Secondary radial nerve injury Distal humeral fractures Polytrauma patient Open fracture of the humeral shaft Irreducible fracture Severe obesity Patient unable to sit Nerve interposition between fragments
12-A2	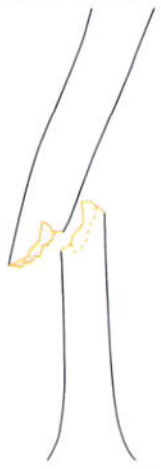	Oblique > 30°	(Applies for all fracture types) Isolated Closed fracture Cooperative patient Alignment nearly anatomical Elderly patients	
12-A3	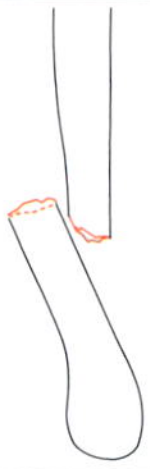	Transverse < 30°		

Authors   Richard Kdolsky, Clemens Dumont

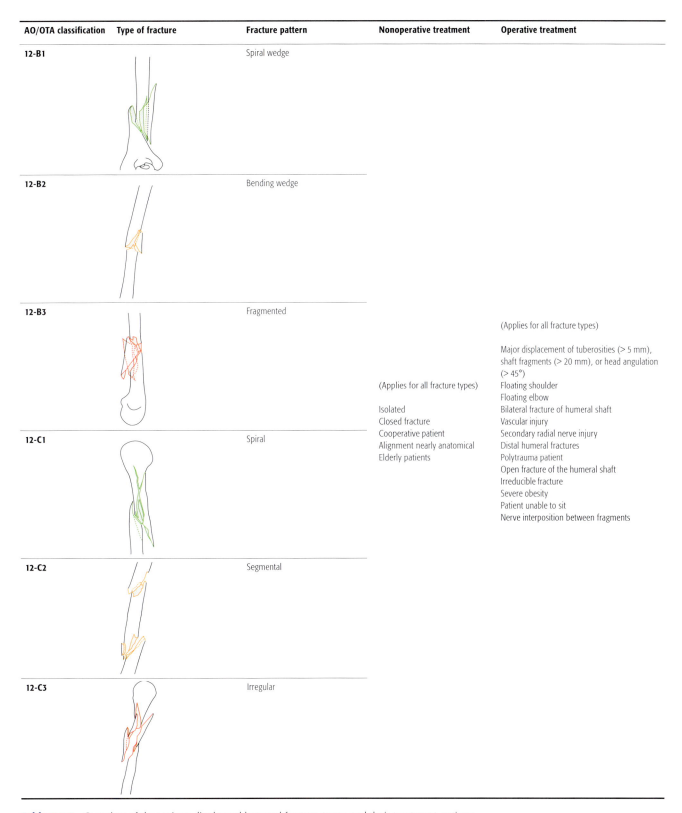

AO/OTA classification	Type of fracture	Fracture pattern	Nonoperative treatment	Operative treatment
12-B1		Spiral wedge		
12-B2		Bending wedge		
12-B3		Fragmented		(Applies for all fracture types) Major displacement of tuberosities (> 5 mm), shaft fragments (> 20 mm), or head angulation (> 45°) Floating shoulder Floating elbow
			(Applies for all fracture types) Isolated Closed fracture Cooperative patient Alignment nearly anatomical Elderly patients	Bilateral fracture of humeral shaft Vascular injury Secondary radial nerve injury Distal humeral fractures
12-C1		Spiral		Polytrauma patient Open fracture of the humeral shaft Irreducible fracture Severe obesity Patient unable to sit Nerve interposition between fragments
12-C2		Segmental		
12-C3		Irregular		

Table 9.1-3   Overview of the various diaphyseal humeral fracture types and their treatment options.

4 Elbow and forearm
Richard Kdolsky

4.1 Diagnostics
Follow the sequence of history, physical examination, imaging, and reevaluation after analyzing the x-rays and images.

4.1.1 History
Includes review of the injury (eg, direct or indirect trauma; high or low energy), and concomitant diseases.

4.1.2 Physical examination
Follow the sequence: inspection, palpation, and ROM. Focus on:
- Wounds
- Excoriations
- Swelling
- ROM of wrist and fingers
- Sensory innervation
- Perfusion.

4.1.3 Imaging
X-rays should be taken as follows:
- Elbow: volo-dorsal and radio-ulnar
- Forearm: with the elbow and the wrist in two planes.

Computed tomography (CT) is used for the detailed evaluation of joint fracture dislocations.

4.1.4 Reevaluation
Includes the findings of history, physical examination, imaging, concomitant injuries, and evaluation of the patient (age/profession/diseases). The treatment options can then be defined and presented to the patient.

4.2 Elbow dislocations
Simple elbow dislocations are treated nonoperatively if closed reduction is successful and no redislocation occurs between 0-30-90° (neutral-0-method). Therefore, a correct lateral x-ray has to be taken after reduction in order not to overlook any subluxation. Then the cast (see chapter 15.1 Long arm splint using plaster of Paris; and 15.2 Long arm splint using synthetic) is applied and again x-ray review is required. If a circular cast is applied, it has to be split completely (see topic 5 in chapter 3 Principles of casting; 15.3 Long arm cast using plaster of Paris; and 15.4 Long arm cast using plaster of Paris).

In addition to the circulatory and neurological check on day 1, another x-ray review is mandatory as the danger of redislocation is highest on the first day. Cast fixation is maintained in pronation and 90° flexion for 2–3 weeks.

Today, complex elbow dislocations are regularly treated operatively. Nevertheless, as was shown [11] in selected cases with the "terrible triad", ie, posterior dislocation of the elbow joint with fracture of both the radial head and coronoid process, or even in divergent dislocations, nonoperative treatment can also be successful.

4.3 Olecranon fractures
Olecranon fractures with minimal displacement (< 5 mm) are treated nonoperatively, especially in elderly patients. The cast is applied in 115° position for 3 weeks (modified in 115° angulation) (see chapters 15.1 Long arm splint using plaster of Paris; and 15.2 Long arm splint using synthetic).

4.4 Radial-head fractures
Radial-head fractures with impaction zone < 30% or displacement < 2 mm do not need operative treatment. However, a CT scan in order to detect the amount of displacement is recommended. A cotton-wool bandage or an elastic bandage (see chapter 18.5 Elbow bandage) is applied for 3–5 days. As an alternative, a dorsal upper-arm splint or cast may be used (see chapters 15.1 Long arm splint using plaster of Paris; 15.2 Long arm splint using synthetic; 15.3 Long arm cast using plaster of Paris; and 15.4 Long arm cast using plaster of Paris).

4.5 Forearm fractures
Fractures of the ulnar shaft with displacement of < 1/3 of diameter can be treated by cast fixation [12]. An above-elbow cast is applied for 2 weeks (see chapters 15.1 Long arm splint using plaster of Paris; 15.2 Long arm splint using synthetic; 15.3 Long arm cast using plaster of Paris; and 15.4 Long arm cast using plaster of Paris), and subsequently exchanged for a forearm brace for another 4–6 weeks (see chapters 15.11 Short arm cast using plaster of Paris; 15.12 Short arm cast using synthetic, combicast technique; modified).

As an alternative, functional treatment with a forearm brace can be chosen, ie, a modification of the method described in chapter 15.20 Short arm cast including two or more fingers using synthetic, combicast technique, however, without including the fingers.

4.6 Indications for nonoperative treatment
An overview of the various types of elbow and forearm fractures and their treatment options is presented in **Table 9.1-4**.

Authors   Richard Kdolsky, Clemens Dumont

AO/OTA classification	Type of fracture	Fracture pattern	Nonoperative treatment	Operative treatment
Elbow dislocation		Dislocation	Stable after reduction	Complex dislocations of elbow
Olecranon **21-A1**		Extraarticular	Displacement < 5 mm	Displacement > 5 mm
Radial-head fracture **21-A2**		Extraarticular	Impaction zone < 30% Displacement < 2 mm	Impaction zone > 30% Displacement > 2 mm
Olecranon + radial head **21-A3**		Fractures of radius and ulna	Nondisplaced	All others
Olecranon **21-B1**		Articular single bone	Stable, nondisplaced or minimally displaced fracture Functional extensor mechanism Very low-demand patient High surgical and anesthetic risk (multimorbidity)	Displaced Open fracture Loss of extensor function
Radial-head fracture **21-B2**		Articular one bone	Fracture < 30% of the radial head Nondisplaced or displacement < 2 mm	Displaced fracture < 70% pronation and supination Open fracture Severe soft-tissue injury
21-B3		Articular one bone and extraarticular at the other bone	Nondisplaced	Recommended

9.1

AO/OTA classification	Type of fracture	Fracture pattern	Nonoperative treatment	Operative treatment
21-C1		Simple	Exceptional High surgical and anesthetic risk (multimorbidity)	Majority
21-C2		Olecranon multifragmentary, radial head, simple	Exceptional High surgical and anesthetic risk (multimorbidity)	Majority
21-C3		Three fragments of each bone	Exceptional High surgical and anesthetic risk (multimorbidity)	Majority
22-A1		Ulna fractured, radius intact, oblique ulna	Nondisplaced fractures, < 25% displacement Low-demand, compliant patients multimorbidity	Open fracture Multiple trauma Chain injury (ipsilateral fracture) Active patient > 25–50% displacement ± 10–15° malalignment
22-A2		Radius fracture, ulna intact, oblique radius	Nondisplaced fractures, < 25% displacement Low-demand, compliant patients Multimorbidity	Open fracture Compartment syndrome Neurovascular injury Relevant soft-tissue injury Multiple trauma Chain injury (ipsilateral fracture) Active patient, > 25 % displacement
22-A3		Simple fracture, both bones	Nondisplaced fractures	Golden standard of all displaced forearm fractures

Authors   Richard Kdolsky, Clemens Dumont

AO/OTA classification	Type of fracture	Fracture pattern	Nonoperative treatment	Operative treatment
22-B1		Ulna fractured, radius intact, oblique ulna	Nondisplaced fractures < 25% displacement Low-demand, compliant patients Multimorbidity	Open fracture Compartment syndrome Neurovascular injury Relevant soft-tissue injury Multiple trauma Chain injury (ipsilateral fracture) Active patient, > 25% displacement
22-B2		Radius fractured, ulna intact	Nondisplaced fractures < 25% displacement Low-demand, compliant patients Multimorbidity	Open fracture Compartment syndrome Neurovascular injury Relevant soft-tissue injury (Gustilo type I, II) Multiple trauma Chain injury (ipsilateral fracture) Active patient > 25% displacement > 20° malalignment, rotation instability
22-B3		One bone with wedge fracture, other simple or wedge	Nondisplaced fractures	Golden standard of all displaced forearm fractures
22-C1		Ulna complex, radius simple	Rare: Nondisplaced fracture	Golden standard of all displaced forearm fractures
22-C2		Radius complex, ulna simple	Rare: Nondisplaced fracture	Golden standard of all displaced forearm fractures
22-C3		Both bones complex	Rare: Nondisplaced fracture	Golden standard of all displaced forearm fractures

Table 9.1-4   Overview of the various types of elbow and forearm fractures and their treatment options.

All Monteggia fractures (proximal ulna fractures with dislocation of the head of the radius), Galeazzi fractures, and Essex-Lopresti lesions are indications for operative treatment. Therefore, in isolated fractures of the ulna, the physician must focus attention on the elbow joint not to overlook a Monteggia lesion. The same is to be mentioned with isolated fractures of the radius and the distal radioulnar joint (Galeazzi).

For the detection of an Essex-Lopresti lesion, the accurate physical examination of the elbow and the wrist is crucial and gives the first track for diagnosis.

5   Wrist   Clemens Dumont

In regards to distal radius fractures, there is more than one way to achieve the objective of functional restoration of the wrist. The required effort and benefit for the patient, ie, the pros and cons, have to be evaluated in accordance with the patient's needs and expectations. Factors such as the patient's age, functional demands, and concomitant diseases have to be taken into consideration in order to find the best treatment option, both in the short and in the long term, in consensus with the patient [13].

5.1   Etiology
Regardless of age, gender, and osteoporosis, the tendency to fall and the manner of falling, especially in elderly people, has an effect on the incidence and fracture type of the distal radius [14].

The annual incidence rate of distal radius fractures is about 195–290 per 100,000 people, with great local variance depending on the area observed and the age of the inhabitants [15–17].

5.2   Diagnostics
Diagnosis is determined by following the sequence of history, physical examination, x-ray, and reevaluation after analyzing the x-ray.

5.2.1   History
History includes review of the cause of the fall, if there was direct or indirect trauma, the degree of force, and concomitant diseases.

5.2.2   Physical examination
Physicians should follow the sequence of inspection, palpation, and range of motion, and look for the following indications:
- Swelling and wounds
- Vascularity and capillary perfusion of the fingers
- Location of sore spot (most patients are able to state precisely where it is located in the hand)
- Sensory innervation, in particular assessment of the median nerve
- Hoffmann-Tinel sign
- Tendon function.

5.2.3   Imaging
The standardized x-ray is performed in two planes and analyzed. Evaluate the x-ray according to the clinical findings and identify the fracture pattern.

If available, CT scanning is a helpful tool in verifying fractures and in assessing bony details, eg, extent of articular involvement. A CT scan is the preferred method for judging fracture patterns, intraarticular involvement, and intraarticular dimension of the fracture.

5.2.4   Reevaluation
Clinical and diagnostic findings should be congruent. If they are not, a second clinical investigation is required. If this alone does not lead to congruity of the findings, further radiological diagnostics are necessary.

5.3   Indications for nonoperative treatment
Classification of fracture types is useful in standardizing the treatment of verified fractures. Even though there is evidence that reproducibility of these classifications is limited [18], and that fracture classification according to the AO/OTA Fracture and Dislocation Classification—long bones, does not correlate to long-term outcomes [19], this classification is still widely used in clinical practice. Criteria describing fracture patterns are helpful for subsequent decision making in regard to fracture prognosis and fracture treatment options.

An overview of the various types of wrist fractures and their treatment options is presented in **Table 9.1-5**.

Authors   Richard Kdolsky, Clemens Dumont

AO/OTA classification	Type of fracture	Fracture pattern	Nonoperative treatment	Operative treatment
Extraarticular				
23-A1		Extraarticular fracture of the ulna	Stable radioulnar joint	Irreducible Comminuted fracture Unstable distal radioulnar joint (DRUJ)
23-A2		Extraarticular fracture of the radius, simple/impacted	Reducible Stable Acceptable/slight secondary displacement	Unstable Secondary displacement
23-A3		Extraarticular fracture of the radius, multifragmentary	Reducible Stable Serious risk of redisplacement	Irreducible Unacceptable shortening or dorsal inclination Secondary displacement
Partial articular				
23-B1		Partial articular fracture of the radius, sagittal	Nondisplaced	Displaced Secondary displacement
23-B2		Partial articular fracture of the radius, dorsal (Barton)	Nondisplaced	Displaced
23-B3		Partial articular fracture of the radius, palmar (reverse Barton)	Nondisplaced No radiocarpal subluxation	Irreducible Unstable Secondary displacement
Partial articular				
23-C1		Complete articular fracture of the radius Articular, simple Metaphyseal, simple	Reducible	Irreducible Unstable Secondary displacement
23-C2		Complete articular fracture of the radius Articular, simple Metaphyseal, multifragmentary	Serious risk of redisplacement	All C2 fractures
23-C3		Complete articular fracture of the radius Articular, multifragmentary Metaphyseal, multifragmentary	Serious risk of redisplacement	All C3 fractures

Table 9.1-5 Overview of the various types of wrist fractures and their treatment options.

Listed below are various other classification systems, which were developed in the past and have become known by each author's proper name (**Table 9.1-6**).

Fracture type	Localization	Treatment
Colles'	Extraarticular fracture with dorsal dislocation	Cast or operatively
Smith	Extraarticular fracture with palmar dislocation	Mostly operatively Cast: Palmar flexion
Barton's, dorsal	Dorsal articular fragment, unstable	Mostly operatively
Barton's, palmar	Palmar articular fragment, unstable	Mostly operatively
Chauffeur	Radial-styloid fracture	Cast or operatively

Table 9.1-6 Fracture type and proper name for fracture classification. Note: While the term "Colles' fracture" in the strict sense is applied to an extraarticular fracture type, it is often also used for dorsally displaced extra- and intraarticular fractures.

Another useful classification for radius fractures was established by Melone [20] (**Table 9.1-7**) and refers to the ulnar aspect of the articular surface in particular, the so-called "medial complex".

However, since there still is a lack of fracture classifications providing 3-D fracture patterns based on CT scans, and that also include the quality of bone stock, the following steps will help physicians in decision making:
- They should note that in dorsal fracture dislocation type fractures, the Colles' type predominates
- They should assume that about 50% of the fractures of the distal radius are intraarticular fractures
- They should consider the age of the patient (bone stock) as an important prognosis factor in regard to the risk of redisplacement
- They should analyze the medial complex in case of doubt with the CT scan.

When evaluating the diagnostic x-rays of radius fractures, two questions arise:
- Is the fracture nondisplaced or displaced? This can be answered by x-ray or CT scans
- Is the fracture stable or unstable? The answer to this question will more likely be provided by experience than by evidence.

5.3.1 Criteria for instability in distal radius fractures
Instability is to be looked for, and the direction of instability – dorsal, radial, ulna, or palmar is to be recognized.

The criteria for instability [21, 22] comprises:
- Radial shortening
- Radial inclination
- Palmar tilt
- Dorsal comminution
- Fracture of the ulnar styloid
- Age of patient.

Physicians should be sure to classify seemingly "stable" fractures that can only be reduced in extreme positions as "unstable", and assume that they have to be operated.

5.4 What is feasible with nonoperative treatment?
Treatment goals include restoration of the radial length, the radial and palmar angulation, and the stepless restoration of the radiocarpal articulation.

Nonoperative treatment of distal radius fractures is still predominant compared with operative treatment [23]. However, the risk of residual stiffness due to immobilization needs to be balanced with operation risks.

During the period of nonoperative treatment and x-ray checkups, it must be verified that nonoperative treatment was the correct decision, or in cases of secondary redisplacement, changeover to operative treatment has to be considered.

5.5 Nonoperative treatment of nondisplaced fractures
Nondisplaced distal radius fractures are treated in a short arm plaster of Paris cast or in a semirigid synthetic cast for 4–5 weeks depending on the extent of the fracture and the quality of the bone stock (see chapters 15.6 Dorsopalmar (radial) short arm splint using plaster of Paris; 15.7 Dorsopalmar (radial) short arm splint using synthetic; 15.8 Palmar short arm splint using plaster of Paris; 15.9 Palmar short arm splint using synthetic; 15.10 Dorsal short arm splint using synthetic; 15.11 Short arm cast using plaster of Paris; and 15.12 Short arm cast using synthetic, combicast technique). At first, in order to avoid complications from swelling, both materials have to be split completely (see topic 5 in chapter 3 Principles of casting; and chapter 6 Properties of cast materials).

Authors   Richard Kdolsky, Clemens Dumont

Melone classification	Fracture type	Description
Type I		Nondisplaced or variable displacement of the medial complex, stable
Type II		"Die-punch", moderate or severe displacement of the medial complex, unstable
Type III		"Spike" fracture, displacement of the medial complex as a unit and an additional spike fragment from the radius shaft, unstable
Type IV		Split fracture, medial complex severely comminuted, wide separation of fragments, unstable
Type V		Explosion injuries

Table 9.1-7   Melone classification of radius fractures [20].

5.6 Nonoperative treatment of displaced fractures

In adult patients, closed reduction should be carried out if the radius fracture is displaced, regardless of being stable or unstable. For example, **Fig 9.1-9** shows that according to the degree of displacement, either nonoperative (blue) or operative (gray) treatment is recommended.

5.7 Closed fracture reduction

In adult patients, closed reduction is usually performed under infiltration anesthesia of the fracture zone (chapter 14.1 Overview of cast, splint, orthosis, and bandage techniques). For children, closed reduction is recommended with general anesthesia. There are several ways to achieve closed reduction depending on fracture displacement, impaction, fracture type, and bone quality. After closed reduction, plaster of Paris (POP) should be used instead of synthetic.

Closed reduction of the fracture can either be performed by manual traction or by a longitudinal traction device with finger traps (**Fig 9.1-10**) (see chapter 15.15 Short arm cast using plaster of Paris with traction and reduction). Longitudinal traction by itself can restore physiological radial length, but manual force is preferred, since this maneuver facilitates palmar translation and ulnar inclination of the midcarpus, if assistance is available [14].

Additional things to consider:
- Avoid performing closed reduction a second time, as the risk of complex regional pain syndrome increases
- If the fracture is displaced a second time, operative treatment is recommended.

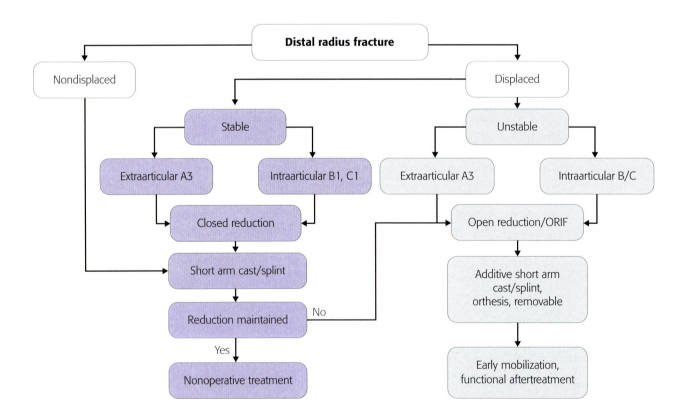

Fig 9.1-9 Treatment algorithm for distal radius fractures.
(Blue = mostly nonoperative, gray = mostly operative) (modified from [13, 24]).

Authors   Richard Kdolsky, Clemens Dumont

5.8   Contraindications for nonoperative treatment

Absolute contraindications for nonoperative treatment include:

- Open fractures
- Fractures with severe soft-tissue trauma with nerve or vascular lesion
- Compartment syndrome
- Perilunate dislocations
- These injuries should be operated immediately if permissible by the patient's condition.

Relative contraindications include:

- Unstable or irreducible fractures
- Fracture-associated ligament injuries (radiocarpal or intercarpal).

5.9   Postoperative protection and aftertreatment

From the author's clinical experience, postoperative cast protection, or preferably, a palmar synthetic splint, is helpful even after angle-stable plate osteosynthesis (see chapter 15.9 Palmar short arm splint using synthetic). A POP splint can also be used (see chapter 15.8 Palmar short arm splint using plaster of Paris).

Things to consider:

- Recommended amount of time for postoperative cast protection with daily mobilization of the fingers out of the splint/cast: 2 weeks for extraarticular distal radius fractures and 4 weeks for intraarticular fractures
- X-ray checkups are recommended after closed reduction, on days 3, 7, 14, 28, and 42
- Independent exercise subsequent to immobilization is recommended. Physical therapy can be added, while occupational therapy has not proved to be superior after surgical therapy [25].

Patients need to be informed about the risk of swelling and increasing pain during the first hours after the injury. A return visit by the patient on the next day is mandatory in order to check soft-tissue reaction and cast position (for more detailed information see topic 11 in chapter 3 Principles of casting).

During the period of immobilization, the patient has to mobilize the uninjured finger joints, the elbow joint, and shoulder joint as far as pain allows and as instructed. Aftertreatment needs to be adapted in accordance with fracture type, quality of bone, and the type of osteosynthesis.

5.10   Risks and complications

Distal radius fractures can be associated with a lesion of the triangular fibrocartilage complex and carpal ligament injuries. During and after reduction, the analysis of the x-ray and CT scan should especially focus on the position of the scaphoid, lunate, and ulna in both planes and the width of the scapholunate distance and integrity of Gilula's lines (**Fig 9.1-11**).

A subluxation of the DRUJ can be difficult to assess on plain x-rays. If a subluxation is suspected, CT scans of both wrist joints in pronation and supination will be helpful.

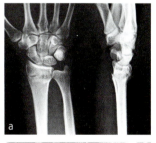
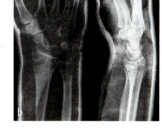
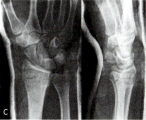

Fig 9.1-11a–c   Example of a distal radius fracture.
a X-ray on the day of the accident.
b X-ray after closed reduction.
c X-ray after 4 weeks.

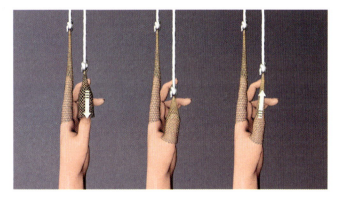

Fig 9.1-10   Finger trap traction.

9.1

6   Hand

Clemens Dumont

The final two topics in this chapter are structured according to fracture localization. Beginning with carpal fractures, the focus of topic 6 is on the scaphoid. Then, topic 7 examines metacarpal and phalangeal fractures.

6.1   Carpal fractures with special regard to scaphoid fractures

Carpal bone fractures are usually the consequence of falling on the hand. The most common carpal bone fracture is the scaphoid fracture, which constitutes up to 60% of carpal bone fractures [26]. Scaphoid fractures typically result from sports or high-speed injuries in younger patients. If overlooked, scaphoid fractures can lead to nonunion or avascular necrosis with degenerative changes in the carpal joints and carpal collapse.

6.2   Diagnostics
6.2.1   Physical examination

Patients with a scaphoid fracture usually present with the feeling of pain and tenderness. Depending on fracture localization, tender areas are the anatomical snuffbox, the proximal dorsal scaphoid, the palmar scaphoid tubercle, or

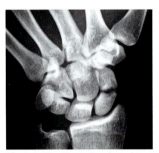

Fig 9.1-12   X-ray: Stecher view.

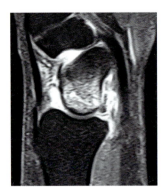

Fig 9.1-14   An MRI of an obvious scaphoid fracture in the proximal third of the sagittal plane.

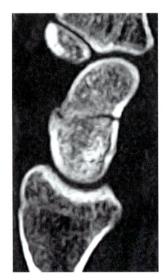

Fig 9.1-13   A CT scan of an obvious scaphoid fracture in the middle third of the sagittal plane.

tenderness during axial compression along the first ray or the thumb. Nevertheless, pain caused by scaphoid fractures can be moderate and one of the reasons why this type of fracture is frequently overlooked.

6.2.2   Imaging

The standardized x-ray images include the following projections: dorsopalmar, lateral, and Stecher view (dorsopalmar plane with clenched fist and ulnarduction) (**Fig 9.1-12**).

In regard to prognosis and adequate fracture treatment, exact fracture classification is necessary. For scaphoid fracture classification, CT diagnostics is necessary and recommended whenever available (**Fig 9.1-13**).

An MRI can also be helpful in detecting a hidden scaphoid fracture (**Fig 9.1-14**). However, the exact fracture morphology is often easier to evaluate in CT scans.

6.3   Indications for nonoperative treatment

Scaphoid fractures are grouped in accordance with the results of the CT scan. In the Herbert or modified Krimmer/Herbert classification, they are described as stable (type A) or unstable (type B) (**Table 9.1-8**) [27, 28].

Fractures of the scaphoid tubercle (type A1) are best immobilized in a splint (see chapters 15.13 Thumb spica splint using plaster of Paris; and 15.14 Thumb spica splint using synthetic) for 4 weeks. Nondisplaced middle and distal third fractures of the scaphoid without displacement can best be treated nonoperatively by immobilization for 6–8 weeks (see chapters 15.13 Thumb spica splint using plaster of Paris; 15.14 Thumb spica splint using synthetic; and 15.16 Short arm scaphoid cast using synthetic, combicast technique).

6.4   Acute scaphoid fractures—what is the evidence?

So far, no general regime exists for acute nondisplaced scaphoid fractures in the middle third (type A2) that would conclusively recommend nonoperative or operative treatment. In a meta-analysis and review of the literature, Buijze et al [29] compared surgical and nonoperative treatment of nondisplaced or minimally displaced acute scaphoid fractures. Buijze showed that results of functional outcome and time off work were favorable in the surgical group (class of evidence I II) whereas the complication rate was higher compared with the nonoperatively treated group [29].

Dias observed no difference in medium-term results in functional or radiological outcome between the operatively treated and the nonoperatively treated group (class of evidence I–II) of patients with acute scaphoid fractures [30].

Authors   Richard Kdolsky, Clemens Dumont

Vinnars et al saw no long-term differences between surgical and nonoperatively treated patients [31].

Initial x-rays of the scaphoid can be without finding. If no CT scan is available and typical clinical signs of a scaphoid fracture persist, a second x-ray in Stecher view after 1 week is recommended. In the meantime, immobilization with a scaphoid splint is indicated (see chapters 15.13 Thumb spica splint using plaster of Paris; and 15.14 Thumb spica splint using synthetic).

Herbert classification	Type of fracture	Fracture pattern	Nonoperative treatment	Operative treatment
Type A Stable fractures				
A1		Fracture of the tubercle	Indicated	Possible
A2		Nondisplaced fracture in the medial or distal third	Indicated	Can be treated operatively in order to reduce the period of immobilization
Type B Unstable fractures				
B1		Long oblique scaphoid fracture	Not indicated	Best treated operatively
B2		Displaced or angulated fracture	Not indicated	Best treated operatively
B3		Fracture of the proximal pole/proximal third	Not indicated	Best treated operatively
B4		Transscaphoidal fracture as part of a complex perilunate dislocation	Not indicated	Best treated operatively

Table 9.1-8   Herbert classification of scaphoid fractures [27, 28].

7 Metacarpals and phalanges
Clemens Dumont

Metacarpal bones are involved in about 42–45% of fractures of the hand [32, 33]. Subcapital fractures account for more than half of the fractures of the metacarpals [33].

7.1 Diagnostics
7.1.1 Physical examination
Patients with metacarpal or phalangeal fractures most often present clinical signs such as swelling, tenderness, and limited function. Physicians should check for malrotation, which becomes obvious in a clenched fist, for axial deviation, and shortening of the fingers. They should also check perfusion and sensation sensitivity in the fingers.

7.1.2 Imaging
General x-rays should be centered on the area of the hand where the fracture is suspected. The two standard planes (AP and lateral view) are necessary for phalangeal fractures and for suspected metacarpal fractures complemented by an additional x-ray in the oblique plane.

Shortening of the metacarpals can be identified by drawing a line along the metacarpal heads III–V. Changes in the carpometacarpal joint space can be proven by an "M-line" that normally will not show in cases of carpometacarpal subluxation or luxation.

7.2 Indications for nonoperative treatment—metacarpal I (thumb)

Table 9.1-9 gives an overview of the fracture patterns of metacarpal I as well as the indications/contraindications for nonoperative treatment.

Type of fracture	Fracture pattern	Nonoperative treatment	Operative treatment
Metacarpal I–Stable fractures			
Winterstein			
	Extraarticular fracture of metacarpal I base	Stable (seldom) No palmar angulation No malrotation	Unstable Comminuted fracture Palmar angulation
Bennett			
	Intraarticular fracture of the metacarpal I base, oblique	Stable (seldom) Serious risk of redisplacement No malrotation	Unstable Dislocation Secondary displacement
Rolando			
	Intraarticular fracture of the metacarpal I base, multifragmentary	Nondisplaced (extremely seldom) No malrotation	Displaced Secondary displacement

Table 9.1-9 Metacarpal fracture localization and recommended treatment.

Authors   Richard Kdolsky, Clemens Dumont

Extraarticular fractures of the first metacarpal (type Winterstein) without displacement can be treated nonoperatively in a forearm/thumb splint or cast for 3–4 weeks (see chapters 15.13 Thumb spica splint using plaster of Paris; 15.14 Thumb spica splint using synthetic; and 15.16 Short arm scaphoid cast using synthetic, combicast technique).

7.3   Contraindications for nonoperative treatment—metacarpal I (thumb)

Intraarticular fractures of the first metacarpal (type Bennett) and especially multifragmentary fractures (type Rolando) are most often displaced. Therefore, an operative treatment regime is recommended for these types of fractures.

7.4   Indications for nonoperative treatment—metacarpals II–V

Most metacarpal fractures are best treated nonoperatively [34]. A nonoperative treatment regime is indicated for nondisplaced and stable fractures without articular involvement. Shaft fractures of the metacarpals III or IV—without displacement and supported by the intact metacarpal ligaments of the neighboring rays—are especially treated nonoperatively. Subcapital fractures with palmar angulation < 20° for metacarpal II and III and < 30° for metacarpal IV and V can be treated nonoperatively.

Table 9.1-10 gives an overview of fracture patterns of metacarpals II–V and indications/contraindications for nonoperative treatment.

It is safe to assume that about 80% of all fractures of the metacarpals II–V can be treated nonoperatively.

Nonoperative treatment examples are found in the following chapters: 15.17 Dorsopalmar (ulnar gutter) short arm splint including two or more fingers using plaster of Paris; 15.18 Dorsopalmar (ulnar gutter) short arm splint including two or more fingers using synthetic; 15.19 Palmar short arm splint including the fingers using plaster of Paris; 15.20 Short arm cast including two or more fingers using synthetic, combicast technique; and secondarily 15.20 Short arm cast including two or more fingers using synthetic, combicast technique.

7.5   Contraindications for nonoperative treatment—metacarpals II–V

Contraindications for nonoperative treatment are rotational deviation of the fractured metacarpal, considerable displacement, and shortening of > 2 mm.

7.6   Indications for nonoperative treatment—phalanges

Phalangeal and metacarpal fractures that are stable or stable after reduction, nondisplaced or nearly nondisplaced fractures, as well as extraarticular fractures without malrotation, can all be treated nonoperatively.

Phalangeal fracture localization and recommended treatment is specified in **Table 9.1-11**.

With phalangeal fractures, splint or cast immobilization for 3 weeks is sufficient in most cases (see chapters 15.17 Dorsopalmar (ulnar gutter) short arm splint including two or more fingers using plaster of Paris; 15.18 Dorsopalmar (ulnar gutter) short arm splint including two or more fingers using synthetic; 15.19 Palmar short arm splint including the fingers using plaster of Paris; 15.20 Short arm cast including two or more fingers using synthetic, combicast technique; and 15.20 Short arm cast including two or more fingers using synthetic, combicast technique).

7.7   What is feasible with nonoperative treatment

Treatment goals include restoration of metacarpal and phalangeal length, the angulation and restoration of the articular surface without a step, and restoration of finger and hand function.

7.8   Contraindications for nonoperative treatment—phalanges

Unstable fractures, displaced fractures, intraarticular fractures, and multifragmentary fractures are best treated operatively.

7.9   Postoperative protection and aftertreatment

Operatively treated metacarpal fractures, depending on the method of retention, require postoperative protection (see chapter 15.23 Metacarpal glove using synthetic, combicast technique).

Postoperative cast protection with daily mobilization of the fingers out of the splint/cast is recommended for a period of 2–3 weeks (see chapters 15.17 Dorsopalmar (ulnar gutter) short arm splint including two or more fingers using plaster of Paris; 15.18 Dorsopalmar (ulnar gutter) short arm splint including two or more fingers using synthetic; 15.19 Palmar short arm splint including the fingers using plaster of Paris; 15.20 Short arm cast including two or more fingers using synthetic, combicast technique; and 15.23 Metacarpal glove using synthetic, combicast technique). Early functional therapy should be started as soon as fracture morphology allows.

9.1

GUIDELINES

Type of fracture	Fracture pattern	Nonoperative treatment	Operative treatment
Metacarpal			
Head			
	Extraarticular fracture of metacarpal head	Stable Dislocation < 30° No malrotation	Unstable Comminuted fracture Dislocation > 30°
	Intraarticular fracture of the metacarpal head	Stable Acceptable/slight secondary displacement	Unstable Secondary displacement
Shaft			
	Extraarticular fracture of the metacarpal diaphysis, oblique	Reducible Stable Serious risk of redisplacement	Irreducible Unacceptable shortening or palmar inclination Secondary displacement
	Extraarticular fracture of the metacarpal diaphysis, multifragmentary	Reducible Stable Serious risk of redisplacement	Irreducible Unacceptable shortening or dorsal inclination Secondary displacement
Base			
	Intraarticular fracture of the metacarpal base	Nondisplaced	Displaced Secondary displacement

Table 9.1-10 Metacarpal fracture localization and recommended treatment.

Authors   Richard Kdolsky, Clemens Dumont

Type of fracture	Fracture pattern	Nonoperative treatment	Operative treatment
Phalanx			
Head			
	Articular fracture of the phalanx, oblique, unicondylar	Stable	Irreducible Comminuted fracture Unstable DRUJ
	Articular fracture of the phalanx, bicondylar	Reducible Stable Acceptable/slight secondary displacement	Unstable Secondary displacement
Shaft			
	Extraarticular fracture of the phalanx, transvers	Reducible Stable Serious risk of redisplacement	Irreducible Unacceptable shortening or palmar inclination Secondary displacement
	Extraarticular fracture of the phalanx, multifragmentary	Reducible Stable Serious risk of redisplacement	Irreducible Unacceptable shortening or dorsal inclination Secondary displacement
Base			
	Articular fracture of the phalanx, oblique, unicondylar	Nondisplaced	Displaced Secondary displacement
Base of the distal phalanx			
	Articular fracture of the distal phalanx	Reducible Stable Fragment < 30% of the articular surface	Subluxation Unstable Gross dislocation

Table 9.1-11   Phalangeal fracture localization and recommended treatment.

131

7.10 Risks and complications

Prolonged immobilization can lead to functional impairment. The proximal interphalangeal joint is especially at risk. Immobilization of uninjured fingers can also lead to functional deficits. Malrotation of metacarpal fractures is a frequent risk and clinical investigation demands paying special attention. Furthermore, in metacarpal and phalangeal fractures, the general risks with bone healing, eg, nonunion exist.

8 Summary
Richard Kdolsky, Clemens Dumont

- Fractures and dislocations in the upper extremity can be successfully treated nonoperatively, particularly if there is little to no fracture fragment displacement
- Fractures of the clavicle and scapula, and acromioclavicular and shoulder dislocations, are initially treated with a sling or Gilchrist bandage, but fractures of the glenoid fossa, or any danger of perforation by displaced bone fragments, are typically indications for operative treatment
- Most proximal humeral fractures, particularly if minimally or nondisplaced, will heal without surgery, and are immobilized by securing the upper arm to the chest until the patient is largely free of pain
- Diaphyseal fractures of the humerus can be treated nonoperatively with a Desault's, Velpeau, or Gilchrist bandage or cast for 2 weeks and subsequent change to a Sarmiento brace
- Simple elbow dislocations can be treated nonoperatively although complex elbow dislocations are regularly treated operatively
- Radial head fractures and forearm fractures with only slight displacement can both be treated with cast fixation
- Proximal ulna fractures with dislocation of the head of the radius, or isolated fractures of the radius with dislocation at the distal radioulnar joint are both indications for operative treatment
- In the wrist, nonoperative treatment of distal radius fractures is more common, yet physicians must consider any risk of residual stiffness due to immobilization, and ensure the stability of the fractures/joints
- In the hand, scaphoid fractures can lead to nonunion, avascular necrosis, and even carpal collapse, so fractures of the scaphoid bones should typically be treated nonoperatively only if they are classified as stable
- Phalangeal and metacarpal fractures that are stable or nondisplaced, as well as extraarticular fractures without malrotation, can all be treated nonoperatively.

Authors   Richard Kdolsky, Clemens Dumont

9   References

1. **Cheung A, Van Rensburg L, Tytherleigh-Strong GM**. Surgical versus conservative interventions for treating fractures of the middle third of the clavicle. *Cochrane Database Syst Rev.* 2008; (3).

2. **Canadian Orthopaedic Trauma Society**. Nonoperative treatment compared with plate fixation of displaced midshaft clavicular fractures. A multicenter, randomized clinical trial. *J Bone Joint Surg Am.* 2007 Jan; 89(1):1–10.

3. **Andersen K, Jensen PO, Lauritzen J**. Treatment of clavicular fractures. Figure-of-eight bandage versus a simple sling. *Acta Orthop Scand.* 1987 Feb; 58(1):71–74.

4. **Nordqvist A, Petersson C, Redlund-Johnell I**. The natural course of lateral clavicle fracture. 15 (11-21) year follow-up of 110 cases. *Acta Orthop Scand.* 1993 Feb; 64(1):87–91.

5. **Kdolsky R, Kollmitzer J, Berlakovits R, et al**. Biomechanics of operative treatment in floating shoulder injuries. *Osteo Int.* 2000; (8):216–219.

6. **Fjalestad T, Hole MØ, Hovden IA, et al**. Surgical treatment with an angular stable plate for complex displaced proximal humeral fractures in elderly patients: a randomized controlled trial. *J Orthop Trauma.* 2012 Feb; 26(2):98–106.

7. **Olerud P, Ahrengart L, Ponzer S, et al**. Internal fixation versus nonoperative treatment of displaced 3-part proximal humeral fractures in elderly patients: a randomized controlled trial. *J Shoulder Elbow Surg.* 2011 Jul; 20(5):747–755.

8. **Zyto K, Ahrengart L, Sperber A, et al**. (1997) Treatment of displaced proximal humeral fractures in elderly patients. *J Bone Joint Surg Br.* 1997 May; 79(3):412–417.

9. **Sarmiento A, Latta LL**. Funktionelle Behandlung bei Humerusschaftfrakturen [Humeral diaphyseal fractures: functional bracing]. *Unfallchirurg.* 2007 Oct; 110(10):824–832. German.

10. **Gosler MW, Testroote M, Morrenhof JW, et al**. Surgical versus non-surgical interventions for treating humeral shaft fractures in adults. Cochrane Database Syst Rev. 2012 Jan 18; 1:CD008832. doi: 10.1002/14651858.CD008832. pub2.

11. **Guitton TG, Ring D**. Nonsurgically treated terrible triad injuries of the elbow: report of four cases. *J Hand Surg Am.* 2010 Mar; 35(3):464–467.

12. **Kwasny O**. [Lower arm shaft fractures in adults: Anatomical-biomechanics of lower-arm torsion. Fundamentals for therapy selection and clinical results]. 1st ed. Wien: Facultas wuv Universitätsverlag; 1990. German.

13. **Wolfe SW**. Distal radius fractures. Wolfe SW, Hotchkiss RN, Pederson WC, et al (eds). *Green's Operative Hand Surgery— Vol 1.* 6th ed. Philadelphia, PA: Churchill Livingstone Elsevier; 2011: 561–638.

14. **Fernandez DL, Jupiter JB**. Epidemiology, Mechanism, Classification. Fernandez DL, Jupiter JB (eds). *Fractures of the Distal Radius: A Practical Approach to Management.* 2nd ed. New York: Springer-Verlag; 2002:24–52.

15. **Melton LJ 3rd, Amadio PC, Crowson CS, et al**. Long-term trends in the incidence of distal forearm fractures. *Osteoporos Int.* 1998; 8(4):341–348.

16. **Court-Brown CM, Caesar B**. Epidemiology of adult fractures: A review. *Injury.* 2006 Jun; 37(8):691–697.

17. **Thompson PW, Taylor J, Dawson A**. The annual incidence and seasonal variation of fractures of the distal radius in men and women over 25 years in Dorset, UK. *Injury.* 2004 May; 35(5):462–466.

18. **Kural C, Sungur I, Kaya I, et al**. Evaluation of the reliability of classification systems used for distal radius fractures. *Orthopedics.* 2010 Nov 2; 33(11):801.

19. **Földhazy Z, Törnkvist H, Elmstedt E, et al**. Long-term outcome of nonsurgically treated distal radius fractures. *J Hand Surg Am.* 2007 Nov; 32(9):1374–1384.

20. **Melone CP Jr**. Articular fractures of the distal radius. *Orthop Clin North Am.* 1984; 15(2):217–236.

21. **Leone J, Bhandari M, Adili A, et al**. Predictors of early and late instability following conservative treatment of extra-articular distal radius fractures. *Arch Orthop Trauma Surg.* 2004 Jan; 124(1):38–41.

22. **Nesbitt KS, Failla JM, Les C**. Assessment of instability factors in adult distal radius fractures. *J Hand Surg Am.* 2004 Nov; 29(6):1128–1138.

23. **Court-Brown CM, Aitken S, Hamilton TW, et al**. Nonoperative fracture treatment in the modern era. *J Trauma.* 2010 Sep; 69(3):699–707.

24. **Dresing K, Stürmer KM**. Leitlinien der Deutschen Gesellschaft für Unfallchirurgie: Distale Radiusfraktur. [Guidelines of the German Society for Trauma Surgery: Distal radius fractures]. Available from: www.awmf.org/uploads/tx_szleitlinien/012-0151_S2_Distale_Radiusfraktur_2008.pdf. [Accessed October 2011]. German.

25. **Souer JS, Buijze G, Ring D**. A prospective randomized controlled trial comparing occupational therapy with independent exercises after volar plate fixation of a fracture of the distal part of the radius. *J Bone Joint Surg Am.* 2011 Oct 5; 93(19):1761–1766.

26. **Haisman JM, Rohde RS, Weiland AJ, et al**. Acute fractures of the scaphoid. *J Bone Joint Surg Am.* 2006 Dec; 88(12):2750–2758.

27. **Herbert TJ, Fisher WE**. Management of the fractured scaphoid using a new bone screw. *J Bone Joint Surg Br.* 1984 Jan; 66(1):114–123.

28. **Moser VL, Krimmer H, Herbert TJ**. Minimal invasive treatment for scaphoid fractures using the cannulated Herbert screw system. *Tech Hand Up Extrem Surg.* 2003 Dec; 7(4):141–146.

29. **Buijze GA, Doornberg JN, Ham JS, et al**. Surgical compared with conservative treatment for acute nondisplaced or minimally displaced scaphoid fractures: a systematic review and meta-analysis of randomized controlled trials. *J Bone Joint Surg Am.* 2010 Jun; 92(6):1534–1544.

30. **Dias JJ, Dhukaram V, Abhinav A, et al**. Clinical and radiological outcome of cast immobilisation versus surgical treatment of acute scaphoid fractures at a mean follow-up of 93 months. *J Bone Joint Surg Br.* 2008 Jul; 90(7):899–905.

31. **Vinnars B, Pietreanu M, Bodestedt A, et al**. Nonoperative compared with operative treatment of acute scaphoid fractures. A randomized clinical trial. *J Bone Joint Surg Am.* 2008 Jun; 90(6):1176–1185.

32. **Feehan LM, Sheps SS**. Treating hand fractures: population-based study of acute health care use in British Columbia. *Can Fam Physician;* 2008 Jul; 54(7):1001–1007.

33. **Stanton JS, Dias JJ, Burke FD**. Fractures of the tubular bones of the hand. *J Hand Surg Eur Vol.* 2007 Dec; 32(6):626–636.

34. **Poolman RW, Goslings JC, Lee JB, et al**. Conservative treatment for closed fifth (small finger) metacarpal neck fractures. *Cochrane Database Syst Rev.* 2005 Jul 20; (3):CD003210.

10   Further reading

Richard Kdolsky, Clemens Dumont

AO Surgery Reference. Casting. *Colton CL, Schatzker J, Trafton P* (eds). AO Foundation. Available at http://www.aosurgery.org. [Accessed July 2011].

Atkin DM, Bohay DR, Slabaugh P, et al. Treatment of ulnar shaft fractures: A prospective, randomized study. *Orthopedics.* 1995 Jun; 18(6):543–547.

Bishop JA, Crall TS, Kocher MS. Operative versus nonoperative treatment after primary traumatic anterior glenohumeral dislocation: expected-value decision analysis. *J Shoulder Elbow Surg.* 2011 Oct; 20(7):1087–1094.

Dimitroulias A, Molinero KG, Krenk DE, et al. Outcomes of nonoperatively treated displaced scapular body fractures. *Clin Orthop Relat Res.* 2011 May; 469(5):1459–1465.

Gerard F, Garbuio P, Tropet Y, et al. [Functional treatment of isolated fractures of the ulnar shaft in adults. A prospective study apropos of ten cases and review of the literature]. *Ann Chir Main Memb Super.* 1997; 16(3):252–257. French.

Giannoudis PV, Tzioupis C, Papathanassopoulos A. Articular step-off and risk of post-traumatic osteoarthritis. Evidence today. *Injury.* 2010 Oct; 41(10):986–995.

Hovelius L, Olofsson A, Sandström B, et al. Nonoperative treatment of primary anterior shoulder dislocation in patients forty years of age and younger: a prospective twenty-five year follow-up. *J Bone Joint Surg Am.* 2008 May; 90(5):945–952.

Jahna H, Wittich H. *Konservative Methoden in der Frakturbehandlung.* [*Conservative methods in bone fracture treatment*]. 1st ed. Wien, München, Baltimore: Urban & Schwarzenberg;1985. German.

Ismail AA, Pye SR, Cockerill WC, et al. Incidence of limb fracture across Europe: results from the European Prospective Osteoporosis Study (EPOS). *Osteoporos Int.* 2002 Jul; 13(7):565–571.

Lichtman DM, Bindra RR, Boyer MI, et al. American Academy of Orthopaedic Surgeons clinical practice guideline on: the treatment of distal radius fractures. *J Bone Joint Surg Am.* 2011 Apr; 93(8):775–778.

Loeffler BJ, Brown SL, D'Alessandro DF, et al. Incidence of False Positive Rotator Cuff Pathology in MRIs of Patients with Adhesive Capsulitis. *Orthopedics.* 2011 May; 34(5):362.

Mnif H, Koubaa M, Zrig M, et al. Transverse divergent dislocation of the elbow in adults: A 9-year follow-up. *Eur J Orthop Surg Traumatol.* 2009; 19(7):495–498.

Pieske O, Dang M, Zaspel J, et al. Die Klavikulaschaftfraktur – Klassifikation und Therapie. [Midshaft clavicle fractures—Classification and therapy. Results of a survey at German trauma departments]. *Unfallchirurg.* 2008 Jun; 111(6):387–394. German.

Prasas G, Rafee A, Chougle A. Divergent dislocation of the elbow treated with a cast brace: case report. *Eur J Orthop Surg Traumatol.* 2006; 16:360–361.

Sárváry A, Baranyi G, Tóth A, et al. Die konservative Behandlung der Oberarmfraktur. [Conservative treatment of fractures of the humeral shaft]. *Akt Traumatol.* 2000; 30:191–194. German.

Schleikis A. [*Plaster cast and synthetic orthosis: Conventional fixation and functional stabilization*]. 2nd ed. Darmstadt: Steinkopff Verlag; 2007. German.

Van Dyck P, Gielen JL, Veryser J, et al. Tears of the supraspinatus tendon: assessment with indirect magnetic resonance arthrography in 67 patients with arthroscopic correlation. *Acta Radiol.* 2009 Nov; 50(9):1057–1063.

Wallny T, Sagebiel C, Westermann K, et al. Comparative results of bracing and interlocking nailing in the treatment of humeral shaft fractures. *Int Orthop.* 1997; 21(6):374–379.

Windolf J, Rueger JM, Werber KD, et al. [Treatment of metacarpal fractures. Recommendations of the Hand Surgery Group of the German Trauma Society]. *Unfallchirurg.* 2009 Jun; 112(6):577–588. German.

9.2 Fractures, dislocations, and subluxations of the lower extremity

Rami Mosheiff, Juan Manuel Concha

9.2

GUIDELINES

Authors   Rami Mosheiff, Juan Manuel Concha

9.2 Fractures, dislocations, and subluxations of the lower extremity

1   Introduction   Rami Mosheiff, Juan Manuel Concha

Most unstable or intraarticular fractures with movement constitute an indication for surgical treatment. This kind of treatment allows for anatomical reduction, stable fixation, and early mobilization. But despite the progress in medicine and technology, there are still patients or medical situations that necessitate nonoperative treatment. This kind of treatment is complex, especially in fractures of the lower extremity, for it deprives the patient of mobility for a long period of time, and the necessary compromises can cause permanent disability in the future.

In the foot, for example, injuries are common. Some of them are very obvious but others are difficult to diagnose and must have a high index of clinical suspicion as they can go unnoticed. Some foot injuries can be treated orthopedically, yet others must be immobilized while the condition of the soft tissue improves and the fixation is performed.

Yet, regardless of fracture location and severity, familiarity with nonoperative treatment is essential, and taking particular care of proper reduction, fixation, and mobility, according to the patient's condition, is critical for the successful treatment of fractures of the lower extremities.

2   Diagnostics   Rami Mosheiff, Juan Manuel Concha

The precise identification of the skeletal injury and diagnosis of the fracture type are performed in the same manner as with a common surgical treatment of fractures of the lower extremities. Images are used, from the outset, as the basis for the identification of the injury (it should be noted that the images should include the entire affected bone as well as its adjacent joints, both proximally and distally). If there is a doubt as to the presence of an intraarticular injury, or if there is a need of a more precise understanding of the injury, more sophisticated methods are used, such as CT.

In the foot, the deformity and pain indicate the injured area and accordingly, diagnostic aid should be requested. X-rays are the mainstay of the images, however, taking into account the overlapping bone and foot tri-dimensional settings, CT and three-dimensional images can be helpful to better understand the various injuries. Exceptionally, MRI is required in the acute stage.

3   Proximal femur   Rami Mosheiff

Fractures of the hip still present a major cause of morbidity and mortality all over the world. A significant number of patients that have sustained hip fractures will die within one year. From the socioeconomic point of view, the economic cost to families, patients, and society is substantial.

Most fractures pertaining to the femoral neck and intertrochanteric region occur in elderly patients due to osteoporotic bone and/or muscular incoordination leading to a fall. If a young patient suffers such a fracture, it is often the result of significant trauma and is associated with further fractures and injuries.

3.1 Indications for nonoperative treatment

It is now universally agreed that intertrochanteric or pertrochanteric fractures of the femur are best treated by operative internal fixation, whenever this is feasible. Whenever the risks of surgery and anesthesia are too great, it may not be advisable to operate the patient. The "predictors of mortality" as classified by the American Society of Anesthesiologists (ASA) indicate the level of risk [1]. In the case of an intracapsular fracture, which requires hemiarthroplasty, there is an additional risk of dislocation, and the full cooperation of the patient is vital. If the patient is senile and suffers from dementia, and is therefore not able to cooperate, nonoperative treatment would be indicated.

3.2 Nonoperative treatment

If such fractures occur in elderly patients, their general medical condition should be assessed, especially since these patients are often suffering from dehydration. The surgeon must also look out for other medical conditions, ie, a stroke and/or other hypertensive episodes as well as cardiac conditions. The nursing requirements should also be evaluated because many of these patients are in an advanced state of senility, sometimes complicated by dementia and incontinence, and the nonoperative treatment of these fractures presents formidable nursing difficulties. Nonoperative treatment of hip fractures should always be considered an option, and it is therefore necessary to decide which technical prerequisites are of importance, both in regard to the comfort of the patient and the convenience of the nursing staff.

Balanced traction (a suspension system that supports traction in the treatment of lower-extremity fractures) is often the best form of nonoperative treatment because treatment by a plaster hip spica is not appropriate in old and senile patients. **Table 9.2-1** provides an overview of the various types of proximal femur fractures and the available treatment options.

3.2.1 Traction (skeletal versus adhesive)

In order to guarantee good results in a manner most comfortable to the patient and most convenient for the nursing staff, skeletal traction (where a pin or wire is surgically inserted into bone) is applied to the tibial tubercle. This is recommended over skin adhesive traction (using adhesive straps on the skin).

AO/OTA classification	Type of fracture	Fracture pattern	Nonoperative treatment	Operative treatment
31-A				
31-A1		Simple pertrochanteric	Rarely Bed-ridden ± debilitated patients Severe soft-tissue problems in surgical area	Standard treatment
31-A2		Pertrochanteric multifragmentary	Rarely Bed-ridden ± debilitated patients Severe soft-tissue problems in surgical area	Standard treatment
31-A3		Intertrochanteric	Rarely Bed-ridden ± debilitated patients Severe soft-tissue problems in surgical area	Standard treatment

Authors Rami Mosheiff, Juan Manuel Concha

AO/OTA classification	Type of fracture	Fracture pattern	Nonoperative treatment	Operative treatment
31-B				
31-B1		Subcapital with slight displacement	Nonambulatory patients	Recommended treatment
31-B2		Transcervical	Severe soft-tissue problems in surgical area Patients willing and able to risk fracture displacement Extremely high-risk patients Risk of secondary displacement up to 50%	Recommended treatment
31-B3		Subcapital, displaced, nonimpacted	Severe soft-tissue problems in surgical area Patients willing and able to risk fracture displacement Extremely high-risk patients Risk of secondary displacement up to 50%	Recommended treatment
31-C				
31-C1		Split (Pipkin)	Only after complete reduction	Recommended treatment
31-C2		With depression	Minor depression fractures Significant comorbidity	Recommended treatment for (large) depressed fractures
31-C3		With neck fracture	Used rarely	Recommended treatment

Table 9.2-1 Overview of the various types of proximal femur fractures and the available treatment options.

Adhesive traction should never be combined with weight traction. A combination of weight traction with skin adhesive traction will almost inevitably result in the "creeping" of the adhesive strapping. As a result, pressure sores may appear, with excoriation of the skin and concomitant pain. External popliteal paralysis is also a frequent result of adhesive traction because, as the adhesive bandages slide down the leg over time, the surrounding circular turns of cotton bandage may constrict the limb as they pass from the small circumference of the knee to the larger circumference at the head of the fibula. Especially in elderly patients, the decision on which method to use should be in favor of skeletal traction despite the fact that many physicians are wary of this technique, it being an invasive procedure.

A Steinmann pin can easily be inserted under local anesthesia, relieving the patient's discomfort. It is recommended to apply a below-knee plaster cast, over adequate padding, and to incorporate the Steinmann pin in the upper end of the plaster. Having completed the traction unit, it can be suspended from a Balkan beam and a 3 kg traction weight, arranged to give a horizontal pull by means of cords and pulleys (**Fig 9.2-1**).

The Hamilton Russell traction for treating hip fractures can do without the complicated system of pulleys, which are needed for the treatment of shaft fractures. However, suspension of the lower extremity and application of traction along the axis of the femur are required. Hip cases do not call for both forces to be correlated because there is no need for an upward lift which, in shaft fractures, is needed in order to correct the backward angulation.

4 Diaphyseal and distal femur   Rami Mosheiff

The incidence of distal femoral fractures has been found to be ten times less frequent than of proximal femoral fractures [2]. During the period of 1980–1989, approximately 34,000 femoral fractures were reported in Europe for example, and only 6% (2,165) of these involved the distal femur. Distal femoral fractures can result from either high-energy or low-energy trauma. High-energy trauma, from motor vehicle accidents, sports, or pedestrian accidents, occur more often in men between the ages of 15–50, whereas low-energy trauma, such as falls from standing height at home, are more likely to lead to distal femoral fractures in elderly people [2].

Fractures of the distal femur may be extraarticular or include an intraarticular component. Mismanagement of any of these fractures can result in abnormalities of alignment of the load bearing axis of the lower limb and/or rotational deformities. These can have profound biomechanical consequences. In addition, intraarticular fractures can result in joint irregularities, leading to degenerative joint disease.

4.1 Indications for nonoperative treatment
Nonoperative treatment should only be resorted to as a temporary measure. Nonoperative treatment is reserved for exceptional cases, ie, if the general medical condition does not allow safe anesthesia. If nonoperative treatment is chosen, external fixation is recommended. Skeletal or adhesive skin traction may be used as an alternative short-term treatment, in order to minimize limb shortening and to provide some pain relief.

Table 9.2-2 provides an overview of the various fracture types of the distal femur and the available treatment options.

4.2 Nonoperative treatment
Options for nonoperative treatment for these types of fractures of the femur typically include:
- Traction
- Fracture braces.

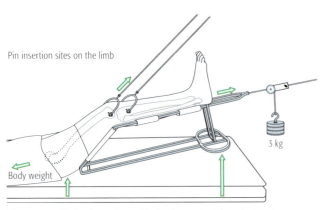

Pin insertion sites on the limb

3 kg

Body weight

Fig 9.2-1   Skeletal traction with the lower limb in a below-knee cast incorporating Steinman pins (extension). The direction of the traction forces is indicated by arrows.

Authors   Rami Mosheiff, Juan Manuel Concha

AO/OTA classification	Type of fracture	Fracture pattern	Nonoperative treatment	Operative treatment
32-A		Simple fractures	Rarely	Recommended treatment
32-B		Wedge fractures	Rarely	Recommended treatment
32-C		Complex fractures	Rarely	Recommended treatment
33-A		Extraarticular	Nondisplaced, no additional knee ligament injury	Recommended treatment
33-B		Partial articular	Rarely	Recommended treatment
33-C		Complete articular	Rarely	Recommended treatment

Table 9.2-2   Overview of the various fracture types of the distal femur and the available treatment options.

4.2.1 Traction

In fractures of the middle third of the femur, the method devised by Thomas (ie, the Thomas splint) is unsuitable because of the difficulty of controlling the proximal fragment. On the other hand, for fractures in the lower third of the femur shaft, nonoperative treatment using the Thomas splint is superior to all other nonoperative methods.

The Thomas splint combines fixed traction with counter traction applied to the ring in the splint, and differs completely from all other conservative methods using combinations of weight traction with counter traction exerted by body weight. The methods using weight traction, subsumed under the term "traction-suspension methods", are numerous, but essentially the splint takes second place to the action of the traction force, and indeed, in some cases, no splint is used at all. The principal methods of using weight traction are described below.

4.2.1.1 Thomas splint

The Thomas splint acts as a cradle. There is no fixed link to the skeleton and, therefore, no influence on controlling the deformity (**Fig 9.2-2**).

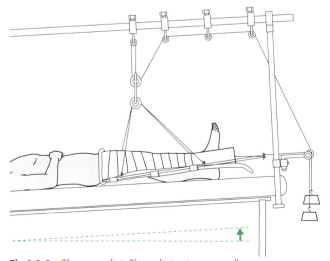

Fig 9.2-2   Thomas splint. The splint acts as a cradle.

4.2.1.2 Traction by Braun frame

In this method, the splint also serves as a cradle for the limb. Moreover, the position of the pulleys cannot be altered, and the size of the splint often does not fit the limb exactly, an additional disadvantage. Lateral bowing often occurs because the splint and the distal fragment are fixed to the frame, whereas the patient and proximal fragment can move away from the frame (**Fig 9.2-3**).

4.2.1.3 Hamilton Russell traction

The most generally used type of traction is known as Hamilton Russell traction or simply Russell traction. Posterior angulation of the distal fragment is controlled by a sling; the lifting force of this sling is linked to the main traction force through the pulleys. No rigid casting is used in this method.

Hamilton Russell devised this system for the treatment of fractures of the femoral shaft. He developed a complicated system of pulleys in order to correlate the traction force necessary to maintain length with the upward lifting force necessary to correct backward angulation at the fracture site. This is accomplished by supporting the fractured limb in a sling under the distal third of the thigh, and using a traction force attached to the sling in order to give an upward lift by an arrangement of pulleys. The same cord that exerts the traction force passes through pulleys, which double its pull along the length of the tibia below the knee. By estimating the direction of the traction force acting on the sling, a parallelogram of forces acting in the axis of the femur may be calculated (**Fig 9.2-4**).

4.2.1.4 Perkins' traction

This method does not use casts/splints. The posterior angulation of the thigh is controlled by a pillow; alignment and fixation completely depend on the action of continuous traction.

4.2.1.5 Fisk traction

Fisk traction is a variation of the Thomas splint, and is arranged to allow 90° of knee movement. It is particularly useful because it allows the active extension of the knee joint. Fixation and alignment entirely depend on weight traction; the splint transfers the motive power for assisted knee movements.

4.2.2 Fracture braces (hinged knee brace)

The high success rate resulting from the ambulatory treatment of patients with a fractured tibia led to a widely accepted similar approach in the treatment of fractures of the femur. The rate of union has been shown to be high. In one report, 150 patients in fracture braces had a mean treatment time of 14.5 weeks and no nonunion. During the same period, a randomized group of 50 patients treated in spica casts had a mean treatment time of 24.7 weeks with 6 cases of nonunion [3].

The longitudinal movement of the femoral fragments when treated with the fracture brace was studied by Connolly and King [4]. They found that the amount of translator motion was related to the fracture type rather than to the weight bearing on the limb. In general, the transverse midshaft fracture moved most, with an average movement of 1.2 cm.

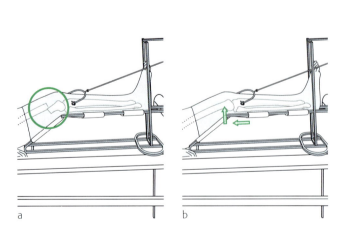

Fig 9.2-3a–b Braun frame. The patient and proximal fragment (**a**) can move away from the frame to allow reduction (**b**).

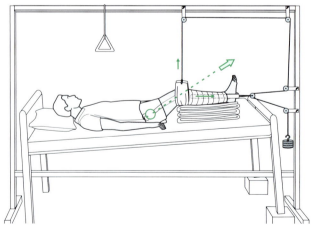

Fig 9.2-4 Hamilton Russell traction. The arrows point out the parallelogram of forces.

Authors   Rami Mosheiff, Juan Manuel Concha

The fragments did not remain in shortened position but returned to their original position during the swing phase. The treatment begins with skeletal traction, applying the usual techniques in order to obtain correct alignment and rotation. The optimal time for applying the fracture brace has yet to be standardized. Some physicians recommend its application after only 1 week of traction, while others wait until the fracture site is no longer tender and no shortening occurs when traction is removed. A period of 3–4 weeks is accepted practice, leaving the transverse midshaft fracture in traction a little longer.

In applying the cast, the area of the thigh is the most critical for an exact fit. To ensure total contact, an elastic stump sock (well-fitting tube bandage) is applied and covered with one layer of cast padding. The patella and joint line are marked on the layer of cast padding in order to provide subsequent positive identification of the joint line. The initial rolls of plaster should be elastic, followed by standard fast-drying plaster rolls. The molding of the thigh should conform to the accepted principles for above-knee sockets. There should be compression with a flat lateral wall for side bearing. Compression should also be applied over the femoral triangle in order to ensure an anteroposterior fit if no quadrilateral socket is used. The supracondylar area should be molded medially in order to achieve better compression and some suspension, and to improve contact with the lateral wall.

A below-knee cast is then applied in the usual manner. The knee joint should be positioned as close to the anatomic axis as possible. This should be about the midpoint of the patella and 2 cm behind the midline.

Polycentric hinges allow slightly more margin for error than single-axis hinges. The hinges should be parallel and on the same joint line (modification of the method described in chapter 16.4 Hinged knee brace with a longer proximal part/sleeve). The major reason for including the foot in the cast is to provide suspension. A pelvic belt is another possible means of suspension if the foot is not incorporated within the cast, or in obese patients.

The most common difficulty encountered is edema of the knee, which is not covered by the cast. Usually, this situation is only annoying, but occasionally it may be so severe as to limit ambulation. Management is symptomatic with an elastic bandage, elevation, and ambulating, with the hinged knee locked. Generally, edema subsides within 10–14 days. The major benefit is to the comfort of the patient and not only to the fracture. The older the patient, the more debilitating a long period of bed confinement may be. The low mortality, decreased morbidity, and more rapid discharge from hospital make fracture bracing treatment attractive for the patient, physician, and hospital, if nonoperative treatment is used.

5 Diaphyseal tibia

Rami Mosheiff

Fractures of the tibial shaft are the most common long bone fractures, and also the most common type of open fractures. Tibial-shaft fractures may affect knee alignment, stability, and strength. Compared to other types of fracture, these fractures are associated with a high incidence of infection, delayed union, nonunion, or malunion. The soft-tissue envelope is the most important component in the evaluation and subsequent care of tibial fractures.

5.1 Indications for nonoperative treatment

Spiral fractures of the tibial diaphysis can be treated nonoperatively. However, some shortening must be expected (the initial x-ray usually showing how much shortening to be expected). Significant displacement or angulation, particularly for distal fractures, indicates an increased risk of secondary displacement with nonoperative treatment. Malrotation is a risk that must be looked for and corrected, particularly during the first week of nonoperative treatment. **Table 9.2-3** provides an overview of the various types of diaphyseal tibial fractures and the available treatment options.

5.2 Nonoperative treatment

Options for nonoperative treatment for diaphyseal tibial fractures include:
- Plaster of Paris cast
- Sarmiento brace.

5.2.1 Plaster of Paris cast

In acute fracture treatment of diaphyseal tibial fractures, plaster of Paris (POP) is the standard cast material. Two grades of initial displacement can be defined:

- Minimal displacement: In these cases the fracture can be brought into an acceptable position simply by correcting angulation. The shortening that will occur is acceptable because the healed bone is stable at this length and will not shorten any further. An intact soft-tissue hinge can usually be predicted on the concave side of the fracture. Union usually will occur without problems and sound consolidation under conservative methods will usually be present within 3 months

- Displacement with overriding: In such cases, the attachment to the interosseous membrane will be ruptured and this important pathway for the bridging by callus of one fragment to the other will be destroyed. Delayed union will most likely occur. Simple correction of angulation does not suffice in this type of fracture. The restoration of length and apposition by at least half diameters is necessary. Mechanical means must be used in order to render the reduced position stable.

In the second group of fractures of both tibia and fibula, the need to prevent redisplacement after reduction is particularly important if the limb is encased in a POP cast. If a fracture of the tibia and fibula has been reduced by applying traction and a POP cast, there will be a grave risk of venous obstruction inside the plaster should the fracture redisplace once the traction is removed (see chapter 4 Thrombosis prophylaxis). Traction both lengthens the leg and makes it narrower, thus when traction is released, the thickness of the limb inside the plaster will increase at the same time it shortens. The vicious circle of venous obstruction, which can result from this type of "plugging", is very dangerous,

AO/OTA classification	Type of fracture	Fracture pattern	Nonoperative treatment	Operative treatment
42-A		Simple fractures	Only in rare cases Nondisplaced Fractures without shortening Fractures with intact fibula, no angulation Low-demand patients	Recommended treatment
42-B		Wedge fractures	Only in rare cases Nondisplaced Fractures without shortening Fractures with intact fibula, no angulation Low-demand patients	Recommended treatment
42-C		Complex fractures	Only in rare cases Nondisplaced Fractures without shortening Fractures with intact fibula, no angulation Low-demand patients	Recommended treatment

Table 9.2-3 Overview of the various types of diaphyseal tibial fractures and the available treatment options.

Authors   Rami Mosheiff, Juan Manuel Concha

especially during the first vital 24 hours after reduction. Most often, attempts to assess the circulation by pressing on a toe in order to observe the return of blood into the blanched area are unreliable. Severe postoperative pain must not be regarded as a normal sequel following the satisfactory reduction and fixation of a fractured tibia. Any patient that despite analgesia is not rendered comfortable after reduction of the fracture might be suffering from serious vascular complications or even compartment syndrome. This must be diagnosed within the first 6 hours after application of the POP cast. The loss of sensation and/or active movement of the toes are both serious signs even in the presence of what may appear to be good circulation when judged by pressure of the finger on the nail bed of a toe (see topic 11 in chapter 3 Principles of casting; and chapters 4 Thrombosis prophylaxis; 16.5 Dorsal long leg splint using plaster of Paris; 16.6 Long leg cast using plaster of Paris; and 16.7 Long leg cast using synthetic, combicast technique).

5.2.2   Sarmiento fracture brace (plaster of Paris or semirigid synthetic)

Immobilization in a skintight long leg cast and immediate weight bearing was first reported by Dehne et al [5]. Other nonoperative weight bearing modifications developed later on. Sarmiento, reasoning that the principle of a below-knee cast/orthosis might be applicable, developed the patella tendon bearing cast for tibial fractures [6] (see chapter 16.8 Sarmiento (patella tendon bearing) cast using plaster of Paris (**Fig 9.2-5**)). The average healing time was 14.5 weeks for closed fractures and 16.7 weeks for open fractures. The average limb shortening in the cast was 6.35 mm. It is now evident that the patella tendon was not carrying as much weight as thought. It is the modeling of the cast as well as pressure considerations—the hydraulic effect—within the leg that provide stability for the fracture fragments.

The functional below-knee orthosis (Sarmiento brace) was the next logical development in the management of tibial fractures. The tibia is stabilized with a covering of thermoplastic material or a semirigid synthetic brace (see chapter 16.9 Sarmiento tibial brace using synthetic, combicast technique), leaving a free ankle joint. The brace is then attached to the foot cast. The results have been shown to be equal to those using the conventional plaster technique [7]. However, the Sarmiento brace, leaving the ankle free, is not applied immediately. In order to avoid problems of edema in the foot and ankle, the entire extremity is conventionally cast for about 2 weeks (see chapters 16.6 Long leg cast using plaster of Paris; and 16.7 Long leg cast using synthetic, combicast technique). During this time, the extremity is intermittently elevated, and the primary consideration is control of swelling. A patella tendon bearing (PTB) total-contact cast is then applied for an additional 2 weeks (see chapter 16.8 Sarmiento (patella tendon bearing) cast using plaster of Paris), and weight bearing is allowed and encouraged. If no edema is present at this time, the cast may be removed and the orthosis applied. The tibia is stabilized with a covering of thermoplastic material or semirigid synthetic cast (see chapter 16.9 Sarmiento tibial brace using synthetic, combicast technique (**Fig 9.2-6**)). Thus, fracture treatment by orthosis begins at about the fifth week.

The advantage of changing to the orthosis is that the ankle can be mobilized. The position of the ankle joint is critical as motion at the fracture site, compelled by differences in the axis of the rotation of the ankle and the orthosis, must be prevented. Wearing of the orthosis is continued until the fracture is healed.

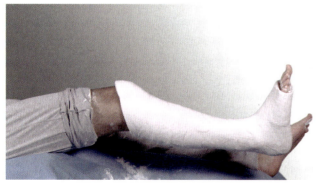

Fig 9.2-5   Example of a Sarmiento (petalla tendon bearing) cast.

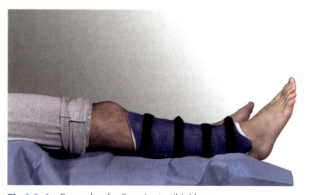

Fig 9.2-6   Example of a Sarmiento tibial brace.

6 Distal tibia

Rami Mosheiff

Distal tibial fractures are primarily located within a square based on the width of the distal tibia. Many fractures of the distal tibia have severe concomitant soft-tissue compromise. It is recommended to assess the soft-tissue condition, sensation, and motor function in the foot as well as to look out for signs of compartment syndrome, which may develop sometime after injury. Grossly displaced fractures and dislocations must be reduced immediately and temporarily stabilized, using a joint-bridging external fixator.

6.1 Indications for nonoperative treatment

Definitive nonoperative treatment with a cast is rarely indicated for distal tibial fractures. The nonoperative treatment may, however, be adequate in nondisplaced or minimally displaced fractures that are stable. Presence of a high surgical risk obviously is another indicator for nonoperative treatment in other fracture types.

Stabilizing the fracture in a cast may be used for initial management until the soft-tissue situation allows open reduction and internal fixation. In highly unstable fractures, the cast may not suffice in order to maintain reduction and prevent shortening. Such fractures will need to be stabilized with an external fixator.

Table 9.2-4 provides an overview of the different types of distal tibial fractures and the available treatment options.

6.2 Nonoperative treatment

Nonoperative treatments for fractures of the distal tibia include:
- Traction
- Manual reduction
- Casts.

6.2.1 Traction

Traction can be used where weight is applied at the calcaneus using a Steinmann pin in order to create reduction (**Fig 9.2-7**).

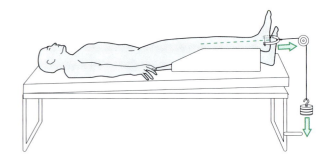

Fig 9.2-7 Traction of the distal tibia.

AO/OTA classification	Type of fracture	Fracture pattern	Nonoperative treatment	Operative treatment
43-A		Extraarticular	Nondisplaced, closed stable fracture Significant comorbidities (high anesthesia risk) Compromising medical conditions (diabetes, neurovascular diseases) Soft-tissue condition preventing surgical intervention Nonambulatory patient	Recommended treatment
43-B		Partial articular	Nondisplaced, closed stable fracture Significant comorbidities (high anesthesia risk) Compromising medical conditions (diabetes, neurovascular diseases) Soft-tissue condition preventing surgical intervention Nonambulatory patient	Recommended treatment
43-C		Complete articular	Nondisplaced, closed stable fracture Significant comorbidities (high anesthesia risk) Compromising medical conditions (diabetes, neurovascular diseases) Soft-tissue condition preventing surgical intervention Nonambulatory patient	Recommended treatment

Table 9.2-4 Overview of the different types of distal tibial fractures and the available treatment options.

Authors   Rami Mosheiff, Juan Manuel Concha

6.2.1.1 The use of gravity in reduction

The importance of recognizing the role of gravity in reduction deformity cannot be better illustrated than by the example of a distal tibial fracture. By holding the foot in one hand with the heel resting in the palm, with the foot and leg held horizontally and in external rotation, the ankle will spontaneously fall into the position of reduction (**Fig 9.2-8**). Only if surgeons truly understand how unnecessary the use of muscular force is, will they really appreciate the mechanics of the fracture and the necessity for patients to present as early as possible after injury. At first, it is important not to reduce any fracture by physical movements but to assess the influence of various mechanical factors on each injury as an individual case.

6.2.2 Manual reduction

Some surgeons instead of using gravity to add positive support in fracture reduction prefer to rearrange the effective forces so that the effect of gravity is eliminated. In an ankle fracture, this can be achieved by carrying out the reduction with the tibia in the vertical position by hanging the lower leg over the end of a table. The physician then holds the foot around its middle section from plantar and medial with one hand and grasping the heel with the other. Reduction is achieved by gentle traction and by aligning the foot to match the axis of the lower leg, thereby also correcting rotation (**Fig 9.2-9**).

6.2.3 Plaster of Paris cast

For the initial purpose of fracture reduction, only sufficient plaster should be applied to be strong enough to maintain reduction temporarily once the plaster has set. Synthetic or semirigid synthetic cast material is not recommended for reduced fractures. During this application, no effort should be spent on the ultimate finish of the upper and lower limits of the plaster, which would only be a waste of time and invite setting of the cast before fracture reduction has been achieved. Having completed the speedy application of the initial plaster bandages, the surgeon now takes over from the assistant and "feels" the fracture by moving it about inside the wet plaster; from the previous analysis of the fracture, he or she again should be able to recognize the sensation of reduction, although these impressions may now be a little muffled by the plaster (see chapter 16.10 Dorsal short leg splint using plaster of Paris). Having recognized the sensation of reduction, the physician now holds the reduction without any further movement until the plaster has set. During this time, using gravity, the assistant maintains the foot and leg in external rotation while the surgeon supports the foot with his or her hand below the heel. The cast is completed by finishing the top and bottom, and applying extra casting material in order to increase the thickness, if necessary.

In regard to finishing the POP cast at the toes, it is usually best to leave the toes free by stopping the plaster at the metatarsophalangeal joints. A platform under the toes, unless made very carefully, often produces a cramped position.

In secondary treatment, synthetic material can also be used (see chapters 16.11 Dorsal short leg splint using synthetic; 16.12 Short leg cast using rigid synthetic; and 16.13 Short leg cast using synthetic, combicast technique).

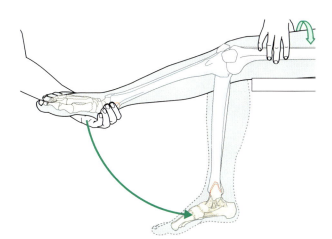

Fig 9.2-8   Making use of gravity in order to help reduce the fracture. This is only possible if treatment is carried out on the day of injury, with the fracture in typical deformity and before swelling has set in. Adequate anesthesia must be administered.

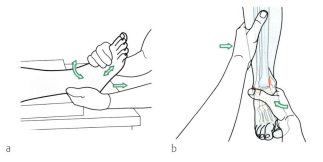

a   b

Fig 9.2-9a–b   Manual reduction is performed on the hanging leg, with the knee flexed in order to reduce the pull on the Achilles tendon. Reduction is achieved by gentle traction (**a**) and by aligning the foot to match the axis of the lower leg, thereby also correcting rotation (**b**).

7   Foot

Juan Manuel Concha

Bone and ligament injuries that affect the foot are common, resulting especially from sports activities, job accidents, and high-energy trauma caused by traffic accidents. Establishing a proper diagnosis is crucial in order to determine the most appropriate treatment.

7.1   Hindfoot

The most frequent injuries of the hindfoot include fractures of the talus, calcaneus, and subtalar dislocations.

7.1.1   Talus fractures

Fractures of the talus are rare, yet the integrity of the talus is essential for proper foot function. Even small fracture displacements, through their effects on joint function and alignment, may cause foot deformity, arthrosis, and significant functional impairment. Soon after injury, soft tissues must be evaluated carefully, as the pressure on the skin from bony deformity, and associated edema, may lead to skin necrosis, slough, and secondary infection. Displaced fractures of the talar neck are associated with avascular necrosis of the talar body, but the urgency of fracture fixation has recently been called into question [8]. Nonetheless, it is important to reduce dislocations (subtalar and ankle) as soon as possible.

Hawkins classification [9] describes four types of talus fractures according to the degree of displacement, and also provides the available therapeutic options (see **Table 9.2-5a–c**).

Hawkins classification	Type of fracture	Fracture pattern	Nonoperative treatment	Operative treatment
Talar neck fracture				
Type I		Nondisplaced	Only completely nondisplaced	Recommended treatment
Type II		Displaced ±multifragmentary	Not indicated	Recommended treatment
Type III		Displaced ±multifragmentary	Not indicated	Recommended treatment
Type IV		Displaced ±multifragmentary	Not indicated	Recommended treatment

Table 9.2-5a   Overview of the four types of talus fractures according to Hawkins and the available treatment options [9].

Authors   Rami Mosheiff, Juan Manuel Concha

AO/OTA classification	Type of fracture	Fracture pattern	Nonoperative treatment	Operative treatment
Talar body fracture C1		Ankle joint involvement	Not indicated	Recommended treatment
C2		Subtalar involvement	Not indicated	Recommended treatment
C3		Ankle + subtalar involvement	Not indicated	Recommended treatment

Table 9.2-5b   Overview of the C-type talar body fractures according to the AO/OTA Fracture and Dislocation Classification.

Lateral + posterior process fractures	Type of fracture	Fracture pattern	Nonoperative treatment	Operative treatment
Lateral process		Nondislocated	Option	Option
Posterior process		Nondislocated	Option	Option
Lateral process		Dislocated	Not indicated	Recommended treatment
Posterior process		Dislocated	Not indicated	Recommended treatment

Table 9.2-5c   Overview of lateral and posterior process fractures and possible nonoperative treatment options.

9.2

GUIDELINES

Only truly nondisplaced type I fractures should be treated nonoperatively by means of immobilization in a nonweight bearing short leg cast, and strict periodic x-ray control. Immobilization splints can initially be used as primary care, and immediately after surgery for comfort as well as to preserve neutral foot alignment until rehabilitation can be initiated [10] (see chapters 16.10 Dorsal short leg splint using plaster of Paris; 16.11 Dorsal short leg splint using synthetic; 16.12 Short leg cast using rigid synthetic; and 16.13 Short leg cast using synthetic, combicast technique).

7.1.2 Calcaneus fractures

The management of calcaneus fractures is still controversial [11]. Recent advances in diagnostics, surgical techniques, soft-tissue care, as well as implants, have helped to achieve better results in the treatment of complex articular fractures of the calcaneus. Displaced tuberosity fractures that carry the threat of skin necrosis are an accepted indication for immediate fracture reduction and fixation.

AO/OTA classification	Type of fracture	Fracture pattern	Nonoperative treatment	Operative treatment
Extraarticular fractures				
A		Avulsion fracture of the calcaneal tuberosity	Nondisplaced	Recommended treatment
B		Involving the anterior process	Nondisplaced	Recommended treatment
C		Articular	Nondisplaced	Recommended treatment
Essex-Lopresti		Joint depression	Not indicated	Recommended treatment
		Tongue type	Not indicated	Recommended treatment

Table 9.2-6 Overview of the various types of calcaneus fractures and the available treatment options.

Authors   Rami Mosheiff, Juan Manuel Concha

Radiographic evaluation, including CT, is useful in order to evaluate and classify the fracture and plan its management. Treatment must be individualized according to:

- Age of the patient
- Activity level
- Bone condition
- Type of fracture
- State of the soft tissues.

Open reduction is recommended in displaced articular fractures, with Böhler's angle inversion, or articular surface displacement [12]. **Table 9.2-6** provides an overview of the various types of calcaneus fractures and the available treatment options.

Immobilization splints are useful at the initial stage of the treatment as well as the postsurgical period. If nonoperative treatment is selected, a splint or cast (see chapters 16.10 Dorsal short leg splint using plaster of Paris; 16.11 Dorsal short leg splint using synthetic; 16.12 Short leg cast using rigid synthetic; and 16.13 Short leg cast using synthetic, combicast technique) to support neutral foot alignment may be used at first, but it should not prevent early mobilization of the ankle and foot (see chapters 16.13 Short leg cast using synthetic, combicast technique), while avoiding weight bearing for 2–3 months.

Application of a foot cast allows unrestricted mobilization of the ankle joint (see chapters 16.18 Foot cast using synthetic, combicast technique; and 16.19 Removable foot cast using synthetic, combicast technique).

7.1.3 Subtalar dislocations

Subtalar dislocations are important injuries generally caused by forced foot inversion or eversion. They affect both the subtalar and talonavicular joints (**Fig 9.2-10**).

Early reduction is important in order to avoid vascular compromise of the soft tissues located above the injury. This maneuver can be done with the knee flexed and with firm longitudinal traction. Generally, the injured joint is stable after reduction. Immobilization is achieved with a splint (see chapters 16.10 Dorsal short leg splint using plaster of Paris; 16.11 Dorsal short leg splint using synthetic; and 16.13 Short leg cast using synthetic, combicast technique) for a few days, followed by active range of motion exercises and, initially, protected weight bearing.

7.2 Midfoot
7.2.1 Minor tarsal bones

Isolated fractures are uncommon and it is important to be on the lookout for the possibility of other associated injuries [13]. Navicular fractures are relevant if the talonavicular articular surface as well as the posterior tibial tendon insertion are compromised. Cuboid fractures are caused by axial force along the lateral foot column and rarely are isolated injuries. Navicular fractures are often induced by high-energy injuries (**Fig 9.2-11**).

X-rays and CT scans are important for the evaluation of midfoot fractures. The management focuses on restoring midfoot alignment and stability, especially preserving the length of the medial and lateral columns.

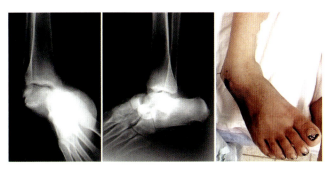

Fig 9.2-10   Subtalar dislocations affect both subtalar and talonavicular joints.

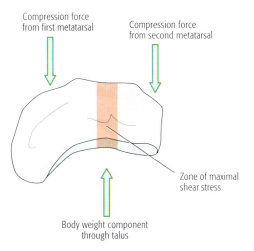

Fig 9.2-11   Traumatic impact on the navicular bone. The zone of maximal shear stress is located at the junction of the middle to the lateral third.

If not displaced, midfoot fractures can be treated nonoperatively, using a short leg cast (see chapters 16.10 Dorsal short leg splint using plaster of Paris; and 16.11 Dorsal short leg splint using synthetic), or with unrestricted movement of the ankle joint (see chapters 16.18 Foot cast using synthetic, combicast technique; and 16.19 Removable foot cast using synthetic, combicast technique), avoiding weight bearing for the first 6 weeks. Displaced fractures or unstable joints should be treated with an open reduction and internal fixation (ORIF).

7.3 Forefoot (metatarsals, phalanges)

The forefoot comprises the tarsometatarsal joint as well as the metatarsals, phalanges, and joints that connect them. The tarsometatarsal joint (TMT), often referred to as Lis-franc's joint in honor of the surgeon that described amputation at that level, is a complex osteoligamentous system that involves the union of the first three metatarsals with the cuneiform bones, and the fourth and fifth with the cuboid.

7.3.1 Tarsometatarsal (Lisfranc's) joint injuries

Lisfranc's TMT joint injuries are usually produced by sudden, violent twists of the forefoot. If deformity or instability is not obvious, these injuries are easily overlooked, with disastrous consequences [14]. Commonly, the patient presents with edema and pain in the dorsal region of the foot. Deformity depends on the degree of displacement. **Table 9.2-7** provides a classification of the various types of TMT joint fractures.

Type of fracture			
Type A	Medial: Lateral:		Total incongruity	All 5 metatarsals together displaced in a dorsolateral direction
Type B1			Homolateral complete	Only the first TMT joint involved.
Type B2			Partial incongruity	Lateral TMTs are also involved.
Type C1			Homolateral incomplete	
Type C2			Partial incongruity	

Table 9.2-7 Classification of the various types of TMT joint fractures (Lisfranc's). The original Lisfranc's classification was done by Quenu and Kuss in 1909 and modified by Myerson and Hardcastle in 1986 [15].

Authors   Rami Mosheiff, Juan Manuel Concha

The x-ray images can vary between subtle injuries, small bone avulsions, and joint space widening (**Fig 9.2-12**) even to major displacements that usually coincide with significant edema and may be associated with vascular lesions (**Fig 9.2-13**).

It is important to check for an increased space between the first and second metatarsal in the anteroposterior view, fractures at the base of the second metatarsal, or subtle bony avulsions that may indicate significantly unstable ligament avulsions. In the lateral and oblique projection, the alignment between the first metatarsal and the first cuneiform must be observed carefully as well as the articulations of the navicular (talonavicular and naviculocuneiform), which may also be involved in a TMT injury.

Only a proper reduction of the fracture and restoration of stability to the injured joints will permit adequate pain-free function [14]. Thus closed treatment is only indicated for stable, accurately reduced, nondisplaced injuries and with no compromise of the soft tissues. If stability of the TMT joint complex is confirmed (stress x-rays), nonoperative treatment is appropriate. This can be done with a well-molded short leg cast (see chapters 16.10 Dorsal short leg splint using plaster of Paris; 16.11 Dorsal short leg splint using synthetic; 16.12 Short leg cast using rigid synthetic; and 16.13 Short leg cast using synthetic, combicast technique) and nonweight bearing immobilization for 6 weeks. The cast should be reapplied if it has loosened due to decreased edema. X-rays must be taken in order to check for further displacement.

Immobilization with a short leg splint instead of a cast plays a role in the initial preoperative treatment as well as postoperative treatment (see chapters 16.10 Dorsal short leg splint using plaster of Paris; and 16.11 Dorsal short leg splint using synthetic), and can be used initially in nonoperative cases with significant swelling [16]. Another option is foot cast immobilization (see chapters 16.18 Foot cast using synthetic, combicast technique; and 16.19 Removable foot cast using synthetic, combicast technique).

7.3.2 Metatarsal fractures

These fractures are frequently produced by a direct blow to the foot, commonly affecting the second, third, and fourth metatarsals. Equally common are avulsion fractures of the base of the fifth metatarsal and neck fractures of the second, third, and fifth metatarsals. Supporting ligaments attached to the proximal and distal ends of the metatarsals usually prevent displacement of shaft fractures of the middle metatarsals. Isolated fractures of the central metatarsals with little displacement can be treated with immobilization in a walking cast for 3 weeks (see chapters 16.12 Short leg cast using rigid synthetic; and 16.13 Short leg cast using synthetic, combicast technique) followed by a semirigid foot cast for another 3 weeks (see chapters 16.18 Foot cast using synthetic, combicast technique; and 16.19 Removable foot cast using synthetic, combicast technique). Moderate displacements in the frontal plane of the central metatarsals are well tolerated. However, significant displacement of the first or the fifth metatarsal requires reduction and percutaneous fixation, or ORIF, as do unstable fractures with shortening in order to prevent maldistribution of weight bearing forces with transfer of pressure to the more prominent metatarsal heads with resulting metatarsalgia [17].

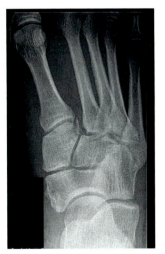

Fig 9.2-12   Small avulsion and joint space widening between the first and second metatarsal bases.

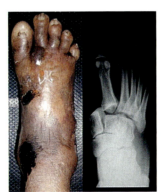

Fig 9.2-13   Severe TMT joint displacement: x-rays and soft-tissue condition.

Fractures of the metatarsal necks are produced by direct trauma and often involve several metatarsals. Usually, it is possible to achieve closed reduction by traction and containment in a walking cast (see chapters 16.12 Short leg cast using rigid synthetic; 16.13 Short leg cast using synthetic, combicast technique; 16.18 Foot cast using synthetic, combicast technique; and 16.19 Removable foot cast using synthetic, combicast technique); otherwise surgical fixation may be required. Improper reductions should not be accepted, as they can affect the support and biomechanics of the foot [18].

Fractures of the fifth metatarsal base deserve special attention. Treatment is based on the location zone (**Fig 9.2-14**):
• Zone 1: Tuberosity
• Zone 2: Metaphyseal-diaphyseal union
• Zone 3: Proximal diaphysis.

Injuries in zone 3 are usually fatigue fractures (see chapter 13 Overload injuries) [18].

Treatment should be individualized, taking into account the site of the fracture as well as the age and activity level of the patient.
• Fractures in zone 1 have a good blood supply and usually heal with partial weight bearing in a comfortable shoe or foot cast (see chapters 16.18 Foot cast using synthetic, combicast technique; and 16.19 Removable foot cast using synthetic, combicast technique)
• Fractures in zone 2 are usually more painful and require immobilization. It is possible to use a short leg POP cast for 3–4 weeks (see chapters 16.10 Dorsal short leg splint using plaster of Paris; 16.11 Dorsal short leg splint using synthetic; 16.12 Short leg cast using rigid synthetic; and 16.13 Short leg cast using synthetic, combicast technique), followed by a functional metatarsal brace/cast until healing is complete (see chapters 16.18 Foot cast using synthetic, combicast technique; and 16.19 Removable foot cast using synthetic, combicast technique)
• Fractures in zone 3 have a greater risk of delayed union or nonunion. Due to this, and in view of the patient's needs, surgical fixation may be an appropriate option [19].

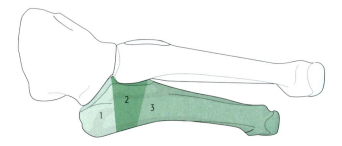

Fig 9.2-14 The location zones for fractures of the fifth metatarsal base.

Authors   Rami Mosheiff, Juan Manuel Concha

7.3.2.1 Metatarsophalangeal joint injuries

Hyperextension sprains of the first metatarsophalangeal (MTP) joint are frequent, especially resulting from sports activities. Treatment is based on rest, cooling (ice), analgesics, and perhaps taping of the first to the second toe. Usually discomfort is diminished by the second or third week and activity can progressively be resumed as tolerated.

Jahss classified the dislocations of the first MTP joint into three types (**Table 9.2-8**) [20].

Type II lesions can be treated by closed reduction and immobilization for 3–4 weeks in a short lower-leg cast (see chapters 16.10 Dorsal short leg splint using plaster of Paris;

16.11 Dorsal short leg splint using synthetic; 16.12 Short leg cast using rigid synthetic; and 16.13 Short leg cast using synthetic, combicast technique) or a foot cast (see chapters 16.18 Foot cast using synthetic, combicast technique; and 16.19 Removable foot cast using synthetic, combicast technique).

Metatarsophalangeal dislocations of the lesser toes are rare and usually only require closed reduction with traction and immobilization in a semirigid foot cast for 3–4 weeks (see chapters 16.18 Foot cast using synthetic, combicast technique; and 16.19 Removable foot cast using synthetic, combicast technique).

Type of fracture	Nonoperative	Operative
Type I	The sesamoid complex and volar plate block the joint, preventing closed reduction	Requiring open reduction with subsequent protection in a short leg cast
Type IIA	Sesamoid complete ruptures without fracture	Relative indication
Type IIB	Fracture of the sesamoid Radiographically, the increased space between the sesamoids is the key to the classification	Relative indication

Table 9.2-8   Jahss' classification of the dislocations of the first MTP joint.

9.2

7.3.3 Fractures of the phalanges, and interphalangeal dislocations

Fractures of the phalanges of the hallux are usually due to direct trauma. If nondisplaced, they may be treated with semirigid foot cast immobilization for 3–4 weeks (see chapters 16.18 Foot cast using synthetic, combicast technique; 16.19 Removable foot cast using synthetic, combicast technique; and 16.20 First toe orthosis using synthetic, combicast technique). Displaced fractures require closed reduction and percutaneous fixation, or ORIF.

Interphalangeal joint dislocations result from axial forces that displace the distal phalanx dorsally. They should be reduced with longitudinal traction and immobilized to the adjacent toe with an adhesive bandage.

Fractures of the lesser toe phalanges likewise require closed reduction and immobilization to the adjacent toe for 3–4 weeks (**Fig 9.2-15**).

8   Summary   Rami Mosheiff, Juan Manuel Concha

- Fractures of the hip/proximal femur present a major cause of morbidity and mortality all over the world
- In many cases, these fractures are best treated by operative internal fixation, yet whenever the risks of surgery and anesthesia are too great, nonoperative treatment must be considered, and the physician must be familiar with closed reduction methods for different fractures
- A variety of types of balanced traction are the preferred nonoperative treatment for fractures of the hip, such as Hamilton Russell traction
- Treatment of tibia fractures often involves a fracture brace, and treatment using functional (Sarmiento) bracing allows for early weight bearing
- Foot injuries are very common and diagnosis is based on clinical examination of the patient and diagnostic imaging (x-ray and CT)
- Closed management in hindfoot fractures is indicated in nondisplaced fractures and in patients with contraindications to operative treatment
- A high index of suspicion must exist to prevent the Lisfranc´s injury to be overlooked with disastrous consequences for the patient
- Isolated fractures of the central metatarsals with little displacement can be treated with immobilization
- Fractures of the fifth metatarsal base deserve special attention, with treatment based on the location zone
- Fractures of the phalanges, if nondisplaced, can be treated with a short period of immobilization.

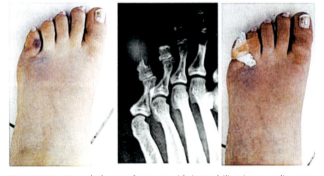

Fig 9.2-15   Toe phalanges fracture with immobilization to adjacent toe.

9 References

Rami Mosheiff, Juan Manuel Concha

1. **Owens WD, Felts JA, Spitznagel EL Jr**. ASA physical status classifications: a study of consistency of ratings. *Anesthesiology.* 1978; 49:239–243.

2. **Wähnert D, Hoffmeier K, Fröber R, et al**. Distal femur fractures of the elderly—different treatment options in a biomechanical comparison. *Injury.* 2011 Jul; 42(7):655–659.

3. **Mooney V, Nickel VL, Harvey JP Jr, et al**. Cast-brace treatment for fractures of the distal part of the femur. A prospective controlled study of one hundred and fifty patients. *J Bone Joint Surg Am.* 1970 Dec; 52(8):1563–1578.

4. **Connolly JF, King P**. Closed reduction and early cast-brace ambulation in the treatment of femoral fractures. An in vivo quantitative analysis of immobilization in skeletal traction and a cast-brace. *J Bone Joint Surg Am.* 1973 Dec; 55(8):1559–1580.

5. **Dehne E, Metz CW, Deffer PA, et al**. Nonoperative treatment of the fractured tibia by immediate weight bearing. *J Trauma.* 1961 Sep; 1:514–535.

6. **Sarmiento A**. A functional below-the-knee cast for tibial fractures. *J Bone Joint Surg Am.* 1967 Jul; 49(5):855–875.

7. **Sarmiento A, Gersten LM, Sobol PA, et al**. Tibial shaft fractures treated with functional braces. *Experience with 780 fractures.* J Bone Joint Surg Br. 1989 Aug; 71(4):602–609.

8. **Vallier HA, Nork SE, Barei DP, et al**. Talar neck fractures: results and outcomes. *J Bone Joint Surg Am.* 2004 Aug; 86-A(8):1616–1624.

9. **Hawkins LG**. Fractures of the neck of the talus. *J Bone Joint Surg Am.* 1970 Jul; 52(5):991–1002.

10. **Metzger MJ, Levin JS, Clancy JT**. Talar neck fractures and rates of avascular necrosis. *J Foot Ankle Surg.* 1999 Mar–Apr; 38(2):154–162.

11. **Kundel K, Funk E, Brutscher M, et al**. Calcaneal fractures: Operative versus nonoperative treatment. *J Trauma.* 1996 Nov; 41(5):839–845.

12. **Sanders R**. Displaced intra-articular fractures of the calcaneus. *J Bone Joint Surg Am.* 2000 Feb; 82(2):225–250.

13. **Dhillon MS, Nagi ON**. Total dislocations of the navicular: Are they ever isolated injuries? *J Bone Joint Surg Br.* 1999 Sep; 81(5):881–885.

14. **Brunet JA, Wiley JJ**. The late results of tarsometatarsal joint injuries. *J Bone Joint Surg Br.* 1987 May; 69(3):437–440.

15. **Myerson MS, Fisher RT, Burgess AR, et al**. Fracture dislocations of the tarsometatarsal joints: End results correlated with pathology and treatment. *Foot Ankle.* 1986 Apr; 6(5):225–242.

16. **Thompson M, Mormino MA**. Injury to the tarsometatarsal joint complex. *J Am Acad Orthop Surg.* 2003 Jul–Aug; 11(4):260–267.

17. **Schenck RC Jr, Heckman JD**. Fractures and Dislocations of the Forefoot: Operative and Nonoperative treatment. *J Am Acad Orthop Surg.* 1995 Mar; 3(2):70–78.

18. **Quill GE Jr**. Fractures of the proximal fifth metatarsal. *Orthop Clin North Am.* 1995 Apr; 26(2):353–361.

19. **Den Hartog BD**. Fracture of the proximal fifth metatarsal. *J Am Acad Orthop Surg.* 2009 Jul; 17(7):458–464.

20. **Jahss MH**. Traumatic dislocations of the first metatarsophalangeal joint. *Foot Ankle.* 1980 Jul; 1(1):15–21.

9.2

GUIDELINES

10   Further reading

Rami Mosheiff, Juan Manuel Concha

AO Surgery Reference. Casting. *Colton CL, Schatzker J, Trafton P* (eds). AO Foundation. Available at http://www.aosurgery.org. [Accessed July 2011].

Bong SC, Lau HK, Leong JC, et al. The treatment of unstable intertrochanteric fractures of the hip: a prospective trial of 150 cases. *Injury.* 1981 Sep; 13(2):139–146.

Cass J, Sems SA. Operative versus nonoperative management of distal femur fracture in myelopathic, nonambulatory patients. *Orthopedics.* 2008 Nov; 31(11):1091.

Clanton TO, Butler JE, Eggert A. Injuries to the metatarsophalangeal joints in athletes. *Foot Ankle.* 1986 Dec; 7(3):162–176.

Connolly JF, Dehne E, Lafollette B. Closed reduction and early cast-brace ambulation in the treatment of femoral fractures. II. Results in one hundred and forty-three fractures. *J Bone Joint Surg Am.* 1973 Dec; 55(8):1581–1599.

Faraj AA. Non-operative treatment of elderly patients with femoral neck fracture. *Acta Orthop Belg.* 2008 Oct; 74(5):627–629.

Hansen FF. Conservative vs. surgical treatment of impacted, subcapital fractures of the femoral neck. *Acta Orthop Scand.* 1994; 65 Suppl:256–259.

Hornby R, Evans JG, Vardon V. Operative or conservative treatment for trochanteric fractures of the femur. A randomised epidemiological trial in elderly patients. *J Bone Joint Surg Br.* 1989 Aug; 71(4):619–623.

Kelley SS. Periprosthetic Femoral Fractures. *J Am Acad Orthop Surg.* 1994 May; 2(3):164–172.

Makwana NK, Bhowal B, Harper WM, et al. Conservative versus operative treatment for displaced ankle fractures in patients over 55 years of age. A prospective randomized study. *J Bone Joint Surg Br.* 2001 May; 83(4):525–529.

Nicoll EA. Fractures of the Tibial Shaft. A survey of 705 cases. *J Bone Joint Surg Br.* 1964 Aug; 46:373–387.

Pakarinen HJ, Flinkkil TE, Ohtonen PP, et al. Stability criteria for nonoperative ankle fracture management. *Foot Ankle Int.* 2011 Feb; 32(2):141–147.

Raaymakers EL, Marti RK. Non-operative treatment of impacted femoral neck fractures. A prospective study of 170 cases. *J Bone Joint Surg Br.* 1991 Nov; 73(6):950–954.

Saltzman C, Marsh JL. Hindfoot Dislocations: When Are They Not Benign? *J Am Acad Orthop Surg.* 1997 Jul; 5(4):192–198.

Sarmiento A, Sinclair WF. Application of prosthetic-orthotics principles to treatment of fractures. *Artif Limbs.* 1967 Autumn; 11(2):28–32.

Witschi H, Omer E Jr. The treatment of open tibial shaft fractures from Vietnam War. *J Trauma.* 1970 Feb; 10(2):105–111.

Zelle BA, Bhandari M, Espiritu M, et al. Treatment of distal tibia fractures without articular involvement: a systematic review of 1125 fractures. *J Orthop Trauma.* 2006 Jan; 20(1):76–79.

9.3 Nonoperative treatment of spinal fractures

Florian Gebhard, Peter Richter, Bastian Scheiderer

9.3

GUIDELINES

Authors   Florian Gebhard, Peter Richter, Bastian Scheiderer

9.3   Nonoperative treatment of spinal fractures

1   Introduction

As was strongly supported by Böhler, spine fractures can be treated nonoperatively. However, some spine fractures, especially if they are unstable, do require surgery [1]. Yet, in some parts of the world, even unstable spine fractures have to be treated nonoperatively because of a complete lack of resources.

Osteoporotic fractures, although generally stable, constitute one of the exceptions. Due to old age and immobility, such patients are prone to suffer from pneumonia and other complications when treated nonoperatively. Therefore, minimally invasive treatment should be the first choice. Vertebral metastases and pathological fractures should also be treated surgically. The high comorbidity of these patients requires fast stabilization and pain reduction in order to allow early mobilization.

2   Diagnostics

When examining spine injuries, the x-ray assessment begins with AP and lateral images. Typically, an additional CT scan is mandatory in order to classify the fracture type and to choose the right treatment. Also, MRIs are increasingly used in order to gain further information.

3   Cervical spine

Many injuries of the cervical spine are treated nonoperatively. Depending on the stability level, treatment options range from immobilization by cervical collars and braces to halo orthosis (**Fig 9.3-1**), or a Minerva or Diadem cast/orthosis (**Fig 9.3-2**). Sternal-occipital-mandibular type immobilizers are the most effective in limiting the upper cervical spine motion of nonhalo devices [2].

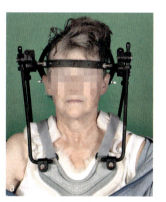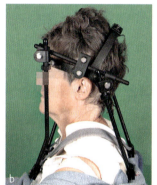

Fig 9.3-1a–b   Halo fixator.

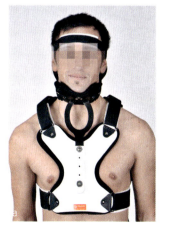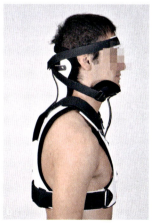

Fig 9.3-2a–b   The Diadem brace. Without the headband, it functions as a Minerva brace.

9.3

3.1 Occipital condyle fractures

Stable occipital condyle fractures with intact alar ligaments (type I and II) are immobilized in a prefabricated hard collar or a semirigid custom-made combicast for 6 weeks. If an avulsion fracture of the alar ligaments exists (type III), this results in increased axial rotation across both the O/C1 and C1/2 joints [3]. In this case, instability is detected and the fracture is treated with either a halo vest, a Minerva/Diadem cast (**Fig 9.3-3**), or internal fixation.

The more frequent atlas fractures occur from axial loading of the occiput that translates into distraction of the lateral masses. This results in ring tension and causes the ring to fail [4]. The treatment of atlas fractures is based on the integrity of the transverse ligament as it plays a major role in determining atlantoaxial stability. Dickman et al reported injuries involving the midportion of the transverse ligament or the insertion point at the tubercle (type I) as unstable [5]. These injuries are incapable of healing with external immobilization alone. In contrast, fractures and avulsions involving the tubercle for insertion of the transverse ligament (type II) have a good chance of healing when treated with a halo vest or Minerva/Diadem cast for 12 weeks. Isolated bony injuries of the atlas are mainly treated nonoperatively with a hard collar for 6–12 weeks. In cases of lateral-mass displacement of more than 7 mm, a halo vest is recommended. In 40–44% of cases, atlas fractures are associated with axis fractures [6–8]. In this case, treatment is based on the type of axis fracture and the integrity of the transverse ligament. External immobilization is recommended unless instability is evident on upright and supine x-rays while the patient is wearing an orthosis (Minerva/Diadem cast).

3.2 Fractures of the C2
3.2.1 Fractures of the odontoid

Fractures of the odontoid process are the most common of all axis fractures and often cause atlantoaxial instability [9]. According to the Anderson-D'Alonzo three-part system (**Table 9.3-1**), type I injuries are treated with a hard collar or semirigid combicast collar for 6 weeks [10]. However, a reevaluation for rotatory atlantoaxial instability should be carried out after 3 months. The management of type II and type III odontoid fractures remains controversial. Müller et al defined fractures that had a fracture gap of less than 2 mm, an initial AP displacement of less than 5 mm, an angulation of less than 11°, and less than 2 mm displacement on lateral flexion/extension views as stable [11]. They showed a fusion rate of 73.7% for type II and 85.7% for type III fractures treated with nonrigid immobilization. A meta-analysis comparing the operative with the nonoperative management of acute type II odontoid fractures showed a significantly

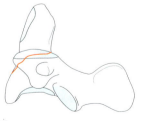

Anderson and D'Alonzo Classification of Odontoid Fractures

Type I Apical (tip) fracture of the dens

Type II Body fracture of the odontoid

Type III Basilar fracture into the body of the axis

Table 9.3-1 The Anderson and D'Alonzo classification of odontoid fractures [10].

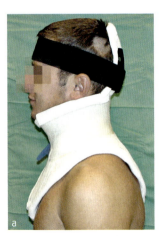 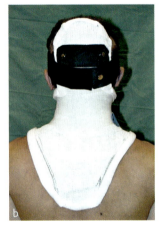

Fig 9.3-3a–b Modified Minerva cast.

Authors   Florian Gebhard, Peter Richter, Bastian Scheiderer

higher fusion rate for operative therapy compared with external immobilization for patients over the age of 44–55. However, the fusion rate was over 80% for patients under the age of 45–55, regardless of treatment modality. The fusion rate in nonoperative management offers comparable results in anteriorly displaced fractures and displacement of less than 4–6 mm [12].

Patients of advanced age show a higher complication rate and lower cervical range of motion when treated with external immobilization [13–15]. The authors advocate that type II fractures with displacement of less than 4 mm and an angulation < 10° should be treated with a halo vest or Minerva/Diadem cast for 6 weeks. Correspondingly, immobilization may be carried out for stable type III odontoid fractures.

3.2.2 Hagman's fracture

The traumatic spondylolisthesis of the axis (Hangman's fracture) is the second most common type of axis fractures (38%) [16]. For therapeutic aspects, the Effendi [17] and Levine [18] classifications have been established (**Table 9.3-2**).

Type I injuries comprise minimally displaced (< 3 mm) fractures of the pars interarticularis. The disc space below the axis is normal and stable. Type II injuries show a displacement of the anterior body (> 3 mm) with an abnormal disc space (the disc at C2/3 is affected). Within the type II group of Effendi et al, Levine identified injuries that have slight or no translation, but severe angulation (type IIA). Hyperextension and axial loading leads to rupture of the disc and the anterior longitudinal ligament, resulting in instability. Type I and type II injuries may be treated with a cervical brace or semirigid combicast collar for 6 weeks. For the reduction of type II injuries, the extension of the cervical spine within the orthosis is essential. Type IIA injuries may be treated with halo immobilization or Minerva/Diadem cast if the alignment can be maintained. The highly unstable type III injuries are relatively rare. Here the facets at C2/3 are dislocated and locked, maintaining the body of C2 in a position of flexion with the disc space at C2/3 open posteriorly. Type III injuries generally require operative stabilization.

3.2.3 C2-body fractures

Isolated fractures of the C2 vertebral body may be treated with a hard collar or semirigid combicast collar for 6 weeks if the fracture orientation is coronal (type I) or sagittal (type II) [19]. Only in highly displaced fractures causing stenosis of the vertebral artery is halo immobilization or a Minerva/Diadem cast required. The teardrop fracture of C2 (type III) generally occurs after high-energy trauma with hyperextension of the cervical spine [20]. Purely anterior fractures of C2 have no impact on stability and can be immobilized with a hard collar or semirigid combicast collar. However, if the fracture continues into the C2/3 intervertebral disc and the common posterior vertebral ligament, leading to C2/3 instability, operative treatment is required. This type of injury should not be confused with teardrop fractures occurring in the lower cervical spine as the result of a compression-flexion mechanism. These fractures are significantly more unstable and, therefore, have to be treated operatively [21].

Effendi Classification of Traumatic Spondylolisthesis of the Axis (as modified by Levine)

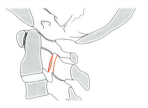

Type I
Nondisplaced fractures and those with up to 3 mm of displacement and no angulation

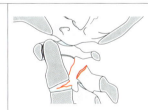

Type II
Displacement greater than 3 mm as well as angulation

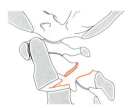

Type IIA
Moderate degrees of displacement combined with severe angulation

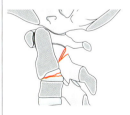

Type III
Unilateral or bilateral facet dislocations in addition to the bilateral posterior element fractures

Table 9.3-2   Effendi classification of traumatic spondylolisthesis of the axis (Hangman's fracture) as modified by Levine [17, 18].

3.2.4 Spinous-process and transverse-process fractures

Spinous-process fractures and transverse-process fractures are stable, and so soft collar immobilization for 6 weeks is sufficient. However, a posterior ligamentous injury might coexist if the spinous-process fracture was caused by a flexion mechanism. In this case, surgical stabilization may even be mandatory. The treatment of lateral-mass fractures depends on the neurological status of the patient. In the case of a spinal-cord injury, the fracture is always considered as unstable and operative treatment is required. In isolated root injuries, nonoperative treatment is possible as long as the fracture does not compromise the neural foramen. Therefore, the patient can be immobilized with a hard collar, sternal-occipital-mandibular immobilizer (**Fig 9.3-4**) or Minerva/Diadem cast. Compression or burst fractures are also possible candidates for external management. However, one should be aware that these injuries tend to result in kyphosis and, therefore, the orthosis must supply a good extension moment and must be rigid [22].

3.2.5 Fractures of the C2 in children

When it comes to fractures of the C2 in children, nonoperative treatment is a good option even with unstable cervical spine fractures or luxation. Minerva/Diadem casts are considered most effective (**Fig 9.3-5**).

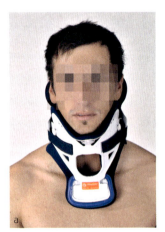
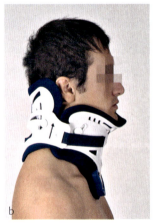

Fig 9.3-4a–b Miami cervical brace (sternal-occipital-mendiobular immobilizer).

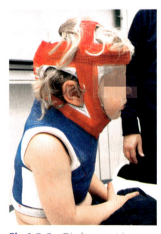

Fig 9.3-5 Diadem cast in a 4-year-old boy.

Authors   Florian Gebhard, Peter Richter, Bastian Scheiderer

4   Thoracic and lumbar spine

Most spine fractures are located in the thoracolumbar area because of the transition zone between the fixed kyphotic thoracic spine and the relatively flexible lordotic lumbar spine.

The majority of thoracic and lumbar spine fractures have to be treated operatively because of their instability and the risk of neurological damage. The goal of every therapy should be pain reduction, early mobilization, avoidance of muscular atrophy, as well as the prevention of neurological damage. Stable fractures without neurological damage should be treated nonoperatively with or without a corset (**Fig 9.3-6**). Kyphoplasty, ie, dorsal and/or ventral stabilization, should be performed when the fractures are unstable.

4.1   Stable fractures

According to the Magerl AO Classification of Spine Injuries [23], stable fractures include the following:

- A1.1 Endplate impaction: This fracture occurs due to axial compression and is often seen in osteoporotic spines. The posterior wall of the vertebra is intact. The spinal canal is not affected. However, the height of the vertebra is reduced

- A1.2 Wedge impaction fractures: This fracture is also due to axial compression. The posterior column wall of the vertebra is intact. The loss of the height can be either located in the upper part of the vertebra, in the inferior part of the vertebra, or anterolaterally

- A2.1 Sagittal split fractures: The vertebral body is split in the sagittal plane with various degrees of displacement. The posterior wall stays unharmed. Depending on the degree of displacement, surgery may be necessary

- A2.2 Coronal split fractures: The vertebral body is split in the coronal plane. The posterior wall stays unharmed. Depending on the degree of displacement, surgery may be necessary.

4.2   Nonoperative treatment

Pain control and mobility restriction are important in the early phase after trauma. For further pain reduction and stabilization of the spine, a corset, eg, a three-point corset, may be worn (see chapters 17.1 Corset using plaster of Paris; 17.2 Corset using synthetic, combicast technique; and 17.3 Removable corset using synthetic, combicast technique) and see **Fig 9.3-7**.

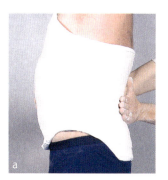
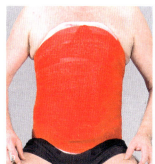
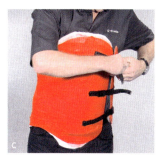
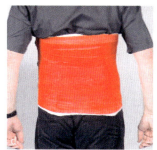

Fig 9.3-7a–d   Immobilization after fracture reduction in vertebral hyperlordosis.

a Corset using plaster of Paris.
b Corset using synthetic, combicast technique.
c–d Removable corset using synthetic, combicast technique.

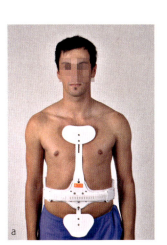
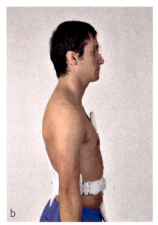

Fig 9.3-6a–b   Thoracolumbar orthosis.

9.3

GUIDELINES

In addition to the stable fractures outlined by Magerl, type A1.3 fractures can also be treated nonoperatively as long as the resources are available, and especially with children and adolescents (**Fig 9.3-8**). However, the fracture must first be reduced in vertebral hyperlordosis. As compression fractures of the lumbar spine often result in kyphosis, by using lumbar hyperlordosis the fractures are reduced, and the retention is then secured by the corset in hyperlordosis.

Radiological reevaluation should be conducted after 7 days, 14 days, and 6 weeks in order to ascertain that the fracture remains stable. This can either be done by x-ray or CT scan. After 6 weeks, full motion is allowed.

Table 9.3-3 provides an overview of the various types of thoracic and lumbar spine fractures and the available treatment options [23].

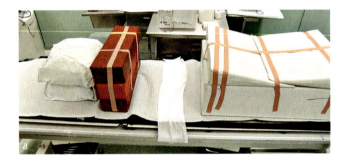
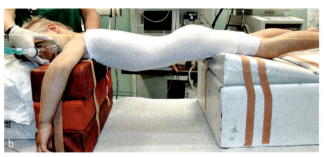
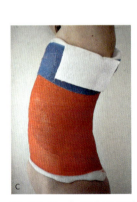
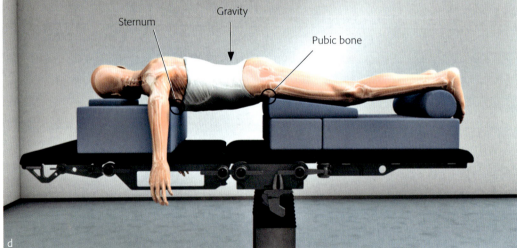

Fig 9.3-8a–d   Patient positioning for cast immobilization after fracture reduction in vertebral hyperlordosis.

a Preparing for a spine corset with simple tools (self-made hyperlordosis table). The entire body will be "sagging".

b Sagging patient positioning.

c Corset in hyperlordosis.

d Image showing the three-point principle at work resulting in the lumbar spine being in hyperlordosis to allow reduction of the vertebral compression fracture.

Authors   Florian Gebhard, Peter Richter, Bastian Scheiderer

Magerl AO Classification	Type of fracture	Fracture pattern	Nonoperative treatment	Operative treatment
A1.1		Wedge pattern, endplate impression stable	Indicated	Not indicated
A1.2		Wedge impaction, stable	Indicated	Limited indication
A1.3		Corpus collapse	Only in special situations	Recommended treatmentw
A2.1		Sagittal split fracture, stable	Only in special situations	Recommended treatment
A2.2		Coronal split fracture stable	Only in special situations	Recommended treatment
A2.3		Pincer fracture	Only in special situations	Recommended treatment
A3.1		Incomplete burst	Only in special situations	Recommended treatment
A3.2		Split burst	Only in special situations	Recommended treatment

Magerl AO Classification	Type of fracture	Fracture pattern	Nonoperative treatment	Operative treatment
A3.3		Complete burst	Only in special situations	Recommended treatment
B1		Flexion-distraction fractures	Only in special situations	Recommended treatment
B2		Flexion-distraction fractures	Only in special situations	Recommended treatment
B3		Flexion-distraction fractures	Not indicated	Recommended treatment
C1		Rotation injuries/fractures	Not indicated	Recommended treatment
C2		Rotation injuries/fractures	Not indicated	Recommended treatment
C3		Rotation injuries/fractures	Not indicated	Recommended treatment

Table 9.3-3 Overview of various types of fractures according to the Magerl AO Classification of thoracic and lumbar spine fractures, and the available treatment options.

Authors   Florian Gebhard, Peter Richter, Bastian Scheiderer

5   Summary

- In contrast to the recommendations made by Böhler, cast immobilization is rarely used for spine fractures in developed countries, yet when nonoperative treatment of spine injuries is indicated, custom-made individually adjusted or removable corsets and orthoses can be used
- In special situations, as well as in developing countries, corsets are a valid alternative to operative treatment
- In the cervical spine, depending on the stability level, treatment options range from immobilization by cervical collars and braces, to halo, Minerva, or Diadem casts/orthoses, with sternal-occipital-mandibular type immobilizers being the most effective in limiting the upper cervical spine motion of nonhalo devices

- Traumatic ruptures of intervertebral discs are indications for operative stabilization
- If not displaced, isolated fractures of the C2 vertebral body can be treated with a hard collar or semirigid combicast collar, including purely anterior fractures of the C2, which have no impact on stability
- Unstable thoracic and lumbar spine fractures must be treated operatively because of the risk of neurological damage, yet some injuries can be treated nonoperatively, especially stable fractures, and fractures in children, once the fracture has first been reduced in vertebral hyperlordosis.

9.3

GUIDELINES

6   References

1. **Böhler L**. [*The Treatment of Fractures*]. Vol 1 and 2. 9th–11th ed. Vienna: Wilhelm Maudrich; 1943. German.
2. **Johnson RM, Hart DL, Simmons EF, et al**. Cervical orthoses. A study comparing their effectiveness in restricting cervical motion in normal subjects. *J Bone Joint Surg Am*. 1977 Apr; 59(3):332–339.
3. **Dvorak J, Schneider E, Saldinger P, et al**. Biomechanics of the craniocervical region: the alar and transverse ligaments. *J Orthop Res*. 1988; 6(3):452–461.
4. **Kakarla UK, Chang SW, Theodore N, et al**. Atlas fractures. *Neurosurgery*. 2010 Mar; 66(3 Suppl):60–67.
5. **Dickman CA, Greene KA, Sonntag VK**. Injuries involving the transverse atlantal ligament: classification and treatment guidelines based upon experience with 39 injuries. *Neurosurgery*. 1996 Jan; 38(1):44–50.
6. **Hadley MN, Dickman CA, Browner CM, et al**. Acute traumatic atlas fractures: management and long term outcome. *Neurosurgery*. 1988 Jul; 23(1):31–35.
7. **Levine AM, Edwards CC**. Fractures of the atlas. *J Bone Joint Surg Am*. 1991 Jun; 73(5):680–691.
8. **Segal LS, Grimm JO, Stauffer ES**. Non-union of fractures of the atlas. *J Bone Joint Surg Am*. 1987 Dec; 69(9):1423–1434.
9. **Denaro V, Papalia R, Di Martino A, et al**. The best surgical treatment for type II fractures of the dens is still controversial. *Clin Orthop Relat Res*. 2011 Mar; 469(3):742–750.
10. **Anderson LD, D'Alonzo RT**. Fractures of the odontoid process of the axis. *J Bone Joint Surg Am*.1974 Dec; 56(8):1663–1674.
11. **Müller EJ, Schwinnen I, Fischer K, et al**. Non-rigid immobilisation of odontoid fractures. *Eur Spine J*. 2003 Oct; 12(5):522–525.
12. **Nourbakhsh A, Shi R, Vannemreddy P, et al**. Operative versus nonoperative management of acute odontoid Type II fractures: a meta-analysis. *J Neurosurg Spine*. 2009 Dec; 11(6):651–658.
13. **Seybold EA, Bayley JC**. Functional outcome of surgically and conservatively managed dens fractures. *Spine* (Phila Pa 1976). 1998 Sep; 23(17):1837–1845.
14. **Lennarson PJ, Mostafavi H, Traynelis VC, et al**. Management of type II dens fractures: a case-control study. *Spine* (Phila Pa 1976). 2000 May; 25(10):1234–1237.
15. **Tashjian RZ, Majercik S, Biffl WL, et al**. Halo-vest immobilization increases early morbidity and mortality in elderly odontoid fractures. *J Trauma*. 2006 Jan; 60(1):199–203.
16. **Ryan MD, Henderson JJ**. The epidemiology of fractures and fracture-dislocations of the cervical spine. *Injury*. 1992; 23(1):38–40.
17. **Effendi B, Roy D, Cornish B, et al**. Fractures of the ring of the axis. A classification based on the analysis of 131 cases. *J Bone Joint Surg Br*. 1981; 63-B(3):319–327.
18. **Levine AM, Edwards CC**. The management of traumatic spondylolisthesis of the axis. *J Bone Joint Surg Am*. 1985 Feb; 67(2):217–226.
19. **Benzel EC, Hart BL, Ball PA, et al**. Fractures of the C-2 vertebral body. *J Neurosurg*. 1994 Aug; 81(2):206–212.
20. **Vialle, R, Schmider L, Levassor N, et al**. [Extension tear-drop fracture of the axis: a surgically treated case]. *Rev Chir Orthop Reparatrice Appar Mot*. 2004 Apr; 90(2):152–155. French.
21. **Kim HJ, Lee KY, Kim WC**. Treatment outcome of cervical tear drop fracture. *Asian Spine J*. 2009 Dec; 3(2):73–79.
22. **Stannard JP, Schmidt AH, Kregor PJ (eds)**. Injuries to the cervicocranium. *Surgical Treatment of Orthopaedic Trauma*. 1st ed. New York: Thieme Medical Publishers; 2007:101–137.
23. **Aebi M, Magerl F**. Classification of injuries of the thoracic and lumbar spine. Aebi M, Arlet V, Webb JK (eds). *AO Spine Manual*. Vol 2. Stuttgart, New York: Thieme Medical Publishers; 2007:41–75

9.4 Pediatric fractures

Thomas Neubauer

9.4

GUIDELINES

Author   Thomas Neubauer

9.4   Pediatric fractures

1   Introduction

Although the number of indications for surgical fixation of pediatric fractures has increased over recent decades, today, more than 90% of all pediatric fractures in industrialized countries are still treated nonoperatively [1]. The skills of nonoperative treatment are still required in order to perform basic therapy if surgical therapy cannot be applied. Therefore, a thorough knowledge of closed fracture reduction and immobilization techniques, as well as their indications, represents a prerequisite for the treatment of the vast majority of children's fractures.

2   Advantages pediatric bones have compared with adult bones

The healing properties of pediatric bones have a number of specific advantages not found in adults, making nonoperative treatment suitable for the majority of fractures in this age group. These include:
- Callus formation is more extensive
- Callus formation is quicker and more reliable
- Callus is quickly degraded
- Spontaneous correction of primary malalignment occurs by growth
- The condition of local soft tissues and vascularity is usually optimal
- Persisting deficits as a result of immobilization are rare.

3   Disadvantages pediatric bones have compared with adult bones

Despite the quicker and more reliable healing properties of young bones, there are, however, a number of disadvantages that need to be considered. These include:
- Due to human growth, a surgeon has to deal with various skeletal developmental stages. This requires a sound knowledge of the adequate therapy for each specific age group. The potential for spontaneous correction must be calculated individually for every fracture in respect to location, growth potential, and corrective mechanisms
- Posttraumatic mechanisms can sometimes cause growth disturbances and aggravate into primary posttraumatic malalignment, a phenomenon that can occur independently of the chosen therapy or the quality of treatment
- Due to the rapid callus formation in pediatric bones, there is a shorter time frame for any successful change in therapy
- In younger children, cooperation between patient and doctor may be restricted, and communication can sometimes become more complex as parents have to be included into the decision making process.

9.4

4 Spontaneous correction and remodeling of bones

The reason that most pediatric fractures can be treated non-operatively is based on the most impressive advantage of the growing skeleton, namely the spontaneous correction of posttraumatic malalignment by growth. The reliability of this remodeling phenomenon depends on several parameters [2]:

- The location: Usually the osteogenic capacity in the metaphyseal area is more pronounced than in the diaphysis. In particular, the contribution of the neighboring physis to growth, which is genetically determined, has a great influence on correction. In the upper extremity, the peripheral physes (proximal humerus, distal radius) contribute considerably to the growth of the bones (usually 80%) (see **Fig 9.4-1**). In contrast, this pattern differs completely in the lower extremity, as here the central physes contribute 80% and the peripheral 20% to growth
- The age of the patient: In general, the corrective potential diminishes continuously from the age of 10–12 years onwards and only minor axial deviations can be tolerated
- The fracture plane: Generally a uniplanar malalignment can be corrected more easily than a multiplanar one. Malalignment situated in the plane of function (eg, sagittal malalignment in fingers) is also corrected more easily by growth than those with an orientation perpendicular to that plane
- The number of interventions: Repeated interventions can cause growth disturbances and, therefore, all invasive interventions as well as manipulations should be kept to a minimum.

Differing results are to be expected in regard to spontaneous correction in different locations depending on the affected bone/epiphysis, age of the patient, and specific orientation of the malalignment.

The local mechanisms of bone remodeling are varied and include specific features as well as completely unspecific processes in which correction occurs by chance through physiological growth mechanisms. These include:

- Fracture angulations: Angulations are corrected by the physis through asymmetric growth as, according to Pauwels, the physis next to a fracture has the disposition to orientate itself perpendicular to the incoming forces [3]. Diaphyseal fracture angulations are corrected by bone apposition onto the concave side of the bone, while on the convex side (tension side) bone is absorbed in accordance with the law of cortical drift (where bones adapt in response to stress/force)
- Posttraumatic overgrowth: It is well known that increased growth activity occurs after trauma, whose effect is more dramatic in the lower extremity. Femoral overgrowth is independent of the fracture level within the bone, age, and position of fracture during healing; it achieves 0.9 cm on average [4]. In contrast, tibial overgrowth is age dependent and less pronounced. However, one theory suggests that posttraumatic hyperemia of a bone and its physes initiates various mechanisms that affect bone length prognosis. Thus, prolonged hyperemia (ie, by intense bone remodeling) produces increased length whenever there is a wide open physis nearby. On the other hand, a paradoxical shortening of the bone may occur in older children as the increased activity contributes to early physeal closure
- Anteversion: Physiological mechanisms such as the development of femoral neck anteversion may show some influence on a rotational malalignment.

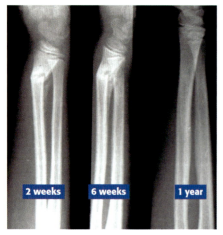

Fig 9.4-1 Distal radial fracture in a young patient, with nonoperative treatment in a plaster cast. Remodeling leads to rebuilding and anatomical change.

Author   Thomas Neubauer

5   Indications for nonoperative treatment

Nonoperative treatment of pediatric fractures, in addition to plaster of Paris and synthetic casts, includes a range of prefabricated and custom-made bandages and devices. However, plaster of Paris (POP) casts cover the majority of indications as it is always available, can be easily applied and contoured to the body surface, and is neither toxic nor inflammable (chapter 6 Properties of cast materials). Due to the quick availability, low cost, and few contraindications for its application, POP is still the working horse in the treatment of pediatric fractures around the world (chapter 7 Socioeconomic considerations). Other options for the nonoperative treatment of pediatric fractures include semirigid synthetic casts or tapes, bandages, and orthoses.

Generally, all articular fractures without primary or secondary displacement (gap < 2 mm, step-off < 2 mm), and well-reduced joint dislocations without additional intraarticular pathology, are eligible for nonoperative treatment.

Metaphyseal fractures are frequently fixed by K-wires or lag screws. Therefore, an additional immobilization is required in order to obtain sufficient stability.

In shaft fractures, nonoperative treatment is applied in nondisplaced fractures and in fractures that do not exceed certain limits of deviation (**Table 9.4-1**). These limits depend on the age of the patient, the power of the local physis, as well as the direction of the deformity. The duration of immobilization for fracture healing differs with age, location, and fracture pattern.

Region		Accepted displacement for nonoperative treatment (age-dependent)	Nonoperative treatment	Duration (on average)	Operative treatment
Humerus, proximal		< 12 years < 40°	Gilchrist Velpeau	3–4 weeks	K-wires
Humerus, shaft		Side to side: shaft width Shortening: < 1 cm Sagittal/frontal: < 10°	Gilchrist Velpeau (brace after 2 weeks)	4 weeks	ESIN[1] (external fixator) (IMN[2])
Humerus, distal	Supracondylar:	Sagittal: < 7 years: 20° > 7 years: none Frontal: none Rotation: none	Collar and cuff: Above-elbow cast	4 weeks	K-wires ESIN[1] (external fixator)
	Radial condyle:	None	Above-elbow cast	4–5 weeks	K-wires Cannulated screws Plates (adolescents)
	Ulnar epicondyle:	None	Above-elbow cast	4 weeks	K-wires Cannulated screws
Forearm, proximal	Radial head:	< 5 years: 60°, 1/2 shaft width < 10 years: 40°, 1/3 shaft width < 14 years: 20° > 14 years: 10°	Above-elbow cast	4 weeks	ESIN[1] K-wires
	Olecranon:	Frontal: none Rotation: none Sagittal: -10°	Above-elbow cast		K-wires Tension-band wiring Screws

9.4

Region		Accepted displacement for nonoperative treatment (age-dependent)	Nonoperative treatment	Duration (on average)	Operative treatment
	Forearm, shaft (proximal and middle third)	Frontal and sagittal: < 5 years: -15° > 5 years: -10° Rotation: none	Above-elbow cast	4–5 weeks	ESIN[1] (plate: if ESIN[1] is contraindicated)
	Forearm, distal	< 12 years: angulations up to 30° Side to side: shaft width > 12yrs: angulations: 10–20° Side to side: ¼ shaft width	Above-elbow cast (both bones) Below-elbow cast (one bone)	3–4 weeks	K-wires (External fixator, plate: diaphyseal/metaphyseal transition zone)
	Proximal femur	≤ 3 years: none	Hip spica cast	4–6 weeks	K-wires Screws
	Femur, shaft	< 3 years: side-to-side: full diameter Shortening: 1 2 cm Varus: 20° Valgus: 10° Antecurvation: 10° Rotation: 20°	Overhead extension (< 15 kg) Hip spica cast	2 weeks	ESIN[1] (external fixator) Adolescent nail
		> 3 years < 10 years: side-to-side: half diameter Sagittal/frontal: none Rotation: 20°	Overhead extension (< 15 kg) Hip spica cast	4 weeks/ 2 weeks after overhead extension	
	Distal femur	Side-to-side: ¼ width Sagittal/frontal: none Rotation: none	Long leg cast	4 weeks	K-wires Screws External fixator
	Patella	None	Long leg cast	4 weeks	K-wires Cerclage wire Screws
	Tibia, proximal	None	Long leg cast	4 weeks	K-wires External fixator Plate

Author   Thomas Neubauer

Region		Accepted displacement for nonoperative treatment (age-dependent)	Nonoperative treatment	Duration (on average)	Operative treatment
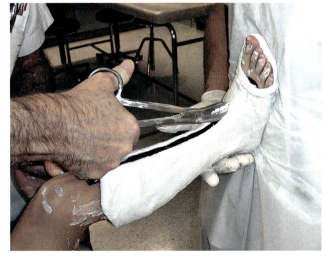	Tibia, shaft	< 10° varus < 5° valgus < 10° re-/antecurvation No shortening No rotation	Long leg cast	4–5 weeks	ESIN[1] Plate External fixator
	Tibia, distal	< 10 years: <10° re-/antecurvation, < 10° varus/valgus; rotation: none > 10 years: anatomic reduction	Short leg cast (long leg cast in small children)	2–3 weeks	K-wires External fixator Screws

[1] Elastic stable intramedullary nailing (ESIN)

[2] Intramedullary nailing (IMN)

Table 9.4-1   Recommendations for nonoperative versus operative treatment in selected pediatric fractures.

6   Contraindications for nonoperative treatment

Application of an immobilizing bandage represents a closed "surgical intervention", especially when combined with reduction maneuvers for a fracture. Sources of complications include an inadequate technique, wrong indications, and bandages not adapted to age group. Some nonoperative techniques, like the wedging of a cast (see topic 12 in chapter 3 Principles of casting) or traction therapy, require a meticulous technique and regular controls in order to prevent complications.

Generally, a closed and circumferential plaster cast should not be applied after acute trauma, immediately postoperatively, or in situations where soft-tissue swelling can be expected. Circular bandages cannot adapt to an increased compartment volume and may provoke compartment syndrome. Therefore, in acute situations, only a well-padded POP splint or a split cast (**Fig 9.4-2**) are allowed in order to achieve immobilization. From a local point of view, contraindications may exist from changes of the soft tissues and/or skin. Allergic reactions to bandages and padding materials are rare.

Fig 9.4-2   Preparation of a split circular cast.

9.4

7 Nonoperative treatment

Generally, most fractures in children can be treated nonoperatively. However, using a nonsurgical procedure must result in a comparable, adequate functional and anatomical outcome. Fractures situated next to a wide open and powerful physis, such as the eccentric physes of the upper extremity or the central physes of the lower extremity, will show more spontaneous correction capacity in response to posttraumatic malalignment. The younger the child, the more reliably these mechanisms will function. Deviations in the main functional axis of the body (sagittal plane) will correct more easily.

In the following paragraphs we present, region by region, the treatment options.

7.1 Proximal humerus

Metaphyseal lesions represent the majority of fractures and, up to an age of 12 years, will heal with excellent correction of posttraumatic deformities (< 40° angulation). Therefore, most fractures can be treated nonoperatively in a Gilchrist (see chapter 18.3 Gilchrist bandage) or Velpeau bandage without prior reduction of the fracture.

7.2 Humerus, shaft

The majority of these fractures occur in adolescents with a low correction potential. Keeping in mind that even low-grade malalignment can represent a distinct cosmetic compromise, it is the current trend to stabilize such fractures operatively, especially in older pediatric patients. If treated nonoperatively, a Gilchrist, Velpeau, or Desault's bandage can be applied (see chapter 18.3 Gilchrist bandage), possibly followed by a Sarmiento brace (see chapter 15.5 Sarmiento humeral brace using synthetic, combicast technique).

7.3 Distal humerus

In supracondylar fractures of the distal humerus, only nondisplaced fractures (grade I) or fractures with uniplanar displacement (grade II) are treated nonoperatively with an above-elbow cast (see chapters 15.1 Long arm splint using plaster of Paris; 15.2 Long arm splint using synthetic; 15.3 Long arm cast using plaster of Paris; and 15.4 Long arm cast using synthetic, combicast technique) or a collar and cuff bandage (**Fig 9.4-3** and **Fig 9.4-4**) (see chapter 18.1 Collar and cuff bandage).

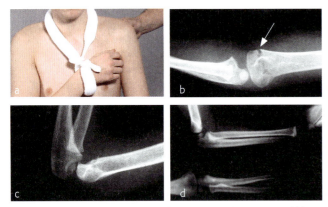

Fig 9.4-3a–d Collar and cuff bandage treatment for a 4-year-old boy.
a Example of a collar and cuff bandage.
b Supracondylar distal humerus fracture (the fracture gap is marked). The patient, a 4-year-old boy, suffered direct trauma on the elbow.
c X-ray after 5 days of immobilization in a collar and cuff bandage, with good anatomical reduction. The Baumann line cuts the capitulum in the middle third.
d The consolidated supracondylar fracture after 5 weeks with good callus formation especially on the radial side.

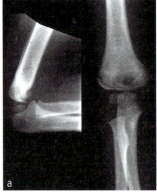
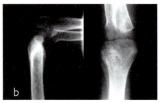

Fig 9.4-4a–b Collar and cuff bandage treatment for a 2-year-old girl.
a Radial epicondyle fracture of a 2-year-old girl, with a small gap at the radial condyle nearly visible.
b Two weeks later, x-ray in collar and cuff, with fracture gap visible, and callus formation on the dorsal and radial aspect of the distal humerus.

Author   Thomas Neubauer

More severe forms (grade III and IV) require operative stabilization with K-wires, with additional postoperative immobilization in an above-elbow cast (see chapters 15.1 Long arm splint using plaster of Paris; 15.2 Long arm splint using synthetic; 15.3 Long arm cast using plaster of Paris; and 15.4 Long arm cast using synthetic, combicast technique), a Gilchrist bandage (see chapter 18.3 Gilchrist bandage), or a Desault's or Velpeau bandage for 4 weeks.

In fractures of the radial condyle, only nondisplaced fractures are treated nonoperatively, while primary or secondarily displaced fractures need to be fixed operatively followed by postoperative immobilization (see chapters 15.1 Long arm splint using plaster of Paris; 15.2 Long arm splint using synthetic; 15.3 Long arm cast using plaster of Paris; and 15.4 Long arm cast using synthetic, combicast technique).

7.4   Radial head
Although its physis contributes little to growth, there are still excellent correction options at this site. However, this area also has very delicate local vascularity, which can easily be disturbed. Therefore, reduction is accomplished only in cases of severe displacement and should be performed in a closed procedure whenever possible. Yet, repeated and frustrated attempts at closed reduction can also damage the physis. The least traumatic manner for reduction of severely displaced fractures is by elastic stable intramedullary nailing (ESIN), which requires no further immobilization of the forearm. All other cases require temporary immobilization with a plaster cast or bandages (see chapters 15.1 Long arm splint using plaster of Paris; 15.2 Long arm splint using synthetic; 15.3 Long arm cast using plaster of Paris; and 15.4 Long arm cast using synthetic, combicast technique) followed by mobilization without physical therapy.

7.5   Forearm, middle and proximal third
With the middle and proximal third of the forearm, only nondisplaced and stable reduced fractures are treated nonoperatively in an above-elbow cast (see chapters 15.1 Long arm splint using plaster of Paris; 15.2 Long arm splint using synthetic; 15.3 Long arm cast using plaster of Paris; and 15.4 Long arm cast using synthetic, combicast technique) as the spontaneous correction is very limited and even small angulations of 10° may cause severe functional impairment. Angulations with narrowing of the interosseous space are especially not acceptable. Thus, most primary displaced fractures at this location are treated operatively with ESIN. In the nonoperative treatment of greenstick fractures in this location, care must be taken in order to achieve a balanced compression of the whole fracture zone during reduction. If not, the concave cortex, which has usually only been fractured partially, will heal more rapidly than the gaping cortex on the convex side, causing a so-called "partial non-union" with an increased risk of causing refracture [5].

7.6   Distal forearm
A very good correction capacity exists in the distal forearm up to the age of 12 years, so most of these fractures are treated nonoperatively. However, while simple buckle fractures can be treated with a removable POP splint, greenstick and complete fractures show a tendency for redisplacement and need continuous radiographic controls and change of cast (see chapters 15.1 Long arm splint using plaster of Paris; 15.2 Long arm splint using synthetic; 15.3 Long arm cast using plaster of Paris; 15.4 Long arm cast using synthetic, combicast technique; 15.6 Dorsopalmar (radial) short arm splint using plaster of Paris; 15.7 Dorsopalmar (radial) short arm splint using synthetic; 15.8 Palmar short arm splint using plaster of Paris; 15.9 Palmar short arm splint using synthetic; 15.10 Dorsal short arm splint using synthetic; 15.11 Short arm cast using plaster of Paris; and 15.12 Short arm cast using synthetic, combicast technique).

7.7 Proximal femur

Most fractures in this area are displaced and represent surgical and orthopedic emergencies. In rare cases of nondisplaced proximal femoral fractures in older children, operative treatment offers great advantages in respect to mobilization and the patient's comfort. If no surgical emergency facilities are available, the immobilization in a hip spica or an overhead extension may be the only option after reduction (**Fig 9.4-5**).

7.8 Femur, shaft

In the shaft of the femur, spontaneous corrections of axial deviations can be expected—even the capacity for some compensation of rotational deformities by growth has been noted. However, remodeling mechanisms may also cause growth disturbances resulting in leg-length discrepancies. This phenomenon should be considered in all displaced fractures and, preferably, these should be reduced and stabilized by osteosynthesis in order to allow mobilization and weight bearing. Theoretically, femoral fractures can be treated in a Pavlik harness (age up to 6 months), by overhead traction of the hips at 90° (age up to 2 maximally 3 years; < 9.1 kg), or by a hip spica cast (**Fig 9.4-5**) (see chapters 16.1 One-and-a-half leg hip spica cast using plaster of Paris; and 16.2 Single leg hip spica cast using synthetic, combicast technique).

Treatment algorithms differ widely according to geographic location. In some countries, femoral shaft fractures are treated with initial overhead extension for 2 weeks followed by a hip spica cast only in infancy (see chapters 16.1 One-and-a-half leg hip spica cast using plaster of Paris; and 16.2 Single leg hip spica cast using synthetic, combicast technique), because with older children, nonoperative treatment is associated with various soft-tissue problems and less reliable realignment.

7.9 Distal femur (supracondylar)

Most fractures of the distal femur are displaced and require reduction. No deviations are to be accepted, because a high rate of secondary malalignment and growth disturbance can be expected. Thus, reduced fractures should be immobilized by K-wires or screws, which are additionally protected by a long leg cast (see chapters 16.5 Dorsal long leg splint using plaster of Paris; 16.6 Long leg cast using plaster of Paris; and 16.7 Long leg cast using synthetic, combicast technique).

7.10 Proximal tibia

There is a tendency for valgus deviation to occur in metaphyseal fractures of the proximal tibia, which is detectable as a growing gape at the medial cortex. Normally, a cast is applied (see chapters 16.3 Cylinder long leg cast using synthetic, combicast technique; 16.5 Dorsal long leg splint using plaster of Paris; 16.6 Long leg cast using plaster of Paris; and 16.7 Long leg cast using synthetic, combicast technique). Normal axial alignment can be restored with reduction or wedging of the cast in light deviation (< 10°) (see topic 12 of chapter 3 Principles of casting).

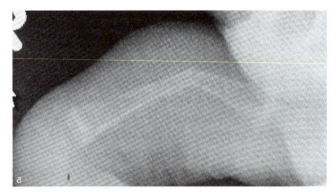

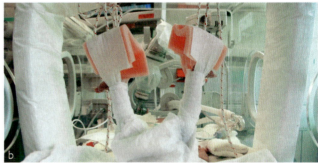

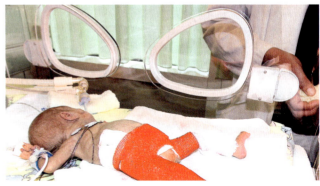

Fig 9.4-5a-c Proximal femur fractures.
a X-ray of a femur in a premature baby.
b Overhead extension in a premature baby.
c Hip spica in a premature baby.

7.11   Tibia, shaft

Most fractures represent isolated fractures of the tibia (70%), which show a tendency for varus displacement, while complete crural fractures (30%) show a tendency for valgus displacement. Isolated tibial fractures are eligible for nonoperative treatment (see chapters 16.5 Dorsal long leg splint using plaster of Paris; 16.6 Long leg cast using plaster of Paris; 16.7 Long leg cast using synthetic, combicast technique; or secondarily 16.8 Sarmiento (patella tendon bearing) cast using plaster of Paris; and 16.9 Sarmiento tibial brace using synthetic, combicast technique). A varus tendency may be corrected by wedging of the cast (see topic 12 in chapter 3 Principles of casting), but care must be taken in order to avoid soft-tissue lesions (**Fig 9.4-6**). Unstable fractures of both crural bones require reduction and stabilization by osteosynthesis.

7.12   Distal tibia (metaphysis)

Spontaneous correction of distal tibial fractures is limited to a range of 10° in the frontal as well as the sagittal plane. In patients older than 10 years, almost no correction is seen. Thus, most displaced fractures are reduced and fixed by K-wires and immobilized in a short leg cast (see chapters 16.10 Dorsal short leg splint using plaster of Paris; 16.11 Dorsal short leg splint using synthetic; 16.12 Short leg cast using rigid synthetic; and 16.13 Short leg cast using synthetic, combicast technique) or long leg cast (see chapters 16.5 Dorsal long leg splint using plaster of Paris; 16.6 Long leg cast using plaster of Paris; and 16.7 Long leg cast using synthetic, combicast technique), while nonoperative treatment is reserved for nondisplaced cases only.

Depending on the location, a short leg cast (see chapters 16.10 Dorsal short leg splint using plaster of Paris; 16.11 Dorsal short leg splint using synthetic; 16.12 Short leg cast using rigid synthetic; and 16.13 Short leg cast using synthetic, combicast technique) or a long leg cast is used (see chapters 16.5 Dorsal long leg splint using plaster of Paris; 16.6 Long leg cast using plaster of Paris; 16.7 Long leg cast using synthetic, combicast technique).

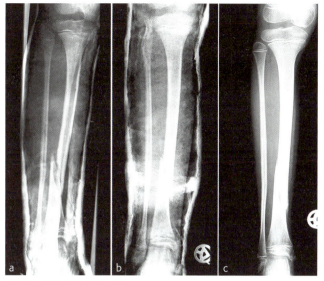
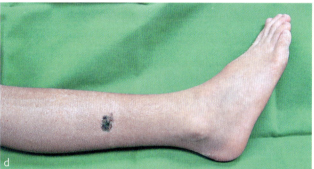
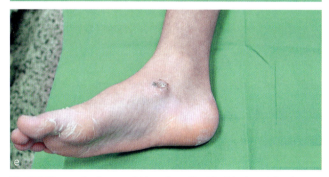

Fig 9.4-6a–e   An 8-year-old female patient that had sustained an isolated fracture of the right tibia while skiing, and who was treated with a plaster of Paris cast.
a X-ray controls at 2 weeks revealing nonacceptable varus displacement of the fragments.
b After wedging of the cast and a further 4 weeks of plaster immobilization, the malalignment was corrected.
c X-rays revealing an orthograde alignment of the healing fracture.
d–e However, after wedging of the cast, the patient complained about pains beneath the cast for one day. At cast removal, a circumscript skin necrosis is visible at the site of the wedge as well as in the area of the medial malleolus.

8 Which types of injury should always be operated?

A few decades ago, nearly all pediatric fractures were treated nonoperatively with only a few exceptions of absolute indications for operative treatment. However, in recent years in industrialized countries, the number of indications for operative stabilization of pediatric fractures increased both in absolute as well as relative indications (**Table 9.4-2**). Next to the socioeconomic demands of patients and parents, children are considered "developed" at an earlier age, and obesity is now a well-known factor needing to be considered even in pediatric patients [6].

However, the decision whether or not to operate is influenced by a wide range of factors, including:
- Type of fracture
- Soft-tissue damage
- Neurovascular status
- General condition
- Age
- Weight
- Bone segment
- Available equipment
- The experience level of the surgeon.

An overview of the indications for surgical fixation of pediatric fractures is given in **Table 9.4-2** [6].

Absolute indication	Relative indication
Open fracture	Ipsilateral, multiple fractures
Neurovascular damage	Bilateral fractures
Severe soft-tissue compromise	"Floating-joint" injury
Displaced intraarticular fracture	Age above 10 years
Irreducible fracture	Pathological fracture
Polytrauma	
Displaced femoral neck fracture	
Unstable forearm fracture	

Table 9.4-2 Indications for surgical fixation of pediatric fractures.

However, the risk of irritating a local physis at the fracture site even more by recurrent manipulation than by operative intervention, and thus affecting the outcome, has to be taken into consideration. Therefore, any reduction maneuver should result in a stable and definitive fracture situation that will persist until fracture healing has been completed. If these goals cannot be achieved by nonoperative treatment, surgical stabilization of the fracture site is then required.

9 Evidence and research

Further studies into pediatric fractures found the following:
- In buckle fractures of the forearm, removable splints achieve the same results as plaster casts [7, 8]
- The risk of redisplacement after distal radius fracture—the most frequently encountered fracture in childhood—is essentially influenced by the initial displacement (> 50% translation, > 30° axial deviation), quality of reduction, isolated radius fracture versus associated ulna fracture at the same level, casting technique, as well as atrophy of soft tissues during immobilization [9, 10, 11]
- Different indices reveal quality of casting and reduction in distal radius and forearm fractures: gap index [12], cast index [13], padding index [14], three-point index (anteroposterior and lateral) [15]
- Although a relatively high rate of redisplacement (approximately 30%) can be expected in distal radius fractures treated nonoperatively, primary pinning of these fractures reveals no superior functional outcome [16] and shows a high rate of pin track infections, therefore, routine pinning cannot be recommended [9]
- Unstable fractures of the diametaphyseal area of the radius are problematic and require transphyseal ESIN osteosynthesis in younger children and volar plating in adolescents [17]
- Nonoperative treatment of femoral shaft fractures is possible and is most often accomplished in infants using overhead traction and/or a hip spica cast. Although nonoperative treatment achieves good long-term functional results and remodeling in younger children [18], operative therapy provides early mobilization, a shorter hospital stay, and less malalignment [19].

Author   Thomas Neubauer

10   Operative and nonoperative treatment in complement

As already mentioned, applying a cast or bandage, with elective reduction of the fracture, represents a "closed surgical" manipulation, which has to be accomplished with the same planning and technical thoroughness as an operative procedure. Additionally, POP casts represent an ideal emergency tool in order to immobilize an extremity and to reduce pain. But nonoperative and operative measures are often not competitive, but complement one another, for instance in metaphyseal fractures fixed with K-wires and additionally stabilized by a plaster cast. The decision between nonoperative and surgical options is essentially influenced by the remaining time until end of growth and the local correction capacity for posttraumatic malalignment. Thus, a sound knowledge of the pathophysiological principles for pediatric fractures is the prerequisite for successful treatment.

Any manipulation under anesthesia should be exclusive. If a stable fracture situation is not obtainable with closed reduction, operative fixation of the fracture should be performed immediately. This has to be taken into consideration in preoperative planning and when informing the parents.

11   Variations in treatment—the influence of environmental, geographic, and socioeconomic factors in industrialized versus developing economies

Although the principles for the treatment of pediatric fractures are based on pathophysiology, the choice of treatment for an individual type of fracture will also be influenced by environmental and geographic factors. These include:

- The individual preference of the treating physician for a specific method
- The tradition of teaching in a specific country
- The skills of treating personnel being limited to some techniques only
- The limited availability of materials due to the developmental and economic situation [20, 21].

In most developing countries, splinting of a roughly reduced limb with POP will be practicable, while surgical treatment is often restricted to when indications suggest there is a need to save the extremity (ie, open fractures). Even in slightly more developed countries, nonoperative treatment will still predominate, as only a few people can afford the costs of an operation on a private basis. In many developing or moderately developed countries, the choice of implants will be reduced to external fixators and K-wires, which are almost always available, and which provide a basic method of stabilization.

In industrialized countries, with their large variety of available implants, the indication for operative treatment is not limited by a lack of resources. This is despite the same indication representing a surgically unsolvable problem in a developing country.

9.4

GUIDELINES

12 Summary

- Nonoperative treatment still represents the appropriate treatment for the vast majority of pediatric patients
- Fractures heal more rapidly in children than in adults, and the adverse effects of immobilization are minimal
- Nonoperative fracture treatment with plaster casts or support bandages is possible in stable diaphyseal and metaphyseal fractures that are nondisplaced or represent an acceptable degree of displacement in respect to local remodeling capacity
- In unstable metaphyseal fractures, casts or support bandages are employed to supplement minimal surgical fixation methods (such as K-wires)

- Articular fractures with less than 2 mm step-off and/or 2 mm gap are considered nondisplaced and can be treated nonoperatively
- Traction therapy should be the exception whenever an adequate operative therapy is available; most often the so-called overhead traction is used for femur fractures in children below the age of 2 years
- The various approaches to treatment are often influenced by regional traditions, socioeconomic factors, and the personal preference of the surgeon.

13 References

1. **Court-Brown CM, Aitken S, Hamilton TW, et al**. Nonoperative fracture treatment in the modern era. *J Trauma.* 2010 Sep; 69(3):699–707.
2. **Wilkins KE**. Principles of fracture remodeling in children. *Injury.* 2005 Feb; 36 Suppl 1:A3–A11.
3. **Pauwels F**. *Gesammelte Abhandlungen zur funktionellen Anatomie des Bewegungsapparates.* Berlin Heidelberg New York: Springer; 1965. German.
4. **Shapiro F**. Fractures of the femoral shaft in children. The overgrowth phenomenon. *Acta Orthop Scand.* 1981 Dec; 52(6):649–55.
5. **Schwarz N, Pienaar S, Schwarz AF, et al**. Refracture of the forearm in children. *J Bone Joint Surg Br.* 1996 Sep; 78(5): 740–744.
6. **Slongo TF**. The choice of treatment according to the type and location of the fracture and the age of the child. *Injury.* 2005 Feb; 36 Suppl 1:A12–A19.
7. **Abraham A, Handoll HH, Khan T**. Interventions for treating wrist fractures in children. *Cochrane Database Syst Rev;* 2008 16(2): CD004576.
8. **Kennedy SA, Slobogean GP, Mulpuri K**. Does degree of immobilization influence refracture rate in the forearm buckle fracture? *J Pediatr Orthop B.* 2010 Jan; 19(1):77–81.
9. **Bae DS**. Pediatric distal radius and forearm fractures. *J Hand Surg Am.* 2008 Dec; 33(10):1911–1923.

10. **Monga P, Raghupathy A, Courtman NH**. Factors affecting remanipulation in paediatric forearm fractures. *J Pediatr Orthop B.* 2010 Mar; 19(2):181–187.
11. **Zamzam MM, Khoshhal KI**. Displaced fracture of the distal radius in children: factors responsible for redisplacement after closed reduction. *J Bone Joint Surg Br.* 2005 Jun; 87(6): 841–843.
12. **Malviya A, Tsintzas D, Mahawar K, et al**. Gap index: a good predictor of failure of plaster cast in distal third radius fractures. *J Pediatr Orthop B.* 2007 Jan; 16(1):48–52.
13. **Chess DG, Hyndman JC, Leahey JL, et al**. Short arm plaster cast for distal pediatric forearm fractures. *J Pediatr Orthop.* 1994 Mar–Apr; 14(2):211–213.
14. **Bhatia M, Housden PH**. Re-displacement of paediatric forearm fractures: role of plaster moulding and padding. *Injury.* 2006 Mar; 37(3):259–268.
15. **AlemdaroÐlu KB, Iltar S, Cimen O, et al**. Risk factors in redisplacement of distal radial fractures in children. *J Bone Joint Surg Am.* 2008 Jun; 90(6):1224–1230.
16. **Miller BS, Taylor B, Widmann RF, et al**. Cast immobilization versus percutaneous pin fixation of displaced distal radius fractures in children: a prospective, randomized study. *J Pediatr Orthop.* 2005 Jul–Aug; 25(4):490–494.

17. **Lieber J, Sommerfeldt DW**. [Diametaphyseal forearm fracture in childhood. Pitfalls and recommendations for treatment]. *Unfallchirurg.* 2011 Apr; 114(4): 292–299. German.
18. **Frech-Dörfler M, Hasler CC, Häcker FM**. Immediate hip spica for unstable femoral shaft fractures in preschool children: still an efficient and effective option. *Eur J Pediatr Surg.* 2010 Jan; 20(1):18–23.
19. **Flynn JM, Luedtke LM , Gangley TJ, et al**. Comparison of titanium elastic nails with traction and a spica cast to treat femoral fractures in children. *J Bone Joint Surg Am.* 2004 Apr; 86-A(4):770–777.
20. **Kirsch TD, Beaudreau RW, Holder YA, et al**. Pediatric injuries presenting to an emergency department in a developing country. *Pediatr Emerg Care.* 1996 Dec; 12(6):411–415.
21. **Ouattara O, Kouame BD, Odehouri TH, et al**. [Results of treatment of forearm fractures in the child]. *Mali Med.* 2007; 22(3):43–46. French.

10 Soft-tissue damage and defects

Clemens Dumont

10

GUIDELINES

GUIDELINES

10

Author   Clemens Dumont

10   Soft-tissue damage and defects

1   Introduction

Soft-tissue damage can occur either isolated or in combination with fractured bone(s), and can be subdivided into blunt or penetrating injuries [1]. Clinical experience shows that there is a tendency to underestimate blunt trauma because, at first glance, it is less striking when compared with a penetrating injury.

Particularly in blunt trauma, it is necessary to search for:
- Vascular injuries [2]
- Nerve injuries and
- Compartment syndrome.

In high-energy traumas, their existence has to be presumed until they have been excluded.

Penetrating injuries can result from:
- Cuts
- Lacerations
- Stabbing
- Bites
- Intrusion of a foreign body.

By way of illustration, in 2008, Clayton and Court-Brown investigated isolated injuries of tendons and ligamentous injuries without fracture in the UK. Their research determined that for the upper extremity, the following incidences occurred that year [3]:
- Forearm/hand extensor tendon injuries (approximately 17.0%)
- Mallet finger (approximately 9.0%)
- Forearm/hand flexor tendon rupture (approximately 4.5%)
- Ulnar collateral ligament injury (approximately 3.2%).

While this chapter broadly explores skin and tissue damage and postoperative protection, more specific details on injuries to the ligaments and tendons, and of nerves, are found in chapters 11.1 Ligament and tendon injuries, and 11.2 Nerve injuries.

2   Diagnostics

Diagnostics in soft-tissue damage starts with history and information about the kind of injury. A standardized approach is strongly recommended. This author suggests, in order, inspection, palpation, perfusion, sensation sensitivity, and function.

Ultrasound is helpful in cases where hematoma is suspected, and can depict and describe the extent of hematoma as well as assist in visualizing the hemorrhage. Fractures are excluded or confirmed by x-ray if bony injury is suggested by history or examination. Computer tomography combined with angiography, if available, is a reasonable tool to localize supposed damage to the vascular system. In contrast to these, magnetic resonance imaging or electromyography play only a secondary role in acute soft-tissue injuries; they are seldom necessary.

3   AO Soft-Tissue Classification

The AO Soft-Tissue Classification quantifies soft-tissue damage and concentrates on the criteria of closed skin lesions (IC=integument closed) and open skin lesions (IO=integument open). Furthermore, in accordance with the AO Soft-Tissue Classification, it is possible to distinguish between muscle-tendon (MT) injury and neurovascular (NV) injury (**see Table 10-1**). Although the illustrations demonstrate soft-tissue injuries of the lower limb, they can be easily transferred to upper-limb tissue injuries.

In the case of severe soft-tissue damage, external fixation and stabilization is the method of choice in order to avoid further damage to the soft tissues. Internal fixation of the upper extremity is indicated whenever soft-tissue coverage is provided, or when flap covering will be available within a few days. On the other hand, casts with windows, or with an external traction device, are not adequate for the treatment of open fractures.

GUIDELINES

10

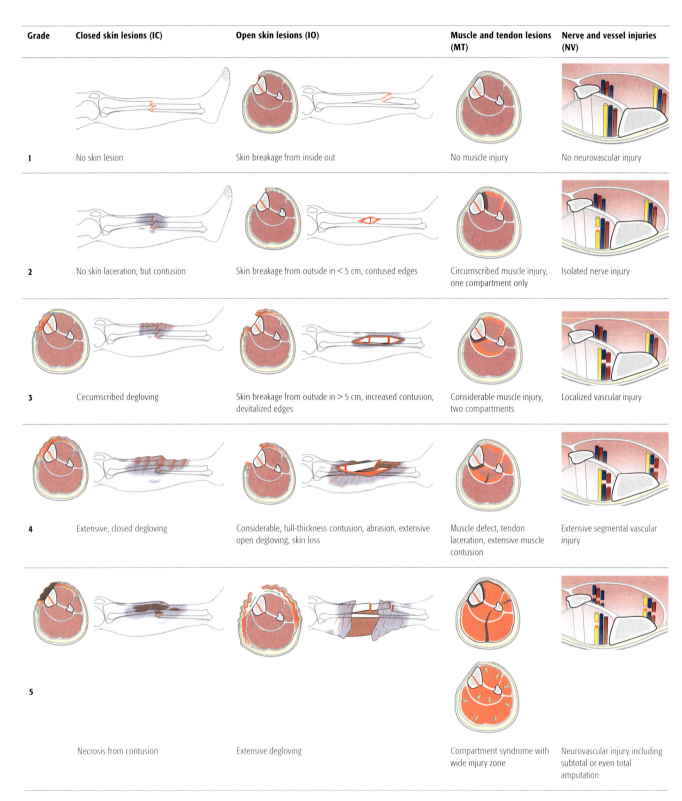

Grade	Closed skin lesions (IC)	Open skin lesions (IO)	Muscle and tendon lesions (MT)	Nerve and vessel injuries (NV)
1	No skin lesion	Skin breakage from inside out	No muscle injury	No neurovascular injury
2	No skin laceration, but contusion	Skin breakage from outside in < 5 cm, contused edges	Circumscribed muscle injury, one compartment only	Isolated nerve injury
3	Circumscribed degloving	Skin breakage from outside in > 5 cm, increased contusion, devitalized edges	Considerable muscle injury, two compartments	Localized vascular injury
4	Extensive, closed degloving	Considerable, full-thickness contusion, abrasion, extensive open degloving, skin loss	Muscle defect, tendon laceration, extensive muscle contusion	Extensive segmental vascular injury
5	Necrosis from contusion	Extensive degloving	Compartment syndrome with wide injury zone	Neurovascular injury including subtotal or even total amputation

Table 10-1 AO Soft-Tissue Classification [4].

Author Clemens Dumont

The following points should always be remembered:
- Do not underestimate soft-tissue injury, especially in the first few days postinjury
- Treat operatively those fractures with open integument in order to avoid further soft-tissue damage that cannot be assessed accurately under a cast or splint
- Treat operatively those fractures with closed integument and severe soft-tissue injury grade II or higher.

Temporary plaster of Paris or synthetic splints are indicated as emergency immobilization until the operative treatment can be initiated.

4 Postoperative protection until wound healing

Overall, a limited postoperative protection for a short period of time can reduce pain and secure the result of the operative therapy (see chapters 15.13 Thumb spica splint using plaster of Paris; 15.14 Thumb spica splint using synthetic; 15.17 Dorsopalmar (ulnar gutter) short arm splint including two or more fingers using plaster of Paris; 15.18 Dorsopalmar (ulnar gutter) short arm splint including two or more fingers using synthetic; 15.19 Palmar short arm splint including the fingers using plaster of Paris; and 15.20 Short arm cast including two or more fingers using synthetic, combicast technique). Yet, depending on the operative technique, postoperative protection and immobilization of thumb or finger joints can carry the risk of stiffness in the hand and especially in the operated finger.

Two further points to remember are:
- During the period of immobilization, patients have to be advised to mobilize the uninjured finger joints, the elbow joint, and shoulder joint as far as pain allows
- In cases of severe soft-tissue injuries, an external fixator is a reliable and secure surgical treatment.

5 Groin flap

Small defects on the dorsal side of the hand can be covered by local flaps. Defects on the palmar side are more complicated because of the firm connection between the skin and the soft tissue. Several microsurgical flaps, developed in recent years, provide more individual and esthetic options. However, pedicled flaps are still in use, and the surgical technique of elevating the groin flap is less demanding in comparison. The pedicled groin flap is based on the superficial circumflex iliac artery that runs parallel to the inguinal ligament, running about 2 cm below it.

The groin flap is a reliable and versatile surgical option for covering larger hand defects. The flap can be selected with a length of about 25 cm and it can be used for defects on either the dorsum (**Fig 10-1, Fig 10-2, Fig 10-3, Fig 10-4**) or palm [5]. The pedicle is cut when the flap has healed in, normally after 3 weeks. Although a long pedicle of the flap is the aim, the disadvantages of using the pedicled groin flap include discomfort for the patient resulting from restricted mobilization of wrist, elbow, and shoulder joints, as well as the impossibility of elevating the hand in order to prevent edema. Further disadvantages include a loss of sensitivity on the dorsum of the hand and the need for a second operation when dividing the flap after 3 weeks, and perhaps a third operation for debulking the flap after 6 months.

5.1 Relative contraindications
The groin flap is not indicated in patients that are:
- Noncompliant
- Restive and stubbornly impatient
- Alcoholic or
- Patients with epilepsy.

In adult noncompliant patients it is recommended to use local flaps or free microsurgical flaps instead of the groin flap.

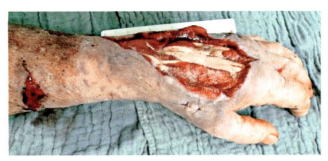

Fig 10-1 A 68-year-old man with a contaminated old wound on the dorsum of the hand.

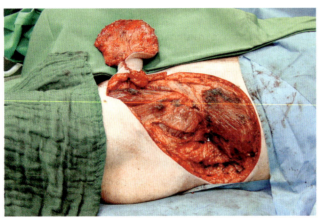

Fig 10-2 Intraoperative picture after elevating the groin flap, which will cover the defect on the dorsal side of the hand. The lower extremity may be immobilized with a special custom-made cast in order to limit motion on the flap during healing.

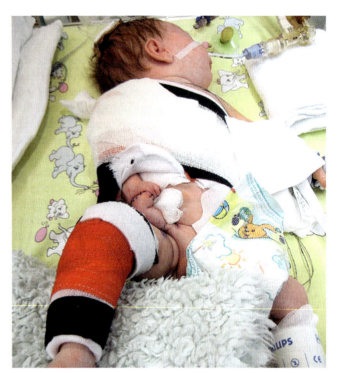

Fig 10-4 The exceptional case of a ventilated premature infant with a necrotic defect of the right hand effectively treated with a groin flap. The custom-made additional thoracic and upper-leg semirigid cast (a modification of the method described in chapter 16.2 Single leg hip spica cast using synthetic, combicast technique) prevented damage to the flap caused by uncontrolled pulling out of the pedicle.

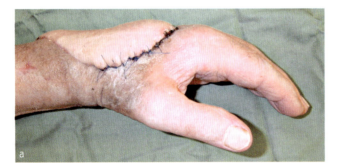

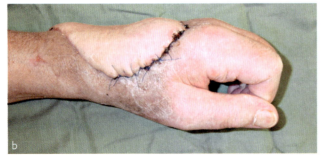

Fig 10-3a–b The same 68-year-old man, 5 weeks after flap covering and 2 weeks after dividing the flap pedicle with restricted function of the fingers in extension (a) and flexion (b).

Author   Clemens Dumont

6   Rupture of muscle fibers

Rupture of muscle fibers of the upper extremity is rare but can result in pain and hematoma. The damaged muscle tissue reacts with swelling and edema. Due to the restriction of the muscle-fascia system, the muscle cannot extend. In the case of pressure buildup within the muscle fibers, the compartment pressure can increase to such a degree that it may even cause compartment syndrome.

In cases of ruptured muscle fibers, an arm cast or splint should be considered (see chapters 15.1 Long arm splint using plaster of Paris; 15.2 Long arm splint using synthetic; 15.3 Long arm cast using plaster of Paris; and 15.4 Long arm cast using synthetic, combicast technique) or a cast or splint for the lower limb (see chapters 16.10 Dorsal short leg splint using plaster of Paris; 16.11 Dorsal short leg splint using synthetic; 16.12 Short leg cast using rigid synthetic; and 16.13 Short leg cast using synthetic, combicast technique). Such immobilization can reduce the pain that normally should decline within the first 2 weeks, at which time the splint can either be removed or, on exceptional occasions, be replaced with a bandage for another 2 weeks.

7   Operative versus nonoperative treatment

Soft-tissue injuries are correlated with several risks of complications. Depending on the severity of the damage, they can result in:
- Seroma
- Hematoma
- Compartment syndrome
- Infection
- Necrosis.

At times, these potential or existing complications, as well as other factors, indicate for operative rather than nonoperative treatment.

7.1   Nonoperative treatment
Treatment with casts or splints, however, can be entirely appropriate in the following instances:
- Ruptured muscles
- Blunt or penetrating tissue injuries
- Select distal tendon injuries, such as mallet finger
- Postoperative protection for surgically treated fractures
- Postoperative protection for select ligament ruptures, such as the ulnar collateral ligament of the thumb
- Postoperative protection for select extensor or flexor tendon injuries.

7.2   Indications for operative treatment
Absolute indications for operative treatment are:
- Significant muscle tear
- Soft-tissue injuries with transection of an artery [6] or nerve [7]
- Open fractures or luxations
- Fractures combined with ligament and/or tendon injuries.

Nevertheless, postoperative immobilization in a cast might be necessary in order to protect the sutures of ligaments, vessels, and/or nerves.

It is therefore then the surgeon's/physician's responsibility that all the factors relating to the type of tissue damage have been considered, the complication risks analyzed, and that the best treatment is implemented for the patient.

Further information on soft-tissue management is available from the AOTrauma publication *Manual of Soft-Tissue Management in Orthopaedic Trauma*.

8 Summary

- Soft-tissue damage, either isolated or combined with fractures, includes blunt and penetrating types of injuries, yet there is a tendency to underestimate blunt trauma as it is not as obvious as a penetrating injury
- External fixation should be considered in cases of severe soft-tissue damage, but internal fixation of the upper extremity is indicated whenever soft-tissue coverage is provided
- The use of a cast can provide postoperative protection until wound healing, as illustrated by the example of a groin flap in a young child
- Operative rather than nonoperative treatment is required in cases of tissue damage with transection of an artery or nerve, open fractures or luxations, or fractures combined with ligament and tendon injuries especially those that require surgical repair to restore function.

9 References

1. **Ficke JR**. Blunt trauma. Volgas DA, Harder Y (eds). *Manual of Soft-Tissue Management in Orthopaedic Trauma*. Stuttgart New York: Georg Thieme Verlag; 2011:28–39.
2. **Rozycki GS, Tremblay LN, Feliciano DV, et al**. Blunt vascular trauma in the extremity: diagnosis, management, and outcome. *J Trauma*. 2003 Nov; 55(5):814–824.
3. **Clayton RA, Court-Brown CM**. The epidemiology of musculoskeletal tendinous and ligamentous injuries. *Injury*. 2008 Dec; 39(12):1338–1344.
4. **Volgas DA**. Classification systems. Volgas DA, Harder Y (eds). *Manual of Soft-Tissue Management in Orthopaedic Trauma*. Stuttgart New York: Georg Thieme Verlag; 2011:66–69.
5. **McGregor IA, Jackson IT**. The groin flap. *Br J Plast Surg*. 1972 Jan; 25(1):3–16.
6. **Franz RW, Skytta CK, Shah KJ, et al**. A five-year review of management of upper-extremity arterial injuries at an urban Level I trauma center. *Ann Vasc Surg*. 2012 Jul; 26(5):655–664.
7. **Sinis N, Kraus A, Papagiannoulis N, et al**. Concepts and developments in peripheral nerve surgery. *Clin Neuropathol*. 2009 Jul–Aug; 28(4):247–262.

11.1 Ligament and tendon injuries

Kamel Afifi

GUIDELINES

Casts, Splints, and Support Bandages—Nonoperative Treatment and Perioperative Protection   Klaus Dresing, Peter Trafton

Author   Kamel Afifi

11.1   Ligament and tendon injuries

1   Introduction

Ligaments and tendons are the body's essential functional connective tissues. Their appearance is often similar, with stout, dense, highly organized collagen fibers. Both are relatively avascular, flexible, and specialized for tensile load bearing. Their relative stiffness in tension allows them to absorb and transmit forces without excessive stretching. This permits ligaments to resist undesirable joint motion, and allows muscular contraction on a tendon to pull on a distant bone, and move or stabilize a joint, and thus to participate in functional activities. The flexibility and gliding properties of ligaments and tendons minimize their interference to desired motion.

Closer assessment reveals that in spite of their similarities, both of these tissues are perfectly adapted to suit their specific function:
- Ligaments are an essential component of joints, providing for constrained functional motion
- Tendons are part of a muscle, and are responsible for transmitting muscle contractile force to an appropriate location.

Ligaments and tendons have to meet several mechanical requirements to fulfill their functional roles satisfactorily. In addition to strength, they must possess appropriate length, sufficient stiffness, and freedom from adhesions that restrict desirable joint motion. A ligament that has been partially torn and stretched beyond its correct length may be unable to keep its joint aligned under load. The same is true when the ligament's elasticity has increased, so that it stretches and allows angular motion and loss of joint surface contact. If an injured ligament has developed scarring and adhesions at the surrounding tissues, joint motion might be restricted, preventing desired activities.

Proper assessment and care of ligament and tendon injuries requires detailed knowledge of local anatomy as well as regionally specific pathology, including symptoms, signs, physical examination, and the spectrum of traumatic and other conditions that involve the region of concern. This chapter offers a general overview of ligament and tendon injuries, and includes select examples to help illustrate the important role played by casts, splints, and support bandages in the care of connective tissue injuries.

2 Diagnostics

Effective diagnosis of ligament and tendon injuries depends significantly upon knowledgeable history and physical examination. Imaging studies (x-rays, MRIs, and/or ultrasonography) play a more subsidiary role, but can be very helpful in selected injury types. The examiner must consider the details of the injury, including possible prior events. Also important is the identification of the severity and timing of any functional deficits after the injury – could activity be continued, and if so with what if any limitations and/or pain. If significant time has elapsed after the injury, what, if any, recovery or deterioration has occurred?

Local pain in the region of a joint or muscle-tendon unit and impaired function of the part are typical of both ligament and tendon injuries. It must be remembered, however, that other structures in the region might be the primary or associated source of pain, and these should be considered as well. Bony tenderness should suggest a fracture, including a growth plate injury in skeletally immature patients. A joint effusion or hemarthrosis may represent internal derangement (torn meniscus or labrum, a torn intraarticular ligament, or an osteochondral fracture). Bursitis, peritendinitis, or intrinsic tendon inflammation (tendinitis) might result from an acute injury or a gradually developing process. Assuming that a painful joint or muscle is simply a minor sprain or strain can be a pitfall that delays diagnosis of a more serious condition. Therefore, pain that increases, and/or fails to improve with rest and simple modalities, should always suggest the need for the reassessment of a painful extremity.

Regarding examination, the crucial issues are:
- Localization of pain and/or tenderness (and swelling)
- Assessment and grading of joint instability
- Strength assessment of each muscle-tendon unit in the involved area
- Neurologic assessment (motor and sensation)
- Peripheral arterial pulses distal to the involved area(s).

In almost all cases of ligament or tendon injury, this thorough assessment, guided by familiarity with the typical regional injuries, will be sufficient for a reliable diagnosis, based upon history and physical examination. Complete ligament ruptures almost always produce gross joint instability. Stress applied to a completely ruptured ligament (eg, inversion stress to an ankle with lateral collateral ligament rupture) results in significant varus tilt and little if any evident resistance. However, muscular contraction and/or intact secondary restraint ligaments can obscure this finding.

3 Ligament and tendon injuries

Ligament and tendon injuries are common in upper and lower extremities. In fact, they account for 30 to 50% of all injuries related to sports activities [1]. Ligament and tendon injuries can be caused by direct or indirect forces, with either open or closed wounds, sometimes with associated local injuries. Many are due to a single traumatic episode, but some are related to repetitive use, and/or preexisting inflammatory or degenerative changes.

Tissue disruption occurs in two forms:
- Partial disruption, as is typical with less-severe injuries, but which are more common
- Complete (or total) disruption, resulting from external lacerations, or from tensile overload that exceeds the failure strength of the injured structure.

Recognition of totally disrupted ligaments and tendons is important as such injuries often require surgical treatment. On the other hand, most partial ruptures of ligaments and tendons (or muscles) will heal satisfactorily with mechanical protection and rehabilitative exercises. Unless an obvious indication for surgical treatment is present, a trial of nonoperative management is appropriate for most patients. Surgery can be deferred until it becomes clear that a satisfactory recovery will not be achieved without it.

Injured ligaments and tendons benefit from mechanical protection from casts, splints, or other supportive devices because partial disruptions weaken these tissues, placing them at risk of complete rupture if significant loading occurs before slowly progressive healing has restored enough strength to withstand the levels of force needed for a relatively sedentary lifestyle, not to mention athletic or risk activities. Reinjury, including complete failure, is a well-known complication after surgical repair of ligaments or tendons, so that immobilization and support are often essential parts of postoperative management. Additionally, motion and loading within tolerated limits actually promotes the healing process, and as with bones, the techniques of immobilization and protection can take advantage of functional rehabilitation – motion and use within safe limits.

Author   Kamel Afifi

3.1   Types of ligament injuries

Ligaments are primarily collagenous tissues that connect the two bones of a joint. Because of their anatomic locations and mechanical characteristics, they limit some types of motion while permitting others, thus determining each joint's normal range of passive motion, including its characteristically stable limits. Ligaments are well innervated, and provide important proprioceptive input. They include cells that are primarily fibroblasts. Their blood supply enters at the boney insertions, and is distributed through an intrinsic microvascular system. Ligaments have more elastin, proteoglycans, and water, but less collagen than tendons, and are more mechanically compliant. Their failure, through sequential rupture of collagen fiber bundles, is more gradual and more likely to be partial than that of the typical tendon.

Ligament injuries are called sprains. They are typically classified into three grades of severity:
• Grade I or mild sprain
• Grade II or moderate sprain
• Grade III or severe sprain.

A grade I or mild sprain has minimal structural damage, but there is some focal hemorrhage, inflammation, and pain with loading.

A grade II or moderate sprain involves partial structural tearing, which results in some mechanical laxity, but there is a firm endpoint to passive stretching during physical examination.

Grade III sprains are severe sprains with complete ligament disruption, confirmable by the absence of an endpoint to stretching. In adults, ligaments typically fail within their midsubstance, while avulsion from bone is more common in children.

3.2   Types of tendon injuries

Tendons are cord-like collagenous structures that cross one or more joints to connect the contractile tissue of a muscle to a discrete insertion site of a bone. They transfer muscular force to the bone to produce or resist joint motion. Tendon tissue is highly organized, with hierarchical bundles of collagen, oriented to the tensile forces applied to the tendon. Two characteristic tendon types should be distinguished. Those covered with paratenon, such as the hamstrings, Achilles, or patellar tendons, have a better blood supply, transmitted via their paratenon, and heal more effectively. Those that lie within sheaths, like the finger flexors, have a poorer blood supply, receiving nourishment in some areas only by diffusion. Tendons have more abundant and more organized collagen than ligaments, and are less viscoelastic. They contain spindle-shaped fibroblasts, which play major roles in tendon healing. Like ligaments, their innervation is significant and contributes essential proprioceptive feedback.

The term strain has long been commonly used to refer to muscle injuries, and is sometimes extended to tendon injuries as well, however, this broad term lacks precision. It is often used for muscular and or tendinous pain resulting from overuse, fatigue, and/or inflammation of muscles, tendons, and surrounding tissues such as tendon sheaths or bursas. A recent sports medicine consensus statement [2] recommended a more precise range of terms to classify muscle and tendon injuries, by separating them into the following two types:
• Functional muscle disorders, without macroscopic tissue disruption
• Structural muscle injuries, referred to as muscle tears, and classified as either partial or total.

Functional muscle disorders, along with minor partial muscle tears and tendinitis, are very common problems, especially in sports medicine. Rest, antiinflammatory measures, and compressive bandages are often recommended for their treatment (see topic 9 RICE regimen). As acute symptoms resolve, rehabilitative exercises often become valuable, and immobilization with a cast or splint is less frequently required.

Structural muscle injuries, involving partial and complete tears, are typically produced by indirect forces opposed to powerful muscle contraction. Such tendon disruptions commonly occur at the myotendinous junction, or at the tendon-bone insertion site. Penetrating injuries with associated tendon lacerations are another common mechanism of tendon injury, especially in the hand and wrist. As many of these types of injuries can be treated successfully with immobilization, this chapter will focus on structural muscle and tendon injuries.

3.3 Principles of ligament and tendon healing

Both ligaments and tendons heal by processes similar to other tissues. However, unlike bone, their healing does not involve regeneration, so that scar tissue, weaker and more viscoelastic than normal tissue, always remains at the site of repair. Maximum strength requires a number of months to be achieved, and is always reduced. Repaired tendons typically only reach two-thirds of normal strength after several years (see **Table 11.1-1** Healing stages of ligaments and tendons).

Knowledge about the factors affecting healing and clinical applications has progressed significantly over the past few decades. Ligaments that are intraarticular (eg, cruciate ligaments of the knee) and have in-substance tears heal poorly with direct repair, which has been discarded in favor of reconstruction with auto- or allografts of similar tissue. On the other hand extraarticular ligaments (eg, knee medial collateral ligament), even with complete tears, heal better, and often achieve satisfactory results with closed nonoperative management. Ligament strength is reduced by immobilization, but excessive stress should be avoided until healing has progressed. Ligament healing is also impaired by increasing age, smoking, nonsteroidal antiinflammatory drugs, diabetes mellitus, and alcohol intake.

With few exceptions, tendons that are completely divided will not heal without surgical repair. For maximum effectiveness, particularly for sheathed tendons, this repair must limit tissue trauma as much as possible, preserve vascularity, approximate tendon ends with minimal gapping, and provide sufficient mechanical strength to permit early gentle (passive) tendon motion, which minimizes function-impairing adhesions and improves the mechanical properties of the healing tissue. It has become well accepted that tendons heal through a combination of both intrinsic and extrinsic processes. Clinically applicable techniques have not yet been shown to promote one healing process over the other.

Injury	Hemorrhage and coagulation occur. These release inflammatory mediators, beginning the processes of repair.	
Inflammation	Accumulation of neutrophils and macrophages Angiogenesis begins Production of type III collagen	1–7 days
Proliferation/organogenesis	Angiogenesis proceeds Inflammation gradually resolves Abundant disorganized collagen accumulates Initially type III, it is gradually replaced by type I Healing ligaments and tendons are weakest during this period	7–21 days
Remodeling	Increased collagen cross-linking Gradual normalization of tissue components and reorganization of structure towards normal	Begins by 2–3 weeks; continues up to 18 months

Table 11.1-1   Healing stages of ligaments and tendons.

Author   Kamel Afifi

3.4   Indications and contraindications for nonoperative treatment

Many ligament and tendon injuries respond well to nonoperative treatment. This is especially true for partial disruptions, which are the majority of injuries. However, surgical repair is preferable for complete tendon disruptions that cause functional impairment, especially those of the hand, knee extensors, and ankle. Achilles tendon ruptures are a somewhat controversial exception, with well documented good outcomes from functional nonoperative care. Many ligaments that experience complete disruption also respond well to nonoperative management, but important exceptions are those that result in joint subluxation or dislocation, and also those involving the intraarticular cruciate ligaments of the knee.

11.1

GUIDELINES

4 Shoulder

Motion of the shoulder occurs primarily at two sites (see **Fig 11.1-1**). The first is between the scapula and the thorax, during which the clavicle pivots upon the sternum, through the sternoclavicular joint. A small amount of motion also occurs normally at the rather stable acromioclavicular joint. The second site of shoulder motion is the much less constrained glenohumeral joint. This ball and socket diarthrodial joint allows generous multiplanar motion, limited at the extremes by thickened regions of its capsule, referred to as capsular ligaments. Concentric alignment of the shoulder is supported by the fibrocartilaginous glenoid labrum, as well as the rotator cuff tendons of teres minor, infraspinatus, supraspinatus, and subscapularis, and also the other regional muscles inserting on the proximal humerus.

A large variety of pathologic processes involve one or more of the shoulder region structures. Because of its mobility and exposure to direct injury as well as indirect leverage forces, this region's joints and associated soft tissues are susceptible to traumatic and repetitive use injuries. Except for injuries to the subcutaneous acromioclavicular (AC) region, precise identification of the cause of shoulder symptoms can be challenging due to the many possible causes of pain and impaired function.

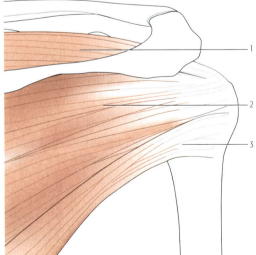

Fig 11.1-1a–c The connective tissue anatomy of the shoulder joint.

a Ligaments.
1 Acromioclavicular ligament/capsule
2 Coracoclavicular ligaments
3 Coracoacromial ligament
4 Coarcohumeral ligament
5 Glenohumeral ligaments/capsule

b Muscles/tendons (anterior).
1 Supraspinatus muscle
2 Subscapularis muscle
3 Long head of biceps

c Muscles/tendons (posterior).
1 Supraspinatus muscle
2 Infraspinatus muscle
3 Teres minor muscle

Author   Kamel Afifi

4.1   Shoulder ligament and tendon injuries

Ligament and tendon injuries of the shoulder are usually identified by the structure(s) involved. The most common shoulder ligament injuries, usually from forces strong enough to stretch and/or tear the ligaments without causing the shoulder to fracture or dislocate, involve the AC joint (**Fig 11.1-2**). However, the capsular ligaments of the glenohumeral (GH) joint, and the fibrocartilaginous glenoid labrum can be injured by dislocation and subluxation. Tears of the labrum are common causes of GH instability and recurrent dislocation, as well as activity-limiting pain. Particularly in middle aged and older individuals, shoulder capsular contracture (or "frozen shoulder") can develop with pain and significantly limited motion. In fact, loss of shoulder motion is common with almost any painful shoulder condition. Prevention of this complication is important and requires gentle passive or assisted range of motion (ROM) exercises, beginning as soon as possible after the onset of the shoulder problem, and repeated several times a day.

Muscle and tendon injuries, whether from acute trauma or repetitive stress, can include damage to the tendons or muscles of the rotator cuff as well as of the biceps or triceps muscles. On occasion, the muscles that attach the upper arm and shoulder to the chest (pectoral muscles), the back (latissimus dorsi, teres major), or those that stabilize the scapula (trapezius, rhomboids) can also be injured. Muscle strains, typically of the functional variety, and sometimes associated with tendinitis and/or bursitis, most commonly occur in the dominant arm and can be the result of a forceful eccentric muscle contraction. The subacromial bursa lies between the superior portion of the rotator cuff tendons and the acromion and lateral clavicle. A common source of pain in this region, aggravated by shoulder abduction and overhead activities, is inflammation of the bursa and adjacent tendons, often related to their being mechanically irritated by pinching (impingement) between the humerus and the overlying coracoacromial arch. Progressive damage to this portion of the rotator cuff, which has a limited local blood supply, leads to attritional tears of the cuff tendons, especially the supraspinatus.

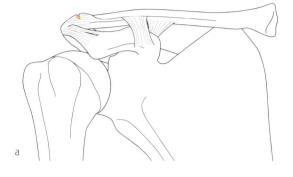

a

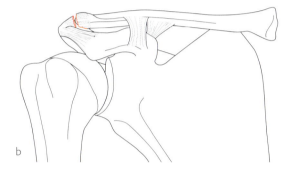

b

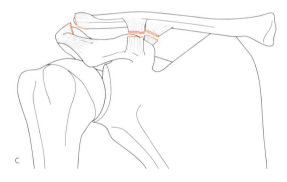

c

Fig 11.1-2   Acromioclavicular joint injuries (Rockwood) [3].

a   Type I, partially torn acromioclavicular ligament without displacement.

b   Type II, tearing and stretching of more ligament fibers, with minimal displacement.

c   Type III complete tears of acromioclavicular and coracoacromial ligaments, allowing significant upward displacement of the lateral clavicle.

4.1.1 Acromioclavicular sprains

Acromioclavicular ligament injuries are graded according to the severity of ligament damage and the resulting amount of joint displacement (prominence of distal clavicle above the acromion) [3]. Rockwood's additional categories (not shown) refer to increased AC displacement. Those injuries are strong indications for surgical reduction and ligament repair or reconstruction. In most cases, nonoperative treatment is recommended for AC injuries unless a rupture of the affected ligament, muscle, or tendon is present resulting in significant instability or weakness of the shoulder.

4.1.2 Acromioclavicular dislocations (separations)

Acromioclavicular dislocations in older patients are typically treated nonoperatively unless the patient engages in heavy overhead work or is very active. Pain reduction may be achieved with a clavicle bandage (see chapter 18.2 Clavicle bandage), or else a sling or Gilchrist bandage (see chapter 18.3 Gilchrist bandage). In the past, various straps and bandage devices were proposed to maintain reduction of an AC dislocation (most of which are easy to reduce with manual pressure but hard to maintain) but nonoperative attempts to maintain reduction all carry the risk of skin breakdown at the shoulder or elbow. Fortunately, for most patients, a prominent lateral clavicle resulting from AC dislocation is largely a cosmetic deformity. If correction is desired, surgical treatment is advised.

4.1.3 Minor and moderate shoulder sprains and strains

Minor and moderate shoulder sprains and muscle and tendon injuries are initially treated with rest, cold therapy, and nonsteroidal antiinflammatory drugs (NSAIDs) in order to help reduce painful symptoms. A sling or Gilchrist bandage (**Fig 11.1-3**) (see chapter 18.3 Gilchrist bandage) can be used for the first few days following injury in order to allow symptoms of acute pain to subside. However, prolonged immobilization can lead to shoulder stiffness and delayed recovery. Early assisted ROM exercises should be performed as tolerated in order to promote healing and reduce the risk of significant stiffness. Although minor injuries will typically heal with nonoperative treatment, grade 2 injuries might additionally require physical therapy in order to improve ROM and promote muscle strengthening.

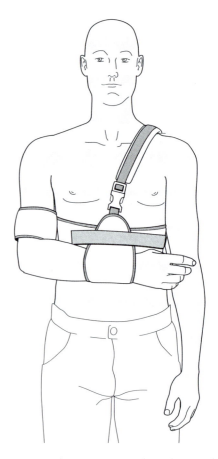

Fig 11.1-3   Example of a commercially available Gilchrist bandage.

Author   Kamel Afifi

4.1.4 Severe shoulder sprains and strains

Severe shoulder sprains and strains can initially be treated with a sling or Gilchrist bandage and cold therapy, but many cases require surgery in order to repair the ruptured ligament, muscle, or tendon.

4.1.5 Other shoulder injuries

Shoulder muscles and tendons of the rotator cuff that have sustained full-thickness tears may require surgery to reattach the ruptured tendon, to trim torn tendon fibers (debridement), or to repair labral cartilage tears (SLAP lesions). Impingement on the supraspinatus tendon by bone or ligament of the coracoacromial arch may also benefit from surgical decompression. Inflammation around the biceps long-head tendon, or rupture of this tendon, might also require either operative or nonoperative treatment.

4.2   Rehabilitation

The goals of rehabilitation are to decrease pain and restore full function with a painless mobile shoulder. Rehabilitation should focus on restoring a full ROM and strength while maintaining independence in activities of daily living. While the goal is to return to the preinjury status, the severity of injury will affect the speed of rehabilitation. Protocols for rehabilitation must consider the type of management (operative versus nonoperative) and should be guided by the treating physician.

After the initial 48 hours, the next phase of rehabilitation should focus on achieving ROM, and then gradually strengthening the involved structures. Modalities such as ice and heat may be used in order to control edema and facilitate participation in physical therapy. In some cases, pain control can also be achieved by using therapeutic ultrasound or iontophoresis [4]. However, in cases of inflamed tendons, ultrasound is contraindicated as it may worsen the injury [5]. Patients should be instructed during early flexibility exercises in order to restore passive followed by active movement in order to prevent the development of shoulder joint stiffness (adhesive capsulitis), which can severely affect recovery. Strengthening exercises are initiated, beginning with isometric exercises and scapulothoracic muscle strengthening, finally progressing to all affected muscles, including the rotator cuff, within painless ROM. Patients are instructed in the proper postural mechanics in regard to reaching activities as well as in exercises to advance proprioception and activity-specific strengthening [5]. A home program should be taught to complement supervised rehabilitation and to be continued after the completion of physical therapy.

4.3   Prognosis

Patients with shoulder sprains and muscular injuries have a good functional outcome with nonoperative treatment in the majority of cases. Studies have shown that successful outcomes with nonoperative treatment for minor and moderate rotator-cuff tears range between 33% and 90% of the time, with older patients requiring longer recovery time. In general, younger patients will more likely have a good outcome than older patients [6]. And while rerupture rates (determined by MRI) following repair of rotator-cuff tears can be as high as 50%, clinically, the majority of these patients remain minimally symptomatic [7]. Biceps tendon lesions, ranging from tendinitis to complete rupture, are commonly associated with rotator-cuff tendon tears. Following biceps tendon rupture and surgical repair, outcomes are usually good, although strength deficits might remain following recovery. If a symptomatic SLAP lesion is also present, satisfactory outcomes generally require arthroscopic surgery in order to repair the torn cartilage.

Severe rotator cuff tears and shoulder sprains have a poorer prognosis, and are associated with a higher degree of continuing disability.

11.1

5 Elbow

The ulnar collateral ligament of the elbow is critical for valgus stability of the elbow and is known as the primary elbow stabilizer [8, 9]. The elbow ulnar collateral ligament (UCL) plays an important role in most throwing sports, including baseball, javelin, racquet sports, and ice hockey. Most of the elbow injuries in young throwing athletes are chronic, with persistent pain and instability from repetitive valgus stress on the elbow with the arm overhead.

Anatomically, the origin of the UCL is the posterior distal aspect of the medial epicondyle; its insertion is at the base of the coronoid process. At 90° flexion, it provides 55% of the resistance to valgus stress at the elbow (**Fig 11.1-4**).

5.1 Elbow ulnar collateral ligament repetitive-use injuries

In many sports activities, the acceleration phase of the overhead throw causes the greatest amount of valgus stress to the elbow [10]. Elbow extension velocities can range up 494° per second and continue to 20° of flexion [11]. During a throw, the forearm lags behind the upper arm and generates valgus stress, with significant tension in the UCL. In this phase of throwing, valgus stress can exceed that tolerated by the UCL in cadavers. This valgus force can cause either chronic microscopic tears or acute rupture of the UCL.

The most common symptom of UCL repetitive-use injury is medial elbow pain in a throwing athlete. Pain can be especially prominent during the acceleration phase of the overhead throw. Pain is often chronic or recurrent, and impairs throwing performance.

A physical examination can disclose the following:
- Medial elbow tenderness and swelling
  - Tenderness is commonly found approximately 2 cm distally to the medial epicondyle. Ulnar collateral ligament tenderness can occasionally be difficult to differentiate from flexor pronator tendinitis, but the pain of flexor pronator tendinitis is aggravated by resisting forearm pronation
- Occasional loss of elbow ROM
- Ecchymosis with acute rupture over the medial elbow
- Pain when clenching the fist
- Valgus stress with the elbow in 25° of flexion (elbow-abduction stress test) generates pain and may cause joint opening. The affected side should be compared with the contralateral elbow as a reference for baseline laxity.

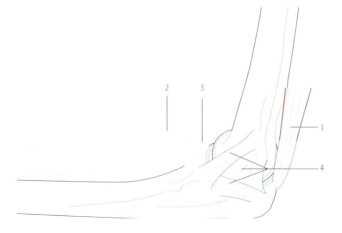

Fig 11.1-4 Anatomical drawing of the elbow joint in 90° flexion: medial view.

1   Triceps brachii tendon.
2   Biceps brachii tendon.
3   Annular ligament.
4   Ulnar collateral ligament.

Author   Kamel Afifi

X-rays may show an avulsion fragment or, in a minority of patients, can reveal secondary findings suggestive of UCL injury, such as ossification of the ligament. X-rays are also helpful in order to exclude other causes of elbow pain, such as epitrochlear osteophytes, medial epicondylar apophyseal abnormalities, loose bodies, or osteochondral fractures, especially of the capitellum [12].

5.2   Nonoperative treatment—acute phase
5.2.1 Immobilization with a cast or splint
A short period of immobilization with a dorsal upper-arm cast or splint (**Fig 11.1-5**) or stabilization with an elbow bandage is recommended (see chapters 15.1 Long arm splint using plaster of Paris; 15.2 Long arm splint using synthetic; 15.3 Long arm cast using plaster of Paris; 15.4 Long arm cast using synthetic, combicast technique; and 18.5 Elbow bandage). Nonsteroidal antiinflammatory drugs may be used briefly for pain relief.

5.2.2 Rehabilitation program
Recommended physical therapy includes:
- Stabilization with elbow bandage or orthosis
- Generally 3–6 months of nonoperative therapy with rest
- Mandatory local physical therapy for improved ROM.

Once pain and swelling have completely resolved and the athlete has returned to a premorbid ROM, usually not before 3 months of treatment, throwing activities can gradually be resumed with careful supervision as duration of training and throwing velocity are progressively increased.

5.3   Nonoperative treatment—maintenance phase
5.3.1 Rehabilitation program
Recommended physical therapy includes:
- Flexibility and strength training of the elbow, which are useful during the maintenance phase in order to prevent recurrent injury
- During the maintenance phase, particular attention to the patient's throwing technique is essential in order to prevent recurrence of injury.

5.4   Prognosis
Proper throwing biomechanics are important for athletes, and should be taught and monitored by coaches, especially for younger players. Thorough warm-up and flexibility exercises are also mandatory to help prevent initial or reinjury.

A return to competitive throwing is possible after successful rehabilitation and reconstruction, if indicated. Before this is considered, the following criteria should be met [13]:
- The athlete is free of pain when throwing
- Elbow and shoulder ROM are within normal limits
- Forearm strength has returned to baseline
- Good throwing biomechanics have been established.

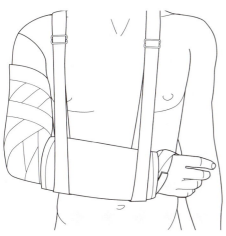

Fig 11.1-5   Dorsal arm splint with sling.

6 Hand

The hand is vital for most human activities. Its motor power is provided by flexor and extensor tendons. Motion in the hand and wrist occurs through a variety of joints: interphalangeal, metacarpophalangeal, metacarpocarpal, intercarpal, and radiocarpal. Each of these is supported by ligaments that provide for both motion and stability in joint-specific planes.

6.1 Hand ligament and tendon injuries

Injuries and disorders of the tendons and of the joints and their ligaments are numerous. Casts and splints play important roles in their care. However, it must be remembered that hand mobility is a crucial part of hand function, and that its preservation and restoration are absolutely vital to the care of hand problems. Thus, any immobilization must be for no longer than necessary, and must be followed by exercises and functional use to restore and maintain mobility. Furthermore, if immobilization is recommended, the hand must be in a position that is as functional as possible, and that avoids shortening of ligaments and loss of joint motion. Mobility of the more proximal upper extremity joints (elbow and especially shoulder) is also at risk when the hand is immobilized, since lack of normal use often results in loss of mobility, especially in older patients and those with arthritis. Therefore, patients should be advised to begin ROM exercises for all nonimmobilized joints whenever a cast or splint is applied to a portion of the upper extremity.

A detailed understanding of hand anatomy and function is required for diagnosis and treatment of significant hand injuries. An excellent further source of information on hand injuries is available on AO Surgery Reference [14]. A selection of common hand and finger injuries and their treatment options is shown as follows.

6.1.1 Ulnar collateral ligament, thumb metacarpophalangeal joint

Rupture of the ulnar collateral ligament of the thumb's metacarpophalangeal joint is not uncommon (**Fig 11.1-6**), and can lead to long-term problems if inadequately treated. Excessive valgus stress applied to the thumb metacarpophalangeal (MCP) joint can injure its UCL, typically by avulsion from its insertion on the base of the proximal phalanx. The avulsion can include a fracture fragment from the phalanx, or can tear the ligament away from the base of the phalanx. The free distal end of the ligament can displace onto the dorsal surface of the adductor pollicis aponeurosis. This displacement (called a Stener lesion) prevents the ligament from healing back to its bony insertion site, and results in persistent MCP instability with weakness of thumb pinch and grasp.

Chronic deficiency of the UCL of the thumb MCP joint was originally described in Scottish gamekeepers, who repeatedly stretched their UCL with occupational tasks. More commonly, the UCL ruptures with an acute injury from a sudden abduction force, as when a skier falls and jams his or her thumb into the snow while continuing forward motion. This injury therefore has two common names:
- Gamekeeper's thumb (chronic)
- Skier's thumb (acute).

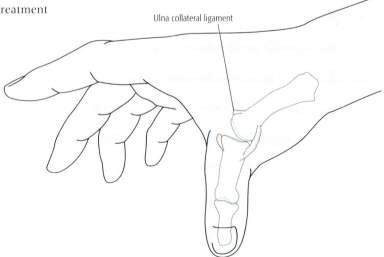

Ulna collateral ligament

Fig 11.1-6 A torn ulna collateral ligament of the thumb MCP joint.

Author   Kamel Afifi

Diagnosis is based on injury mechanism, pain, and swelling and tenderness of the thumb MCP joint, and instability to valgus stress of this joint (**Fig 11.1-7**). If the joint is extremely unstable (compared with the opposite thumb) a complete tear is diagnosed and surgical repair is advisable. If there is less laxity but pain and tenderness, an incomplete tear is likely, and nonoperative treatment is appropriate. An x-ray that shows a nondisplaced avulsion fracture suggests that nonoperative treatment is appropriate. Wide displacement of an avulsed fragment suggests a Stener lesion with need for surgical repair. Absence of an avulsion fragment indicates a purely ligamentous injury, the severity of which is uncertain.

Nonoperative treatment involves use of a thumb spica cast or splint, applied carefully to avoid any tension on the UCL (see chapters 15.13 Thumb spica splint using plaster of Paris; 15.14 Thumb spica splint using synthetic; and 15.16 Short arm scaphoid cast using synthetic, combicast technique). This is left for 4–6 weeks. A similar splint or cast is recommended after surgical repair of the ligament.

6.1.2 Proximal interphalangeal joint sprain
Finger proximal interphalangeal joints are hinge joints with three major ligaments, namely the medial and lateral collateral, which resist varus and valgus forces, and a volar (palmar) ligament, the distal portion of which is fibrocartilaginous and called the volar plate. Sprains and dislocations can damage these ligaments. Avulsion or impaction fractures may coexist, involving the proximal interphalangeal articular surface.

Injuries to the collateral ligaments of the proximal interphalangeal (PIP) joint usually occur through bending or twisting. The result is a swollen joint and point tenderness over the collateral ligament. If the joint opens when stress-tested, the patient has sustained a grade 2 or 3 ligament tear. Fortunately, due to the skeletal configuration of the interphalangeal joint, ligament injuries rarely lead to chronic instability and almost never require surgical intervention.

Treatment consists of short-term immobilization with a splint or cast or by "buddy taping" the injured finger to an adjacent normal one, and active ROM exercises. The buddy taping should be worn full time for 10–14 days or until full ROM has been achieved. Thereafter, if the patient is an athlete, he or she only needs buddy taping when playing for the remainder of the season. The most common long-term consequence of PIP joint injuries is decreased ROM and stiffness. Injured PIP joints will remain swollen for up to 6–8 months, sometimes even permanently. Note that early protected motion is a key part of treatment, to promote recovery of PIP joint motion.

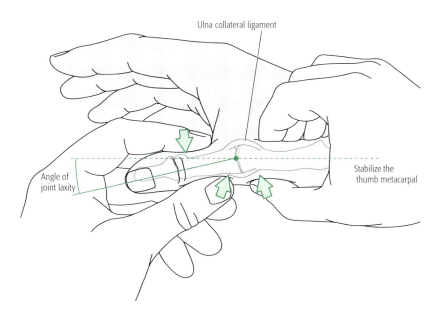

Fig 11.1-7   Stress test for ruptured ulna collateral ligament of the thumb.

Suggested splint/casts include chapters 15.17 Dorsopalmar (ulnar gutter) short arm splint including two or more fingers plaster of Paris; 15.18 Dorsopalmar (ulnar gutter) short arm splint including two or more fingers using synthetic; 15.19 Palmar short arm splint including the fingers using plaster of Paris; 15.20 Short arm cast including two or more fingers using synthetic, combicast technique; and 15.25 Removable finger splint using synthetic.

6.1.3 Volar plate injuries of the fingers

These are caused by hyperextension of the PIP joint. This injury is usually associated with a dorsal dislocation or subluxation of the middle phalanx. The volar plate can fail in two ways: distal rupture of the volar plate, or avulsion of its attachment to the middle phalanx.

If the avulsed fragment is tiny (ie, in the case of a chip fracture) and the joint is congruent, treatment is the same whether or not a chip fracture exists. A variation of dorsal block splinting is the usual regimen (see chapter 15.25 Removable finger splint using synthetic). The PIP joint is blocked 30° from full extension, but the patient is allowed full active flexion. Over the next 3–4 weeks, extension is increased until full extension is achieved. However, if the chip is large and the PIP joint is unstable, surgical intervention is needed.

6.1.4 Flexor tendon lacerations

The long finger flexor tendons begin in the forearm flexor muscles and insert in the finger phalanges. The superficial flexors insert on the base of the middle phalanges, and the deep flexors on the base of the distal phalanges. The thumb has only a single long flexor, which attaches to the base of its distal phalanx. The long flexor tendons run in synovial-lined sheaths in the wrist and proximal palm, and again in the fingers. The digital portion of the flexor tendon sheaths are reinforced by fibrous thickening that act as pulleys, keeping the tendons close to the bone and avoiding "bow-stringing" across flexed joints. The ends of a completely divided flexor tendon will separate within the sheath, pulled apart by flexor muscles and finger extension. Without repair, they will not heal. Incomplete lacerations may result in tendon irregularities that interfere with tendon motion within the sheath, so that they too might benefit from surgery. It is essential to consider the possibility of associated digital artery and nerve injury with any finger flexor laceration.

Surgical repair of a finger (or thumb) flexor tendon laceration is complex because of slow healing, with risk of the repair pulling apart until several weeks have elapsed. Mechanical protection of the repair is thus advisable, but immobilization contributes to formation of adhesions that interfere with tendon gliding and thus limit active finger motion. Healing and ultimate function are enhanced by motion, but excessive tendon tension should be avoided to protect the tendon repair. Kleinert and colleagues devised a dynamic splinting program, using a short arm cast to anchor elastic bands that attach to the nails of involved fingers (**Fig 11.1-8**). The elastics passively flex the fingers, which the patient is able to extend actively against the elastics, thus moving the tendon while keeping its tension at a low level. The use of such a dynamic splint, together with a rigorous supervised therapy program, has become an integral part of optimal flexor tendon repair surgery (see chapters 15.21 Kleinert dynamic splint using plaster of Paris; and 15.22 Kleinert dynamic splint using synthetic, combicast technique).

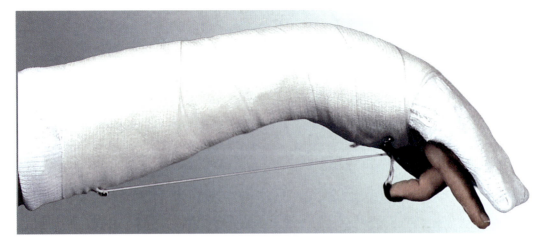

Fig 11.1-8 Example of a Kleinert dynamic splint using plaster of Paris.

Author   Kamel Afifi

6.1.5 Flexor tendon avulsion—rugby finger

The so-called rugby finger injury is an avulsion of the bony insertion of the flexor digitorum profundus tendon into the distal phalanx. The mechanism of injury is a powerful external extension force applied to the distal phalanx against forceful active flexion by the would-be tackler (**Fig 11.1-9**).

Treatment for this injury is surgical, to restore the flexor digitorum profundus (FDP) tendon insertion, as well as to repair the bone defect that often significantly deforms the distal interphalangeal joint surface.

6.1.6 Mallet finger (baseball finger)

A mallet finger or baseball finger is an injury to the terminal slip of the extensor tendon. It is caused by sudden forceful flexion of the distal phalanx (for example, from a fast travelling ball or a forceful impact with a heavy/solid object).

The injury can be one of three types:
* Stretch of the tendon
* Rupture of the tendon
* Avulsion of the bony attachment from the distal phalanx.

The injured patient will feel tenderness on the dorsal aspect of the distal interphalangeal (DIP) joint and be unable to actively extend the distal phalanx, which assumes a mallet-like flexed deformity.

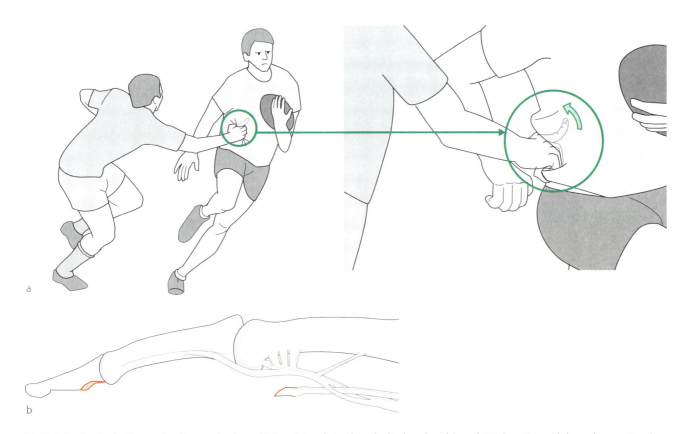

Fig 11.1-9a–b   Rugby finger, showing mechanism of injury (**a**) and significantly displaced avulsion of FDP insertion with bone fragment and the resulting defect (**b**).

11.1

GUIDELINES

An x-ray should be obtained in order to make sure the joint is congruent. Only rarely is this injury not able to be treated with splinting with the finger in extension (**Fig 11.1-10**). However, if volar subluxation of the distal phalanx persists after attempted reduction and extension splinting, typically because of a fracture-dislocation, surgical repair is usually necessary.

Several commercial mallet finger splints are available, or you can make your own (see chapter 15.26 Mallet finger splint using synthetic). The splint should hold the DIP joint in full extension. Excessive hyperextension can compromise blood circulation to the skin over the dorsal aspect of the DIP joint, with possibility of necrosis and skin slough. The splint should not interfere with ROM at the PIP joint. The injured patient must wear the splint 24 hours a day for 6 weeks, then at night for another 2–4 weeks. The joint must be maintained in extension, even when changing the splint. If the splint is removed before healing is adequate, and a flexion deformity recurs, success may still be achievable with another 6 week course of extension splinting.

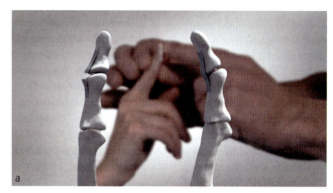
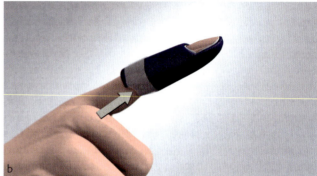

Fig 11.1-10a–b Mallet finger.

a Injury to the terminal slip of the extensor tendon, on dorsal aspect of DIP joint.

b A mallet finger splint is used to maintain the affected finger's DIP joint in full extension.

Author   Kamel Afifi

6.1.7 Traumatic boutonnierre deformity

A boutonnierre deformity can result from an injury to the digital extensor hood. The central slip becomes detached from the base of the middle phalanx, and the lateral bands displace palmarly, so they flex the PIP joint while extending the DIP joint (**Fig 11.1-11**). Prompt treatment with a palmar splint that mildly hyperextends the PIP while allowing active flexion exercises of the DIP is usually successful. This splint is worn for 4–6 weeks with gradual weaning with attention to restoring active PIP flexion range. A splint that applies three-point contact to the finger to maintain PIP extension could also be used. Delayed treatment of a traumatic boutonniere injury may result in permanent deformity and impaired function.

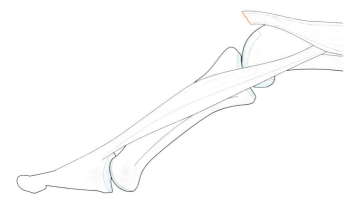

Fig 11.1-11   Boutonniere deformity, showing disruption of extensor hood central slip attachment to the base of the middle phalanx, with palmar displacement of lateral bands so that they exert a flexion force on the PIP joint and hyperextend the DIP joint.

11.1

7 Knee

The knee is the largest joint in the human body and connects the tibia and fibula of the lower leg with the femur, with protection in front by the patella. The main element is the tibiofemoral joint, and stability to this joint is provided by several ligaments (**Fig 11.1-12**, **Fig 11.1-13**, **Fig 11.1-14**):
- Medial collateral ligament
- Lateral collateral ligament
- Anterior cruciate ligament
- Posterior cruciate ligament.

The medial collateral ligament (MCL) resists valgus angulation of the tibia on the femur. It runs between the medial epicondyle of the femur and the anteromedial aspect of the proximal tibia. Its deep portion is attached to the medial meniscus.

The lateral collateral ligament (LCL) resists varus angulation of the tibia on the femur. It runs between the lateral epicondyle of the femur and the head of the fibula. The LCL is closely related to other posterolateral corner structures: the popliteofibular ligament, the posterolateral knee capsule, and the popliteus muscle. These structures are important rotational stabilizers.

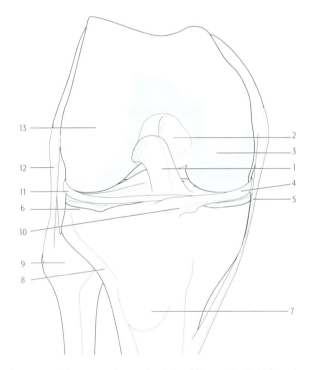

Fig 11.1-12   Knee—cruciate and collateral ligaments. Right knee in flexion (anterior view).

1   Anterior cruciate ligament.
2   Posterior cruciate ligament.
3   Medial condyle of femur (articular surface).
4   Medial meniscus.
5   Medial collateral ligament.
6   Medial condyle of tibia.
7   Tuberosity of tibia.
8   Gerdy's tubercle.
9   Head of fibula.
10   Transverse ligament of knee.
11   Lateral meniscus.
12   Lateral collateral ligament.
13   Lateral condyle of femur (articular surface).

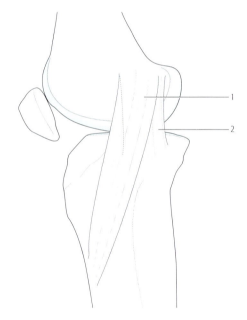

Fig 11.1-13   Knee—medial collateral ligament anatomy.
1   Superficial medial collateral ligament.
2   Deep medial collateral ligament.

Author   Kamel Afifi

The anterior cruciate ligament (ACL) controls rotational movement and prevents forward movement of the tibia in relation to the femur. It runs between the attachments on the anterior aspect of the tibial plateau and the posterolateral aspect of the intercondylar notch of the femur.

The posterior cruciate ligament (PCL) prevents posterior displacement of the proximal tibia relative to the femoral condyles. It runs between the attachments on the posterior part (hence posterior cruciate) of the tibial plateau and the medial aspect of the intercondylar notch of the femur [15–19].

In addition to these ligaments, the knee area includes the base of the quadriceps and the patella tendon. The patellar tendon attaches the distal pole of the patella to the tibial tubercle. It is actually a ligament that connects two different bones, the patella and the tibia. The patella is attached to the quadriceps muscles by the quadriceps tendon (**Fig 11.1-15**). Working together, the quadriceps muscles, quadriceps tendon, and patellar tendon extend the knee [16, 20].

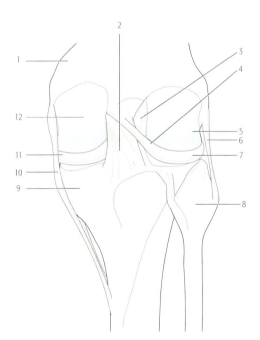

Fig 11.1-14   Knee—cruciate and collateral ligament anatomy. Right knee in extension (posterior view).

1   Adductor tubercle (medial epicondyle of femur).
2   Posterior cruciate ligament.
3   Anterior cruciate ligament.
4   Meniscofemoral ligament.
5   Lateral condyle of femur (articular surface).
6   Lateral collateral ligament.
7   Lateral meniscus.
8   Head of fibula.
9   Medial condyle of tibia.
10   Medial collateral ligament.
11   Medial meniscus.
12   Medial condyle of femur (articular surface).

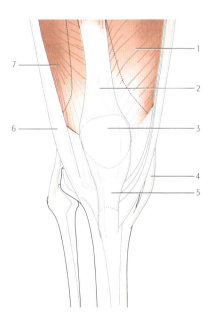

Fig 11.1-15   Quadriceps and patellar tendons.

1   Vastus medialis muscle.
2   Vastus intermedius muscle.
3   Patella.
4   Medial collateral ligament.
5   Patellar ligament.
6   Iliotibial tract.
7   Vastus lateralis muscle.

7.1 Knee ligament and tendon injuries

Knee ligament injuries are but one of many potential causes of disability related to this joint, which is so important for athletics and vocation as well as activities of daily living. A correct diagnosis is very valuable, but not strictly required for every less severe episode of knee discomfort. These will frequently respond to rest, with gradual resumption of activity and perhaps some formal therapeutic exercise without identification of the exact cause. Failure to improve requires reassessment. The diagnostic criteria for ligament injuries (described in topic 2 Diagnostics) will help with their identification: localized tenderness, pain on ligament stress, and laxity varying with injury severity. An intraarticular ligament tear (eg, anterior cruciate ligament) often produces a rapidly developing joint effusion (hemarthrosis). A significant multiligamentous tear may produce swelling, and perhaps ecchymosis, but often no palpable effusion because the capsule is torn and cannot contain fluid.

Minor ligament injuries can be painful and interfere with weight bearing activities, but do not produce mechanical instability. However, pain and muscle inhibition often result in functional instability so that a patient may report that the injured knee feels unstable or untrustworthy. With increasing ligament damage, instability is evident on physical examination, with laxity on maneuvers that stretch the injured ligament, but an end-point is felt. Still more severe knee ligament injuries, with complete ruptures, exhibit laxity without a convincing endpoint. Knee ligament injuries may involve only one ligament, but with increasing severity, multiple ligaments are damaged. This can be associated with evident or occult knee dislocation. It is very important to recognize these highly unstable knee injuries since they might include a popliteal artery disruption or blockage that places the lower leg at risk of ischemic necrosis and amputation. The first indication of such a vascular injury is usually calf pain, with progressive weakness and decreased sensation. Distal pulses are usually reduced or absent, and should always be checked after a knee injury as recognition of an arterial injury and urgent referral may save a leg.

Less severe knee ligament injuries respond well to nonoperative care, especially if they involve only a single collateral ligament. Tears of the ACL that produce significant instability are best treated with surgical reconstruction. The same is true for in-substance complete tears of the PCL, but if the PCL is avulsed from its attachment to the posterior tibial plateau, reattachment with correct tension is often successful. Multiple ligament injuries, with greater instability, are also more often managed surgically if this is available.

Without a strong indication for surgical repair, a trial of nonoperative management is reasonable, followed by delayed reconstruction if functionally significant instability remains. Patients with primarily sedentary job duties and low-demand activities of daily living can be treated nonoperatively with expectation of a good outcome for regaining stability of the joint.

Tendon tears in the knee are described as either partial or complete. Partial tears do not completely disrupt the soft tissue (similar to a rope stretched so far that some of the fibers are torn but the rope remains in one piece). A complete tear separates the tendon tissue into two unconnected pieces, a strong indication for surgery.

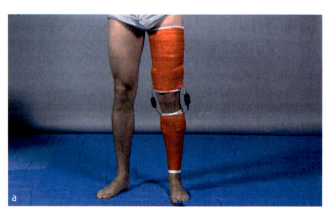

Fig 11.1-16a–c Hinged knee brace.

Author   Kamel Afifi

7.1.1 Collateral ligament sprains

Nonoperative treatment for grade 1 or 2 collateral knee ligament sprains includes the following:

- Rest, ice, compression, and elevation (see topic 9 RICE regimen) and prescription of NSAIDs are the usual treatments during the first 24–72 hours after an injury
- Crutches can be used on a short-term basis in order to prevent weight bearing on the affected knee
- Knee immobilizers are advisable but should be used only for a few days to exclude muscle atrophy (see chapter 16.4 Hinged knee brace) (**Fig 1.11-16**)
- Physical therapy or establishment of a home exercise program can be started after 72 hours to begin ROM and gradual weight bearing
- A brace can also be used for grade 2 sprains for 4–6 weeks in order to prevent reinjury (see chapter 16.4 Hinged knee brace)
- Thrombosis prophylaxis should be considered, especially for higher risk patients (see chapter 4 Thrombosis prophylaxis).

With more severe but isolated collateral ligament injuries, surgery is usually not needed. The patient should remain in a brace for 4–8 weeks and then receive physical therapy to strengthen the muscles that help provide functional joint stability (see chapters 16.3 Cylinder long leg cast using synthetic, combicast technique; and 16.4 Hinged knee brace). Active ROM is initiated early in order to prevent stiffness with concomitant strengthening exercises. Finally, once a patient's strength and proprioception have recovered to levels comparable to the contralateral side, the patient may return to sports activities.

7.1.2 Cruciate ligament sprains

If the clinical findings of a suspected cruciate ligament injury do not indicate a structural ACL or PCL tear or an associated meniscal injury, nonoperative treatment with RICE, physical therapy, and bracing can be introduced (see chapters 16.3 Cylinder long leg cast using synthetic, combicast technique; and 16.4 Hinged knee brace). In nonoperative treatment, progressive physical therapy and rehabilitation can restore the knee to a condition close to its preinjury state. Moreover, the patient should be trained on how to prevent instability. However, many people selecting not to have surgery may experience secondary injury to the knee due to repetitive episodes of instability.

Surgical treatment is recommended in combined ACL injuries (ie, ACL tears in combination with other injuries in the knee). However, deciding against surgery may be reasonable for selected patients. Nonoperative management of isolated ACL tears is likely to be successful or may be indicated in the following patients:

- With partial tears and no instability symptoms
- With complete tears and no symptoms of knee instability during the patient's preferred activities
- Willing to give up high-demand sports
- Doing light manual work or with sedentary lifestyles
- With open growth plates (ie, children) [18, 21, 22].

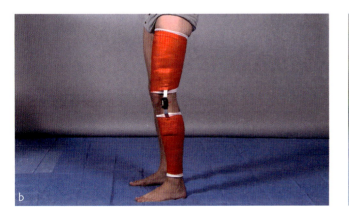

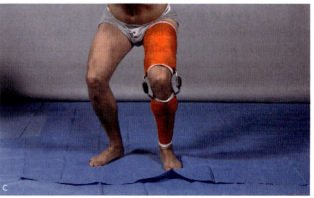

If the PCL only is injured, it can also be treated without surgery. The injury can occur following hyperextension while running, or as a result of a direct blow to the flexed knee, common in some tackling sports. Initially, the RICE regimen can speed recovery. For immobilization, a brace is applied in order to prevent the knee from moving (see chapters 16.3 Cylinder long leg cast using synthetic, combicast technique; and 16.4 Hinged knee brace). To further protect the knee, crutches can be used in order to prevent putting weight on the leg. Physical therapy is recommended, and as the swelling goes down, a careful rehabilitation program is started. Specific exercises will restore function to the knee and strengthen the leg muscles that support it. Strengthening the muscles in the front of the thigh (quadriceps) has been shown to be a key factor in a successful recovery [19, 23].

7.1.3 Patellar tendon tears

The patellar tendon often tears where it attaches to the kneecap, and can break off a piece of the bone as it tears. More distal tears also occur. Swelling, tenderness, and a palpable defect in the tendon help to localize the disruption. A complete tear is likely if the patient is unable to extend the knee fully and keep it straight while lifting the leg off the surface of the exam table (straight leg raising test). This test is also positive in the case of a complete quadriceps tendon tear, or a displaced transverse patellar fracture with associated tears of the patellar retinacula. Taking AP and lateral x-rays of the knee helps with the assessment of quadriceps mechanism injuries.

The type of treatment required for a patellar tendon tear depends on type and size of the tear, the patient's activity level, and age. Very small partial tears respond well to treatment with immobilization of the knee in very slight flexion in an immobilizer or brace (see chapters 16.3 Cylinder long leg cast using synthetic, combicast technique; and 16.5 Dorsal long leg splint using plaster of Paris), and weight bearing limited with crutches. Structural healing is usually achieved within 6 weeks.

Physical therapy, with specific exercises to strengthen the quadriceps muscles, is mandatory, and may begin before unprotected weight bearing. Straight leg raises are often prescribed. After some time, unlocking of the brace is often possible, allowing more freedom of movement with a greater ROM.

Most people with complete or nearly complete patellar tendon tears require surgery in order to regain most of the function in their leg. Surgical repair reattaches the torn tendon to the kneecap, and is usually protected with a cast or splint until the tissues have healed enough to begin progressive rehabilitation.

Author   Kamel Afifi

7.1.4 Quadriceps tendon tears

Quadriceps tendon injuries are partial or complete disruptions of the myotendinous tissue where the quadriceps muscle attaches to the proximal pole of the patella. They often propagate into the medial and lateral patellar retinacula. Like complete patellar tendon tears and displaced patellar fractures, complete quadriceps tears produce a positive straight leg raising test. They require surgical repair, with postoperative cast or splint, and rehabilitation after healing. Incomplete tears, unless large, can be treated similarly to incomplete patellar tendon tears, previously described.

7.2   Prognosis

Knee injuries heal over three phases. Both tendons and ligaments initially experience an acute inflammation phase within the first few days followed by a repair phase of several weeks. Finally, in phase 3 there is remodeling and maturation, which can require many months before there is eventual cross-linking and improved tensile strength.

In most cases, the original strength of the knee is not regained (estimated at 50–70%). Isolated grade 3 ACL and PCL injuries do not heal as they are not contained in a vascularized bed. However, it is important to note that not all injuries lead to functional disability [24, 25].

8   Ankle

There are two diarthrodial joints in the ankle region. The "upper ankle joint" (tibiotalar) is a complex hinge articulation between a socket formed by the distal tibia and fibula, held together by the syndesmotic ligaments and the proximal surfaces of the talus. This joint is supported by its bony architecture and collateral ligaments. The "lower ankle joint" (subtalar) between the talus and the calcaneus, is an obliquely oriented hinge that permits inversion and eversion. Its ligaments are hidden in the space between these bones, except for the ankle lateral collateral ligament's fibulocalcaneal portion, which crosses both joints. The tendons crossing the ankle provide motor power and control for both upper and lower ankle joints, which interact during normal gait.

Ankle stability is conferred by bony architecture and capsular ligamentous structures (**Fig 11.1-17**, **Fig 11.1-18**) and supporting tendons. When the strength of these structures is exceeded, typically by torsional forces produced by the body's kinetic energy acting against the stationary planted foot, injuries occur that damage bone and/or ligaments in patterns that are fairly predictable, depending on the direction of the applied forces. Many of these involve combinations of bone and ligament injuries.

There are three major portions of the ankle lateral collateral ligament complex. These are:
• The anterior talofibular ligament
• The calcaneofibular ligament
• The posterior talofibular ligament.

The anterior talofibular ligament (ATFL) is the weakest of the three, and might be the only portion injured in an inversion sprain.

The calcaneofibular ligament (CFL) is a strong, flat, oval ligament originating from the lateral malleolus, running deep to the fibular tendons and inserting on the posterior aspect of the lateral calcaneus. This ligament resists inversion with the ankle in dorsiflexion and stabilizes both the ankle and subtalar joint.

The posterior talofibular ligament (PTFL) is a very strong ligament that originates on the medial surface of the lateral malleolus and inserts on the posterior surface of the talus. It is the strongest of the lateral ligaments and prevents posterior and rotatory subluxation of the talus.

Additionally, the ankle's tendon and neurovascular structure include five nerves, two major arteries and veins, and 13 tendons that cross the ankle joint. These tendons can be divided according to their locations: anterior, posterior, medial, and lateral. The posterior group includes the Achilles tendon, from the gastrocnemius and soleus muscles. It is the most powerful plantar flexor of the ankle and is particularly important for stabilizing the position crural segment during stance-phase weight bearing on the forefoot.

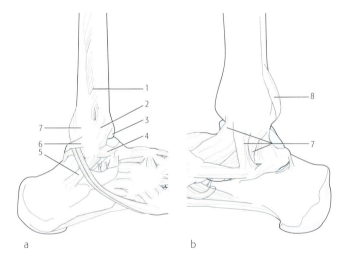

a   b

Fig 11.1-17   Collateral ligament complexes of the ankle.
a   The lateral collateral ligament complex (4–6).
b   The medial collateral ligament complex (deltoid ligament).
1   Interosseous membrane.
2   Anterior tibiofibular ligament.
3   Anterior tibial tubercle (tubercle of Tillaux-Chaput).
4   Anterior talofibular ligament.
5   Calcaneofibular ligament.
6   Posterior talofibular ligament.
7   Deltoid ligament.
8   Posterior tibiofibular ligament.

Author   Kamel Afifi

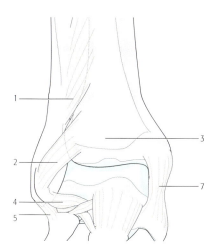

a

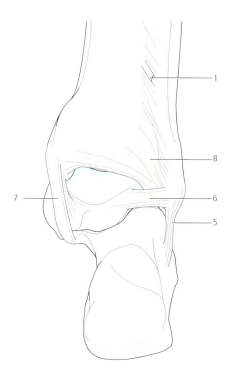

b

Fig 11.1-18   Anterior and posterior views of the ankle joint.
a   Anterior view.
b   Posterior view.
1   Interosseous membrane.
2   Anterior tibiofibular ligament.
3   Anterior tibial tubercle (tubercle of Tillaux-Chaput).
4   Anterior talofibular ligament.
5   Calcaneofibular ligament.
6   Posterior talofibular ligament.
7   Deltoid ligament.
8   Posterior tibiofibular ligament.

8.1   Ankle ligament and tendon injuries

Soft-tissue ankle injuries are common, particularly among athletes. In fact a wide range of injuries from various causes can affect the ankle and its ligaments and tendons.

Forcible inversion of the ankle and foot can cause partial or complete disruption of the lateral collateral ligament. This common "ankle sprain" is the most frequent injury in the ankle region, and varies greatly in severity depending upon the degree of ligament disruption. Ligamentous laxity is hard to assess because inversion through the subtalar joint is normally present. Inversion stress can produce tilting of the talus in the ankle mortise, but an x-ray taken with inversion stress is required to demonstrate this and distinguish it from normal inversion of the calcaneus through the subtalar joint.

Ankle syndesmosis sprains also occur, but are less common. The ankle syndesmosis is composed of three short stout ligaments that firmly unite the distal tibia and fibula, just proximal to the tibiotalar joint (anterior and posterior inferior tibiofibular, and interosseous ligaments). Only very slight motion normally occurs at the syndesmosis. However, forcible rotation of the leg with weight bearing around the fixed talus can spread the tibia and fibula apart, stretching and tearing the syndesmotic ligament fibers and causing a "high ankle sprain". The location of maximal tenderness helps distinguish these two types of ankle sprains. Ankle syndesmosis injuries also occur in association with malleolar ankle fractures, especially bimalleolar and trimalleolar fractures, in which the fibula is fractured above the syndesmosis. Sometimes a purely ligamentous syndesmotic injury produces radiographically visible widening of the ankle mortise. As with ankle fractures that show similar widening, surgical repair is required to reposition the fibula correctly in the tibia's incisural notch and hold it there for the several months, which is required for stable healing. Lesser degrees of syndesmotic sprain usually heal satisfactorily with nonoperative treatment, but these high ankle sprains heal much more slowly than those of the lateral collateral ligament.

Ruptures of the Achilles tendon typically occur in middle aged or older individuals during running activities, and are often preceded by degenerative changes in the tendon (tendinopathy or tendinitis). They are usually complete, which may be hard to appreciate because active plantar flexion, although weak, is preserved due to the integrity of other posterior tendons (long flexors and peroneals).

8.1.1 Lateral ankle sprains

Sprains of the lateral ligaments of the ankle are the most common musculoskeletal injury in sports [26] and occur when the ankle is forcefully inverted. The ATFL is the weakest but resists anterior subluxation of the talus in plantar flexion of the ankle. Its integrity and laxity can be assessed with an "anterior drawer" force applied manually through the foot while stabilizing the lower leg with the opposite hand.

Lateral ankle ligament injuries can be classified into three grades: minor (grade 1), moderate (grade 2), and severe (grade 3). The latter is usually considered to represent complete disruption of a significant portion of the LCL, with resulting inversion instability.

Other possible diagnoses should always be considered:
- Syndesmotic injury
- Peroneal tendon subluxation
- Posterior tibial tendon tear
- Achilles tendon tear
- 5th metatarsal base fracture
- Midfoot injuries
- Lateral talar process fracture
- Anterior process of calcaneus fracture
- Osteochondral talar fracture.

The initial care of a lateral collateral ankle sprain typically follows the RICE regimen, including using an elastic wrap/bandage (see chapter 18.6 Ankle and foot bandage), and protected weight bearing.

For grade 1 sprains, start mobilization, ROM, and isometric exercises early. For grade 2 ankle sprains, an external support such as an air-stirrup or an ankle splint/orthosis (see chapter 16.15 Removable ankle splint using synthetic, combicast technique) as well as early ROM and isometric exercises are advised. The most common methods used to manage grade 3 acute lateral ankle-ligament injury are cast immobilization and functional rehabilitation (see chapters 16.10 Dorsal short leg splint using plaster of Paris; 16.11 Dorsal short leg splint using synthetic; 16.12 Short leg cast using rigid synthetic; and 16.13 Short leg cast using synthetic, combicast technique). Surgical repair is usually reserved for chronic ankle instability.

Cast immobilization typically entails a period of 4–6 weeks in a below-knee walking cast (see chapters 16.12 Short leg cast using rigid synthetic; and 16.13 Short leg cast using synthetic, combicast technique), followed by proprioceptive rehabilitation, functional management, early mobilization with external support, and RICE. This is followed by a rehabilitation program consisting of ROM exercises, strengthening, proprioception rehabilitation, and activity-specific training. Proprioception training, which is essential for the recovery of balance and postural control, consists of a series of progressive drills on devices such as wobble boards and trampolines. In addition to providing mechanical stability, external supports also provide proprioceptive feedback and thus aid in rehabilitation.

In lateral ankle sprains, regaining full ROM, strength, and neuromuscular coordination are paramount during rehabilitation. Isometrics and open-chain ROM exercises can be carried out by patients not allowed to bear weight. Range of motion exercises should focus on dorsiflexion and plantar flexion and be performed passively and actively as tolerated. During early rehabilitation, towel stretches, and wobble-board ROM exercises should be introduced as tolerated.

Author   Kamel Afifi

8.1.2 Syndesmosis sprains of the ankle

Syndesmotic sprains are less frequently encountered. The interosseous ligaments between the tibia and fibula will be ruptured with or without a fibular fracture and with or without frank diastasis. However, immediate and spontaneous reduction usually occurs, making the diagnosis challenging. Many of these so-called high ankle sprains probably go undiagnosed and will cause chronic ankle pain. Injuries to the syndesmotic ligaments often take months to heal. Tibiofibular syndesmotic ligamentous injuries are slower to recover than any other ligamentous ankle injury and can benefit from a more restrictive approach to initial management.

Patients with a significant syndesmotic sprain should typically be immobilized in a short leg nonweight bearing cast for 4–6 weeks after injury (see chapters 16.10 Dorsal short leg splint using plaster of Paris; 16.11 Dorsal short leg splint using synthetic; 16.12 Short leg cast using rigid synthetic; and 16.13 Short leg cast using synthetic, combicast technique). The cast and avoidance of weight bearing minimize stresses on the syndesmosis, and helps avoid separation of the distal tibia and fibula, a motion that imposes stress on the interosseous tibiofibular ligament between the distal tibia and fibula. The prescription lasts for 4–6 weeks, allowing the interosseous tibiofibular ligament to heal. This is followed by use of a protective, modified, articulated ankle-foot orthosis that eliminates external rotation stress on the ankle for a variable period, depending on the functional needs and sports activities of the patient (see chapter 16.15 Removable ankle splint using synthetic, combicast technique).

More severe syndesmotic injuries with displacement of the fibula and tibia require surgical treatment, unless a totally anatomical closed reduction can be confirmed.

8.1.3 Achilles tendon ruptures

The Achilles tendon is the largest tendon of the human body. It lacks a true synovial sheath and instead is enclosed in the paratenon, with visceral and parietal layers permitting approximately 1.5 cm of tendon glide. It receives its blood supply from three sources:
- The musculotendinous junction
- The osseous insertion
- Multiple mesotenal vessels on the anterior surface of the tendon.

Unlike most other complete tendon injuries, which usually have a gap between the free tendon ends, the Achilles tendon ends usually remain in proximity particularly if the foot is allowed to fall into plantar flexion (the position produced by gravity without any additional force). Perhaps because of this, complete Achilles tendon ruptures can often be treated successfully without surgical repair, but this requires a prolonged period of immobilization to ensure that tensile strength has returned to the tendon before significant loading is applied. Complete ruptures of the other ankle flexor and extensor tendons should usually be considered for surgical repair.

Most Achilles tendon problems are related to overuse injuries and are multifactorial or degenerative. The principal factors include host susceptibility and mechanical overload. The spectrum of injury ranges from paratendonitis to tendinosis to acute rupture. In a trauma setting, a true rupture is the most common presentation. This is usually complete, with a palpable defect in the tendon. Sometimes, partial rupture can occur. To distinguish between partial and complete ruptures, Thompson's test is recommended. With the patient lying prone on the table with his or her foot extended beyond the end of the table the examiner squeezes the calf. A normal noninjured response to this maneuver is slight plantar flexion of the ankle, but a lack of ankle plantar flexion may indicate a rupture of the Achilles tendon.

The treatment goals for a ruptured Achilles tendon are to restore normal musculotendinous length and tension and thereby optimize ultimate strength and function of the gastrocnemius-soleus complex. While nonoperative treatment usually results in increased muscle-tendon length (ie, increased dorsiflexion range and reduced calf muscle bulk), the functional results of properly managed nonoperative treatment for Achilles tendon ruptures are similar to those of surgery, without its complications, thus this approach deserves serious consideration for many patients.

11.1

GUIDELINES

Some important indications and risks should be considered:

- Approximation of the ruptured tendon ends, which can be documented with ultrasonography in gravity equinus position
- Older, sedentary patients
- Patients with increased risk of soft-tissue complications
  - Insulin-dependent diabetes mellitus
  - Smokers
  - Vascular disease.

In regards to nonoperative treatment, a lower-leg cast is applied with the ankle in plantar flexion:

- The cast is progressively brought out of equinus over a period of 8–10 weeks
- Walking (in the cast) is allowed at 4–6 weeks
- Return to sports usually requires at least 4–6 months
- Alternatively, the use of a functional brace may be considered, starting in 45° of flexion
- Following the period of cast immobilization, a 2 cm heel lift is worn for an additional 2–4 months
- It can take 12 months to regain maximal plantar flexion power.

8.2 Prognosis

Literature reviews show that the majority of patients with acute ankle sprains report full recovery within 36 months, independent of the initial grade of sprain, with most recovery occurring within the first 6 months [27, 28]. After 12 months, the risk of recurrent ankle sprain returns to preinjury levels [29]. However, some patients report resprains from 2 weeks up to 96 months after the initial injury, and after 3 years, patients can still report residual pain and instability. One risk factor for residual symptoms seems to be participation in competitive sports [27]. Nevertheless, if a ligament injury is treated early, and appropriate rehabilitation is initiated, the prognosis is still excellent with nonoperative treatment.

Author   Kamel Afifi

9   RICE regimen (Rest, Ice, Compression, and Elevation)

Combined elevation, gentle compression, cooling, and rest of the injured part have long been recommended for initial care of muscle and joint injuries of the extremities. A splint or cast is often added, especially for more painful or more severe injuries. Mild to moderate elevation helps to reduce interstitial edema without lowering perfusion pressure, as might happen with extreme elevation. Maintaining elevation, in a sitting or recumbent position, necessitates reduced activity, which reduces mechanical stress on the injured area, rendering it less painful as well as less likely to sustain additional trauma. While strong evidence may not support faster or more significant healing [30], the advice is sound with regard to prevention of reinjury as well as for pain control. Icing does lower intramuscular temperature and decreases blood flow to the injured area. Studies have shown that cryotherapy is effective in decreasing pain associated with muscle injury [31].

Compression may help decrease local interstitial fluid accumulation, in combination with elevation of the injured part. In practice, the first 1–3 days usually after a ligament or muscle-tendon injury should be devoted to the RICE regimen. Cryotherapy accompanied by compression should be applied for 15–20 minutes at a time with 30–60 minutes between applications. During this period of time, the affected region should be kept relatively immobile in order to allow for appropriate healing and to prevent further injury (see appropriate extremity immobilization throughout section 2 Guidelines). Once significant swelling has clearly begun to resolve, an initial splint can be exchanged for tighter immobilization. For example, a short leg splint might be replaced with a weight bearing cast.

The use of NSAIDs can be beneficial for reducing pain and may allow earlier return to activity. As the long-term effects of NSAIDs in muscle strains are yet unknown, recent reviews recommend only a short 3–7 day period after muscle strains. In contrast, the use of corticosteroids is definitely discouraged based on research demonstrating delayed healing and reduced biomechanical strength of injured muscle.

The acute phase of treatment with RICE is followed by an active phase of management once the injured part is recovering well. This phase usually begins approximately 3–5 days after the initial injury, depending on severity. Stretching, strengthening, ROM exercises, maintenance of aerobic fitness, proprioceptive exercises, and functional training are important components of rehabilitation during this phase to preserve overall fitness while facilitating recovery of the injured structures. Stretching should be performed carefully and always just to the point of discomfort, but not pain. Various techniques can be used including passive, active-passive, dynamic, and proprioceptive neuromuscular facilitation stretching. Generally, ballistic stretching is discouraged until healing is well advanced due to the risk of retearing the muscle fibers. An active warm-up should always precede any type of rehabilitation exercises as it has been shown to activate neural pathways within the muscle and reduce muscle viscosity. Strengthening exercises can begin gradually and progress sequentially through isometric, isotonic, isokinetic, and functional exercises.

All strengthening exercises should be performed through a painless ROM. Advancing through each type of strengthening regimen depends on the level of soreness and pain created by each type of exercise. For example, for a knee injury, once isometric straight leg raises at 0°, 20°, and 40° can be completed without experiencing pain or subsequent soreness, isotonics can be initiated. Maintaining aerobic fitness during rehabilitation is important and can be accomplished by resorting to activities like swimming and biking. Once again, these activities should not increase the level of pain in the injured area and should be performed within a painless ROM [24, 32, 33].

11.1

GUIDELINES

10 Summary

- Ligaments and tendons consist of a hierarchy of highly aligned collagen composed of fibrils, fascicles, fibers, and the tissue itself; they are some of the strongest tissues in the body and must withstand some of the greatest applied forces
- The healing of ligament and tendon injuries is generally slow, going through three phases of repair comprising an immediate inflammatory phase, an organogenesis phase, and a remodeling phase, which can continue for many months
- Shoulder sprains and strains result from forces strong enough to stretch and/or tear ligaments and tendons in the AC and GH joints without causing the shoulder to fracture or dislocate, yet these injuries can often be successfully treated nonoperatively using a range of support bandages, cold therapy, and rehabilitation
- The ulnar collateral ligament of the elbow is the primary elbow stabilizer and plays an important role in throwing sports, but it can respond favorably to nonoperative treatment following an injury, particularly when involving a program of stabilization with support bandaging, rest, nonsteroidal antiinflammatory drugs, and appropriate physical therapy
- The hand is susceptible to a wide range of ligament and tendon injuries from such actions as twisting, overload/overuse, and hyperextension or forceful flexion of fingers and joints during contact sports, yet in many cases these injuries can also be successfully treated nonoperatively

- The knee experiences instability (abnormally increased ROM) due to ligamentous, capsular, meniscal, cartilage, or bone injury/abnormality. While severe ligament injuries deserve consideration for surgical repair or reconstruction, less severe injuries, including many medial collateral or isolated cruciate ligament tears, as well as injuries sustained by patients with primarily sedentary job duties and low-demand activities of daily living, can be treated nonoperatively with a good chance of regaining a stable joint and acceptable function
- The ankle joint, comprising syndesmotic ligaments, lateral collateral ligaments, and medial collateral ligaments, as well as a number of important tendons such as the Achilles, is susceptible to sprain and strain injuries particularly during sport, however, most patients can be successfully treated using nonoperative immobilization
- In most ligament and tendon injuries, the RICE regimen, being rest, ice, compression, and elevation, is an essential part of treatment, particularly during the first few days after the injury.

11 References

1. **Woo SL, Renstrom P, Arnoczky SP (eds)**. *Tendinopathy in Athletes.* Malden: Blackwell Publishing; 2007: xi–xii.

2. **Mueller-Wohlfahrt HW, Haensel L, Mithoefer K, et al**. Terminology and classification of muscle injuries in sport: the Munich consensus statement. *Br J Sports Med.* 2013 Apr; 47(6):342–350.

3. **Rockwood CA Williams GR, Youg DC**. Disorders of the acromioclavicular joint. Rockwood CA, Matsen FA (eds). *The Shoulder.* Philadelphia: Saunders; 1998:483–553.

4. **Stretanski MF**. Biceps tendon rupture. Frontera WR, Silver J, Rizzo TD Jr (eds). *Essentials of Physical Medicine and Rehabilitation—Musculoskeletal Disorders, Pain, and Rehabilitation.* 2nd ed. Philadelphia: Saunders Elsevier; 2008:59–62.

5. **Malanga GA, Bowen JE**. Rotator Cuff Tear. Frontera WR, Silver J, Rizzo TD Jr (eds). *Essentials of Physical Medicine and Rehabilitation—Musculoskeletal Disorders, Pain, and Rehabilitation.* 2nd ed. Philadelphia: Saunders Elsevier; 2008:77–82.

6. **Quintana EC, Sinert R**. Rotator Cuff Injuries. *eMedicine.Medscape.* 2007. Available from: http://emedicine.medscape.com/article/827841-overview. [Accessed March 2009].

7. **Snyder SJ, Banas MP, Karzel RP**. An analysis of 140 injuries to the superior glenoid labrum. *J Shoulder Elbow Surg.* 1995 Jul-Aug; 4(4):243–248.

8. **Hechtman KS, Tjin-A-Tsoi EW, Zvijac JE, et al**. Biomechanics of a less invasive procedure for reconstruction of the ulnar collateral ligament of the elbow. *Am J Sports Med.* 1998 Sep–Oct; 26(5):620–624.

9. **Lee ML, Rosenwasser MP**. Chronic elbow instability. *Orthop Clin North Am.* 1999 Jan; 30(1):81–89.

10. **Fleisig GS, Andrews JR, Dillman CJ, et al**. Kinetics of baseball pitching with implications about injury mechanisms. *Am J Sports Med.* 1995 Mar–Apr; 23(2):233–239.

11. **Harwood B, Davidson AW, Rice CL**. Motor unit discharge rates of the anconeus muscle during high-velocity elbow extensions. *Exp Brain Res.* 2011 Jan; 208(1):103–113.

12. **Safran MR**. Ulnar collateral ligament injury in the overhead athlete: diagnosis and treatment. *Clin Sports Med.* 2004 Oct; 23(4):643–663.

13. **Curl LA**. Return to sport following elbow surgery. *Clin Sports Med.* 2004 Jul; 23(3):353–366.

14. **AO Surgery Reference**. Hand. Fricker R, Kastelec M, Nuñez F. AO Foundation. Available from: http://www.aosurgery.org. [Accessed July 2014].

15. **Wheeless CR**. Medial collateral ligament. *Wheeless' textbook of orthopaedics.* 2012. Available from: http://www.wheelessonline.com/ortho/medial_collateral_ligament. [Accessed October 2012].

16. **Scotney B**. Sports knee injuries—assessment and management. *AustFam Physician.* 2010; 39(1–2):30–34.

17. **Wheeless CR**. Lateral collateral ligament. *Wheeless' textbook of orthopaedics.* 2012. Available from: http://www.wheelessonline.com/ortho/lateral_collateral_ligament. [Accessed October 2012].

18. **Wheeless CR**. Anterior cruciate ligament. *Wheeless' textbook of orthopaedics.* 2012. Available from: http://www.wheelessonline.com/ortho/anterior_cruciate_ligament. [Accessed October 2012].

19. **Wheeless CR**. Posterior cruciate ligament. *Wheeless' textbook of orthopaedics.* 2012. Available from: http://www.wheelessonline.com/ortho/posterior_cruciate_ligament. [Accessed October 2012].

20. **Garrett WE Jr**. Muscle strain injuries. *Am J Sports Med.* 1996; 24(6 Suppl):S2–S8.

21. **Gammons M, Schwartz E**. Anterior Cruciate Ligament Injury. *eMedicine. Medscape.* 2012. Available from: http://emedicine.medscape.com/article/89442-overview. [Accessed October 2012].

22. **Biau DJ, Tournoux C, Katsahian S, et al**. Bone-patellar tendon-bone autografts versus hamstring autografts for reconstruction of anterior cruciate ligament: meta-analysis. *BMJ.* 2006 Apr 29; 332(7548):995–1001.

23. **Peterson CS, Agesen T**. Posterior Cruciate Ligament Injury. *eMedicine. Medscape.* 2012. Available from: http://emedicine.medscape.com/article/90514-overview. [Accessed October 2012].

24. **Cross TM, Gibbs N, Houang MT, et al**. Acute quadriceps muscle strains: magnetic resonance imaging features and prognosis. *Am J Sports Med.* 2004 Apr-May; 32(3):710–719.

25. **Jacobson KE, Chi FS**. Evaluation and treatment of medial collateral ligament and medial-sided injuries of the knee. *Sports Med Arthrosc.* 2006 Jun; 14(2):58–66.

26. **Garrik JG**. The frequency of injury, mechanism of injury, and epidemiology of ankle sprains. *Am J Sports Med.* 1977 Nov–Dec; 5(6):241–242.

27. **Van Rijn RM, van Os AG, Bernsen RM, et al**. What is the clinical course of acute ankle sprains? A systematic literature review. *Am J Med.* 2008 Apr; 121(4):324–331.

28. **Verhagen RA, de Keizer G, van Dijk CN**. Long-term follow-up of inversion trauma of the ankle. *Arch Orthop Trauma Surg.* 1995; 114(2):92–96.

29. **Verhagen E, van der Beek A, Twisk J, et al**. The effect of a proprioceptive balance board training program for the prevention of ankle sprains: a prospective controlled trial. *Am J Sports Med.* 2004 Sep; 32(6):1385–1393.

30. **Kaminski TW**. I thought everyone knew that RICE is effective in treating acute ankle sprains. *Athletic Training & Sports Health Care.* 2012; 4:247

31. **Hubbard TJ, Denegar CR**. Does cryotherapy improve outcomes with soft tissue injury? *J Athl Train.* 2004 Sep; 39(3):278–279.

32. **Young JL, Laskowski ER, Rock MG**. Thigh injuries in athletes. *Mayo Clin Proc.* 1993 Nov; 68(11):1099–1106.

33. **Hasselman CT, Best TM, Hughes C, et al**. An explanation for various rectus femoris strain injuries using previously undescribed muscle architecture. *Am J Sports Med.* 1995 Jul-Aug; 23(4):493–499.

12 Further reading

Alexy C, De Carlo M. Rehabilitation and use of protective devices in hand and wrist injuries. *Clin Sports Med.* 1998 Jul; 17(3):635–655.

American Academy of Orthopaedic Surgeons. Common Shoulder Injuries. 2009. Available from: http://orthoinfo.aaos.org/topic.cfm?topic=A00327. [Accessed October 2012].

Anandacoomarasamy A, Barnsley L. Long term outcomes of inversion ankle injuries. *Br J Sports Med.* 2005 Mar; 39(3):e14; discussion e14.

Apfel E, Sigafoos GT. Comparison of range of motion constraints provided by splints used in the treatment of cubital tunnel syndrome—a pilot study. *J Hand Ther.* 2006 Oct-Dec; 19(4):384–392; quiz 392.

Aronowitz ER, Leddy JP. Closed tendon injuries of the hand and wrist in athletes. *Clin Sports Med.* 1998 Jul; 17(3):449–467.

Beumer A, van Hemert WL, Niesing R, et al. Radiographic measurement of the distal tibiofibular syndesmosis has limited use. *Clin Orthop Relat Res.* 2004: 227–234.

Bowers AL, Dines JS, Dines DM, et al. Elbow medial ulnar collateral ligament reconstruction: clinical relevance and the docking technique. *J Shoulder Elbow Surg.* 2010 Mar; 19(2 Suppl):110–117.

Bowers WH. The proximal interphalangeal joint volar plate. II: A clinical study of hyperextension injury. *J Hand Surg Am.* 1981 Jan; 6(1):77–81.

Bowers WH, Wolf JW Jr, Nehil JL, et al. The proximal interphalangeal joint volar plate. I: An anatomical and biochemical study. *J Hand Surg Am.* 1980 Jan; 5(1):79–88.

Boytim MJ, Fischer DA, Neumann L. Syndesmotic ankle sprains. *Am J Sports Med.* 1991; 19:294–298.

Brown KW, Morrison WB, Schweitzer ME, et al. MRI findings associated with distal tibiofibular syndesmosis injury. *Am J Roentgenol.* 2004; 182:131–136.

Buck FM, Zoner CS, Cardoso F, et al. Can osseous landmarks in the distal medial humerus be used to identify the attachment sites of ligaments and tendons: paleopathologic-anatomic imaging study in cadavers. *Skeletal Radiol.* 2010 Sep; 39(9):905–913.

Bushnell BD, Anz AW, Noonan TJ, et al. Association of maximum pitch velocity and elbow injury in professional baseball pitchers. *Am J Sports Med.* 2010 Apr; 38(4):728–732.

Corley FG Jr, Schenck RC Jr. Ligament injuries of the proximal interphalangeal joint. *Op Tech Sports Med.* 1996; 4:248–256.

Dahlin LB. Nerve injuries. *Curr Orthop.* 2008; 22(1):9–16.

Dattani R, Patnaik S, Kantak A, et al. Injuries to the tibiofibular syndesmosis. *J Bone Joint Surg Br.* 2008; 90:405–410.

Demirel M, Turhan E, Dereboy F. Surgical treatment of skier's thumb injuries: case report and review of the literature. *Mt Sinai J Med.* 2006 Sep; 73(5):818–821.

Derscheid GL, Garrick JG. Medial collateral ligament injuries in football. Nonoperative management of grade I and grade II sprains. *Am J Sports Med.* 1981 Nov–Dec; 9(6):365–368.

Doyle JR. Anatomy of the finger flexor tendon sheath and pulley system. *J Hand Surg Am.* 1988 Jul; 13(4):473–484.

Ebraheim NA, Lu J, Yang H, et al. Radiographic and CT evaluation of tibiofibular syndesmotic diastasis: a cadaver study. *American Orthopaedic Foot and Ankle Society-Foot and Ankle International J.* 1997; 18:693–698.

Ebrahim FS, De Maeseneer M, Jager T, et al. US diagnosis of UCL tears of the thumb and Stener lesions: technique, pattern-based approach, and differential diagnosis. *Radiographics.* 2006 Jul–Aug; 26(4):1007–1020.

Edwards GS Jr, DeLee JC. Ankle diastasis without fracture. *Foot Ankle.* 1984 May-Jun; 4(6):305–312.

Fraser B, Veitch J, Firoozbakhsh K. Assessment of rotational instability with disruption of the accessory collateral ligament of the thumb MCP joint: a biomechanical study hand. *Hand (NY).* 2008 Sep; 3(3):224–228.

Freeman MA. Instability of the foot after injuries to the lateral ligament of the ankle. *J Bone Joint Surg Br.* 1965 Nov; 47(4):669–677.

Green DP. General principles. Wolfe SW, Hotchkiss RN, Pederson WC, et al (eds). *Green's Operative Hand Surgery.* Vol 1. 6th ed. Philadelphia: Churchill Livingstone Elsevier; 1999:3–24.

Hale SA, Hertel J, Olmsted-Kramer LC. The effect of a 4-week comprehensive rehabilitation program on postural control and lower extremity function in individuals with chronic ankle instability. *J Orthop Sports Phys Ther.* 2007 Jun; 37(6):303–311.

Halinen J, Lindahl J, Hirvensalo E et al. Operative and nonoperative treatments of medial collateral ligament rupture with early anterior cruciate ligament reconstruction: a prospective randomized study. *Am J Sports Med.* 2006 Jul; 34(7):1134–1140.

Halinen J, Lindahl J, Hirvensalo E. Range of motion and quadriceps muscle power after early surgical treatment of acute combined anterior cruciate and grade-3 medial collateral ligament injuries. A prospective randomized study. *J Bone Joint Surg Am.* 2009 Jun; 91(6):1305–1312.

Harris C Jr, Rutledge GL Jr. The functional anatomy of the extensor mechanism of the finger. *J Bone Joint Surg Am.* 1972 Jun; 54(4):713–726.

Hersh CK. Pitfalls in athletic hand injuries. *Op Tech Sports Med.* 1996; 4(4):268–274.

Ho SSW, Erikson S. Lateral Collateral Knee Ligament Injury. eMedicine.Medscape. 2012. Available from: http://emedicine. medscape.com/article/89819-overview. [Accessed October 2012].

Hoffman DF, Schaffer TC. Management of common finger injuries. *Am Fam Physician.* 1991 May; 43(5):1594–1607.

Hughes C, Hasselman CT, Best TM, et al. Incomplete, intrasubstance strain injuries of the rectus femoris muscle. *Am J Sports Med*. 1995 Jul–Aug; 23:500–506.

Indelicato PA. Isolated medial collateral ligament injuries in the knee. *J Am Acad Orthop Surg*. 1995 Jan; 3(1):9–14.

Idler RS. *The Hand: Examination and Diagnosis*. 3rd ed. New York: Churchill Livingstone; 1990:5–113.

Jacobson MD, Plancher KD. Evaluation of hand and wrist injuries in athletes. *Op Tech Sports Med*. 1966; 4(4):210–226.

Kim TK, Queale WS, Cosgarea AJ et al. Clinical features of the different types of SLAP lesions: an analysis of one hundred and thirty-nine cases. *J Bone Joint Surg Am*. 2003 Jan; 85-A(1):66–71.

Lairmore JR, Engber WD. Serious, often subtle, finger injuries: avoiding diagnosis and treatment pitfalls. *Phys Sportsmed*. 1998 Jun; 26(6):57–69.

Langford SA, Whitaker JH, Toby EB. Thumb injuries in the athlete. *Clin Sports Med*. 1998; 17(3):553–566.

Lundberg M, Messner K. Long-term prognosis of isolated partial medial collateral ligament ruptures. A ten-year clinical and radiographic evaluation of a prospectively observed group of patients. *Am J Sports Med*. 1996 Mar–Apr; 24(2):160–163.

Lynch SA. Assessment of the injured ankle in the athlete. *J Athl Train*. 2002; 37:406–412.

Lynch SA, Renström PA. Treatment of acute lateral ankle ligament rupture in the athlete. Conservative versus surgical treatment. *Sports Med*. 1999 Jan; 27(1):61–71.

Maloney MD, Mohr KJ, el Attrache NS. Elbow injuries in the throwing athlete. Difficult diagnoses and surgical complications. *Clin Sports Med*. 1999 Oct; 18(4):795–809.

Mastey RD, Weiss AP, Akelman E. Primary care of hand and wrist athletic injuries. *Clin Sports Med*. 1997 Oct; 16(4):705–724.

Miyamoto RG, Bosco JA, Sherman OH. Treatment of medial collateral ligament injuries. *J Am Acad Orthop Surg*. 2009 Mar; 17(3):152–161.

Nielson JH, Gardner MJ, Peterson MG, et al. Radiographic measurements do not predict syndesmotic injury in ankle fractures: an MRI study. *Clin Orthop Relat Res*. 2005: 216–221.

Noyes FR, DeMaio M, Mangine RE. Evaluation-based protocols: a new approach to rehabilitation. *Orthopedics*. 1991 Dec; 14(12):1383–1385.

O'Donoghue A. *Treatment of Injuries to Athletes*. 2nd ed. Philadelphia: WB Saunders; 1970.

Palmer RE. Joint injuries of the hand in athletes. *Clin Sports Med*. 1998 Jul; 17(3):513–531.

Reider B, Sathy MR, Talkington J, et al. Treatment of isolated medial collateral ligament injuries in athletes with early functional rehabilitation. A five-year follow-up study. *Am J Sports Med*. 1994 Jul-Aug; 22(4):470–477.

Rettig AC. Epidemiology of hand and wrist injuries in sports. *Clin Sports Med*. 1998 Jul; 17(3):401–406.

Rijke AM, Goitz HT, McCue FC, et al. Stress radiography of the medial elbow ligaments. *Radiology*. 1994 Apr; 191(1):213-216.

Ross SE. Noise-enhanced postural stability in subjects with functional ankle instability. *Br J Sports Med*. 2007 Oct; 41(10):656–659; discussion 659.

Ross SE, Arnold BL, Blackburn JT, et al. Enhanced balance associated with coordination training with stochastic resonance stimulation in subjects with functional ankle instability: an experimental trial. *J Neuroeng Rehabil*. 2007 Dec 17; 4:47.

Roy A, Dahan THM, Bélair M, et al. Rotator Cuff Disease. eMedicine.Medscape. 2006. Available from: http://emedicine. medscape.com/article/328253-overview. [Accessed October 2012].

Sasaki J, Takahara M, Ogino T, et al. Ultrasonographic assessment of the ulnar collateral ligament and medial elbow laxity in college baseball players. *J Bone Joint Surg Am*. 2002 Apr; 84-A(4):525–531.

Sclafani SJ. Ligamentous injury of the lower tibiofibular syndesmosis: radiographic evidence. *Radiology*. 1985; 156:21–27.

Seade LE, Bartz RL, Josey R. Acromioclavicular Joint Injury. *eMedicine Medscape*. 2008. Available from: http://emedicine. medscape.com/article/92337-overview. [Accessed October 2012].

Smith RJ. Post-traumatic instability of the metacarpophalangeal joint of the thumb. *J Bone Joint Surg Am*. 1977 Jan; 59-A:14–21.

Sport Medicine Institute – University of Minnesota. Valgus Stress test. Knee Ligament Injuries. Available from: www. sportsdoc.umn.edu. [Accessed September 2010].

Timmerman LA, Schwartz ML, Andrews JR. Preoperative evaluation of the ulnar collateral ligament by magnetic resonance imaging and computed tomography arthrography. Evaluation in 25 baseball players with surgical confirmation. *Am J Sports Med*. 1994 Jan–Feb; 22(1):26–31; discussion 32.

Tischer T, Salzmann GM, El-Azab H, et al. Incidence of associated injuries with acute acromioclavicular joint dislocations types III through V. *Am J Sports Med*. 2009 Jan; 37(1):136–139.

Vogl TJ, Hochmuth K, Diebold T, et al. Magnetic resonance imaging in the diagnosis of acute injured distal tibiofibular syndesmosis. *Invest Radiol*. 1997; 32:401–409.

Williams GN, Jones MH, Amendola A. Syndesmotic ankle sprains in athletes. *Am J Sports Med*. 2007; 35:1197–1207.

Zook EG. The perionychium: anatomy, physiology, and care of injuries. *Clin Plast Surg*. 1981 Jan; 8(1):21–31.

11.1

GUIDELINES

227

11.2 Nerve injuries

Endre Varga

Author Endre Varga

11.2   Nerve injuries

1   Introduction

Nerve injury involves damage to the nervous tissue, and peripheral nerve injuries are a major contributor of chronic disability. In recent decades, significant time and resources have been spent to make progress in nerve repair techniques and to invent tools to assist in the diagnosis and mapping of neural injury. This cannot be said, however, of the resources invested in researching rehabilitation strategies after neurorrhaphy (nerve suture). There are also controversial topics such as the timing of nerve repair.

Dagum recognized this, stating that "the question of how long to immobilize an extremity, and hence a nerve, after repair has never been properly addressed" [1]. For example, digital nerve injuries in the hand are frequent and can result in significant impairment and functional restriction. Despite this, only a relatively small number of papers are devoted to this topic, particularly with respect to postoperative rehabilitation. Splinting after repair, with the idea to protect the repaired nerve from excessive stretching, is still commonly used. Studies of anatomical specimens indicate postoperative rehabilitation is not necessary with resections of up to 2.5 mm [2].

A randomized controlled trial was undertaken to determine whether splinting after isolated fifth-degree digital nerve transection was in fact required [3]. Twenty six subjects were recruited over a 2-year period and randomized to either 3 weeks of hand-based splinting or free active motion. Analysis of covariance indicated no differences in sensitivity at 6 months between the two groups. Subjects also reported their greatest functional limitations were because of hyperesthesia [3]. Although this study is underpowered, these limited results suggest splinting may not be obligatory postoperatively.

In general, however, splints and casts are applied to injured limbs to support and protect bones and soft tissue. The cast helps to reduce pain, swelling, and muscle spasms following the injury. If a bone is fractured, a cast or splint can be used to stabilize the fracture. If a nerve has also been injured and surgically repaired, the cast holds the joint in an appropriate position in order to avoid suture tension. Following the suture of a lacerated nerve, casts generally remain in place until nerve healing has occurred (typically 3–6 weeks).

2   Diagnostics

In assessing for a potential nerve injury, accurate diagnosis of nerve injury type can be difficult. If the injury is open, differential diagnosis is easy because the definitive nerve injury is evident. However, with closed nerve injuries (eg, blunt injuries, crushing) the correct immediate diagnosis is much more difficult. Regular observation and electrodiagnostic tests, such as a nerve conduction study, could be required.

2.1   Electrodiagnostic tests

A nerve conduction study (NCS) is a diagnostic test frequently used to evaluate the function of the motor and sensory nerves, principally using electrical conduction. Nerve conduction velocity is a common measurement made during this test. The term nerve conduction velocity (NCV) is often used to mean the actual test, but this can be misleading, since velocity is only one measurement in the test suite.

For the motor nerves, nerve conduction studies are performed by electrical stimulation of a peripheral nerve and recordings from a muscle supplied by this nerve. The time it takes for the electrical impulse to travel from the stimulation to the recording site is measured. This value is called the latency, and is measured in milliseconds (ms). The size of the response, called the amplitude, is also measured. Motor amplitudes are measured in millivolts (mV). By stimulating two or more different locations along the same nerve, the NCV can be determined across different segments. Calculations are performed using the distance between the different stimulating electrodes and the difference in latencies.

11.2

GUIDELINES

Sensory NCS are performed by electrical stimulation of a peripheral nerve and recordings from a purely sensory portion of the nerve, such as on a finger. Like the motor studies, sensory latencies are on the scale of milliseconds. Sensory amplitudes are much smaller than the motor amplitudes, usually in the microvolt (µV) range. The sensory NCV is calculated based upon the latency and the distance between the stimulating and recording electrodes.

3   Types of peripheral nerve injuries

Peripheral nerves (**Fig 11.2-1**) can suffer injury in a variety of ways, and these injuries are classified as being one of the following three types [4]:

- Neurapraxia
- Axonotmesis
- Neurotmesis.

Neurapraxia is the least form of nerve injury where there is temporary or incomplete interruption of nerve transmission down the nerve fiber. The nerve and sheath remain intact and complete recovery is expected.

Axonotmesis is a more serious injury and exists when the axon nerves and the myelin sheaths are injured but the epineurium, endoneurium, and perineurium are intact. Axonotmesis is usually the result of a more severe crush or contusion than neuropraxia, but can also occur when the nerve is stretched (without damage to the epineurium). Regeneration occurs over weeks to years.

Neurotmesis is the most severe lesion with a much smaller potential for recovery as the nerve and nerve sheath are completely interrupted. It occurs following severe contusion, stretching, and laceration injuries. Both the axon and encapsulating connective tissue lose their continuity. Denervation changes recorded by NCS are the same as those seen with axonotmetic injury. There is a complete loss of motor, sensory, and autonomic function. If the nerve has been completely divided, axonal regeneration causes a neuroma to form in the proximal stump.

While the prognosis can often be good for significant or complete recovery for the first two nerve injury categories, complete interruption rarely achieves complete return of sensation and motor function [5]. Immobilization is typically used after repair of a neurotmesis, but it can also be helpful for patients with neurapraxias or axonotmeses.

4   Protection of nerves from tension

4.1   Physiologic limits

When nerves are elongated within physiologic (normal) limits, adequate neural blood flow is maintained, but only up to the point where the normal vascular protective mechanisms are preserved. Maintenance of intraneural blood flow during neural elongation is accomplished by the blood vessels in nerves containing undulations and coils. When nerves are loose, these vascular convolutions are accentuated. However, if the nerve is lengthened, the vascular coils follow the nerve elongation and are pulled taut. Furthermore, the lumen (internal space) of the vessels is reduced and occlusion (blockage) can occur, particularly when the nerve is stretched beyond the limit of protection [6]. The blood vessels are then strangled, intraneural blood flow is compromised, and nerve function deteriorates [7]. If the stretch is taken only slightly beyond the protective limits, and for a brief period, nerve function is likely to rapidly return to normal [8]. However, if the strain in the nerve is particularly severe or sustained, the alterations in nerve function will be permanent. The relevance of intraneural blood flow is that excessive mechanical stress can cause anoxia and nerve damage, leading to heightened mechanosensitivity and pain. In these circumstances, movements that mechanically stress the neural tissues may evoke symptoms.

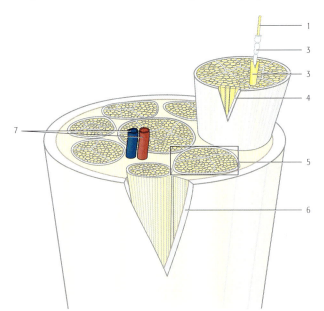

Fig 11.2-1   Peripheral nerve anatomy.
1 Axon.
2 Myelin sheath.
3 Endoneurium.
4 Perineurium.
5 Fascicle.
6 Epineurium.
7 Intraneural blood vessels.

Author   Endre Varga

4.2   Postoperative protection

During the early phase of healing, it is important to protect a sutured nerve from tensile stress. Repairing nerves under significant tension is undesirable and axonal conduction and neural regeneration can be placed at risk. Intraneural hemorrhage from suture-line tension invites scar tissue to occur between the nerve ends. Maturing scar tissue can shrink and constrict the nerve fibers and, therefore, retard axonal maturation and prevent proper myelination. Lundborg stated "slight physiologic tension (intraoperatively) is probably no disadvantage, as longitudinally oriented stress lines may provide useful contact guidance to the advancing axons" [9].

The tension placed on a nerve also depends on the nerve's location and the joint position. For example, a radial nerve is relaxed by elbow flexion but the posteriorly located ulna nerve is stretched by elbow flexion and relaxed by elbow extension. Immobilization using casts, splints, or orthoses temporarily places the limb into a position that avoids stretching those repaired nerves until the repair can withstand the usually applied forces.

5   Indications for preoperative and postoperative immobilization

Immobilization bandages are indicated in the treatment of nerve injuries for a variety of reasons, and are ideal for helping to achieve the following goals [10]:

- To keep surgically repaired nerve(s) limp in order to prevent tension that could interfere with nerve healing at the suture site
- To avoid joint positions/motions that could aggravate a compressed nerve
- To reduce pain and paresthesia caused by nerve entrapment
- To improve hand dexterity by compensating for weak/paralyzed muscles
- To avoid overstretching of denervated muscles
- To prevent shortening of unopposed innervated muscles
- To prevent joint contractures
- To retain tendon and nerve glide
- To permit joint motion in order to optimize joint cartilage nutrition and health
- To prevent the development of maladaptive compensatory/substitution prehension patterns.

6   Upper extremity (radial nerve)

Orthotic intervention, casts, or splinting for radial nerve paralysis should deal with both the functional (occupational) needs of the patient and biological needs of the tissue.

6.1   Static volar wrist-hand splints

A static volar wrist-hand splint (see chapters 15.8 Palmar short arm splint using plaster of Paris; 15.9 Palmar short arm splint using synthetic; and 15.19 Palmar short arm splint including the fingers using plaster of Paris) is commonly provided for night use to optimally position the wrist, thumb, and fingers and to prevent contractures. For daytime function, various orthotic designs have been documented. They vary according to the force system used (static, dynamic, or tenodesis) and to the number of joints incorporated:

- Wrist only (see chapters 15.8 Palmar short arm splint using plaster of Paris; 15.9 Palmar short arm splint using synthetic)
- Wrist and fingers (15.19 Palmar short arm splint including the fingers using plaster of Paris)
- Wrist, fingers, and thumb (15.13 Thumb spica splint using plaster of Paris; 15.14 Thumb spica splint using synthetic)
- Fingers and thumb.

Static splints maintain the wrist alone and can be volar (see chapters 15.8 Palmar short arm splint using plaster of Paris; 15.9 Palmar short arm splint using synthetic), dorsal (15.10 Dorsal short arm splint using synthetic), or circumferential (15.11 Short arm cast using plaster of Paris; 15.12 Short arm cast using synthetic, combicast technique). They can be either custom-made or prefabricated.

6.2   Dynamic splints

Dynamic splints use energy-storing materials, such as elastic, springs, or spring wire, to pull affected joint(s) in one direction while allowing active-resisted movement in the opposite direction of the dynamic force [11]. The most commonly provided orthotic design for high or intermediate radial nerve paralysis is composed of a static support for the wrist (across the palmar arch), whereas the fingers and thumb have dynamic extension assists via cuffs around the proximal phalanges. Other designs provide dynamic extension assistance to the fingers, thumb, and wrist.

The provision of dynamic extension power generally requires an outrigger, formed either from wire or thermoplastic that projects above the dorsal surface of the hand for the fingers and above the radial surface for the thumb. Construction of such an outrigger often requires arduous wire cutting and bending and very secure attachment to the dorsal forearm base.

6.3   Tenodesis splints

Tenodesis splints harness active wrist flexion to create passive finger metacarpophalangeal joint extension and conversely harness active metacarpophalangeal (MCP) joint flexion in order to produce passive wrist extension. An advantage of tenodesis splints over dynamic splints is that metal tenodesis components closely follow the contours of the hand, thus taking up less space. However, the drawbacks are:

- The finger MCP joints flex or extend as a unit, thus independent MCP joint motion is not possible
- The thumb is often excluded unless a separate dynamic component is added
- The entire weight of the hand is suspended by cuffs around the proximal finger phalanges, which can be tiring when continuously in use during the day.

High-level and intermediate-level radial nerve injuries require a forearm-based splint because the wrist needs support. A low-level injury involving only the posterior interosseus nerve (the deep motor branch of the radial nerve) might not require wrist support/assistance. A hand-based design providing dynamic finger and thumb extension assistance could be adequate. Correspondingly, in a high-level injury when the radial nerve has regenerated sufficiently to restore wrist extension power, a hand-based design can be substituted for a forearm-based design. Many patients with high radial nerve palsies find that a simple short arm splint that holds the wrist dorsiflexed permits fairly functional use of fingers with less encumbrance than either a dynamic or a tenodesis splint (**Fig 11.2-2**) (see chapter 15.8 Palmar short arm splint using plaster of Paris; and 15.9 Palmar short arm splint using synthetic).

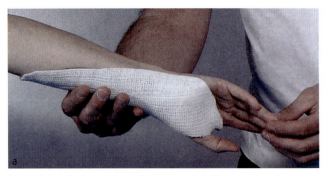 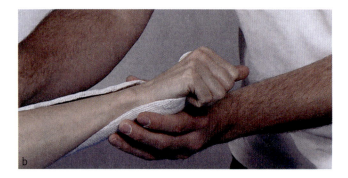

Fig 11.2-2a–b   In a palmar short arm splint, the carpus and metacarpus on the palmar side of the wrist are supported, which can help treat nerve palsy.

6.4 Patient outcomes and patient preferences

Hannah and Hudak conducted a single-subject study on a patient that had sustained a subglenoid shoulder dislocation [12]. After a brachial plexopathy, she experienced full recovery of the biceps, triceps, supinator, and pronator-teres muscles but residual impairments included lack of wrist, finger, and thumb extension (ie, radial nerve palsy). Their study examined hand function and patient preference, comparing three orthotic designs:

- Static volar wrist
- Dorsal forearm-based dynamic finger and thumb MCP joint assistive extension
- Dorsal forearm-based tenodesis with dynamic thumb assistive extension.

Three standardized functional outcome measures statistically showed that both the dynamic and tenodesis splints enabled considerably improved hand function, whereas the static volar wrist splint did not. When given the choice, one female patient at no stage used the tenodesis splint. She wore the static volar wrist splint more often than the dynamic splint because it provided support and was less evident. Thus, some patients seem to prefer to sacrifice better hand function in favor of wearing a splint that draws less attention.

Alsancak explored satisfaction among 83 subjects with radial nerve injury that were fitted with dorsal dynamic wrist-hand splints [13]. All patients were very happy with the support, functionality, and ease of taking on and off, but were dissatisfied with the appearance until the design was modified to a lower-profile, more rationalized style, which fitted more closely to the hand.

7 Lower extremity (fibular nerve)

Fibular nerve malfunction could stem from disc herniation, pelvic fractures, acetabular fractures, knee dislocations, open injuries, and compression [14]. It is important to keep in mind that an inappropriate cast can itself be a cause of fibular nerve damage. Care must be taken to fashion a properly molded cast, especially near the fibular-head region.

Fibular nerve palsy does not always resolve spontaneously; if it is left untreated, the loss of dorsiflexion of the ankle and persistent paresthesias can result in severe functional disability. Therefore, if nonoperative immobilization does not lead to improvement within 2 months, operative decompression might need to be considered [15].

In chronic fibular nerve palsy, an orthosis or splint may be indicated (see chapters 16.10 Dorsal short leg splint using plaster of Paris; and 16.11 Dorsal short leg splint using synthetic) in order to lift the forefoot and avoid stumbling.

11.2

GUIDELINES

8 Complications

Compartment syndrome is particularly hard to recognize in patients with peripheral nerve injuries as severe pain is typically absent, and the progressive impairment of sensation and motor function might already exist when the patient presents. It is also one of the most serious complications following an inappropriately applied cast and can occur when a cast is too tight. As the affected limb swells, the cast acts as a closed compartment, tightly compressing both nerves and blood vessels. Compartment syndrome can cause permanent nerve damage or loss of limb due to decreased circulation and oxygen supply to the tissues.

Patients should be instructed to call the physician at once if one or more of the following signs or symptoms appear:
- Increased pain combined with the feeling that the cast is too tight
- Numbness and tingling in the hand or foot, or an inability to actively move the fingers or toes
- Burning and stinging sensations
- Extreme swelling of the limb below the cast
- Progressive impairment of sensation and motor function.

9 Summary

- Nerve injuries involve damage to the nervous tissue and are a major contributor of chronic disability
- Nerve injuries are classified into three types: neurapraxia, the least severe form of injury, where the structure of the nerve remains intact; axonotmesis, the result of a more severe crush injury, contusion, or stretch injury, where regeneration occurs over weeks to years; and neurotmesis, the most severe lesion, with axon and connective tissue losing continuity, resulting in complete loss of function
- When nerves are recovering from injury or treatment, immobilization using casts, splints, or orthoses temporarily places the limb into a position that avoids stretching the repaired nerves, until the repair can withstand the usually applied forces
- Nonoperative and postoperative treatment for radial nerve injuries include static splints (to help prevent contractures), dynamic splints (using energy-storing materials such as elastic or springs), and tenodesis splints (allowing wrist and MCP joint movement)
- Nonoperative treatment using casts and splints can also be indicated for fibular nerve injuries of the lower extremity
- Compartment syndrome is a serious potential complication following an inappropriately applied cast, occurring when a cast is too tight, compressing both nerves and blood vessels.

Author   Endre Varga

10   References

1. **Dagum AB**. Peripheral nerve regeneration, repair and grafting. *J Hand Ther.* 1998; 11(2):111–117.
2. **Chao RP, Braun FA, Ta KT, et al**. Early passive mobilization after digital nerve repair and grafting in a fresh cadaver model. *Plast Reconstr Surg.* 2001; 108(2):386–391.
3. **Vipond N, Taylor W, Rider M**. Postoperative splinting for isolated digital nerve injuries in the hand. *J Hand Ther.* 2007 Jul–Sep; 20(3):222–231.
4. **Seddon HJ**. Classification of nerve injuries. *Br Med J.* 1942 Aug 29; 2(4260):237–239.
5. **Vordemvenne T, Langer M, Ochman S, et al**. Long-term results after primary microsurgical repair of ulnar and median nerve injuries: a comparison of common score systems. *Clin Neurol Neurosurg.* 2007 Apr; 109(3):263–271.
6. **Lundborg G, Rydevik B**. Effects of stretching the tibial nerve of the rabbit. A preliminary study of the intraneural circulation and the barrier function of the perineurium. *J Bone Joint Surg Br.* 1973 May; 55(2):390–401.
7. **Ogata K, Naito M**. Blood flow of peripheral nerve effects of dissection, stretching and compression. *J Hand Surg Br.* 1986 Feb; 11(1):10–14.
8. **Lundborg G, Gelberman RH, Minteer-Convery M, et al**. Median nerve compression in the carpal tunnel – functional response to experimentally induced controlled pressure. *J Hand Surg Am.* 1982 May; 7(3):252–259.
9. **Lundborg G.** Neurotropism, frozen muscle grafts and other conduits. *J Hand Surg Br.* 1991 Dec; 16(5):473–476.
10. **Apfel E, Sigafoos GT**. Comparison of range-of-motion constraints provided by splints used in the treatment of cubital tunnel syndrome – a pilot study. *J Hand Ther.* 2006 Oct–Dec; 19(4):384–392.
11. **Parry CB, Harper D, Fletcher I, et al**. New types of lively splints for peripheral nerve lesions affecting the hand. *Hand.* 1970 Mar; 2(1):31–38.
12. **Hannah SD, Hudak PL.** Splinting and radial nerve palsy: a single-subject experiment. *J Hand Ther.* 2001 Jul–Sep; 14(3):195–201.
13. **Alsancak S.** Splint satisfaction in the treatment of traumatic radial nerve injuries. *Prosthet Orthot Int.* 2003 Aug; 27(2):139–145.
14. **Mihalko WM, Rohrbacher B, McGrath B.** Transient peroneal nerve palsies from injuries placed in traction splints. *Am J Emerg Med.* 1999 Mar; 17(2):160–162.
15. **Mont MA, Dellon AL, Chen F, et al**. The operative treatment of peroneal nerve palsy. *J Bone Joint Surg Am.* 1996 Jun; 78(6):863–869.

11   Further reading

Dahlin LB. Techniques of peripheral nerve repair. *Scand J Surg.* 2008; 97(4):310–316.

Fess EE, Gettle KS, Philips CA, et al. *Hand and Upper Extremity Splinting: Principles and Methods.* 3rd ed. St Louis: Elsevier Mosby; 2005.

Gibson G. Peripheral Nerve Injuries. Cameron MH, Monroe LG (eds). *Physical Rehabilitation: Evidence-Based Examination, Evaluation, and Intervention.* St Louis: Saunders Elsevier; 2007:473–513.

McKee P, Nguyen C. Customized dynamic splinting: orthoses that promote optimal function and recovery after radial nerve injury: a case report. *J Hand Ther.* 2007 Jan–Mar; 20(1):73–88.

11.2

GUIDELINES

12 Indications for nonoperative treatment of infections

Matej Cimerman

Author   Matej Cimerman

12   Indications for nonoperative treatment of infections

1   Introduction

Inflammation of bone is called "osteitis" and infection of the bone channel is classically called "osteomyelitis". The root words osteon (bone) and myelo (marrow) are combined with itis (inflammation). The term was first used by the French surgeon Eduard Chassaignac in 1852 [1], who defined the disease as an inflammatory process accompanied by bone destruction and caused by an infecting microorganism. This definition still applies today. The septic inflammation of the joint is called "septic arthritis". Osteomyelitis is a complex disease and can differ with regard to duration, etiology, pathogenesis, extent of bone involvement, and the type of host the respective patient represents. Despite new diagnostic tools, operative techniques, and antimicrobial agents, it remains difficult to treat and the consequences can be devastating.

2   Pathogenesis

Osteomyelitis can be one of two types, depending on its source of infection:

- Hematogenous, when it originates from bacteremia in the blood
- Contiguous, when it originates from an infection of nearby tissue.

Hematogenous osteomyelitis mainly occurs in children, but can also be found among the adult population. In childhood, the metaphysis of long bones (tibia and femur) is most frequently involved. Hematogenous infection starts in the metaphysis and is caused by microinfarction in the metaphyseal-epiphyseal junction where nutritional blood flow is relatively poor. The incidence of acute hematogenous osteomyelitis in children has not varied over recent decades. A single infection is most common, and staphylococcus aureus remains the main organism causing it [2].

In contiguous osteomyelitis, the pathogenic organism is either directly inoculated into the bone by the trauma itself (open fractures), by surgery (internal fixation of fractures), or reaches the bone from adjacent infected soft tissue (especially in cases of generalized vascular insufficiency and diabetes). The bacteriology in contiguous infection is more diverse, but in this type of osteomyelitis, staphylococcus aureus is also the most common and important microorganism [3]. The incidence of osteomyelitis due to direct inoculation is increasing [4]. This is probably due to the rising number of high-energy fractures and the increasing use of orthopedic fixation devices.

Acute osteomyelitis is a suppurative infection of the bone, accompanied by edema, vascular congestion, and small-vessel thrombosis. Once the inflammation progresses, vascular supply to the bone decreases and the infection will also extend into the surrounding soft tissue. Once areas of dead bone are formed (sequestra), the disease becomes chronic and is difficult to treat and eradicate. Therefore, acute osteomyelitis should be treated as soon as possible in order to prevent the formation of dead bone and the progression to its chronic form.

In the pathogenesis of bone infection, it is very important to understand the role of biofilm. Some important microorganisms in bone infection, including staphylococcus aureus, epidermidis, streptococci, and pseudomonas aeruginosa, grow as biofilms. Biofilm is a highly structured heterogeneous community of sessile bacteria surrounded by hydrated extracellular matrix attached to a surface of inert material (implant) or nonvital bone. The characteristics of biofilm bacteria make them difficult to eradicate. This derives from a combination of phenotypic, mechanical, and metabolic mechanisms. For example, the sessile microorganisms within a biofilm are up to 1,000 times more resistant to antimicrobial agents than their free-living (planktonic) counterparts [5]. Another way in which bacteria elude host defenses and cause bone infection is by gaining access to the interior of the cell. This was demonstrated with staphylococci in human osteoblasts and osteocytes as well as in vitro [6].

12

3 Diagnostics

3.1 Physical examination

Children with hematogenous osteomyelitis may present with acute signs of infection including fever, lethargy, pain, and local signs of infection. In older children, pain is more localized and the child refuses to bear weight. Normal body temperature does not exclude osteomyelitis [7]. In contrast, adults with hematogenous osteomyelitis present with vague symptoms consisting of nonspecific pain and a low-grade fever over a period of 1–3 months. Patients with contiguous or posttraumatic osteomyelitis may present with localized bone and joint pain, erythema, swelling, and drainage around the site of trauma or surgery. Signs of bacteremia such as fever, chills, and night sweats may be present in the acute phase, but not in the chronic phase. Both hematogenous and contiguous osteomyelitis can progress to a chronic infection. This can often present with pain, chronic skin changes, purulent drainage through fistulas, sequestration, and possible instability. When this occurs, diagnosis is easy but treatment will be much more difficult than if infection is found early.

3.2 Laboratory studies

Basic laboratory tests that should routinely be obtained in cases of suspected osteomyelitis include:
- White blood cell count
- Erythrocyte sedimentation rate
- C-reactive protein.

White blood cell count (WBC) may be elevated with acute infection but is often normal with chronic osteomyelitis. Erythrocyte sedimentation rate (ESR) is usually elevated both in acute and chronic osteomyelitis and decreases after successful treatment. The ESR is a sensitive but nonspecific measure of inflammation because it can be influenced by numerous factors such as age, fluid disbalance, nutritional status, and hormonal disorders. The patient's ESR also rises after major operative procedures and returns to normal within months. The level of C-reactive protein (CRP) also rises in acute and chronic osteomyelitis. It is an "acute-phase" reactant, rising within 6 hours in response to tissue damage and inflammation, and then decreasing rapidly. A transient rise in the level of CRP is seen after surgery, with its peak at about 2 days, and decline over the next few days, reaching its baseline by 3 weeks. If the ESR and CRP levels return to normal during the course of treatment it is a favorable prognostic sign, but in compromised hosts, these laboratory values are not reliable because these patients are constantly challenged by other illnesses and peripheral lesions that can elevate these indices as well [8].

Although not routinely used, the serum-procalcitonin level can be a helpful diagnostic marker in order to differentiate infectious from noninfectious fever more reliably after orthopedic surgery [9]. Further laboratory tests should be requested in order to monitor the systemic and local status of the patient.

3.3 Imaging
3.3.1 X-rays

Conventional x-rays remain the basic initial imaging technique and should be made whenever acute or chronic osteomyelitis is suspected because they are simple, economical, easily available, and usually effective. The x-rays should be scrutinized for the following:
- Discrete periosteal elevation
- Endosteal scalloping
- Areas of demineralization
- Hardware loosening.

Physicians should be aware that these changes occur relatively later, after the onset of osteomyelitis and are not seen during the first 2 weeks.

3.3.2 MRI

Magnetic resonance imaging should be requested if the diagnosis is doubtful. Magnetic resonance imaging (MRI) is especially useful in the diagnosis of hematogenous osteomyelitis in childhood, distinguished by high sensitivity and specificity with no radiation burden. If an MRI is not feasible due to the presence of hardware, bone scintigraphy should be performed.

3.3.3 CT scan and PET

Additional imaging includes computed tomography and positron emission tomography. Computed tomography (CT) scans can be used to help establish a surgical plan both for acute and chronic osteomyelitis with excellent presentation of possible sequestra [6] (**Fig 12-1**).

Positron emission tomography (PET) with its high sensitivity and specificity is used more frequently in the diagnosis of osteomyelitis (**Fig 12-2**), however, it may not be available everywhere.

3.4 Cultures

Identifying the causative organism(s) of osteomyelitis is helpful in making a definitive diagnosis and selecting the appropriate antibiotic regimen. Specimens for cultures should optimally be obtained from bone or from blood (in acute hematogenous osteomyelitis). Sinus tract cultures are generally unreliable and specimens from soft-tissue aspiration

Author   Matej Cimerman

do not correlate well with bone cultures [10]. Whenever possible, cultures should be obtained before antimicrobial therapy has been started. At least three intraoperative tissue areas should be sampled and paired for microbiology and histopathology. Biopsies and cultures should be repeated during each surgical procedure until the end of the treatment. In the case of removed implants, sonication of implants is recommended and the sonication fluid should be cultured. This improves the sensitivity of detecting biofilms.

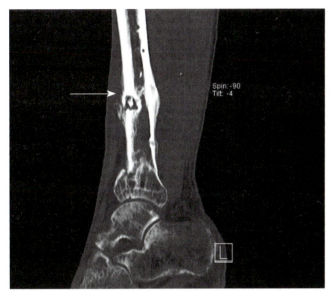

Fig 12-1   CT scan. Multiplanar reconstruction of a chronic tibial osteomyelitis with a sequestra (arrow) and thickening and irregularity of the tibial cortex.

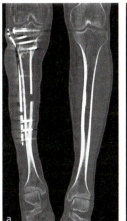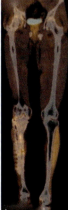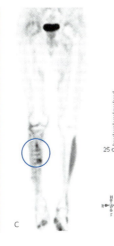

4   Classification

The most popular and currently accepted classification for osteomyelitis was proposed by Cierny and Mader [11] (**Fig 12-3**). It is based on the degree of bone involvement and on the physiological state of the patient or host. The classification combines four anatomic stages (of the disease) with three physiological classes (of the host) to define the final clinical stage.

The anatomical stages are:

Stage I
• Medullary osteomyelitis: The primary lesion is endosteal. Hematogenous osteomyelitis and early infection after intramedullary fixation are typical examples.

Stage II
• Superficial osteomyelitis: The problem is localized on the surface of the bone. This is a true contiguous focus lesion. Stage II, or localized osteomyelitis, is a full-thickness lesion with sequestration and a stable bone segment.

Stage III
• Localized osteomyelitis: It involves the cortical and medullary bone.

Stage IV
• Diffuse osteomyelitis: It involves the entire thickness of the bone with loss of stability, as in an infected nonunion.

Fig 12-2a–c   CT and PET images: traffic accident patient.
a CT scan: leg AP.
An AP x-ray of the leg (including knee and ankle joint) of a 28-year-old male patient, 14 months after a traffic accident. The patient was a pedestrian when rolled over by a car, suffering grade III open tibia and fibula fractures, and was treated with a primary external fixator, multiple soft-tissue revision surgeries, followed by a plate osteosynthesis. There were multiple revision procedures because of osteomyelitis with fistula at the region of the former external fixator pins. This x-ray was taken after partial resection of the tibia.
b PET.
The PET (positron emission tomography) showing enhanced activity in the glucose metabolism in metaphysis and diaphysis as signs of osteomyelitis.
c Fusion of CT and PET.
Fusion of the CT scan and the PET showing activity (black spots) in the diaphysis and the metaphysis of the tibia: osteomyelitis. In the resection of the tibia, followed by callus distraction using an Ilizarov device, the pathologist found active osteomyelitis with fistula.

This system includes all types of osteitis, including septic arthritis, by which a septic joint is classified as superficial osteomyelitis (osteochondritis).

The host is classified as either type A, B, or C:

Type A host
- The patient shows a normal physiological response to infection and therapy.

Type B host
- The patient is compromised either locally (type BL) or systemically (type BS).

Type C host
- Whenever the treatment of the disease is more compromising for the patient than the disability caused by osteomyelitis itself, the patient is classified as a type C host.

This classification is of great value for preoperative planning and for comparison of clinical results.

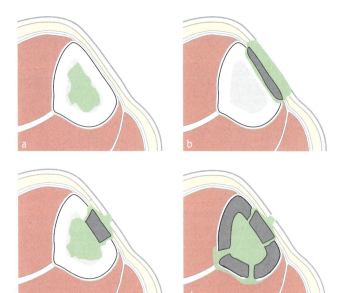

Fig 12-3a–d   Osteomyelitis classification according to Cierny and Mader.

a Stage I—Medullary osteomyelitis. The infection is within the medullary cavity.
b Stage II—Superficial osteomyelitis. The infection is on the surface of cortical bone.
c Stage III—Localized osteomyelitis. Full-thickness cortical sequestration, bone stability is maintained.
d Stage IV—Diffuse osteomyelitis. Circumferential lesion of the bone with impaired stability.

5   Treatment

Complete understanding of the extent of the disease as well as the nature of the host is necessary before any decisions can be made. In practice, this means complete clinical staging according to Cierny-Mader. In most cases, the treatment should be carried out as a team effort, with internists optimizing host status, infectious disease consultants managing antibacterial treatment, and surgeons (orthopedic, plastic, vascular) addressing any operative treatments [12]. Moreover, functional impairment caused by the disease or reconstruction operations as well as the metabolic consequences of aggressive therapy may influence the selection of the appropriate therapy. Basic therapy of osteomyelitis comprises the administration of antibiotics and surgery [12]. Although osteomyelitis first of all is a disease that is treated surgically, many cases may instead be treated with antibiotics alone. Acute hematogenous osteomyelitis in children should be treated by antibiotic therapy. The treatment starts with parenteral antibiotics, which clears the staphylococcus aureus infection, the main causative microorganism. As soon as all involved organisms are isolated, the treatment should be adjusted and optimized. The classic duration of antibiotic treatment is 4–6 weeks [7], although there is no general agreement on the duration of therapy [7, 13].

Limb immobilization is an adequate adjuvant in treating infections of bone and soft tissue. A short-term splinting of neighboring joints in the acute phase is also advisable [14].

5.1   Nonoperative treatment

Sometimes, osteomyelitis can be treated nonoperatively. **Table 12-1** offers a summary of the advised cast treatment for the various cases of osteomyelitis.

Author   Matej Cimerman

Site of infection	Nonoperative treatment
Upper arm	15.1 Long arm splint using plaster of Paris 15.2 Long arm splint using synthetic 18.3 Gilchrist bandage
Forearm	15.1 Long arm splint using plaster of Paris 15.2 Long arm splint using synthetic
Wrist/hand/finger	15.6 Dorsopalmar (radial) short arm splint using plaster of Paris 15.7 Dorsopalmar (radial) short arm splint using synthetic 15.8 Palmar short arm splint using plaster of Paris 15.9 Palmar short arm splint using synthetic 15.10 Dorsal short arm splint using synthetic 15.17 Dorsopalmar (ulnar gutter) short arm splint including two or more fingers using plaster of Paris 15.18 Dorsopalmar (ulnar gutter) short arm splint including two or more fingers using synthetic 15.19 Palmar short arm splint including the fingers using plaster of Paris
Upper leg (distal)	16.5 Dorsal long leg splint using plaster of Paris
Lower leg	16.5 Dorsal long leg splint using plaster of Paris
Ankle/foot	16.10 Dorsal short leg splint using plaster of Paris 16.11 Dorsal short leg splint using synthetic

Table 12-1   Recommended nonoperative treatments for cases of osteomyelitis.

Site of arthritis	Nonoperative treatment
Shoulder	18.3 Gilchrist bandage
Elbow	15.1 Long arm splint using plaster of Paris 15.2 Long arm splint using synthetic
Wrist	15.6 Dorsopalmar (radial) short arm splint using plaster of Paris 15.7 Dorsopalmar (radial) short arm splint using synthetic 15.8 Palmar short arm splint using plaster of Paris 15.9 Palmar short arm splint using synthetic 15.10 Dorsal short arm splint using synthetic
Fingers	15.17 Dorsopalmar (ulnar gutter) short arm splint including two or more fingers using plaster of Paris 15.18 Dorsopalmar (ulnar gutter) short arm splint including two or more fingers using synthetic 15.19 Palmar short arm splint including the fingers using plaster of Paris
Hip	Adults: no indication Pediatric: 16.1 One-and-a-half leg hip spica cast using plaster of Paris 16.2 Single leg hip spica cast using synthetic, combicast technique
Knee	16.5 Dorsal long leg splint using plaster of Paris
Ankle/foot	16.10 Dorsal short leg splint using plaster of Paris 16.11 Dorsal short leg splint using synthetic

Table 12-2   Recommended nonoperative treatments in cases of acute septic arthritis.

5.2   Acute septic arthritis

Acute septic arthritis is treated with appropriate antibiotics and regular irrigation of the joint through a needle, either by arthroscopy or arthrotomy. Splinting and immobilization of the joint are only necessary in acute phases; early motion is paramount in preserving long-term joint function [15]. **Table 12-2** offers a summary of the advised cast treatments in cases of acute septic arthritis.

Antibiotics are usually given intravenously for 2 weeks, followed by oral administration for 4 weeks [16]. The surgical treatment of osteomyelitis includes adequate drainage, thorough debridement, dead space management, soft-tissue and bone reconstruction procedures, and stabilization, if necessary [6].

In Cierny-Mader stages I, II, and III, stabilization is not usually necessary. In these cases, a short period of immobilization of the neighboring joints may be advisable for pain relief and patient comfort. After the reconstruction of soft-tissue defects with free flaps, 1 week of immobilization in order to protect the anastomosis is recommended. The splints should be custom-made in order not to compromise problematic soft tissues [17]. The suggested duration of antibiotic treatment is 6 weeks after implant removal or after the last surgical procedure, and 3 months in cases of device retention [18]. When surgical treatment is not possible because of the bad general conditions of the patient (type C host), long-term antibiotic therapy is advised.

12

6   Summary

- Despite modern techniques and new antimicrobial agents, osteomyelitis and other infections and inflammation of the bones and joints are difficult to manage
- A fast and correct diagnosis, and identification of the causative agent(s) are of utmost importance
- Immobilization is one of the main principles in treatment of infections
- In adults, the principal treatment consists of a combination of antibiotics, surgery, and immobilization

- In children, acute hematogenous osteomyelitis is treated with antibiotics and immobilization
- In developing countries, conservative management of infections is often the only treatment available, which means: antibiotics and immobilization
- An interdisciplinary approach to the disease is highly recommended.

7   References

1. **Chaissaignac E**. [About osteomyelitis]. *Bull Mem Soc Chir.* 1852; 431–436. French.
2. **Gutierrez K**. Bone and joint infections in children. *Pediatr Clin North Am.* 2005 Jun; 52(3):779–794.
3. **Lew DP, Waldvogel FA**. Osteomyelitis. *N Engl J Med.* 1997 Apr 3; 336(14):999–1007.
4. **Gillespie WJ**. Epidemiology in bone and joint infection. *Infect Dis Clin North Am.* 1990 Sep; 4(3):361–376.
5. **Stewart PS, Costerton JW**. Antibiotic resistance of bacteria in biofilms. *Lancet.* 2001 Jul 14; 358(9276):135–138.
6. **Lazzarini L, Mader JT, Calhoun JH**. Osteomyelitis in long bones. *J Bone Joint Surg Am.* 2004 Oct; 86-A(10):2305–2318.
7. **Weichert S, Sharland M, Clarke NM, et al**. Acute haematogenous osteomyelitis in children: is there any evidence for how long we should treat? *Curr Opin Infect Dis.* 2008 Jun; 21(3):258–262.
8. **Lew DP, Waldvogel FA**. Osteomyelitis. *Lancet.* 2004 Jul 24–30; 364(9431):369–379.

9. **Hunziker S, Hügle T, Schuchardt K, et al**. The value of serum procalcitonin level for differentiation of infectious from noninfectious causes of fever after orthopaedic surgery. *J Bone Joint Surg Am.* 2010 Jan; 92(1):138–148.
10. **Mackowiak PA, Jones SR, Smith JW**. Diagnostic value of sinus-tract cultures in chronic osteomyelitis. *JAMA.* 1978 Jun 30; 239(26):2772–2775.
11. **Cierny G 3rd, Mader JT, Penninck JJ**. A clinical staging system for adult osteomyelitis. *Clin Orthop Relat Res.* 2003 Sep; (414):7–24.
12. **Rao N, Ziran BH, Lipsky BA**. Treating osteomyelitis: antibiotics and surgery. *Plast Reconstr Surg.* 2011 Jan; 127 Suppl 1:177S–187S.
13. **Pääkkönen M, Peltola H**. Antibiotic treatment for acute haematogenous osteomyelitis of childhood: moving towards shorter courses and oral administration. *Int J Antimicrob Agents.* 2011 Oct; 38(4):273–280. doi: 10.1016/j.ijantimicag.2011.04.007. Epub 2011 Jun 2.

14. **Dietz HG, Bachmeyr A, Joppich I**. [Osteomyelitis in children]. *Orthopade.* 2004 Mar; 33(3):287–296. German.
15. **Donatto KC**. Orthopedic management of septic arthritis. *Rheum Dis Clin North Am.* 1998 May; 24(2):275–286.
16. **Mathews CJ, Weston VC, Jones A, et al**. Bacterial septic arthritis in adults. *Lancet.* 2010 Mar; 375(9717):846–855.
17. **Caulfield RH, Maleki-Tabrizi A, Birch J, et al**. A novel splinting technique to protect free flaps in major limb trauma. *J Trauma.* 2008 Mar; 64(3):E44–46.
18. **Trampuz A, Zimmerli W**. Diagnosis and treatment of infections associated with fracture-fixation devices. *Injury.* 2006 May; 37 Suppl 2:S59–66.

13 Overload injuries

Miles Francis T Dela Rosa

13

GUIDELINES

Author   Miles Francis T Dela Rosa

13   Overload injuries

1   Introduction

The term "overload injuries" encompasses a spectrum of musculoskeletal infirmities resulting from events beyond the physiologic limits of adaptation. Such failures are often the result of repetitive microtrauma, which explains why they are sometimes also called "overuse injuries" in the literature.

2   Pathomechanics of injury

Overload injuries occur due to excessive force loads and are determined by such intrinsic factors as age, flexibility, strength, previous injuries, and limb alignment, or extrinsic factors such as the environment of the sports event, and specific biomechanical demands of the sport. The nature of the injury implies chronic sequelae of repetitive insults causing a progressive intensity of injury to the end organ involved. These repetitive injuries result in local tissue damage in the form of cellular and extracellular degenerative changes. On the cellular level, repetitive overload of tissues that fail to adapt to new or increased demands may lead to tissue breakdown and overuse injury. Stress or fatigue fractures occur when the bone does not adapt adequately to the mechanical load [1]. Physiologically, bone responds to strain with remodeling. In overload situations, the osteoclasts first resorb the lamellar bone, causing cavities, which are then refilled with denser bone by osteoblasts. Because of the imbalance between the activities of osteoclasts and osteoblasts, the result is the weakening of the bone, which will fracture. If the load is decreased, the bone may form denser bone mass. However, if the load continues, the microdamage results in stress fractures. One of the risk factors is the existence of a previous stress fracture [2].

Failure of adaptation is the result of an excessive load when executing maximal physical effort (**Fig 13-1**). These injuries are generally seen in relation to physical activity covering sports and work-related activities of the lower and upper extremities as well as the lower back. Approximately 50% of all sport injuries are the result of overuse [1].

3   Prevention of injury

The most important step in injury prevention is to establish the limits of performance in relation to the desired goal. The intrinsic risk factors must be considered, such as age, strength, and flexibility, while taking into account the nature of the sport and the environment in which the sport is carried out. The next step is to plan a systematic process of adaptation, which is referred to as a training program. This will define the goals of improving the body physique to meet the performance level desired, similar to the weight category a boxer intends to compete in [3–5].

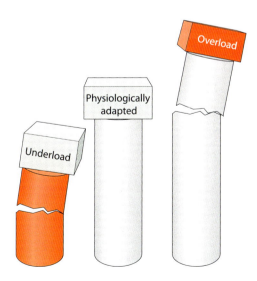

Fig 13-1   Training and adaptation.

4   Soft-tissue injuries

The following paragraphs outline some of the common overload related soft-tissue injuries.

4.1   Little-league elbow syndrome

This is a valgus overuse syndrome, resulting from repetitive throwing motions causing overload injuries to the medial elbow. A major factor contributing to this is the long and intense period of training for these young athletes. The ulnar collateral ligament is placed at risk, with injuries ranging from an injury to the ligament, avulsion of the condyle, to nerve compression. The use of temporary immobilization reduces pain [6–9].

4.2   Quadriceps tendonitis

Quadriceps tendonitis is an overload injury causing inflammation of the quadriceps located at the insertion of the ligament on top of the patella. This is commonly found in weightlifters or older athletes and is mainly due to the high strain on the muscle during the deep squats. Symptoms present as constant pain during and after exercise, which is at its worst during contraction of the quadriceps. Pain can also be elicited by applying anterior pressure on the patella, or after standing up from a crouched position [10] (**Fig 13-2**).

4.3   Osgood Schlatter disease

This is a traction injury of the tibial tubercle apophysis, which causes a painful lump below the knee cap noted during the growth-spurts phase of adolescence. The injury is precipitated by sports such as running or jumping, which inflict excessive tension forces on the tibial tubercle. The underlying pathology affects the vulnerable epiphyseal plate, which becomes inflamed and prone to injury [3, 7] (**Fig 13-3**).

4.4   Ruptured Achilles tendon

This is a common injury associated with badminton, squash, and highly demanding sports that call for agility, speed, and abrupt direction shifts (**Fig 13-4**). A second group comprises athletes involved in running sports [1]. Injury often results from extrinsic factors such as improper warm-up or the use of inappropriate footwear for the playing field or track. There are also a number of intrinsic factors that can influence the injury:

- Biomechanical malalignment of hindfoot and foot, eg, hyperpronation
- Varus deformity of the forefoot
- Increased inversion of the hindfoot
- Length discrepancies of the legs
- Restricted mobility in ankle and subtalar joint
- Decreased ankle dorsiflexion.

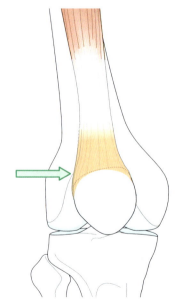

Fig 13-2   Quadriceps tendonitis (arrow).

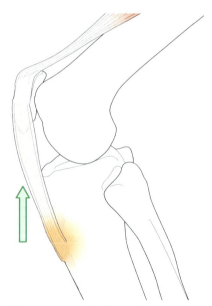

Fig 13-3   Osgood Schlatter disease, commonly caused from excessive tension force on the tibial tuberosity (arrow).

Author   Miles Francis T Dela Rosa

4.5   Retrocalcaneal bursitis

Retrocalcaneal bursitis frequently affects runners and is often mistaken for Achilles tendonitis. The pathology is inflammation of the bursa, located between the Achilles tendon and calcaneus. This is a result of repetitive microtrauma to the heel area brought about by inadequate cushioning during heel strike. Proper foot wear, technique, and terrain are important factors that need to be considered in order to prevent this injury [3] (**Fig 13-5**).

4.6   Dance injuries

There are intrinsic factors related to the specific dance regimens. In contemporary jazz dance for example, injuries are often related to weight and age, and it is therefore not recommended for heavy individuals [11]. Classical ballet and tap dancing injuries typically arise from the extensive amount of practice, therefore, training regimens must be regulated in order to achieve performance goals without causing injury. For classical ballet, an essential technique called "turnout" requires that the knee and foot are turned outward. This often results in overload injuries in the foot, ankle, and metatarsals, such as tendonitis and stress fractures [12].

4.7   Chronic compartment syndrome

Unlike acute compartment syndromes, this is not a surgical emergency. It is often precipitated by athletic exertion, ie, overload, and thus is also known as exertional compartment syndrome. It is related to repetitive athletic motions like running, biking, or swimming. Mostly, it is observed in the thigh and/or the medial compartment of the foot. Symptoms can include:

• Cramping during exercise
• Numbness
• Difficulty in moving the foot
• Occasionally muscle bulging.

The symptoms usually subside as the activity is discontinued. This syndrome must be differentiated from intermittent claudication [3, 13, 14].

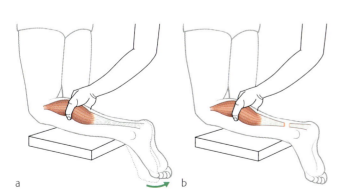

Fig 13-4a–b Ruptured Achilles tendon.
a Pressure on the gastrocnemius muscles transfers movement to the calcaneus via the Achilles tendon.
b If the tendon is ruptured, no movement of the hindfoot occurs.

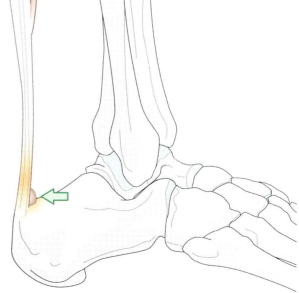

Fig 13-5 Retrocalcaneal bursitis (arrow).

13

5 Stress fractures

In fatigue or stress fractures, correct diagnostics are essential. Often the initial x-rays will show no fracture. However, focal periosteal thickening may be the first clue. An MRI can often confirm the diagnosis long before an x-ray can [15].

5.1 Stress fractures, medial tibia

The patient will experience shin pain under repetitive or excessive loading of the posteromedial lower third of the tibia. With removal of the load, with or without a cast, the tenderness will disappear within 4–8 weeks [15].

5.2 Stress fractures of the anterior tibial cortex

These fractures are especially dangerous as they can result in a delayed union or even nonunion. The first choice of treatment is rest or immobilization, preferably in a cast. In cases of nonhealing, further treatment such as autologous bone grafting or drilling of the fracture may be indicated [3, 14].

5.3 Stress fractures of the calcaneus

These are often localized at the upper posterior margin of the calcaneus. The x-ray will show typical density or sclerosis in lateral view, but MRI diagnostics are more sensitive. The appropriate treatment is load bearing restriction and, preferably, immobilization in a cast [1].

5.4 Stress fractures of the metatarsals

This injury is also known as a "march fracture" as it is generally seen in army recruits having to march for long periods of time. It usually involves the second, third, and fourth metatarsals as they absorb the greatest stress during push off. In the x-ray, partial or complete bone fractures can be documented. Risk factors associated with this injury typically are periods of transition where there is an increased frequency and duration of activity with limited intervals of rest. Other contributing factors are comorbid conditions, such as rheumatoid arthritis, and diabetic foot neuropathy [3, 15] (**Fig 13-6**).

6 Nonoperative treatment

A range of immediate and longer term treatments can be considered following an overload injury. These include:
- Nonoperative treatment, by applying the basic principles of rest and cooling (ice) as well as compression and elevation of the limb in order to control edema, pain, and hemorrhage
- Administering antiinflammatory drugs when necessary
- Identifying any risk factors or precipitating events causing the injury
- Bracing and casting when applicable for protection and immobilization in order to restrict a certain type of movement
- Implementing a well-planned physical therapy/rehabilitation program centered on a progressive functional exercise regimens with the objective of returning to the preinjury level of activity
- However, surgical management is indicated in cases of failed conservative treatment in addressing issues of persistent pain, instability, or nerve compression.

Table 13-1 provides an overview of the various types of overload injuries and the chapters covering the appropriate nonoperative treatment options.

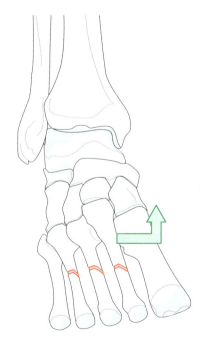

Fig 13-6 Stress fractures can occur in metatarsals II–IV as these absorb the greatest stress during push off (arrow).

Author   Miles Francis T Dela Rosa

Overload injury	Nonoperative treatment
Little-league elbow syndrome	15.1 Long arm splint using plaster of Paris 15.2 Long arm splint using synthetic
Quadriceps tendonitis	16.3 Cylinder long leg cast using synthetic, combicast technique
Osgood Schlatter disease	16.3 Cylinder long leg cast using synthetic, combicast technique
Ruptured Achilles tendon	16.10 Dorsal short leg splint using plaster of Paris 16.11 Dorsal short leg splint using synthetic 16.12 Short leg cast using rigid synthetic 16.13 Short leg cast using synthetic, combicast technique
Retrocalcaneal bursitis	Not indicated
Dance injuries	16.10 Dorsal short leg splint using plaster of Paris 16.11 Dorsal short leg splint using synthetic 16.12 Short leg cast using rigid synthetic 16.13 Short leg cast using synthetic, combicast technique 16.15 Removable ankle splint using synthetic, combicast technique 16.16 Fifth metatarsal cast using synthetic, combicast technique 16.17 Removable fifth metatarsal cast using synthetic, combicast technique 16.18 Foot cast using synthetic, combicast technique 16.19 Removable foot cast using synthetic, combicast technique
Chronic (exertional) compartment syndrome	Not indicated

Overload injury	Nonoperative treatment
Stress fractures medial tibia	16.10 Dorsal short leg splint using plaster of Paris 16.11 Dorsal short leg splint using synthetic 16.12 Short leg cast using rigid synthetic 16.13 Short leg cast using synthetic, combicast technique
Stress fracture of the anterior tibial cortex	16.10 Dorsal short leg splint using plaster of Paris 16.11 Dorsal short leg splint using synthetic 16.12 Short leg cast using rigid synthetic 16.13 Short leg cast using synthetic, combicast technique
Stress fracture of the calcaneus	16.11 Dorsal short leg splint using synthetic 16.12 Short leg cast using rigid synthetic 16.13 Short leg cast using synthetic, combicast technique 16.14 Antirotation short leg cast using synthetic, combicast technique 16.18 Foot cast using synthetic, combicast technique 16.19 Removable foot cast using synthetic, combicast technique
Metatarsal stress fractures	16.16 Fifth metatarsal cast using synthetic, combicast technique 16.17 Removable fifth metatarsal cast using synthetic, combicast technique 16.18 Foot cast using synthetic, combicast technique 16.19 Removable foot cast using synthetic, combicast technique

Table 13-1   Overview of the various types of overload injuries and the chapters covering appropriate treatment.

13

7 Summary

- Overload injuries occur due to excessive force loads, and are influenced by intrinsic factors (age, flexibility, strength, previous injuries) and extrinsic factors (the demands of the specific sport/work activity)
- While bones and soft-tissue can adapt to the various forces, repetition of the activity can lead to a failure in adaptation, resulting in tissue breakdown and overuse injury

- Common overload related soft-tissue injuries include little-league elbow syndrome, quadriceps tendonitis, ruptured Achilles tendon, dance injuries, and stress fractures
- While nonoperative treatment can be used to treat most forms of overload injury, the most important step in injury prevention is to have previously established the individual's limits of performance.

8 References

1. **Wilder RP, Sethi S**. Overuse injuries: tendinopathies, stress fractures, compartment syndrome, and shin splints. *Clin Sports Med*. 2004 Jan; 23(1):55–81.
2. **Van Oers RF, Van Rietbergen B, Ito K, et al**. Simulation of trabecular remodeling and fatigue: is remodeling helpful or harmful? *Bone*. 2011 May; 48(5):1210–1215.
3. **Rouzier P, White T, Gilfilan T, et al**. *The Sports Medicine Patient Advisor*. 3rd ed. Amherst, USA: SportsMedPress; 2010:3, 44, 79, 202, 326.
4. **West RV, Fu FH**. Soft-tissue physiology and repair. Vaccaro AR (ed). *AAOS Orthopaedic Knowledge Update 8*. 1st ed. Rosemont, USA: American Academy of Orthopaedic Surgeons; 2005:15–27.
5. **Duca M**. Medical care of athletes. *AAOS Orthopaedic Knowledge Update 8*. 1st ed. Rosemont, USA: American Academy of Orthopaedic Surgeons; 2005:149–158.
6. **Bernstein J, Pepe M, Kaplan L**. Shoulder and elbow disorders in the athlete. Flynn J (ed). *AAOS Orthopaedic Knowledge Update 10*. 1st ed. Rosemont, USA: American Academy of Orthopaedic Surgeons; 2011:315–324.
7. **Cassas KJ, Cassettari-Wayhs**. Childhood and adolescent sport-related overuse Injuries. *American Family Physician*. 2006 Mar 15; 73(6):1014–1022.

8. **Li X, Heffernan MJ, Mortimer ES**. Upper extremity stress fractures and spondylosis in an adolescent baseball pitcher with an associated endocrine abnormality: a case report. *Journal Pediatric Orthopedics*. 2010 Jun; 30(4):339–43.
9. **Safran M, Ahmad CS, Elatrache NS**. Ulnar collateral ligament of the elbow. *Arthroscopy*. 2005 Nov; 21(11):1381–1385.
10. **Snider R, Green W, Johnson T, et al.** Essentials of musculoskeletal care. *AAOS Orthopaedic Knowledge Update 9*. 1st ed. Rosemont, USA: American Academy of Orthopaedic Surgeons; 2010:46, 136, 356, 387.
11. **Campoy FA, Coelho LR, Bastos FN, et al.** Investigation of risk factors and characteristics of dance injuries. *Clin J Sport Med*. 2011 Nov; 21(6):493–498.
12. **Khan K, Brown J, Way S, et al.** Overuse injuries in classical ballet. *Sports Med*. 1995 May; 19(5):341–357.
13. **Chhabra A, Katolik L, Pavlovich R Jr.** Sports medicine. Miller MD (ed). *Review of Orthopaedics*. 4th ed. Philadelphia: Saunders Elsevier; 2004:228–230.
14. **Hart J, Baumfield J, Miller M**. Sports medicine. Miller MD (ed). *Review of Orthopaedics*. 5th ed. Philadelphia: Saunders Elsevier; 2008:263–264.
15. **Patel DS, Roth M, Kapil N**. Stress fractures: diagnosis, treatment, and prevention. *American Family Physician*. 2011 Jan 1; 83(1):39–46.

9 Further reading

Craig DI. Current developments concerning medial tibial stress syndrome. *Phys Sportsmed*. 2009 Dec; (4):39–40.

Roehrig GJ, Baumhauer JF, Giordano BD, et al. Disorders of the foot and ankle. Miller MD (ed). *Review of Orthopaedics*. 5th ed. Philadelphia: Saunders Elsevier; 2008:359–402.

Shea K, Ganley T. Injuries and conditions of the pediatric and adolescent athlete. *AAOS Orthopaedic Knowledge Update 10*. 1st ed. Rosemont, USA: American Academy of Orthopaedic Surgeons; 2011:783–793.

Story J. Cymet TC. Shin splints: painful to have and to treat. *Compr Ther*. 2006 Fall; 32(3):192–195.

TECHNIQUES

Casts, splints, and support bandages—techniques

Techniques

14.1 Overview of cast, splint, orthosis, and bandage techniques

Klaus Dresing, Jos Engelen

Authors Klaus Dresing, Jos Engelen

14.1 Overview of cast, splint, orthosis, and bandage techniques

1 Introduction

In this third and final section, the techniques for preparing and applying casts, splints, orthoses, and support bandages are presented. It outlines the individual steps for 55 casting and immobilization procedures, covering the upper extremity, the lower extremity, and the spine. But just as with any invasive procedure, preparation and planning is mandatory before beginning to apply a noninvasive immobilization bandage. It is therefore recommended that prior to the procedure the caregiver obtains the relevant materials and has a full understanding of the following:

- The sequence for examination and treatment
- Resources and staffing needs
- The various types of immobilization
- The various types of materials
- Pain relief
- Fracture reduction
- Patient and limb positioning
- Applying and handling cast materials
- Bandaging techniques
- Cast splitting and cast removal
- Patient information and consent
- Controls and reviews
- Duration of immobilization.

The process of applying a cast, splint, or orthosis is initiated by the physician's decision that some form of immobilization is indicated, as a part of nonoperative or perioperative care. If immobilization is necessary, the required resources must be prepared. These may include assistance and appropriate facility, but appropriate supplies and equipment are always required. Since the various cast materials have different properties, the professional user must select the material that will best fit the type of fracture or lesion, the body region, or the age of the patient. The medical indications for immobilization have been spelled out in section 2 Guidelines.

Skillful application of the cast by the trauma or orthopedic resident or surgeon is essential for good results [1]. The physician confirming that immobilization is indicated should of course also be able to personally apply the cast, splint, orthosis, or support bandage themselves.

> Only this experience and understanding will enable the surgeon to assess casts applied by residents, cast technicians, or other caregivers. And only with this knowledge and experience will he/she be able to obtain the comprehensive informed consent and provide an informed discharge for the patient (see chapter 3 Principles of casting).

This chapter therefore provides the reader with an essential overview and technique tips for the effective and safe application of immobilization bandages.

14.1

TECHNIQUES

2   Sequence of examination and treatment

In the case of nonoperative fracture care, the sequence of examination and treatment is as follows:
- Examination and diagnosis
- Fracture reduction
- Application of casting materials
- Assessment of reduction and immobilization
- Documentation.

2.1   Examination

In the previous section Guidelines, the process for examination and diagnosis is outlined for each of the extremities. Typically, the first step in any treatment is the medical history, including mechanism of injury, followed by a complete medical examination and relevant diagnostic tools.

When examining the injured extremity and body region, look for the following signs:
- Localized tenderness, swelling, deformity, or instability
- Unwillingness or inability to move or use the part normally
- Visible bone injury in an open wound
- Abnormal mobility at suspected fracture site
- Bony crepitus
- Fracture evident by x-ray.

This is followed by examination of the fracture region and distal extremity for:
- Traumatic skin lesion
- Hematoma
- Soft-tissue injury
- Vascular injury
- Nerve lesion.

2.2   Fracture reduction

The sequence of fracture reduction is nearly the same in all extremities, and should follow this sequence:
- Effective elimination of pain, with analgesia or anesthesia
  - Local
  - Regional
  - General
- Traction (extension) in longitudinal axial direction
- "Hooking-together" of the fragments, when the fracture pattern permits
- Alignment along the anatomical axis (rotation and angulation).

2.3   Cast procedure

The order and steps for applying the cast or splint are as follows:
- Lining layer over the skin, using tube bandage (stockinette)
- Padding
- Application of plaster of Paris or synthetic cast material
- Molding
- Splitting of the cast (in primary fracture care this is mandatory)
- Anchoring, with gauze or elastic bandage.

Take care to protect the patient's clothing against contact with plaster or synthetic cast material.

2.4   Documentation

These vital steps should be followed (see the topics Pretreatment medical information and informed consent, and Posttreatment patient information and cast check in chapter 3 Principles of casting):
- All results of the medical examination should be documented in writing
- All reduced fractures will be documented with x-ray review
- If a patient is unable to sign or give informed consent due to his/her injury, the information is documented by the physician.

Documentation of the neurovascular status and x-ray review at the end of the cast/splint procedure is mandatory before the patient is allowed to leave the emergency department.

Each of the elements in the sequence for casting is further detailed in this chapter.

Authors   Klaus Dresing, Jos Engelen

3   Cast room preparation

For the application of plaster of Paris (POP) and synthetic immobilization bandages, the specially equipped room called a cast room is recommended (**Fig 14.1-1**) (see chapter 5 Logistics and resources in the cast room). While other nonoperative and bandaging activities can also take place in this room, it is specially designed for efficient cast application, including safety measures for patient and staff.

Prior to an immobilization procedure, ensure that all necessary materials, instruments, and equipment are readily available. Check monitoring equipment, energy, lighting, and water supply, and prepare image viewing equipment, if needed. Prepare the cast cart (trolley) and move it into place within easy reach. Similarly, prepare the cast table, cushions to support extremities, and other furniture so that the patient can be positioned appropriately before beginning the procedure. Remember that the materials have a limited working and setting time, so it is important not to interrupt the procedure.

The cast room must have an appropriate plaster sink and trap. When using plaster of Paris, plaster is lost into the water. Without separating this plaster from the wastewater, the outlet pipes will soon clog with hardening plaster sludge. A bucket or plaster basin can be used for dipping and wetting plaster closer to the patient, but these should always be emptied into an appropriately drained plaster sink. Appropriate waste disposal containers should be readily available for both contaminated and nonmedical waste.

Normally a cast technician is the person applying the casts but operating room personnel or nursing staff may also be trained to apply casts and bandages. Every trauma or orthopedic surgeon should also be trained and able to apply casts and bandages. Fracture reduction, however, is always the task of the surgeon.

4   Types of immobilization

When considering what type of immobilization is required, the physician must assess the stage and severity of the injury, the potential for instability, the risk of complications, and the patient's functional requirements (see also chapter 3 Principles of casting) [2].

A cast is applied in a circumferential manner around the extremity. Split casts are often used in primary fracture care after reduction of complex fractures, but nonsplit casts are rarely indicated in definitive fracture care. A cast is the first choice in cases involving noncompliant patients because casts are more difficult for patients to remove by themselves. In special indications, primary definitive fracture care with semirigid synthetic cast materials could be considered. Boyd et al summarized that "casts provide more effective immobilization, but require more skill and time to apply and have a higher risk of complications if not applied properly" [2].

A splint does not circumferentially surround the extremity and therefore allows soft-tissue expansion during the posttraumatic inflammatory phase. Splints are often used in initial fracture care, as well as for sprains, tendon injuries, soft-tissue injuries, nerve injuries, and postoperatively. Splints make it easier to examine or redress the wound, because they are easier to remove than a fully circular (closed) or split plaster cast.

Orthoses, removable casts, and support bandages allow much easier access to the limb, but provide less stability. Their use is particularly indicated when functional therapy is considered appropriate.

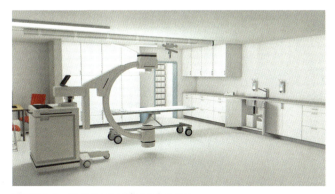

Fig 14.1-1   Cast room with equipment.

4.1 Primary fracture care

The initial (primary) treatment of a fractured bone is reduction (if necessary), retention, and immobilization of the extremity. In primary fracture care, a splint is often used after reduction of the fracture because of the likelihood of soft-tissue swelling. Another immobilization method is the application of a POP cast that is mandatorily split to allow widening of the cast, again in expectation of soft-tissue swelling. Normally, this initial split cast or splint is then replaced by a final definitive cast after 2-3 weeks.

4.2 Primary definitive fracture care

In special indications, a cast is applied only once at admission in hospital, and no replacement is needed (hence it is called the definitive cast). For these indications, such as nondisplaced fractures, or pediatric greenstick fractures, the patient is treated with a split synthetic cast (eg, semirigid or using the combicast technique). After the swelling has decreased (normally after one week) the split cast is further reduced in diameter by cutting away a strip of cast material. The cast is then closed using another roll of semirigid cast material or by fixing it with an elastic bandage or velcro strips. This process also permits tightening of a cast that has become loose once swelling resolves.

5 Types of materials

As outlined in chapter 6 Properties of cast materials, casts, splints, and orthoses all follow the same modular construction:
- Lining material ie, tube bandage (stockinette)
- Padding
- Casting material.

Note that you should always read the instructions of use from the cast and padding material carefully before working with the material.

5.1 Tube bandage (stockinette)

Adapt the tube bandage diameter to the extremity or body region (**Table 14.1-1**). Do not tighten or stretch the tubular bandage too much as this can lead to high skin pressure and can result in compartment syndrome if not cut open at the end of the application. Once the first layer is applied, keep the joint and limb in the desired position. Avoid wrinkles, as they can lead to pressure sores beneath the cast or splint.

Site of cast	Diameter of tube bandage[1]
Finger	Approximately 2–2.5 cm
Upper extremity	Approximately 5–7.5 cm
Lower extremity	Approximately 7.5–10 cm

[1] Depending on the brand of the tube bandage.

Table 14.1-1 Recommended diameter of tube bandage in relation to body region.

Authors   Klaus Dresing, Jos Engelen

5.2   Cast padding and the protection of bony prominences

Cast padding acts as a protection layer between the cast material, skin, and soft tissue (see also chapter 6 Properties of cast materials). The recommended width of rolled cast padding in relation to the body region is outlined in **Table 14.1-2**.

Site of cast	Recommended padding width
Hand	Approximately 5 cm
Upper extremity	Approximately 5–7.5 cm
Foot	Approximately 5 cm
Lower extremity	Approximately 10–15 cm

Table 14.1-2   Recommended width for cast padding rolls in relation to body region.

The padding should usually extend beyond the intended edge of the cast or splint by 1–2 fingers breadth. Cast padding is normally applied using the "half-overlapping technique" (see topic 10 Bandaging techniques in this chapter).

Padding is normally only applied after the desired joint position, usually the neutral (or "functional") position, has been achieved (see topic 8 Patient positioning in this chapter). Do not apply padding around joints, for example, the elbow joint, before the final position is reached. If this is not done carefully, poorly fitted padding can compress the concave region, and cause pressure that might cause swelling from venous compression, skin injury, nerve palsy, or ischemia.

If fingers or toes are included in a cast or splint, the interdigital space should be protected against maceration with additional tube bandages or padding (**Fig 14.1-2**). More padding layers can also be used if soft-tissue swelling, to a large extent, is to be expected.

A layer of water-resistant crepe paper bandage can be used over the padding before wet plaster or synthetic cast materials are applied. This can be used to "snug-up" and secure the padding for smooth, gentle compression. Underwrap is necessary to allow an even compression of the padding layers and to separate the dry padding from the wet POP. This layer also keeps water and dissolved plaster from wetting the padding layers, resulting in hardening of the padding and the potential for pressure sores.

At times, extra padding, typically as a focal patch instead of circumferentially, has to be applied at the "bony prominences" and vessels. A bony prominence is a part of a bone that sticks out or protrudes, such as a knobby knee or shoulder blade, and they are often not well covered by soft tissue or are positioned immediately under the skin surface. Bony prominences are areas with a high risk of developing pressure sores or other damage. Additionally, nerves running directly along the bone near the prominences are also in danger of suffering injury, such as nerve palsy.

In the upper limb, the prominences include the inner epicondyle of the humerus, the tip of the elbow, and the styloid process at the wrist. In the lower limb, areas requiring extra protection include the heel, malleoli, the patella, the head of the fibula, and the greater trochanter. Prominences of the torso include the sacrum/coccyx, the anterior superior iliac spines or iliac crest, and the ischial tuberosity of the spinal process. Particularly with synthetic casts, additional pieces of foam or felt padding to cover these sensitive places are recommended. **Fig 14.1-3** indicates the most sensitive locations, and these are further highlighted in each of the casting technique demonstrations in chapters 15 to 18.

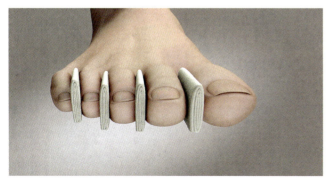

Fig 14.1-2   Extra protection of the interdigital space between the fingers or toes is sometimes required.

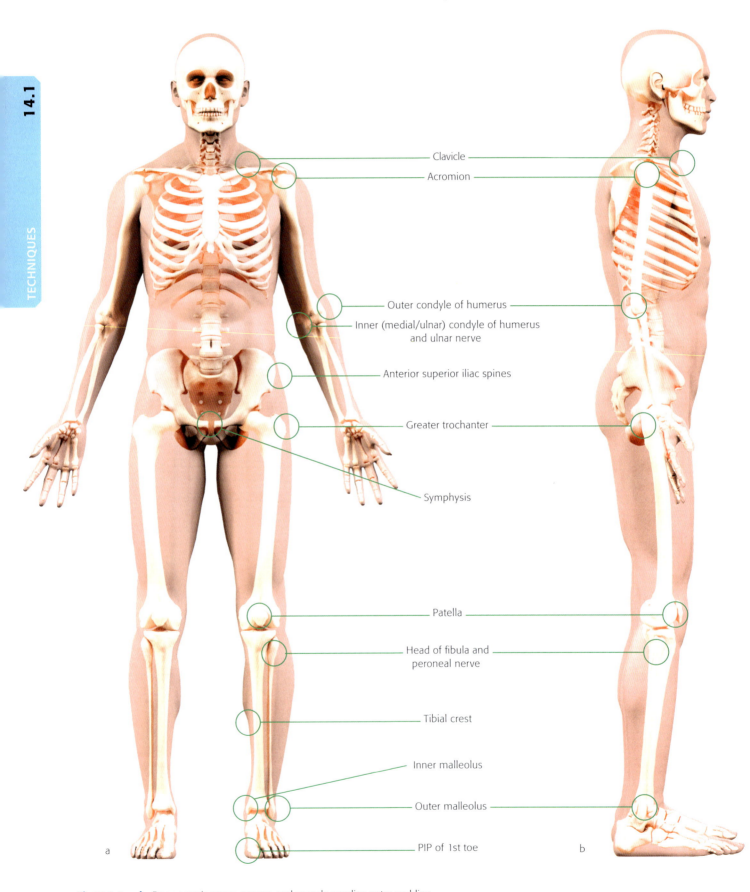

Clavicle

Acromion

Outer condyle of humerus

Inner (medial/ulnar) condyle of humerus and ulnar nerve

Anterior superior iliac spines

Greater trochanter

Symphysis

Patella

Head of fibula and peroneal nerve

Tibial crest

Inner malleolus

Outer malleolus

PIP of 1st toe

a   b

Fig 14.1-3a–d   Bony prominences, nerves, and vessels needing extra padding.

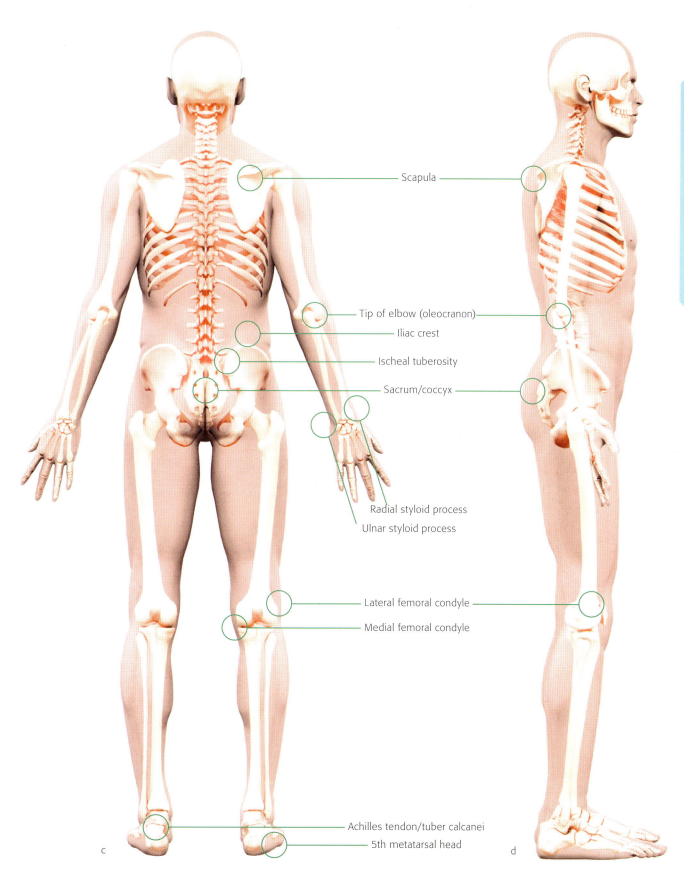

Scapula

Tip of elbow (oleocranon)

Iliac crest

Ischeal tuberosity

Sacrum/coccyx

Radial styloid process

Ulnar styloid process

Lateral femoral condyle

Medial femoral condyle

Achilles tendon/tuber calcanei

5th metatarsal head

c

d

TECHNIQUES

5.3 Cast material
5.3.1 Plaster of Paris

The main advantage of plaster of Paris is its pliability and moldability (see also chapter 6 Properties of cast materials). **Table 14.1-3** provides a list of the appropriate dimensions for POP cast material in relation to the respective area of application.

Site of cast	Recommended width of plaster of Paris cast rolls
Hand	6–8 cm
Upper extremity	8–10 cm
Foot	6–8 cm
Lower extremity	10–15 cm

Table 14.1-3 Width recommendations for plaster of Paris cast material in relation to body region.

5.3.2 Synthetic

The advantages of synthetic cast material are its stability, water resistance, low weight, and shorter setting and hardening time (see also chapter 6 Properties of cast materials) in comparison to POP. **Table 14.1-4** provides a list of the appropriate dimensions for synthetic cast material in relation to the respective area of application.

Site of cast	Recommended width of synthetic cast rolls
Hand	2.5–5 cm
Upper extremity	5–7.5 cm
Foot	5–7.5 cm
Lower extremity	7.5–10 cm

Table 14.1-4 Width recommendations for synthetic cast material in relation to body region.

Authors   Klaus Dresing, Jos Engelen

6   Pain relief

Acute fractures are normally quite painful. For fracture reduction, and sometimes even for cast application without fracture manipulation, some form of analgesia and/or anesthesia is needed. Fracture reduction, or even just splint application, are procedures that can temporarily increase pain. For patient comfort, and muscle relaxation to facilitate fracture manipulation, an anesthetic is recommended typically in addition to analgesic medications.

While an anesthetic may not be required, a strong analgesic can still make the procedure more tolerable, and improves the patient's ability to relax and cooperate. Consider analgesia alone if the fracture is stable, when manipulation is not necessary, or if a recent injury's pain has significantly resolved. Use some form of anesthesia for more severe pain, and if relaxation is necessary for the reduction. In any case, it is essential to assess the patient's need for pain relief and provide it adequately. This may require a change in plans if discomfort proves more than anticipated. While a given procedure may be satisfactorily tolerated by an adult with analgesia plus local or regional anesthesia, a child is usually more comfortable with a general anesthetic.

It is essential for the surgeon to be aware of the available medications and their pharmacologic aspects, as well as his/her institution's pain management policies and the necessary safety precautions. Patient allergies must be identified. Awareness of maximal allowable doses of any local anesthetic is important. Particularly if given rapidly, the possibility of causing a seizure must be considered when using a so-called hematoma block (see below), since an injection into a bone's intramedullary space is essentially an intravenous injection. Antidotes for reversal of narcotics and benzodiazepines should be available. Whenever intravenous sedation is used, an emergency cart is required. This must contain devices for suction, positive pressure breathing, and airway establishment. All members of the treatment team must be aware of how to request an emergency resuscitation team ("code call").

6.1   Anesthetics

Anesthetics are classified according to route of administration as:

- Local anesthesia, injected into the involved area
- Regional anesthesia
  - Neuraxial: spinal or epidural, or
  - Peripheral: via plexus or single nerve blocks
  - Another form of regional anesthesia, available in some institutions, is an intravenous regional or Bier block, used with an arterial tourniquet
- General anesthesia, with inhalation and or intravenous medications.

In many hospitals, surgeons will administer local and sometimes regional anesthetics, while anesthesiologists or nurse anesthetists manage more complex regional as well as general anesthetics. In some situations, other techniques of anesthesia/analgesia are used during fracture treatment, such as a mixture of nitrous oxide and oxygen which is administered to the patient with a self-controlled inhalation device. So-called "conscious sedation" is another technique used during procedures, and is often applicable for nonoperative fracture care. This involves intravenous administration of sedative and analgesic drugs, at a level that depresses consciousness but allows the patient to maintain their airway, independently and continuously. It requires a trained nurse or physician, and comprehensive continuous monitoring by an assigned member of the treating team with no other responsibilities. There should be a pulse oximeter, electrocardiographic monitor, and facilities for measuring and recording blood pressure, pulse, and level of consciousness, as well as a complete emergency cart with all necessary resuscitation equipment and supplies. Yet another technique involves the use of ketamine, a dissociative anesthetic with less respiratory and cardiac depression, but frequent dysphoric effects in adults. Its major use is for children.

14.1

TECHNIQUES

14.1

6.1.1 Local anesthesia

The hematoma block is often a good alternative to more complex anesthesia, if the fracture is fresh and the hematoma is still liquid. Premedication with systemic analgesics is helpful. Sterile technique is required. The fracture is localized by palpation or with x-ray under the C-arm. After subcutaneous application of a small deposit of local anesthetic, followed by an appropriate reaction time, the needle is inserted into the gap between the main fragments (**Fig 14.1-4**).

After bone contact with the needle, aspiration of blood confirms that the needle is correctly located within the hematoma (**Fig 14.1-5**). The aspiration of fat droplets is additional evidence of correct positioning of the needle (**Fig 14.1-6**). Inject 5–10 ml of anesthetic (for example, 0.5% or 1% lidocaine without epinephrine) stepwise after aspiration of as much hematoma as possible. This may be easier with a larger bore needle, after the initial injection with a smaller one. Hematoma removal may decrease the pressure in the fracture gap.

During the creation of a hematoma block, the patient can become anxious, in which case muscle spasms are common. Sufficient time should be allowed for the patient to adapt to the situation and for the drug to act. The surgeon should inform the patient of all steps of treatment; he or she should calm the patient and create a professional atmosphere for treatment. With pain relief, the muscles will be more relaxed and fracture reduction can be performed more easily and effectively.

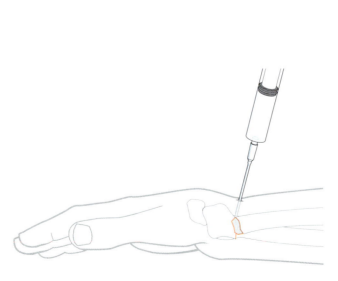

Fig 14.1-4   A needle with local anesthetic is inserted into the gap between the main fracture fragments.

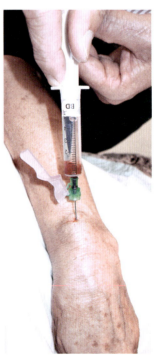

Fig 14.1-5   After subcutaneous injection of a small deposit of local anesthesia, the needle is guided into the fracture hematoma. The aspiration of blood into the syringe is proof of correct positioning of the needle into the fracture gap.

Authors   Klaus Dresing, Jos Engelen

6.1.2 Regional anesthesia

Peripheral regional anesthesia is achieved by injection of an appropriate volume of local anesthetic adjacent to the nerves supplying the anatomic region for which anesthesia is desired. If a structural sheath envelopes the nerves (eg, brachial plexus) the injection should fill and distend this structure. A successful regional anesthetic should eliminate sensation and motor function in the distribution of the blocked nerves, through its inhibition of nerve membrane depolarization. Normally, serious complications from regional anesthesia are exceedingly rare.

There are a number of nerve blocks commonly used in clinical practice:

- Upper extremity: interscalene block, axillary (brachial plexus) block, medial, ulnar, and digital blocks
- Lower extremity: femoral, sciatic, saphenous, sural and ankle blocks
- Digital nerve blocks are frequently used in the emergency department for finger injuries and distal infections (felons and paronychiae).

6.1.3 General anesthesia

General anesthetics offer advantages for children, especially pain-free induction, reliable anesthesia, good muscle relaxation, and amnesia for the procedure. They should be considered whenever fracture reduction is being planned for a young child [3]. A general anesthetic is certainly an option for any significant fracture manipulation in an adult as well. Sometimes the combination of a regional anesthetic with a lower level of general anesthesia nicely balances the benefits of both techniques. Collaboration with an anesthesiologist is often helpful in choosing the most appropriate means of pain control, and is highly recommended when patients have complicating medical issues. The surgeon should discuss with the anesthesiologist the planned procedure, its steps (such as the need to assess x-rays before awakening the patient), the need for muscle relaxation, and other relevant details.

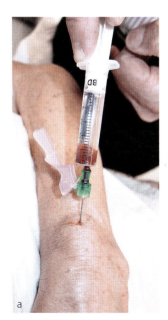
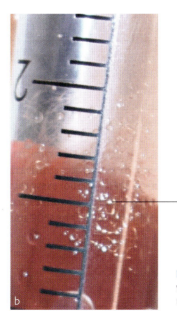

Note the many fat droplets aspirated from the medullary space.

Fig 14.1-6a–b   Hematoma with fat droplets indicates correct needle placement.

14.1

TECHNIQUES

6.2   Analgesia

Analgesia for fracture manipulation can be provided using oral premedication with a well-absorbed narcotic or nonsteroidal antiinflammatory agent. Alternatively, a parenteral analgesic can be given, via intramuscular or intravenous routes. Parenteral analgesics are often needed initially. Intravenous medications can be given with a patient-controlled device, or titrated with repeated small doses to achieve relief without excessive sedation or respiratory depression. Intramuscular administration is slower to take effect, and harder to control, but lasts longer.

Typically, it is the procedure itself that is painful, with relief after the cast has been applied and is hard enough to be an effective splint. Sufficient medication to permit a fracture reduction can result in over-sedation after the procedure is finished. Whenever significant analgesic doses are used, they should be appropriate for the patient's age, weight, and metabolism.

Strong analgesics are typically needed for the pain of a fresh fracture, at least for the first few days after injury [3]. Adequate fracture splinting aids significantly with pain control. Muscle spasms aggravate fracture pain. Muscle relaxants (for example, benzodiazepines) are sometimes added to analgesics, but they do not themselves relieve pain, and, in combination with narcotics, can produce excessive sedation.

Significant fracture pain often persists for a week or two, especially with nonoperative treatment. Thus, every patient should receive an analgesic prescription for use in the post-fracture and post-reduction periods. In addition, patients should be instructed to consult the surgeon immediately if the pain does not ease with time and/or rest, and especially if it increases in spite of analgesics. A compartment syndrome could be the cause of severe, increasing pain.

Authors   Klaus Dresing, Jos Engelen

7   Reducing the fracture

The anatomical realignment of fractures is called reduction. In diaphyseal fractures, restoration of axis, bone length, and anatomical rotation are the goals. While this might be sufficient for metaphyseal fractures, displaced articular fractures cannot be anatomically reduced successfully without surgical reduction and fixation. In most anatomic regions, rotation and angular alignment of diaphyseal fractures can be achieved with manipulation, and often maintained with a cast. Successful maintenance of length can be more difficult, unless the ends of two major fracture fragments can be hooked onto one another so that, stabilized by external immobilization, they do not redisplace and shorten. Fractures that are comminuted, spiral, or significantly oblique cannot be hooked together in a way that produces length stability. If they are significantly shortened, even if temporarily restored to appropriate length, they can be expected to return to the degree of shortening evident on initial unreduced x-rays.

While some shortening of the humerus is well tolerated, forearm diaphyseal fractures must be fixed anatomically, and only slight shortening of the tibia or femur can be accepted without compromise of gait.

Closed reduction of a displaced fracture, in an adult, typically requires initial distraction, to permit correction of the deformity, and/or to allow hooking-on and restoration of length stability. To distract the fracture site, gravity can be used to great advantage (**Fig 14.1-7** and **Fig 14.1-8**) (see chapters 9.2 Fractures, dislocations, and subluxations of the lower extremity; and 15.15 Short arm cast using plaster of Paris with traction and reduction).

The amount of force needed to realign the fragments depends on displacement, relaxation, and the location of the fracture, but especially upon the viscoelasticity of the fracture site. Sustained, sufficient, but relatively gentle force can gradually stretch the soft tissues surrounding a fresh fracture so that overlapping is eliminated, and a gap develops between the fracture ends (see also topic 7 Reduction of bone fractures in chapter 3 Principles of casting).

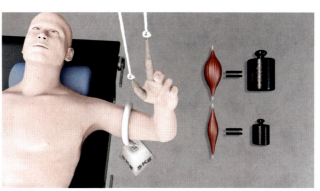
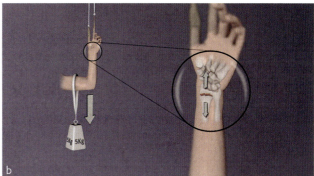

Fig 14.1-8a–b   Gravity and fracture reduction.

a   The amount of weight to be used in traction depends on the patient's muscle volume and strength.

b   The relevant weight is used to disimpact the fracture.

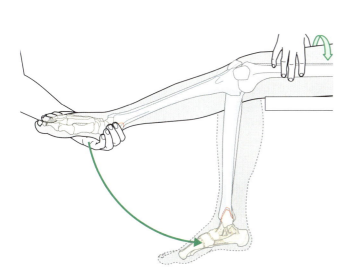

Fig 14.1-7   The effect of using gravity in order to achieve fracture reduction.

If the fragments are impacted (truly crushed into each other, as typically occurs in corticocancellous metaphyseal bone), the surgeon will try to disimpact the fracture. Since x-rays are two dimensional, it is important to remember that apparent "impaction" may only represent overlapping fragments. To correct true impaction, the fragments must be mobilized so they can be moved independently. One way to do this is to apply forces in the direction of those that caused the fracture ("reproduce the injury"), and then correct the fracture deformity. For example, with a typical, dorsally displaced and angulated distal radius fracture, one

may begin by increasing dorsal angulation, increasing deformity, and then, with distracting force, correct the dorsal displacement and restore palmar angulation. To help us understand this, Charnley described the "gear-wheel" mechanism, pointing out that disengagement of the improperly "meshed gears" was necessary before deformity could be corrected (**Fig 14.1-9**) (and see chapter 15.15 Short arm cast using plaster of Paris with traction and reduction) [4].

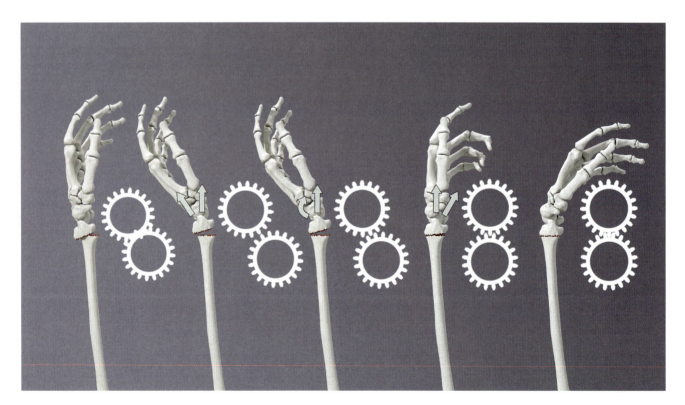

Fig 14.1-9   "Gear-wheel" mechanism illustration of the radius, according to Charnley [4]. Note that first impaction and then displacement must be corrected before reduction is possible.

Authors   Klaus Dresing, Jos Engelen

7.1   X-ray review during reduction

An x-ray is mandatory to assess and confirm a successful fracture reduction. Although x-rays are potentially dangerous, for both patient and medical personnel, this is the only way to verify the anatomical position of the fractured limb. Normally, a C-arm imaging apparatus is used in the emergency department or cast room. Surgeons and staff should wear protective clothing during x-ray exposure: thyroid shield, gown, and, if possible, lead goggles, and lead gloves. Increasing the distance from an x-ray source is the best way of limiting x-ray exposure for the surgeon and staff, especially considering the inverse square law. Duration of x-ray exposure must also be considered. Manipulation with the fluoroscope running continuously results in greater radiation exposure than if brief single-shot images were obtained instead. These are almost always the most appropriate choice of image acquisition [5] (**Fig 14.1-10**).

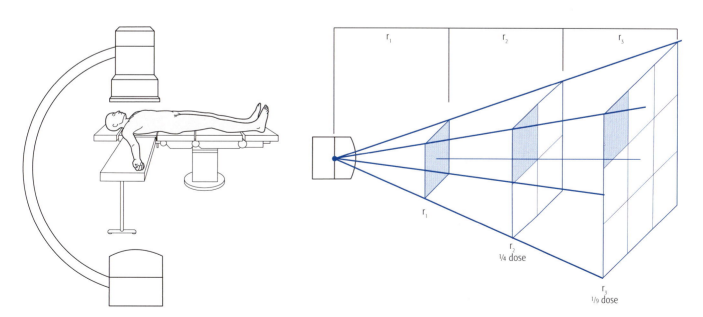

Fig 14.1-10   The inverse square law. The dose is reduced by the power of two of the distance to the x-ray source.

14.1

TECHNIQUES

Fracture reduction performed directly over the tube is the worst position of the C-arm with the highest radiation exposure to the surgeon and staff [5]. However, positioning the x-ray tube above the patient is dangerous as most of the scattered radiation is reflected off the patient's body towards the team. Exposure to radiation, especially scattered radiation, can be reduced by positioning the image intensifier over the top, ie, having a short distance between the image intensifier and above the patient, and a long distance between the patient and the x-ray tube (**Fig 14.1-11**). By posi-

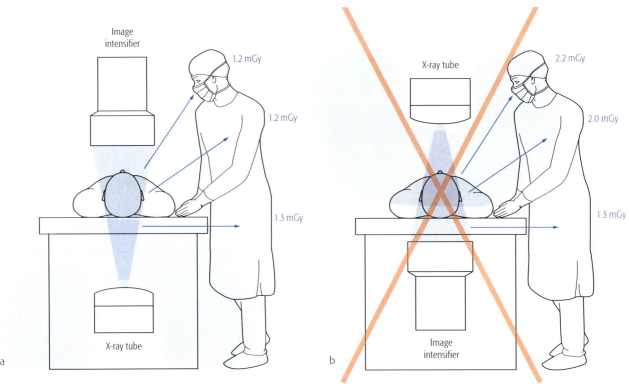

Fig 14.1-11a–b   Scattered radiation from imaging.

a   By positioning the C-arm in the recommended position below the operating table, the scattered radiation that comes from the x-ray tube will mostly stay under the table (indicated by the blue radiation cloud). A Gray is the physical quantity of radiation, with 1 Gray (Gy) being the deposit of a joule of radiation energy in a kg of matter or tissue. With the x-ray tube placed under the table, between 1.2 and 1.3 mGy are scattered towards the surgeon's eyes, sternum, and pelvic region.

b   Positioning the x-ray tube above the operating table and patient reflects the radiation off the patient's body towards the team. It also increases high-dose radiation rates to the eyes. With the x-ray tube in this position, the amount of radiation that is scattered towards the eyes and sternum regions nearly doubles (ie, 2.0 to 2.2 mGy) compared to **Fig 14.1-11a**.

Authors   Klaus Dresing, Jos Engelen

tioning the x-ray tube below the operating table there is the further advantage of reducing high-dose radiation rates to the eye lenses and thyroid gland by a factor of three or more [5–7].

In lateral projection, the surgeon should be on the image intensifier (receiver) side because scattered radiation exposure, from the beam hitting the patient, can be as much as ten times less than if on the other side [6] (**Fig 14.1-12**).

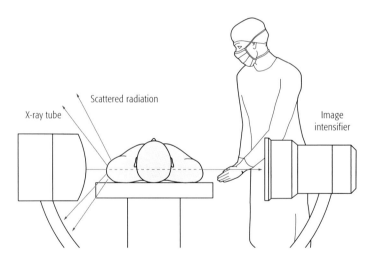

Fig 14.1-12   The exposure to scattered radiation is approximately ten times less on the amplifier side than the x-ray tube side.

14.1

TECHNIQUES

8   Patient positioning

Joint angulation and positioning of the affected limb are important considerations when beginning the immobilization procedure. Depending on the affected limb, the patient should be sitting or lying comfortably, with the affected limb resting on the table. Specific information on patient positioning is outlined in each of the demonstrations in chapters 15 Upper extremities; 16 Lower extremities; 17 Spine; and 18 Support bandages.

8.1   Joint position

In the functional position of a joint, the antagonistic muscle groups are balanced, with less deforming tension across the fracture. Additionally, should joint stiffness develop, the recommended functional position is the one that least interferes with the important activities of daily life. Therefore, immobilization of the joint in the functional position benefits functional recovery.

8.2   Shoulder position

When beginning immobilization for the shoulder, the shoulder position should be 80° flexion, 40° abduction, 20° external rotation, and 20° elevation of the forearm (**Fig 14.1-13**).

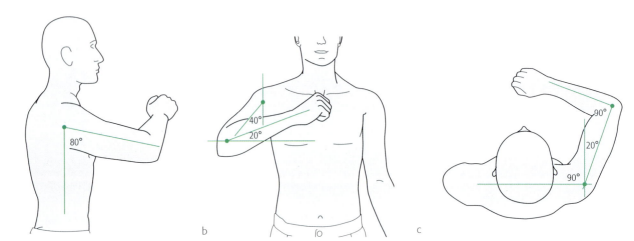

Fig 14.1-13a–c   Optimal shoulder position for cast immobilization.
a   Shoulder in frontal plane, with 80° flexion.
b   Shoulder in sagittal plane, with 40° abduction and 20° forearm elevation.
c   Shoulder in transverse plane, with 20° external rotation of the arm and 90° flexion of the elbow.

8.3   Elbow position

The functional position of the elbow is in 90° flexion (see **Fig 14.1-14**).

8.4   Position of proximal and distal radioulnar joints

The functional position of these joints is 10° pronation (see **Fig 14.1-15**).

8.5   Wrist position

Functional position of the wrist is 20–30° dorsal flexion with full fist closure possible (**Fig 14.1-16**).

8.6   Position of fingers and hand
8.6.1 Thumb position

With the thumb, there should be slight flexion of 15–20° in the metacarpophalangeal joint and 10° in the interphalangeal joint. It should be opposed to the fingers, rather than in the same plane with them (**Fig 14.1-17**).

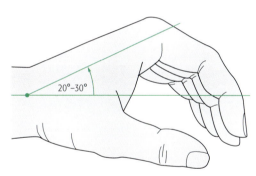

Fig 14.1-16   Functional position of the wrist.

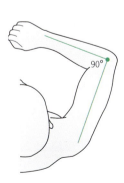

Fig 14.1-14   Elbow in 90° flexion.

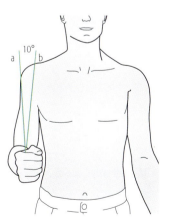

Fig 14.1-15   Functional position of the radioulnar joints.

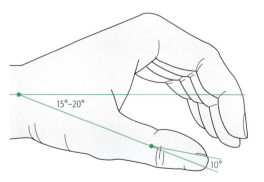

Fig 14.1-17   Functional position of the thumb.

8.6.2 Position of fingers II–V

The functional position of the metacarpophalangeal (MCP) joints is 45–50° flexion with the interphalangeal (IP) joints in 20 to 30° flexion. The fingers are positioned as if they are holding a bottle (**Fig 14.1-18**).

8.6.3 Intrinsic-plus position

The intrinsic-plus position allows better preservation of finger function, particularly regarding metacarpophalangeal flexion range, than the previously described functional position. In the intrinsic-plus position, the MCP joints are in 70–90° flexion with the IP joints in extension. This places the collateral ligaments of the MCP joints under tension so they do not contract while immobilized. The proximal interphalangeal and distal interphalangeal joints, immobilized in full extension, have less risk of developing flexion contractures (**Fig 14.1-19**). Rotational alignment of metacarpal of proximal phalangeal fractures is correct if all injured fingers point to the scaphoid in flexion (**Fig 14.1-20**).

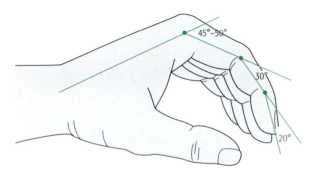

Fig 14.1-18 Functional position of the fingers.

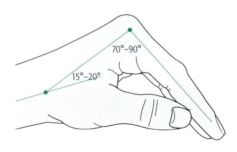

a

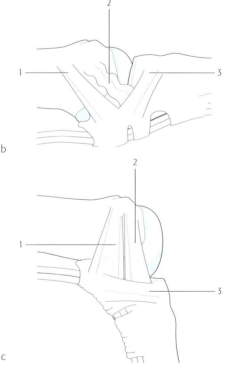

b

c

Fig 14.1-19a–c Intrinsic-plus position of fingers for cast immobilization.

a Correct position of fingers and hand for cast immobilization.

b In extension of the proximal interphalangeal (PIP) joints, the collateral ligaments are without tension and would shorten during immobilization in this position.

c In flexion of the PIP joints, the ligaments are under tension and will not shorten during immobilization in this position.

1 Accessory collateral ligament.

2 Collateral ligament.

3 Phalango-glenoidale ligament

Authors   Klaus Dresing, Jos Engelen

8.6.4 Thumb carpometacarpal

For the thumb carpometacarpal (trapeziometacarpal or saddle joint), the functional position is with the thumb opposed, as when you are holding a bottle.

8.7 Hip position

The functional position of the hip joint is 15° flexion, with neutral abduction and approximately 30° of external rotation (**Fig 14.1-21**).

8.8 Knee position

The functional position of the knee in a cast is 10–20° flexion. In a weight bearing cast, knee flexion should be closer to 10° in order to achieve better walking function.

8.9 Ankle position

For the ankle, a functional position corresponding to 90° flexion is advised. Keep in mind that when relaxed, the foot falls into the "drop foot" position (supination and plantar flexion). It is important to preserve a plantigrade foot position, with the plantar surface parallel to the ground when the tibia is upright.

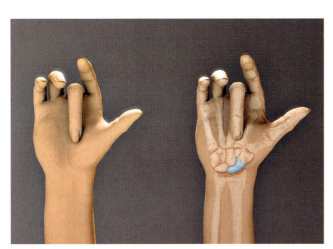

Fig 14.1-20   Correct rotation. In flexion, all fingers point to the scaphoid.

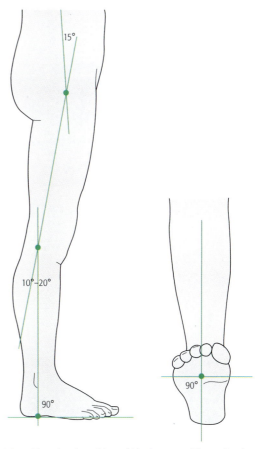

Fig 14.1-21   Functional position of hip, knee, and lower leg for cast immobilization.

14.1

TECHNIQUES

8.10   Foot joints

In standing position, all joints of the foot are in the functional position.

8.11   Dynamic splinting after Kleinert

In "dynamic splinting" (see chapters 15.21 Kleinert dynamic splint using plaster of Paris; and 15.22 Kleinert dynamic splint using synthetic, combicast technique) the position of the joints are changed in comparison to the functional position. This special splint avoids flexor tension while allowing motion as the digit is actively extended against elastic resistance. With relaxation of extensors, the elastic passively restores finger flexion.

8.11.1 Thumb

In cases of tendon flexion injuries of the thumb, dynamic Kleinert splinting is carried out in a 30° wrist position and 30° position of the basic joint and thumb end joint (**Fig 14.1-22**).

8.11.2 Fingers II–V

In cases of tendon flexion injuries of the fingers, dynamic Kleinert splinting is carried out in a 30–40° wrist position and 50–70° finger flexion (**Fig 14.1-23**).

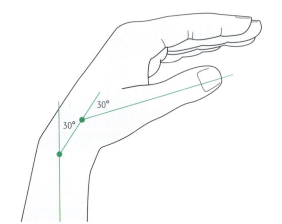

Fig 14.1-22   Position of thumb and wrist for dynamic Kleinert splinting in cases of tendon flexion injury of the thumb.

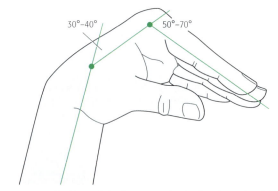

Fig 14.1-23   Position of the fingers and wrist for dynamic Kleinert splinting after flexor tendon repairs.

Authors   Klaus Dresing, Jos Engelen

9 Applying and handling cast material

There are pronounced differences among POP, rigid synthetic, and semirigid synthetic cast materials (see chapter 6 Properties of cast materials). These differences affect both the application process and the end result.

9.1 Applying plaster of Paris

Before beginning the casting procedure, prepare a container of water at room temperature (at or around 20° C). The correct water temperature is important to avoid allow sufficient time for cast application, and to excessive heat and due to the normal exothermic reaction of the setting cast (see chapter 6 Properties of cast materials). A higher temperature of the dipping water will accelerate setting, and shorten molding working time. Increased heat within the cast might result in burn injuries. Furthermore, in hot water, plaster will detach from the textile layer or dissolve into the water, a process that will result in reduced stability (**Fig 14.1-24**). It must also be remembered that that cast thickness also contributes to heating of a setting cast. Thus the more cast layers that are used, the higher the temperature during setting.

Water in the cast basin or sink should be clean and changed routinely several times during the day.

9.1.1 Plaster of Paris roll

Rolled plaster bandages will become wet rapidly if submerged into water in the correct way. The best way is to hold the POP roll between thumb and fingers during the dipping process (**Fig 14.1-25**), with the axis of the roll more or less vertical in the water. The POP bandage roll lies in the palm of the hand, the thumb rests on the roll without much pressure, while the free end of the bandage is supported by the long fingers. This way "the eyes can look into the bandage" as it is unrolled onto the patient's limb (**Fig 14.1-26**). Dipping the plaster roll without leaving the first layer free causes the cast layers to stick together, and interferes with identifying the free end (**Fig 14.1-27**).

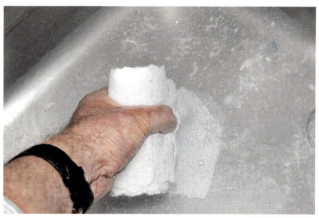

Fig 14.1-25   Holding the POP roll correctly during the dipping process allows you to quickly identify the free end of the roll, and begin applying the cast.

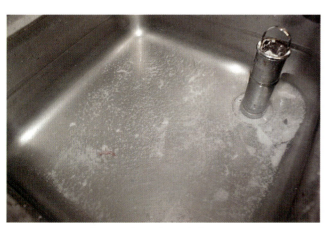

Fig 14.1-24   Cast basin with residues of plaster material.

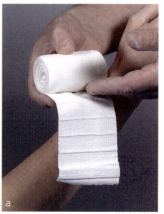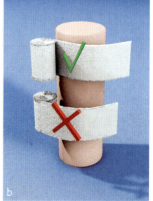

Fig 14.1-26a–b The caregiver must be able to look into the space between the roll and the end being wrapped around the patient.

When dipping plaster rolls, the depth of the water should be at least 20–30 cm. When rolls are dipped as described above, air bubbles will escape through the core of the roll, allowing the water to saturate all layers of plaster uniformly. After a few seconds, when the bubbling ceases, the plaster is adequately wet (**Fig 14.1-28**). A gentle squeeze eliminates excess water (**Fig 14.1-29**). Then, the free end is applied to the patient's limb and the roll material is wrapped onto the limb while the roll itself remains in contact with the cast padding. Plaster of Paris rolls are applied using the half-overlapping technique (see topic 10 Bandaging techniques) so that at least half of each preceding wrap is covered by the following turn. When rolling plaster over an angled region, for example the ankle joint, plaster overlaps halfway over the heel while much greater overlapping is accepted anteriorly.

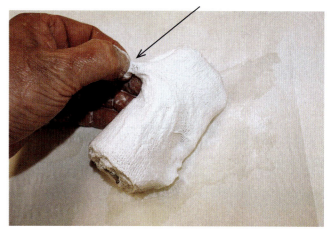

Fig 14.1-27   Plaster roll that was dipped incorrectly, without keeping the end free.

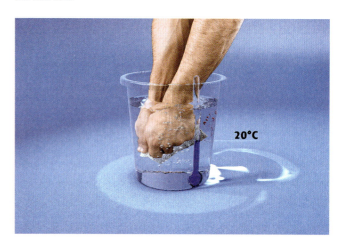

Fig 14.1-28   If dipped correctly into 20–30 cm water depth, air bubbles escape from the POP roll.

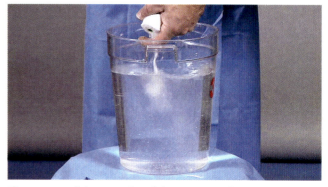

Fig 14.1-29   Slight squeezing of the wet POP roll.

Authors   Klaus Dresing, Jos Engelen

9.1.2 Plaster of Paris splints (longuettes)

Plaster of Paris splints (longuettes) are folded and dipped into water at an angle of 45° in order to let the air bubbles escape (**Fig 14.1-30**). A water column of 20–30 cm produces enough pressure to expel air bubbles from between the layers. The immersion time is approximately 3 seconds or until bubbling ceases. The excess water is then squeezed out as it is with plaster rolls (**Fig 14.1-31**). Hold each end separately, so that they can readily be separated to preserve correct alignment of the splint layers.

The layers of the splint (longuette) are now stuck together by manual longitudinal compression "massage" on a flat, easily cleanable surface of a counter or the cast cart (**Fig 14.1-32**).

Dry spots or dry POP layers reduce the quality and strength of the cast. Insufficiently soaked plaster will result in delaminated, uncompounded plaster, resulting in so-called puff pastry plaster (**Fig 14.1-33**).

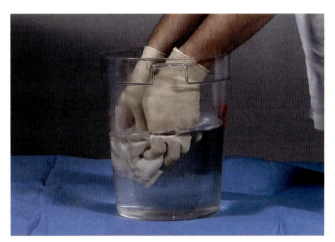

Fig 14.1-30   Dipping the dry folded POP splint (longuette) into water.

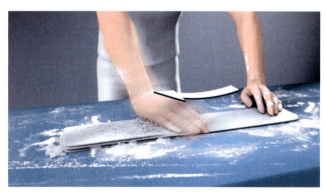

Fig 14.1-32   Splint (longuette) is stretched and smoothed out, molding the layers together and releasing the air bubbles trapped inside the material.

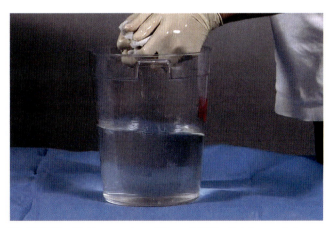

Fig 14.1-31   Slight squeezing of the wet POP splint (longuette).

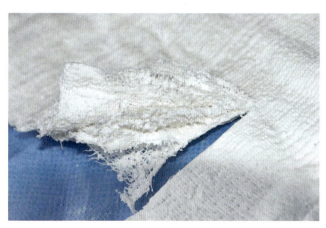

Fig 14.1-33   Puff pastry plaster.

14.1

After having smoothed the plaster splints (longuettes), they are applied where desired, and the smoothing process is repeated manually on the extremity, rubbing them into previously applied plaster, or onto the padding if an end-product splint rather than a circumferential cast is intended. This smoothing process should result in wrinkleless POP cast material, positioned as chosen on the extremity, which remains in the desired functional position without wrinkles or weak spots in the plaster, and without irregularities in the padding. While the plaster is still soft, it is molded to the extremity, with smooth broad appropriately located pressure surfaces to maintain fracture reduction and limb alignment.

During the application and molding of POP, avoid creating finger-tip pressure points (indentations) by using only the heel and flat surface of the hand ("flat hand technique") (**Fig 14.1-34**).

9.2   Applying synthetic

Synthetic cast material is normally (according to its accompanying instructions) dipped into cold water at room temperature of around 20 degrees. However, synthetic material can actually be applied either wet, or using a dry application technique.

9.2.1   Wet application

With the standard wet application, dip the synthetic material into water with an immersion time of approximately 3 seconds and a water depth of 20–30 cm. Submerging the material in water begins the polymerization process (**Fig 14.1-35**).

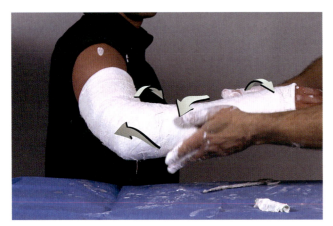

Fig 14.1-34   Flat hand technique. Correct manner of applying and molding the plaster by only using the heel of the palm, not the fingers.

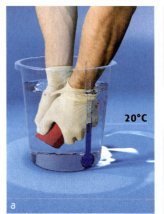
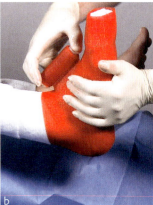

Fig 14.1-35a-b   Dipping synthetic material in water starts the polymerization process.

Authors   Klaus Dresing, Jos Engelen

9.2.2 Dry application

Synthetic material can also be applied dry, without previous dipping into water. This increases the working time, before the cast can no longer accept molding. This application technique is recommended for inexperienced users or in complex cases where more time is needed, as well as on occasions when an assistant is not available. After dry application of synthetic cast material, polymerization can be accelerated by wrapping the cast temporarily with a wet elastic cloth bandage (**Fig 14.1-36**). Like POP, synthetic cast rolls are applied using the half-overlapping technique.

9.3 Number of cast material layers

The thickness (number of cast material layers) required depends on the following:

- The casting material used (POP or synthetic)
- The patient's weight
- Body region (lower or upper extremity and anticipated loading)
- Expected patient compliance.

More layers will provide greater strength but will also increase the weight and cost of the cast or splint. **Table 14.1-5a** and **Table 14.1-5b** provide a list of the required number of cast material layers (thickness) in relation to body region.

Body region	Number of layers for plaster of Paris cast material	Number of layers for synthetic cast material
Upper extremity	8–10 layers	4–6 layers
Lower extremity	8–10 layers	6–8 layers

Table 14.1-5a Number of cast material layers within a cast in relation to body region.

Body region	Number of layers for plaster of Paris cast material	Number of layers for synthetic cast material
Upper extremity	8–10 layers	6–8 layers
Lower extremity	12–16 layers	9–12 layers

Table 14.1-5b Number of cast material layers within a splint in relation to body region.

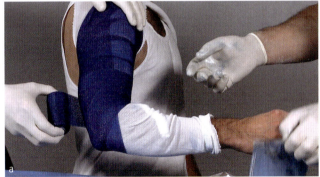
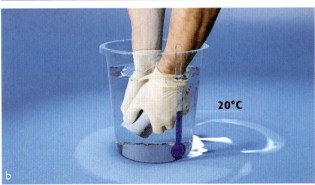
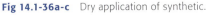
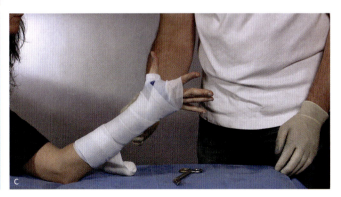

Fig 14.1-36a-c   Dry application of synthetic.

a   Synthetic cast material being applied using a dry application.

b–c   After applying the synthetic material, an elastic bandage can be dipped in water, then wrapped around the material to accelerate the setting.

9.4   Trimming and molding of cast edges

The length of a cast or splint should be enough for optimal support, without impinging on the flexed surface of an adjacent nonimmobilized joint. The adequate length of splints and casts has to be determined in order to avoid insufficient immobilization on one side and unnecessary restriction of joint motion on the other side (**Fig 14.1-37**). By folding back the padding and tube bandage, smooth edges will result, which will protect both soft tissues and bones from pressure and sharp edges (**Fig 14.1-38**).

9.5   Working and setting time

An overview of working and setting times for POP and synthetic cast materials is provided in **Table 14.1-6**. When using dry synthetic material, the setting time can be shortened by wrapping a wet bandage around the dry cast or splint in order to speed up the polymerization rate.

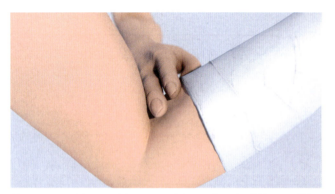

Fig 14.1-37   When applying a cast, joint motion should be possible without any restriction. During flexion, a gap of two fingers breadth (approximately 2-3 cm) should exist between the proximal cast and the proximal limb segment, as shown here for the elbow. On the extensor side, the cast can approach the joint line, but still should be checked for impingement with the joint in full extension.

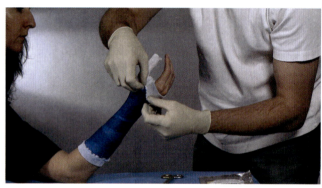

Fig 14.1-38   Folding the padding and the tube bandage back over the edge of the cast results in smooth padded edges and protects the soft tissue during motion.

Type of cast material / application	Working time	Setting time	Weight bearing permissible after
Plaster of Paris	3–5 minutes[1]	10–12 minutes[2]	24–48 hours[3] (if allowed)
Synthetic cast material:			
Wet application	2–4 minutes	6-8 minutes	30 minutes
Dry application	5–7 minutes	8-10 minutes	30 minutes

Legend

[1] Depending on water temperature and cast material (brand).

[2] For the initial period of hardening.

[3] Complete period of time for setting and possibility of weight bearing depends on the thickness of the cast or splint.

Table 14.1-6   Overview of working and setting times for POP and synthetic cast materials.

Authors   Klaus Dresing, Jos Engelen

9.6   Cast fenestration (windowing)

Sometimes it is indicated to cut a "window" into the cast to permit wound examination and care while the cast is maintained on the limb (**Fig 14.1-39**). After marking the window, and cutting the hardened cast with a saw, the cast window and padding are removed, and the tube bandage is cut to allow access to the wound. The tube bandage can be turned back over the window edges to secure the remaining padding. After treatment and dressing of the wound, the cast segment that was removed is repadded, and replaced into the window, to cover the wound and apply uniform gentle pressure to minimize swelling of soft tissues into the window (window edema). The window cover is secured with elastic or adhesive bandage, with the goal of restoring uniform pressure over the windowed area. Plastic foam padding, with adhesive backing, if available, is ideal for this purpose.

If a cast window is desired, it must be positioned perfectly over the wound, and large enough to permit dressing removal and reapplication. Planning ahead will include an appropriately sized and applied dressing, and often a bump or mound of rolled cast padding over the dressing so it is easily located before the window is cut. Too large a window weakens a cast, especially if wound drainage is significant. Strength and patient compliance can be augmented by overwrapping the window with cast material (plaster or synthetic). To avoid its adherence to the underlying cast, a layer of cast padding can be applied first. This permits removal of the overwrap with a cast saw, without adding undesirable additional cast thickness, or weakening the cast by trying to find the covered window.

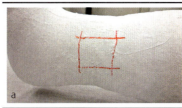

Planning of the fenestration and marking with a felt tip marker or wax crayon.

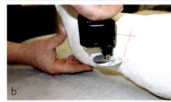

Cutting of the cast window with the oscillating cast saw.

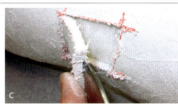

Using a cast knife to lever out the cast window.

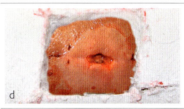

View of the soft tissue after removing padding and undercast material. The wound can now be examined and the treatment can take place.

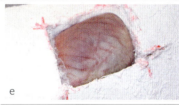

Swelling of the soft tissue results in a window edema. The photograph shows blanched areas of skin suggesting impaired perfusion.

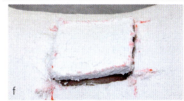

This image shows the window edema preventing the reinsertion of the cast window to the same level (niveau) of the adjacent cast material.

Fig 14.1-39a–f   Cast fenestration to view soft tissues during casting.

14.1

TECHNIQUES

10   Bandaging techniques

The most common bandage wrapping techniques include the following:
- Half-overlapping technique
- Criss-cross technique
- Stretch-relax technique
- Figure-of-eight wrapping technique.

10.1   Half-overlapping technique
Elastic bandages and casting materials are often applied using the half-overlapping technique, where the bandage is overlapped by about half of its width on each wrap. When applying the half-overlapping technique (see **Fig 14.1-40**) the soft tissues are compressed in order to decrease swelling and edema.

10.2   Criss-cross technique
The criss-cross technique is used on a tapered extremity, where there is an increasing or decreasing diameter as you progress proximally or distally along a limb. Begin by anchoring the bandage, then wrap around the extremity at a slight angle away from the joint or injury. Head back towards the joint moving above the previous level of wrapping, then again wrap down away from the joint at a slight angle before moving up again. Slowly, you make your way up the limb, from smaller to larger diameter (**Fig 14.1-41**). This technique is ideal for providing compression when there are variations in the circumference of the extremity, and is therefore effective for longer (see chapter 18.4 Wrist bandage).

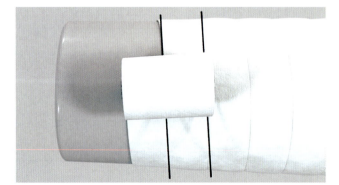

Fig 14.1-40   The half-overlapping technique.

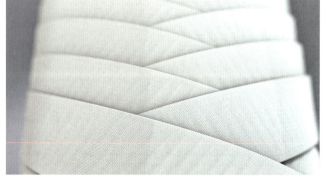

Fig 14.1-41   Criss-cross bandage technique used for tapered extremities.

Authors   Klaus Dresing, Jos Engelen

10.3   Stretch-relax technique

The stretch-relax technique is used for synthetic cast material. Firstly, by pulling the material from the roll, the tension is released. Then, without the tension, the bandage is applied onto the extremity or underlying layers of synthetic cast material (**Fig 14.1-42**). Using too much tension while applying the synthetic material would result in the cast being too tight.

10.4   Figure-of-eight technique

The figure-of-eight technique is used to wrap a joint at an angle, and is principally used for the elbow, knee, or ankle joint. Once anchored (circular wrap) below the joint, the bandage is applied diagonally and anchors to the limb above the joint, before returning to its origin. This step is repeated, making a figure of eight shape. This technique provides support while still allowing movement in the joint.

The most frequent indication for an elastic bandages is the bandage of the ankle joint, and at this location, the figure-of-eight technique is recommended. The complete ankle wrapping technique is described in detail in chapter 18.6 Ankle and foot bandage (**Fig 14.1-43**).

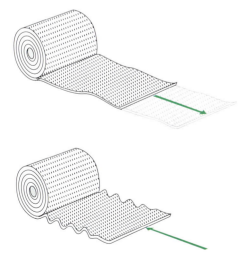

Fig 14.1-42   Stretch-relax technique for synthetic cast materials.

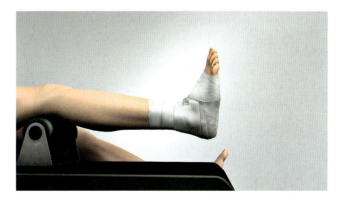

14.1-43   The figure-of-eight technique provides support but avoids excessive material at the joint.

11   Cast splitting techniques and cast removal

Böhler was the first to emphasize the need for splitting casts completely in primary fracture care [8]. In primary care, POP and synthetic casts are always split completely to ensure that swelling can be accommodated. The location of the split should be planned before the cast is cut. If possible, avoid splitting over bony prominences. A good manner is to first mark the line with a felt or grease pen (on POP casts only) or a permanent marker (**Fig 14.1-44**).

In semirigid synthetic casts, the cast is split with scissors. In most rigid synthetic or POP casts, the use of a cast saw is recommended (**Fig 14.1-45**). However, the padding and underlying lining material (ie, tube bandage) are then completely cut using scissors (**Fig 14.1-46**).

11.1   Oscillating cast saw

When using the oscillating cast saw for either cast splitting or for permanent removal at the end of treatment, it is important to explain to the patient how the cast saw works as the blade and saw design can terrify some patients, and the loud noises can be frightening for children. A good sawing technique and ear protectors for the patient can greatly reduce patient anxiety. Cast saw blades, especially if dull, can become hot, and burns as well as lacerations are possible. If the patient complains of pain, sawing should be stopped immediately, and the underlying skin assessed, along with the blade temperature. Very careful resumption of sawing may, of course, be required to expose the possibly injured area.

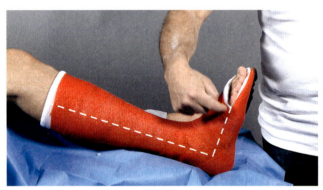

Fig 14.1-44   Before splitting the cast, mark the splitting line with a marker/pen.

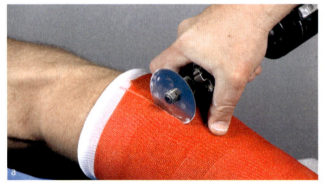

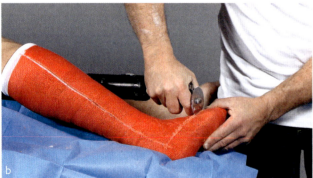

Fig 14.1-45a-b   Cast saw being used to split a leg cast.

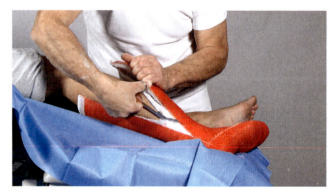

Fig 14.1-46   Cutting the padding and underlying lining material with scissors.

Authors   Klaus Dresing, Jos Engelen

An oscillating saw blade does not rotate like a circular saw but instead vibrates rapidly with very little rotation. The vibrations or oscillations are still enough to allow the blade to cut the rigid cast/plaster material. When the saw gets through the cast, the technician will feel less pressure due to the soft underlying cast padding. At that moment, the saw should be lifted, manually rotated slightly, and reapplied further along the cast (**Fig 14.1-47**). With this technique, there is less risk of burns or skin damage, but the risks are not entirely eliminated, particularly if the skin is dystrophic, as with some elderly patients, or those receiving high doses of adreno-cortical steroids. It is, however, highly recommended to demonstrate the saw harmlessly touching the skin of the operator (**Fig 14.1-48**).

To split or remove the cast, follow these steps:

1   Training: The use of a cast saw is only permitted for trained personal.
2   Heat: Use a sharp saw blade as a blunt blade will get hot much faster.
3   Rotate the blade: Due to the vibrations that occur within the rigid material, the blade will get hot and can cause burning stripes. This effect is reduced/avoided if a sharp saw blade is used and when the saw blade in manually turned slightly by the saw operator, after each step of cutting. With this procedure, another part of the blade is used for cutting resulting in less heat at that part of the blade.
4   Gentle application: Apply the saw blade with a little pressure on the cast. Use the opposite hand or the fingers of the ipsilateral hand for depth regulation.
5   Bony prominences: Ensure the cutting line is not over bony prominences (eg, malleolus or styloid process of radius or ulna).
6   Padding: The padding and tube bandage are cut with blunt-tipped bandage scissors.
7   Bivalving: Sometimes it is necessary to cut the cast at two sides (bivalve it) in order to make removal/opening easier and less harmful to the patient. Careful placement of the two cuts is necessary to ensure easy removal and preservation of the cast if its reapplication is intended.

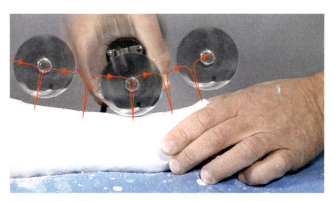

Fig 14.1-47   Lifting the saw blade, rotating the blade slightly by hand, then reapplying the saw further along the cast greatly reduces heat generation.

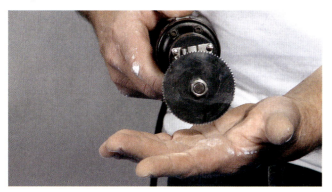

Fig 14.1-48   The saw blade oscillates and does not rotate, so the risk of skin injury is reduced.

14.1

TECHNIQUES

If considerable swelling is expected during primary fracture care, a strip is cut out of the cast (**Fig 14.1-49**). After complete splitting of the underlying layers of padding and tube bandage, the gap is filled with padding in order to avoid gap edema (similar to window edema). The cast is then wrapped with elastic bandage.

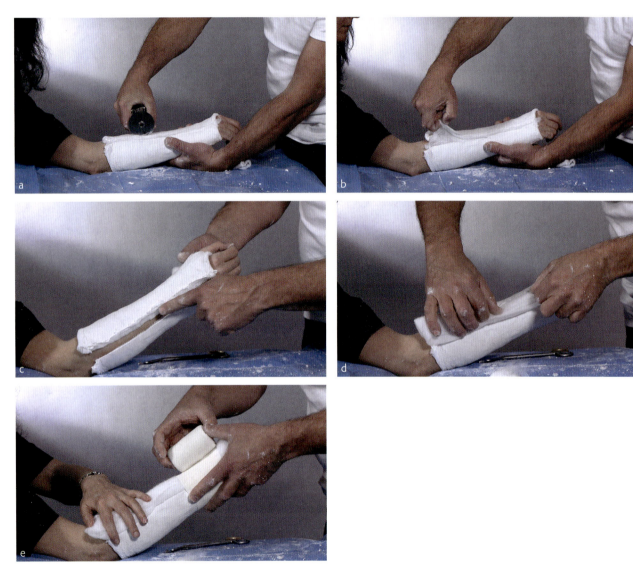

Fig 14.1-49a–e   Removing a strip of cast.
a–b   Splitting and removal of cast material, padding, and tube bandaging.
c–d   The resulting gap is refilled with padding.
e   The cast is then wrapped with an elastic bandage.

Authors   Klaus Dresing, Jos Engelen

When cutting semirigid casts, squeeze the cast by pressing on both sides to bulge the cast away from the patient, as shown. This provides space to insert scissors and helps avoid injury to the patient's skin and soft tissues (**Fig 14.1-50**).

11.2   Refixing the cast

After splitting of the cast, the cast is closed (fixed) with an elastic bandage (**Fig 14.1-51**).

In special situations, it is advisable not to split the cast completely all at once but to split and fix the cast in stages (step-by-step) in order to avoid affecting the fracture reduction. This involves cutting a part of the cast, then wrapping that section with bandage, then cutting a little more of the cast, followed by a little more bandaging, etc. **Fig 14.1-52** shows the step-by-step splitting and fixing technique.

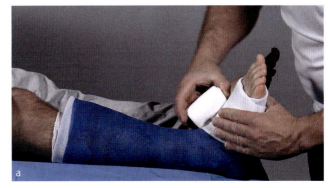

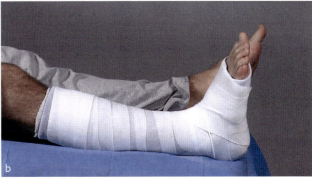

Fig 14.1-51a–b   Applying the elastic fixation bandage around the split cast.

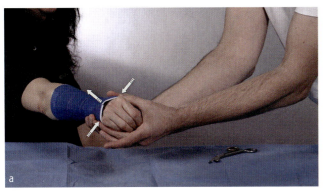

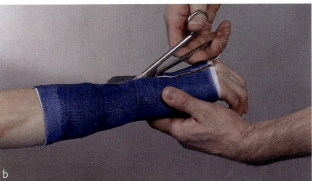

Fig 14.1-50a–b   Pressing on both sides of the cast with the hand creates a small bulge for inserting the scissors.

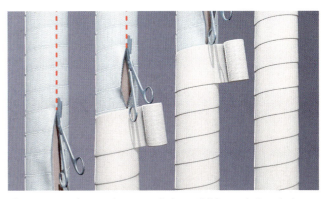

Fig 14.1-52   The step-by-step splitting and fixing technique helps to prevent loss of reduction.

14.1

TECHNIQUES

12   Patient information

The surgeon should inform the patient about the diagnosis and treatment options, as well as provide sufficient, specific information about any planned intervention (see topic 6 in chapter 3 Principles of casting). Before leaving the emergency department, the patient should receive information on how to deal with potential problems or complications related to the injury and its treatment, including the cast or bandage (see topic 11 in chapter 3 Principles of casting). A well-accepted method is to give the patient not only verbal but also written information (Appendix 1) before he or she leaves the treatment center. This should include instructions for when and how to call for help should any problems arise.

Patients should be scheduled to return the following day for cast review and re-assessment.

13   Review and assessment

The day after application of the cast, a medical review is mandatory. It is very important that the following items are checked:
- Circulation with
    - Pulse assessment
    - Capillary refill assessment
- Sensation
- Motor function
- Swelling
- Level of pain.

Authors   Klaus Dresing, Jos Engelen

14   Duration of immobilization

The duration of immobilization varies depending on the type of fracture or injury, patient's age, if surgery was involved, joint stability, and patient compliance. More specific information on duration of immobilization is provided in the chapters of section 2 Guidelines.

15   Summary

- Physicians responsible for selecting and managing nonoperative fracture care should also be able to apply any cast, splint, orthosis, or support bandage themselves
- In primary fracture care, a splint is often initially used after reduction of the fracture because of the likelihood of soft-tissue swelling; the splint can later be replaced with a cast
- Primary definitive fracture care occurs when, in special circumstances, the initial cast or splint does not need to be replaced
- Before applying any form of immobilization bandage, the caregiver should have a thorough understanding of the properties, recommended sizes, working and setting times, and wrapping and cutting techniques for the various types of paddings and casting materials
- Before conducting an immobilization procedure, the caregiver should be fully prepared with the relevant materials, casting and monitoring equipment, instrumentation, and ideally, a specific cast room
- Apart from the actual bandaging techniques, the surgeon is also responsible for other important elements including pain relief, fracture reduction, patient information and consent, and reviews and assessment post-immobilization
- Only when the surgeon has the full understanding of performing nonoperative immobilization can he or she confidently assess the casts applied by residents, cast technicians, or other caregivers.

14.1

TECHNIQUES

14.1

TECHNIQUES

16   References

1. **Bhatia M, Housden PH**. Re-displacement of paediatric forearm fractures: role of plaster moulding and padding. *Injury.* 2006 Mar; 37(3):259–268.
2. **Boyd AS, Benjamin HJ, Asplund C**. Principles of casting and splinting. *Am Fam Physician.* 2009 Jan 1; 79(1):16–22.
3. **Brown JC, Klein EJ, Lewis CW, et al**. Emergency department analgesia for fracture pain. *Ann Emerg Med.* 2003 Aug; 42(2):197–205.
4. **Charnley J**. *The Closed Treatment of Common Fractures.* 4th ed. United Kingdom. Cambridge University Press; 2010.
5. **Dresing K**. Intraoperative imaging. Babst R, Bavonratanavech S, Pesantez R (eds). *Minimally Invasive Plate Osteosynthesis.* 2nd ed. Stuttgart New York: Georg Thieme Verlag; 2012:75–88.
6. **Rampersaud YR, Foley KT, Shen AC, et al**. Radiation exposure to the spine surgeon during fluoroscopically assisted pedicle screw insertion. *Spine.* 2000 Oct 15; 25(20):2637–2645.
7. **Fuchs M, Schmid A, Eiteljörge T, et al**. Exposure of the surgeon to radiation during surgery. *Int Orthop.* 1998, 22(3):153-156.
8. **Böhler L**. [*The Treatment of Fractures*]. 9th–11th ed. Wien: Wilhelm Maudrich; 1943. German.

14.2 Overview of cast, splint, orthosis, and bandage techniques—demonstration format and icons

Klaus Dresing, Jos Engelen

14.2

TECHNIQUES

Authors   Klaus Dresing, Jos Engelen

14.2   Overview of cast, splint, orthosis, and bandage techniques—demonstration format and icons

1   Introduction

In the following chapters (chapters 15 to 18) a total of 55 cast, splint, orthosis, and support bandage procedures are demonstrated. Each demonstration provides a wide range of information outlining the preprocedure planning, step-by-step immobilization instructions, and postprocedure review and assessment. In most cases, a uniform sequence and structure of presentation is used in these demonstrations in order to facilitate reference and understanding. However, not all demonstrations contain the same information, for example, additional instructions on cast removal are included when it is an especially sensitive procedure, and alternative steps are sometimes included for the same procedure when this is considered appropriate. Nevertheless, the topics and subject headings used in each demonstration clearly outline the steps required for each procedure.

2   Headings and instructions

The 55 immobilization demonstrations typically comprise the following topic headings and information:

- Indications and goals
- Equipment list
- Personnel
- Patient positioning
- Special things to keep in mind
- Procedure
- Final assessment
- Cast splitting and/or cast removal

To further support learning, a number of images and graphics have been added throughout each demonstration. These additional elements are in the form of pictographs, 3-D illustrations, or snap shots from the actual demonstration video and are particularly useful to show complex procedures, the recommended limb and patient positioning angles, or to provide other viewing angles in addition to the camera.

2.1   Indications and goals

In each demonstration, the indications and goals of treatment are presented.

INDICATION

- Fracture of the forearm or elbow
- Epicondylitis

GOAL

- Stabilization of the forearm and elbow

Additionally, a picture of the end result of the immobilization procedure is shown (**Fig 14.2-1**).

As an additional aid to learning, a pictograph has also been developed to represent the affected body region (**Fig 14.2-2**). This image is placed on the top right hand side of the chapter pages to assist with speedy referencing.

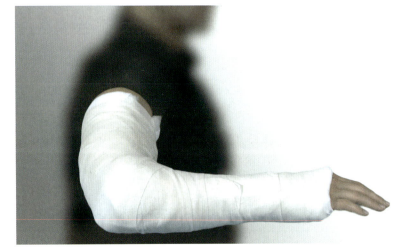

Fig 14.2-1   Cast image.

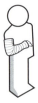

Fig 14.2-2   Pictograph indicating the affected limb.

Authors   Klaus Dresing, Jos Engelen

2.2   Equipment list

An equipment list and photograph of all materials needed for the cast, splint, orthosis, or support bandage is provided. This information outlines whether plaster of Paris or rigid or semirigid synthetic casting materials are to be used. All other materials and equipment, including padding, tube bandages, and any fixing materials such as velcro or tape etc are also listed and shown (**Fig 14.2-3**).

2.3   Personnel

For each demonstration, the number of personnel required to apply the immobilization bandage is indicated with a number and a pictograph. A pictograph of a person with a stethoscope indicates a trained physician/surgeon is required. A person with no markings indicates a cast technician/caregiver is suitable.

These symbols facilitate quick understanding of who is required (**Fig 14.2-4**).

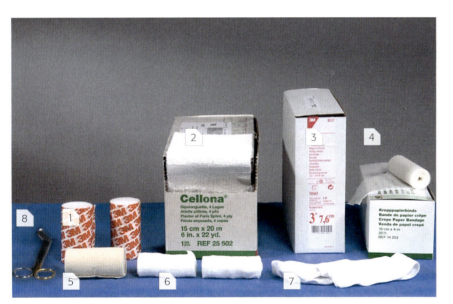

Fig 14.2-3   Equipment and materials.

EQUIPMENT

1 Cast padding
2 Plaster of Paris splint 12 cm, 15 cm, or 20 cm
3 Tube bandage 7.5 cm in dispenser box
4 Crepe paper bandage
5 Elastic bandage
6 Gauze bandage
7 Cut tube bandage
8 Scissors

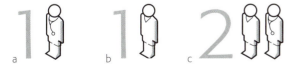

Fig 14.2-4a–c   Personnel.

a   1 surgeon is needed.
b   1 cast technician/caregiver is needed.
c   1 surgeon and 1 cast technician/caregiver are needed.

2.4   Patient positioning

The positioning of the patient is presented in a 3-D illustration and described in detail (**Fig 14.2-5**).

2.5   Special things

A list of special items to keep in mind while performing the procedure is listed (**Fig 14.2-6**). For example, these might include such things as ensuring the protection of bony prominences, reviewing circulation, or ensuring that the cast or splint material does not interfere with the normal movement of the rest of the limb.

POSITIONING

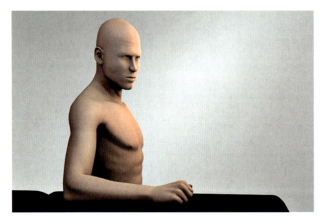

Seat the patient comfortably on a stool.
Place the affected limb on the table, in a functional position, with 90° flexion of the elbow.

Fig 14.2-5   Patient and limb positioning.

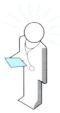

SPECIAL THINGS TO KEEP IN MIND

- The distal palmar crease should remain free
- Protection of the lateral and medial epicondyle
- Protection of the olecranon
- While the splint is setting, the limb should be positioned halfway between supination and pronation

Fig 14.2-6   Special things.

Authors   Klaus Dresing, Jos Engelen

2.6   Procedure

After the equipment list and patient preparation have been outlined, the demonstrations then give a step-by-step outline of the procedure that must take place (**Fig 14.2-7**). The procedure section in each demonstration is regularly supported with additional pictures and illustrations, with each new step providing its own clear descriptive text.

Many of the demonstrations use common steps and techniques (for example, the half-overlapping technique for wrapping, or the dipping process for wetting cast material). Rather than provide a lengthy explanation on these elements in each demonstration, further information on these common techniques (including working times, layers of material, and wrapping techniques) can be found in chapter 14.1 Overview of cast, splint, orthosis, and bandage techniques.

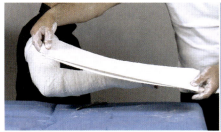

Apply a 4-layer POP splint on the dorsal side for extra stability

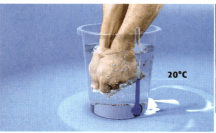

Submerge the splint in water for a few seconds, remove, and squeeze out the excess water

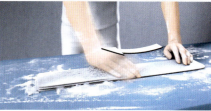

Stretch and smooth out the splint, pressing the layers together, resulting in a compact splint. If this procedure is not done, puff pastry plaster will result, causing an unstable splint

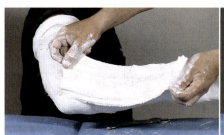

Position the splint and cut at the elbow to allow overlapping

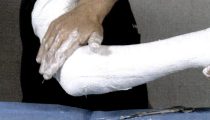

Smooth out the splint

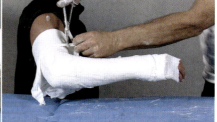

Fold back the tube bandage, proximally and distally, and trim

Fig 14.2-7   The step by step procedure, including graphics and instructions.

2.7   Final assessment

Once the procedure is finished, a final assessment section is provided to summarize the main requirements of the cast, splint, orthosis, or support bandage in order to show the expected range of motion and to avoid complications (**Fig 14.2-8**). Typically, the images for the final assessment indicate what the immobilization bandage should look like, but may also include images of the inside of the cast, after it has been removed, to indicate its form or shape from the inside, or to show other features that could not be seen if it was still on the patient.

2.8   Cast splitting, cast removal

Occasionally, special additional instructions are provided, such as cast removal, where special attention must be paid when removing the cast to avoid bony prominences etc. This is particularly so when the oscillating cast saw is used.

In demonstrations for removable casts and orthoses, additional information is also provided on how to remove the cast, trim the excess material, and attach relevant fixing materials such as velcro, so that the cast can be easily reapplied by the doctor or patient.

3   Summary

- A range of instructions, illustrations, and pictographs have been developed and included into the 55 demonstration videos (and chapters 15–18) for enhanced learning
- Further information on many of the general techniques used in the demonstrations can be found in chapter 14.1 Overview of cast, splint, orthosis, and bandage techniques, and in other earlier chapters of the book.

FINAL ASSESSMENT

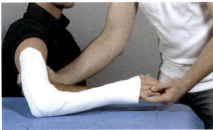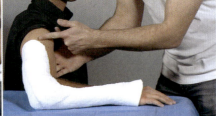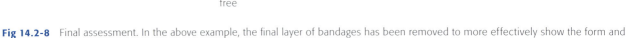

Metacarpal heads remain free to allow free motion of the fingers

The splint should extend to the top of the biceps, and the inside of the elbow remains free

Fig 14.2-8   Final assessment. In the above example, the final layer of bandages has been removed to more effectively show the form and extent of the splint.

TECHNIQUES

15 Upper extremity

15 Upper extremity

15.1 Long arm splint using plaster of Paris

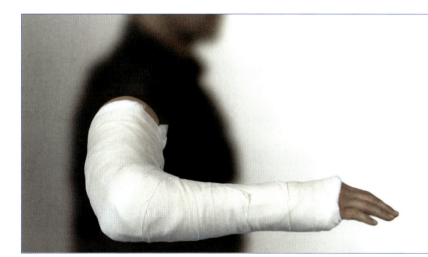

INDICATION

- Fracture of the forearm
- Fracture of the radial head
- Fracture of the distal humerus
- Fracture of the epicondyle
- Epicondylitis

GOAL

- Stabilization of the forearm and elbow

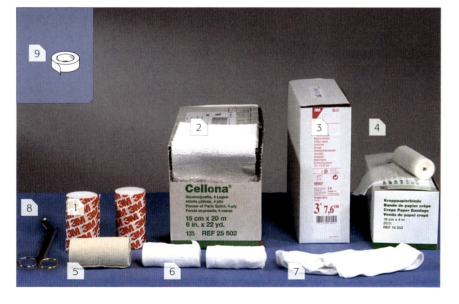

EQUIPMENT

1 Cast padding
2 Plaster of Paris splint 12 cm, 15 cm, or 20 cm
3 Tube bandage 7.5 cm in dispenser box
4 Crepe paper bandage
5 Elastic bandage
6 Gauze bandage
7 Cut tube bandage
8 Scissors
9 Surgical tape or bandage clips

PERSONNEL

POSITIONING

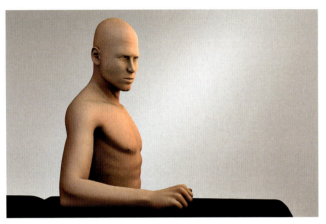

Seat the patient comfortably on a stool.

Place the affected limb on the table, in a functional position, with 90° flexion of the elbow.

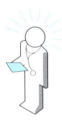

SPECIAL THINGS TO KEEP IN MIND

- The distal palmar crease should remain free
- Protection of the lateral and medial epicondyle
- Protection of the olecranon
- While the splint is setting, the limb should be positioned halfway between supination and pronation

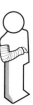

PROCEDURE

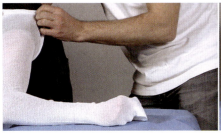

Apply the tube bandage up to the shoulder

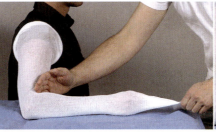

Pull the tube bandage tight to remove any wrinkles

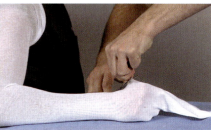

Cut holes in the tube bandage for the thumb

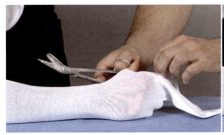

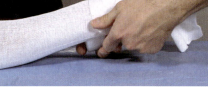

Apply the padding; make a hole for the thumb

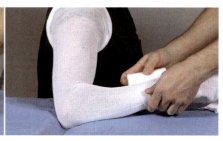

Wrap the forearm using the half-overlapping technique

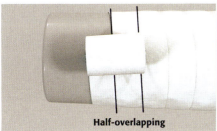

Half-overlapping

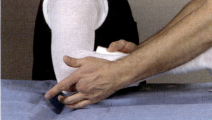

The padding protects the bony prominences

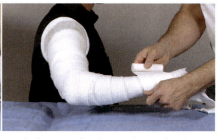

Apply the paper bandage to form a barrier between the dry padding and the wet POP

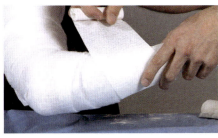

Wrap the forearm using the half-overlapping technique

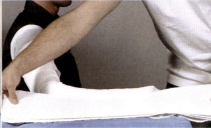

Fold the POP splint in two to make eight layers

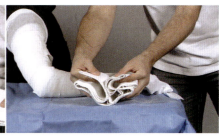

Fold up the splint before submerging in water

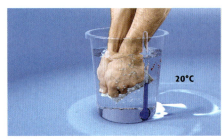

Submerge the splint in water for a few seconds, remove, and squeeze out excess water

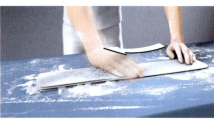

Stretch and smooth out the splint, pressing the layers together, resulting in a compact splint. If this procedure is not done, puff pastry plaster will result, causing an unstable splint

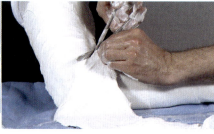

Position the splint and cut at the elbow to allow overlapping

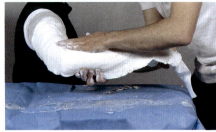

Overlap the cut section of the splint

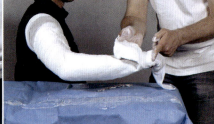

Trim the splint at the level of the MCP joints

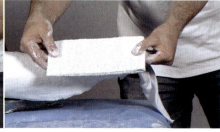

Reinforce the area of the elbow with a short POP splint

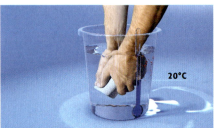

Apply a wet gauze bandage to hold the splint in place

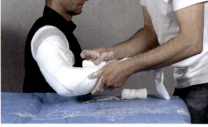

Wrap the forearm using the half-overlapping technique

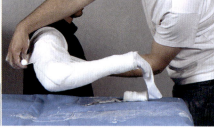

Use the figure-of-eight technique at the elbow to avoid an excessive amount of layers

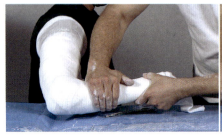

Mold the splint and support the arm until it is set

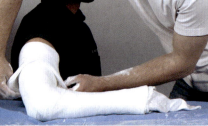

After the splint has set, fold back the tube bandage proximally and distally

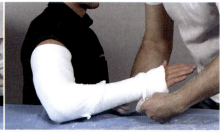

Pass the thumb through the hole in the tube bandage

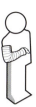

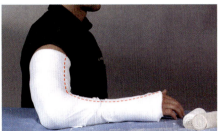

Mark the splitting line

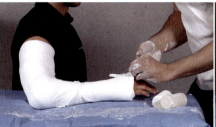

Cut through all layers, beginning distally

Complete the cutting proximally

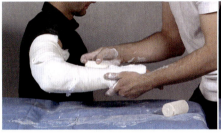

Apply an elastic bandage to hold the splint in place, using the half-overlapping technique

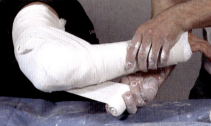

Use the figure-of-eight technique at the elbow to avoid an excessive amount of layers

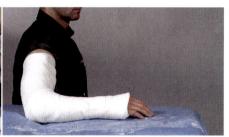

Secure the bandage with surgical tape or bandage clips

FINAL ASSESSMENT

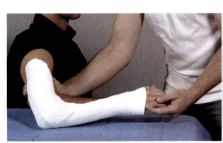

Metacarpal heads remain free to allow free motion of the fingers

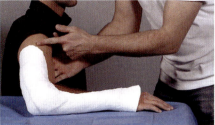

The splint should extend to the top of the biceps, and the inside of the elbow remains free

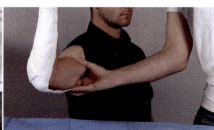

311

15.1

TECHNIQUES

Klaus Dresing, Jos Engelen

15.2 Long arm splint using synthetic

15.2

TECHNIQUES

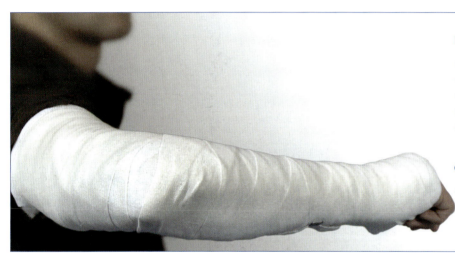

INDICATION

- Fracture of the forearm
- Fracture of the radial head
- Fracture of the distal humerus
- Fracture of the epicondyle
- Epicondylitis

GOAL

- Stabilization of the forearm and elbow

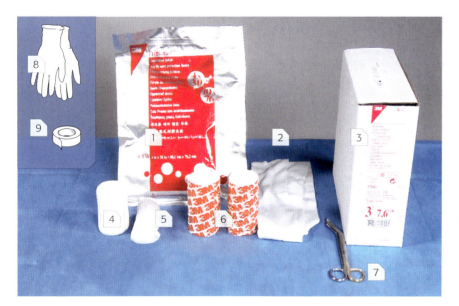

EQUIPMENT

1. Rigid synthetic splint 10 cm x 76 cm
2. Cut tube bandage
3. Tube bandage 7.5 cm in dispenser box
4. Elastic bandage
5. Gauze bandage
6. Cast padding
7. Scissors
8. Gloves
9. Surgical tape or bandage clips

PERSONNEL

15.2

POSITIONING

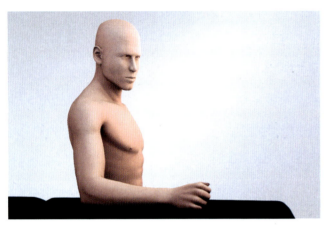

Seat the patient comfortably on a stool.

Place the affected limb on the table, in a functional position, with 90° flexion of the elbow.

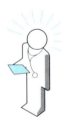

SPECIAL THINGS TO KEEP IN MIND

- The distal palmar crease should remain free
- Protection of the lateral and medial epicondyle
- Protection of the olecranon
- While the splint is setting, the limb should be positioned halfway between supination and pronation

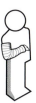
Klaus Dresing, Jos Engelen

PROCEDURE

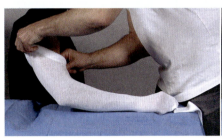

Apply the tube bandage up to the shoulder

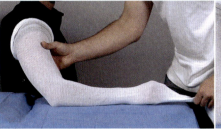

Pull the tube bandage tight to remove any wrinkles

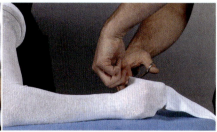

Cut holes in the tube bandage for the thumb

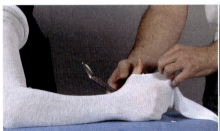

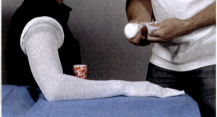

Apply the padding; make a hole for the thumb first

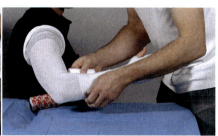

Wrap the forearm using the half-overlapping technique

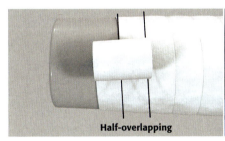

Half-overlapping

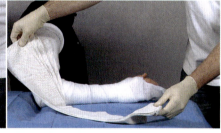

Use the figure-of-eight technique at the elbow to avoid an excessive amount of layers

In order to fit the diameter of the arm, the splint layers must be fanned out proximally

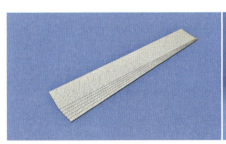

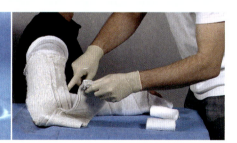

Submerge the splint in water for a few seconds, remove, and squeeze out excess water

Apply the splint; leave the inside of the elbow free

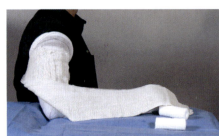

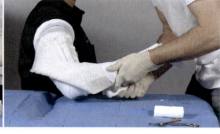

Trim the splint along the MCP joints

Wrap the splint with a gauze bandage, using the half-overlapping technique

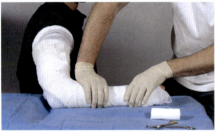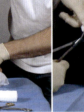

Mold the splint to the arm

Trim the splint proximally and wrap with a gauze bandage

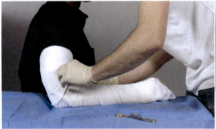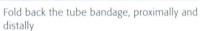

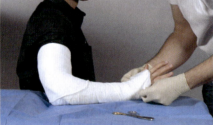

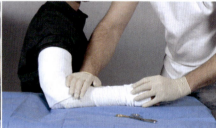

Fold back the tube bandage, proximally and distally

Pass the thumb through the hole in the tube bandage

Hold the splint in the required position until set

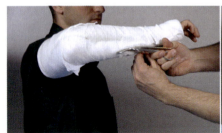

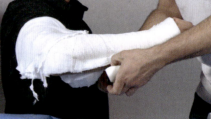

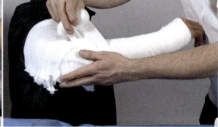

Cut the splint open, either on the inner side, or as shown here on the outer side

Apply an elastic bandage to hold the splint in place, using the half-overlapping technique

Use the figure-of-eight technique at the elbow to avoid an excessive amount of layers

Klaus Dresing, Jos Engelen

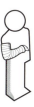

TECHNIQUES

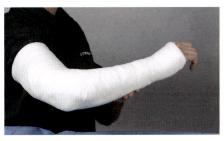

Secure the bandage with surgical tape or bandage clips

FINAL ASSESSMENT

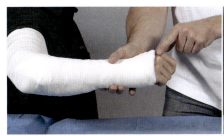

Metacarpal heads remain free to allow free motion of the fingers

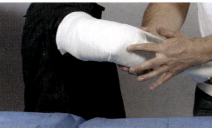

The olecranon remains free of splint

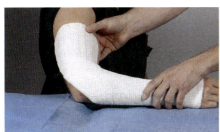

The splint should extend to the top of the biceps

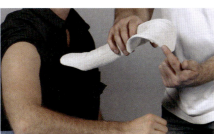

The splint is formed to the shape of the wrist and the upper arm

317

15.3　Long arm cast using plaster of Paris

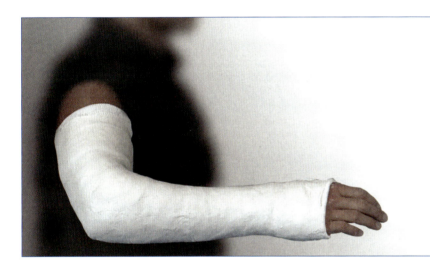

INDICATION

- Fracture of the radius
- Fracture of the ulna
- Fracture of the elbow
- Epicondylitis

GOAL

- Stabilization of the forearm and elbow

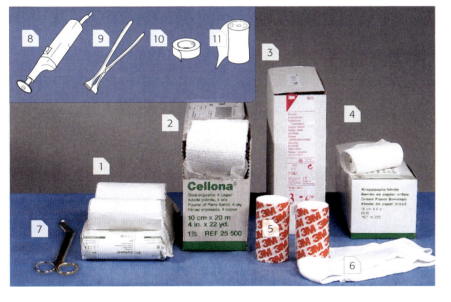

EQUIPMENT

1　Plaster of Paris rolls 10 cm or 12 cm
2　Plaster of Paris splint 10 cm or 12 cm
3　Tube bandage 7.5 cm in dispenser box
4　Crepe paper bandage
5　Cast padding
6　Cut tube bandage
7　Scissors
8　Oscillating saw
9　Cast spreader
10　Surgical tape or bandage clips
11　Elastic bandage

PERSONNEL

15.3

TECHNIQUES

POSITIONING

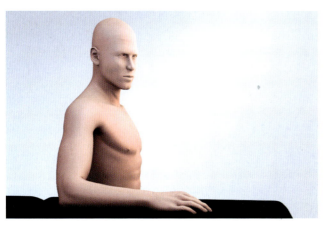

Seat the patient comfortably on a stool.

Place the affected limb on the table, in a functional position, with 90° flexion of the elbow.

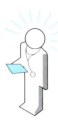

SPECIAL THINGS TO KEEP IN MIND

- The distal palmar crease should remain free
- Protection of the lateral and medial epicondyle
- Protection of the olecranon
- While the splint is setting, the limb should be positioned halfway between supination and pronation
- If necessary, the cast can be split after setting

PROCEDURE

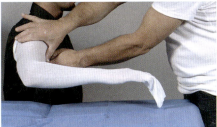

Apply the tube bandage up to the shoulder. Pull the tube bandage tight to remove any wrinkles

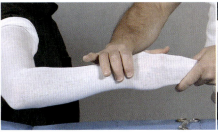

Cut a hole in the tube bandage for the thumb

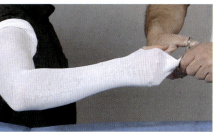

The patient makes a fist to allow the tube bandage to be trimmed, which ensures free movement of the fingers

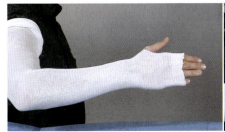

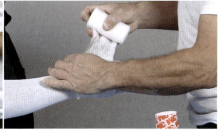

Apply the padding; make a hole for the thumb first

Make a tear in the padding to ensure smooth protection between the thumb and index finger

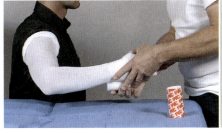

Wrap the forearm using the half-overlapping technique

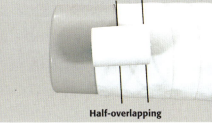

Half-overlapping

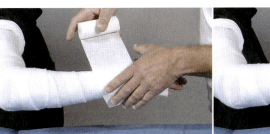

Use the figure-of-eight technique at the elbow to avoid an excessive amount of layers

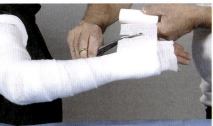

Apply the paper bandage to form a barrier between the dry padding and the wet POP

Cut halfway through the bandage, from proximal to distal, for easy application between the thumb and the index finger

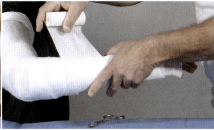

Wrap the forearm using the half-overlapping technique

15.3

TECHNIQUES

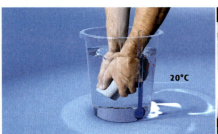

Submerge the roll of POP in water for a few seconds, remove, and squeeze out excess water

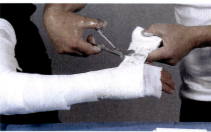

Cut halfway through, from proximal to distal, for easy application between the thumb and the index finger

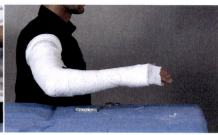

Wrap the arm using the half-overlapping technique

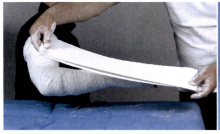

Apply a 4-layer POP splint on the dorsal side for extra stability

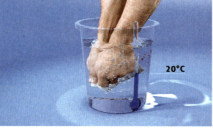

Submerge the splint in water for a few seconds, remove, and squeeze out the excess water

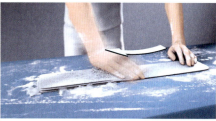

Stretch and smooth out the splint, pressing the layers together, resulting in a compact splint. If this procedure is not done, puff pastry plaster will result, causing an unstable splint

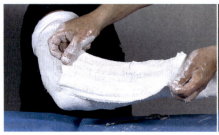

Position the splint and cut at the elbow to allow overlapping

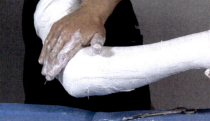

Smooth out the splint

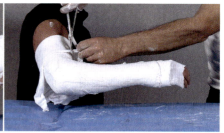

Fold back the tube bandage, proximally and distally, and trim

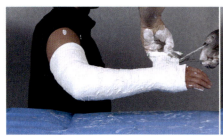

Apply the final rolls of POP

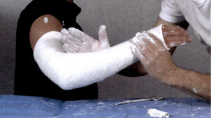

Mold the cast to the desired position of the wrist and elbow

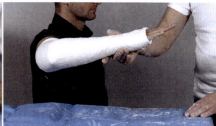

Ensure there is free movement of the shoulder, fingers, and thumb

Klaus Dresing, Jos Engelen

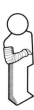

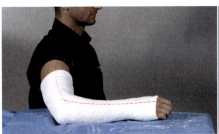

Mark the splitting line

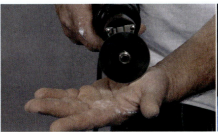

The saw blade oscillates and does not rotate, so there is no direct harm to the skin

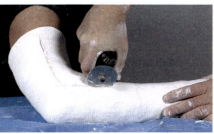

Split the cast with the oscillating saw

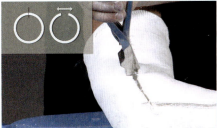

Widen the split with the cast spreader

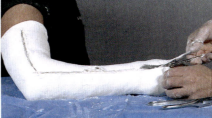

Finish the splitting by cutting the padding and tube bandage completely with scissors

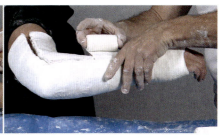

Apply an elastic bandage to secure the split cast. Wrap the arm using the half-overlapping technique

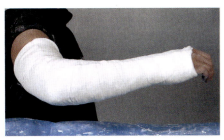

Secure the bandage with surgical tape or bandage clips

15.3

FINAL ASSESSMENT

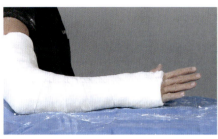

Free flexion of the fingers and thumb at the MCP joints

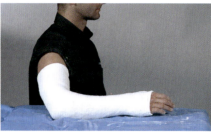

There is two finger's breadth between the cast and the armpit

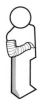

15.4 Long arm cast using synthetic, combicast technique

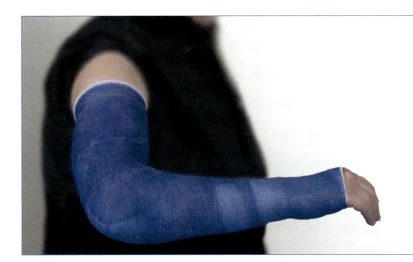

INDICATION

- Fracture of the radius
- Fracture of the ulna
- Fracture of the elbow
- Epicondylitis

GOAL

- Stabilization of the forearm and elbow

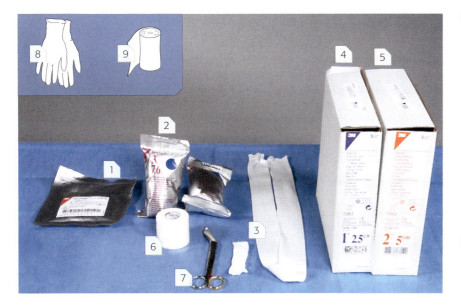

EQUIPMENT

1. Rigid synthetic splint 7.5 cm x 45 cm
2. Semirigid casting tape 7.5 cm
3. Cut tube bandages
4. Tube bandage 2.5 cm in dispenser box
5. Tube bandage 5 cm in dispenser box
6. Elastic foam tape
7. Scissors
8. Gloves
9. Elastic bandage

PERSONNEL

POSITIONING

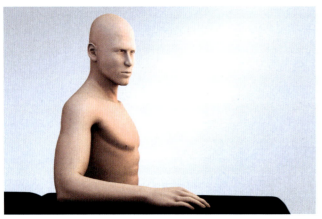

Seat the patient comfortably on a stool.

Place the affected limb on the table, in a functional position, with 90° flexion of the elbow.

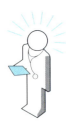

SPECIAL THINGS TO KEEP IN MIND

- The distal palmar crease should remain free
- Protection of the lateral and medial epicondyle
- Protection of the olecranon
- While the splint is setting, the limb should be positioned halfway between supination and pronation
- If necessary, the cast can be split after setting

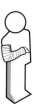

Klaus Dresing, Jos Engelen

15.4

TECHNIQUES

PROCEDURE

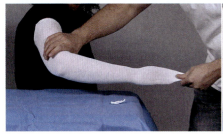

Apply the tube bandage up to the shoulder. Pull the tube bandage tight to remove any wrinkles

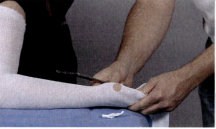

Cut a hole in the tube bandage for the thumb

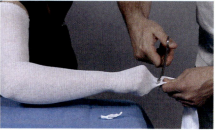

The patient makes a fist to allow the tube bandage to be trimmed, which ensures free movement of the fingers

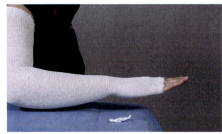

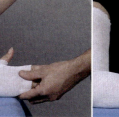

Apply a small tube bandage over the thumb

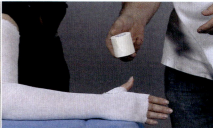

Apply padding over the bony prominences using elastic foam tape

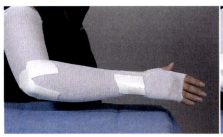

Apply the padding over the radial and ulnar styloid processes, the radial and ulnar epicondyles, and the olecranon

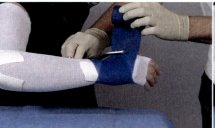

Apply the semirigid casting tape; cut halfway through, proximal to distal, for easy application between the thumb and the index finger

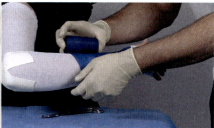

Wrap the forearm using the half-overlapping technique

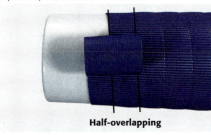

Half-overlapping

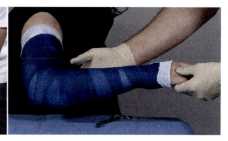

Use the figure-of-eight technique at the elbow to avoid an excessive amount of layers

Fold back the tube bandage, proximally and distally

327

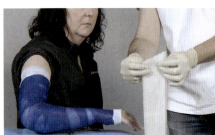

Trim the rigid splint at an angle, distally and proximally

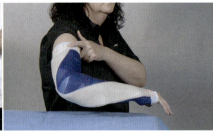

Ensure the splint ends 1 cm short of the semirigid cast, distally and proximally. The patient holds the splint in place proximally

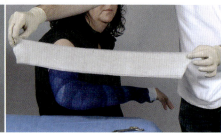

The splint has a trapezoid form

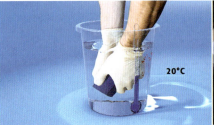

Submerge the semirigid casting tape in water for a few seconds, remove, and squeeze out excess water

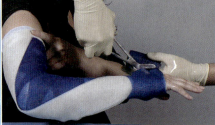

Cut halfway through the semirigid casting tape, from proximal to distal, for easy application between the thumb and the index finger

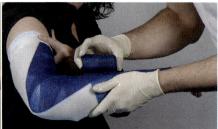

Wrap the forearm using the half-overlapping technique

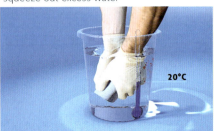

Submerge the elastic bandage in water; using a wet bandage accelerates the setting

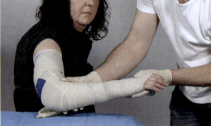

Mold the cast and hold it in 90° flexion at the elbow and in functional position at the wrist until it is set

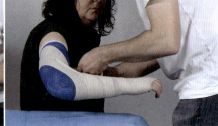

Remove the wet bandage after the cast has set

FINAL ASSESSMENT

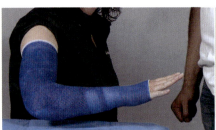

Free flexion of the fingers and thumb at the MCP joints

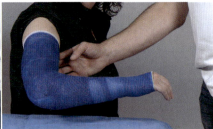

There is two finger's breadth between the cast and the armpit

Klaus Dresing, Jos Engelen

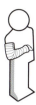

CAST REMOVAL

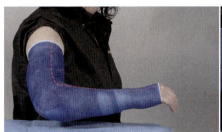

Mark the splitting line

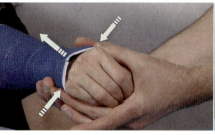

Before splitting the cast, press on both sides of the hand to create a small space for the scissors

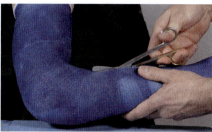

Split all layers, including the padding and the tube bandage

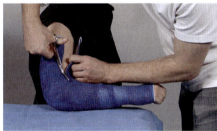

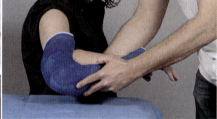

Remove the cast by opening the combicast

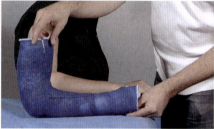

There is 90° flexion at the elbow and functional position of the wrist

15.4

TECHNIQUES

15.5 Sarmiento humeral brace using synthetic, combicast technique

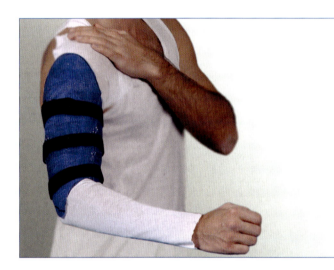

INDICATION

- Diaphyseal fractures of the humerus
- Not recommended for primary fracture care

GOAL

- Stabilization of the humeral shaft

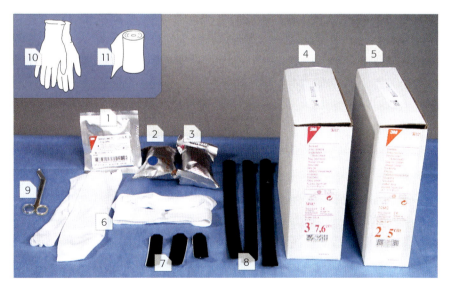

EQUIPMENT

1. Rigid synthetic splint 7.5 cm x 20 cm
2. Semirigid casting tape 5 cm
3. Semirigid casting tape 7.5 cm
4. Tube bandage 7.5 cm in dispenser box
5. Tube bandage 5 cm in dispenser box
6. Cut tube bandages
7. Velcro strips (loop) adhesive
8. Velcro strips (hook) nonadhesive
9. Scissors
10. Gloves
11. Elastic bandage

PERSONNEL

(1 surgeon if needed)

15.5

TECHNIQUES

POSITIONING

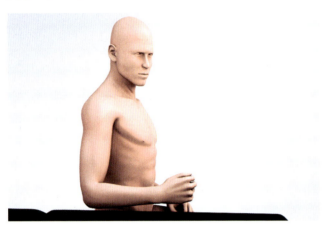

Seat the patient comfortably on a stool.

The affected limb hangs in the air, with 90° flexion of the elbow.

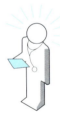

SPECIAL THINGS TO KEEP IN MIND

- Skin irritation under the axilla
- Circulation

PROCEDURE

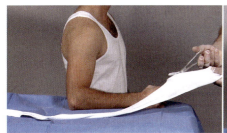

Cut two slits in the tube bandage, one long and one short

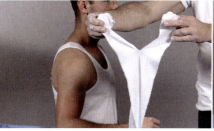

These slits allow application around the neck

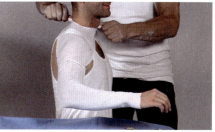

Apply the tube bandage and tie around the neck

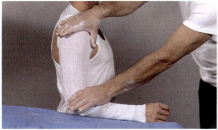

Pull the tube bandage tight to remove any wrinkles

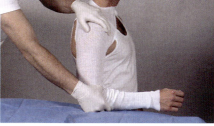

An assistant is needed to hold the shoulder and elbow in position for the rest of the procedure

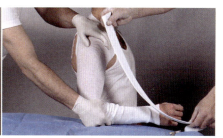

Thread a smaller double-length tube bandage under the first; it will be used later to make splitting the brace easier

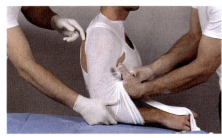

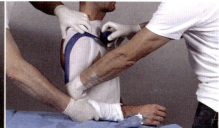

Apply the first layer of semirigid casting tape; the assistant holds the tape at the shoulder

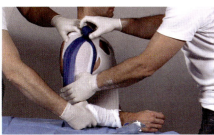

Wrap the semirigid casting tape twice from elbow to shoulder, longitudinally

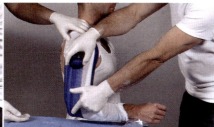

Wrap the semirigid casting tape over the olecranon to hold the elbow at 90° flexion

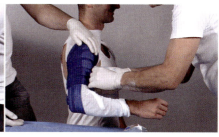

Wrap the rest of the upper arm using the half-overlapping technique

333

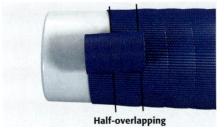

Half-overlapping

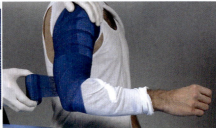

Ensure there are no creases in the tube bandage at the inside of the elbow

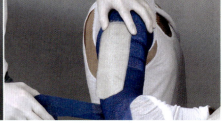

Apply the rigid splint and trim to the required length

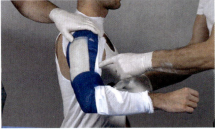

Fold the small tube bandage back over the semirigid casting tape, and hold in place with the next layer of semirigid casting tape

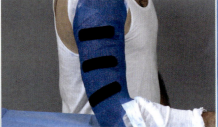

Apply three strips of adhesive velcro (with loops)

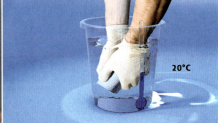

Submerge the elastic bandage in water; using a wet bandage accelerates the setting

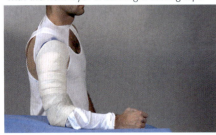

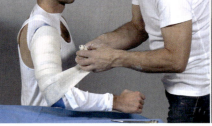

Remove the wet bandage after the brace has set

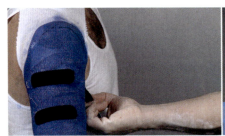

Ensure there is enough space at the armpit and shoulder

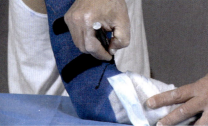

Mark the epicondyles and the fold of the elbow

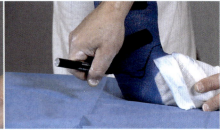

Ensure the olecranon fossa is free

Mark the brace where it needs to be trimmed

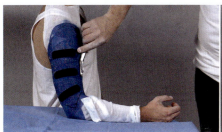

Split the semirigid casting tape using the small tube bandage as a guide

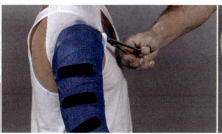

Cut through the small tube bandage proximally

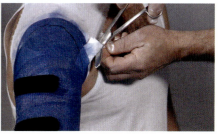

Proximally, slide one blade of the scissors into the outer tube bandage

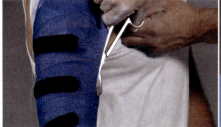

Guide the scissors down the tube bandage and split open the outer layer of semirigid casting tape

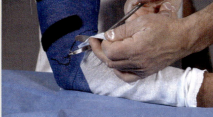

Cut through the tube bandage distally

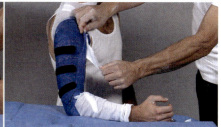

Remove the outer section of the small tube bandage

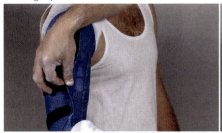

Ensure the split section of semirigid casting tape can be opened

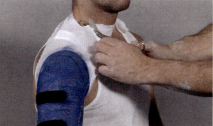

Cut the large tube bandage from around the neck

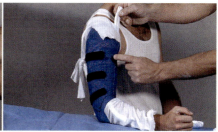

Position the lower tube bandage at the outer side of the flap

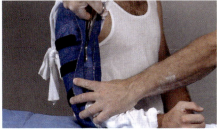

Open the flap, and guide the scissors along the small tube bandage to cut through the lower layer of semirigid casting tape

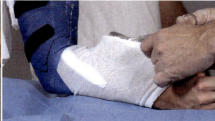

Cut through the large tube bandage

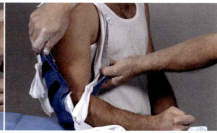

Open the brace and remove it

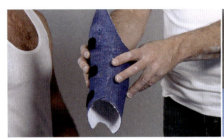

Trim the brace to the desired shape

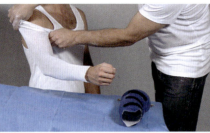

Prepare a new tube bandage and place over the arm before applying the brace

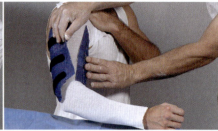

The overlapping sections prevent the skin being trapped between the edges

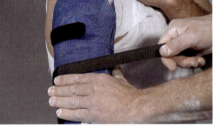

Attach the velcro strips (with hooks); compress the brace slightly and close provisionally with the strips

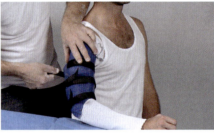

Apply tension to the tube bandage, loosen the velcro strips, place the brace in the final position and re-fasten the strips

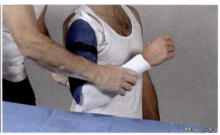

Ensure free flexion and extension of the elbow

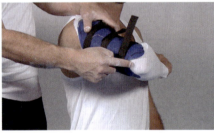

Ensure free movement of the olecranon fossa

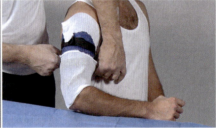

Fold the tube bandage over the brace to provide protection

FINAL ASSESSMENT

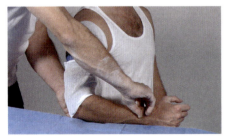

Check that the brace is not too tight by taking the pulse. Check there is no skin irritation

Klaus Dresing, Jos Engelen

15.6   Dorsopalmar (radial) short arm splint using plaster of Paris

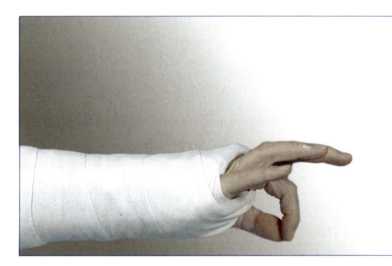

INDICATION

- Fracture of the distal radius

GOAL

- Stabilization of the dorsal forearm and wrist

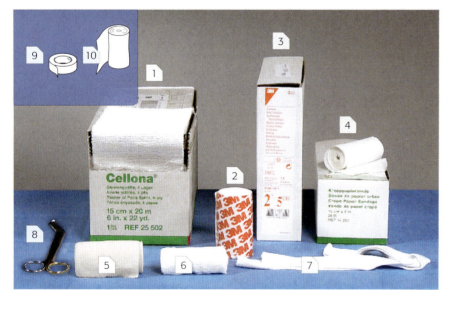

EQUIPMENT

1 Plaster of Paris splint 12 cm, 15 cm, or 20 cm
2 Cast padding
3 Tube bandage 5 cm in dispenser box
4 Crepe paper bandage
5 Elastic bandage
6 Gauze bandage
7 Cut tube bandage
8 Scissors
9 Surgical tape or bandage clips
10 Elastic bandage

PERSONNEL

(1 surgeon in case of reduction)

POSITIONING

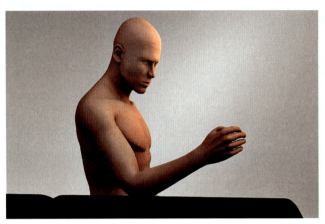

Seat the patient comfortably on a stool.

Place the affected limb on the table, in a functional position.

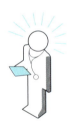

SPECIAL THINGS TO KEEP IN MIND

- The distal palmar crease should remain free
- The metacarpal heads should remain free
- Free flexion of the elbow should be possible
- While the splint is setting, the limb should be positioned halfway between supination and pronation

PROCEDURE

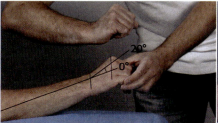

Place the wrist in 20° dorsal flexion

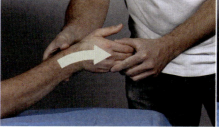

Position the wrist in ulnar abduction

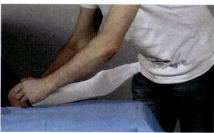

Apply the tube bandage

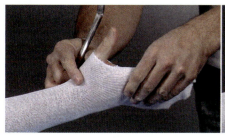

Cut an opening for the thumb

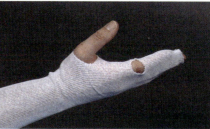

Cut a second opening over the PIP joint of the index finger, to allow the tube bandage to be folded back over the thumb later

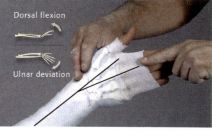

Ensure the wrist is in 20° dorsal flexion and slight ulnar deviation

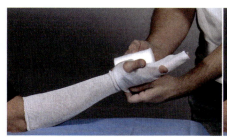

Apply the padding; make a hole for the thumb first

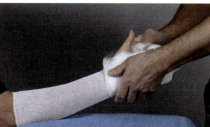

Make a tear in the padding to ensure smooth protection between the thumb and index finger

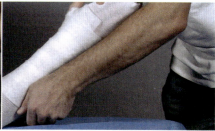

Wrap the forearm using the half-overlapping technique

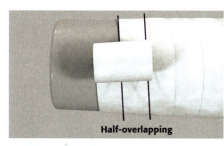

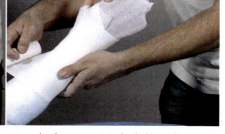

Apply the paper bandage to form a barrier between the dry padding and the wet POP

Wrap the forearm using the half-overlapping technique

339

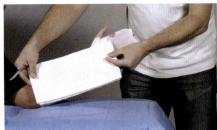

Fold the POP splint to the appropriate length and trim to the required shape

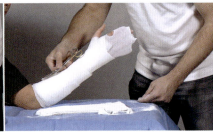

Starting two finger's breadth from the elbow crease, measure a scissor's length, and cut the splint to this point

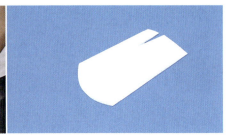

Shape the splint like this

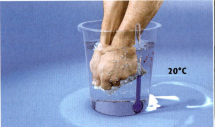

Submerge the splint in water for a few seconds, remove, and squeeze out excess water

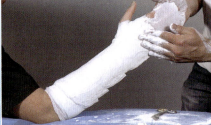

Apply the splint and mold into place

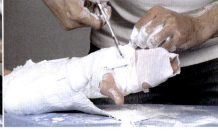

Trim the splint at the palmar crease to ensure free flexion of the fingers, use the thumb as a reference

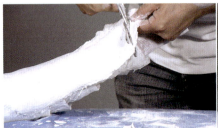

Trim the splint dorsally at the MCP joints to ensure free extension

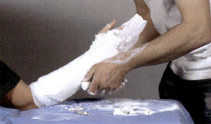

Apply the gauze bandage using the half-overlapping technique

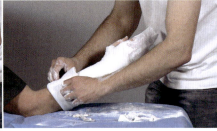

Fold back the tube bandage, proximally and distally

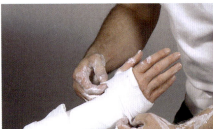

Pass the thumb through the hole in the tube bandage

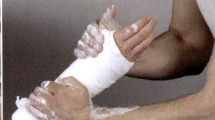

Place the thumb into the desired position and hold in place until the splint is set

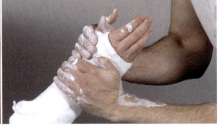

Use the flat hand technique to hold the splint in the correct position

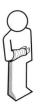

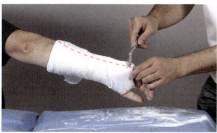 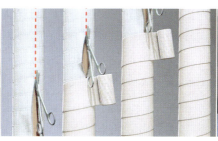

Split the splint completely at the ulnar side. Use the step-by-step splitting and fixing technique to avoid loss of reduction

Cut the gauze bandage and padding starting distally

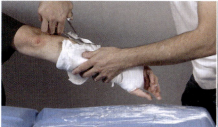 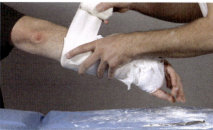 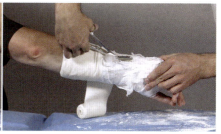

Cut the tube bandage proximally

Apply an elastic bandage proximally to close the splint

Cut another section of the tube bandage and close the splint

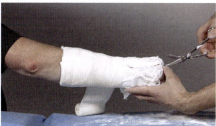 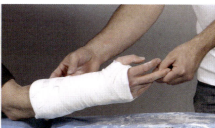

Cut the rest of the tube bandage and close the splint; using this technique avoids loss of reduction

Secure the bandage with surgical tape or bandage clips

FINAL ASSESSMENT

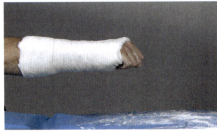

Free flexion of the fingers at the MCP joints

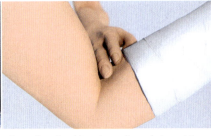

The splint should end two finger's breadth from the elbow crease to allow free flexion of the elbow

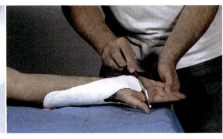

Free movement of the thumb and free palmar crease

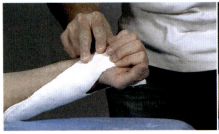

Free movement of the MCP joints

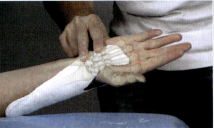

The skeleton illustrates the line of the MCP joints

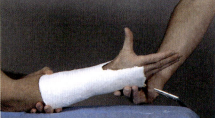

Free movement of the thumb

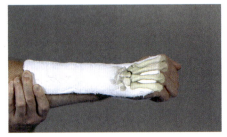

Wrist is in 20° dorsal flexion

15.7   Dorsopalmar (radial) short arm splint using synthetic

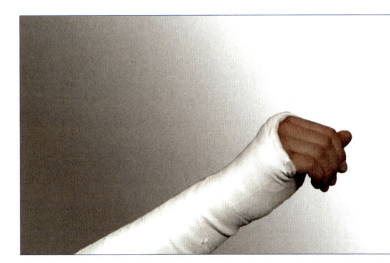

INDICATION

- Fracture of the distal radius

GOAL

- Stabilization of the dorsal forearm and wrist

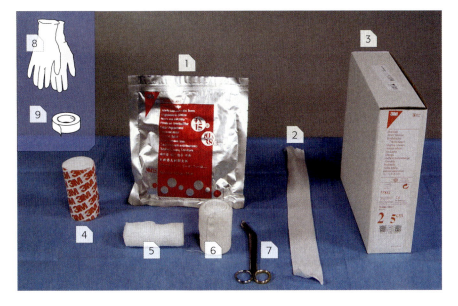

EQUIPMENT

1 Rigid synthetic splint 10 cm or 12.5 cm
2 Cut tube bandage
3 Tube bandage 5 cm in dispenser box
4 Cast padding
5 Gauze bandage
6 Elastic bandage
7 Scissors
8 Gloves
9 Surgical tape or bandage clips

PERSONNEL

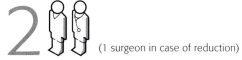

2 (1 surgeon in case of reduction)

343

15.7

TECHNIQUES

POSITIONING

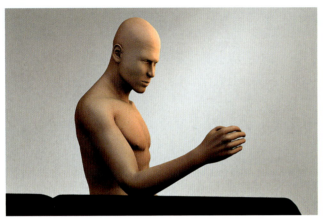

Seat the patient comfortably on a stool.

Place the affected limb on the table, in a functional position.

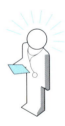

SPECIAL THINGS TO KEEP IN MIND

- The distal palmar crease should remain free
- The metacarpal heads should remain free
- Free flexion of the elbow should be possible
- While the splint is setting, the limb should be positioned halfway between supination and pronation

Klaus Dresing, Jos Engelen

PROCEDURE

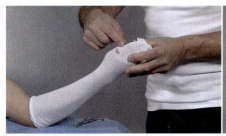

Apply the tube bandage; cut an opening for the thumb

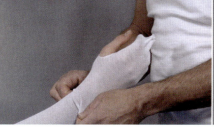

Pull the tube bandage tight to remove any wrinkles

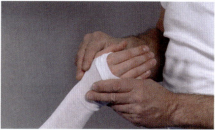

Position the wrist in ulnar abduction

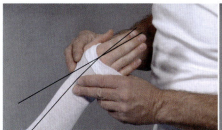

Ulnar abduction is demonstrated

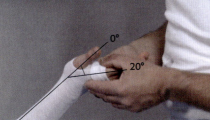

Demonstration of 20° dorsal flexion

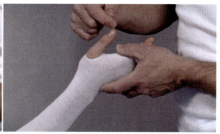

The axis of the thumb is in line with the radius

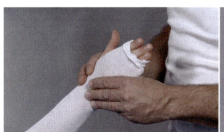

Position the forearm midway between supination and pronation

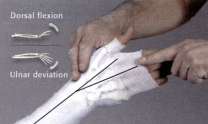

Ensure the wrist is in 20° dorsal flexion and slight ulnar deviation

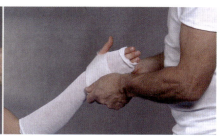

Make a hole in the padding for the thumb

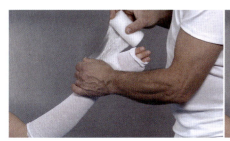

Make a tear in the padding to ensure smooth protection between the thumb and index finger

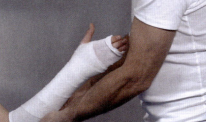

Apply the padding using the half-overlapping technique

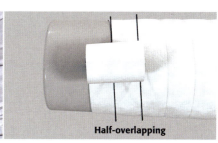

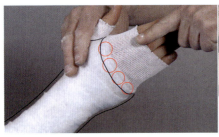

Border of padding and splint at the metacarpal heads

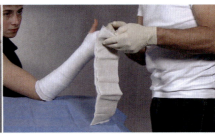

Measure the splint to the appropriate length needed

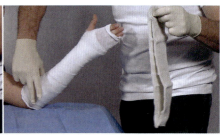

In order to fit the diameter of the forearm, the splint layers must be fanned out proximally and the ends trimmed

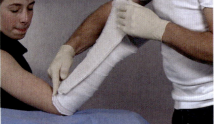

Place the splint two finger's breadth below the elbow crease and trim along the MCP joints

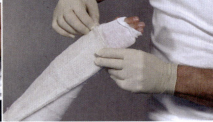

Ensure the metacarpal heads remain free

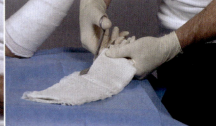

Trim the splint to the desired shape

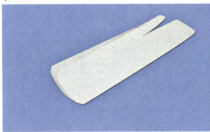

Shape the splint like this to give a small palmar and a large dorsal component

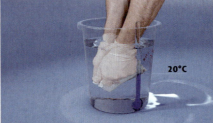

Submerge the splint in water for a few seconds, remove, and squeeze out excess water

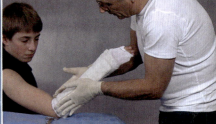

Apply the splint dorsally and mold into place

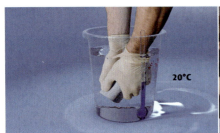

Submerge the gauze bandage in water for a few seconds, remove, and squeeze out excess water

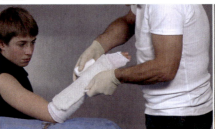

Wrap the gauze bandage around the splint, beginning at the wrist

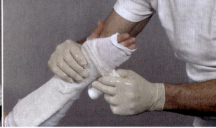

Ensure the palmar component of the splint is on the palmar side

Klaus Dresing, Jos Engelen

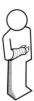

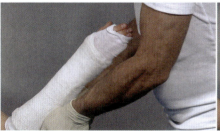

Wrap the forearm using the half-overlapping technique

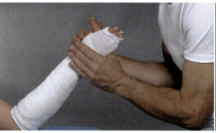

Remove gloves for easier molding of the splint

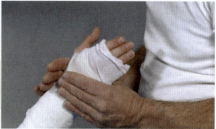

Place the thumb in the required position, and mold the splint in correct dorsal flexion and ulnar abduction while it sets

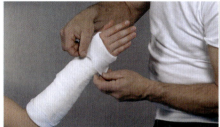

Fold back the tube bandage, distally and proximally

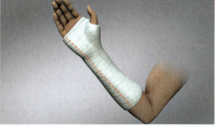

Split the splint on the ulnar aspect after it has set

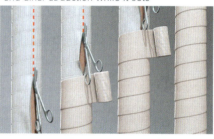

Use the step-by-step splitting and fixing technique to split the splint, and close it with an elastic bandage to avoid loss of reduction

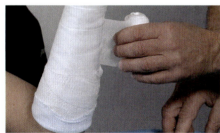

Wrap the forearm using the half-overlapping technique

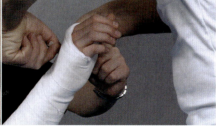

Secure the bandage with surgical tape or bandage clips

15.7

TECHNIQUES

FINAL ASSESSMENT

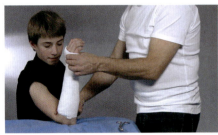

The length of the splint allows free flexion of the elbow.

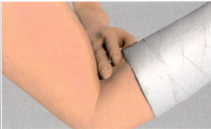

The splint should end two finger's breadth from the elbow crease

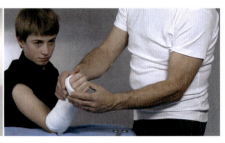

Ensure free movement of the fingers and thumb

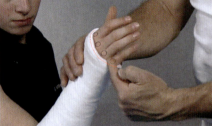

Metacarpal heads should remain free

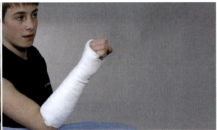

The distal palmar crease is free to allow full motion of the fingers

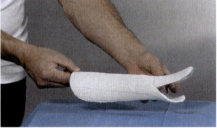

"Shark" design of the splint in lateral view. Exact contouring of the dorsal and radial aspects of the wrist joint can be seen

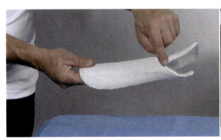

The dorsal extension and the space for the base of the thumb are clearly visible

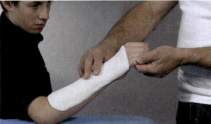

The MCP joints are free dorsally, and the splint wraps far enough around on the ulnar side to give support

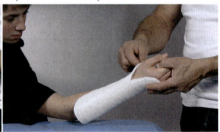

Free movement of the thumb is possible. The splint provides support for the distal radius

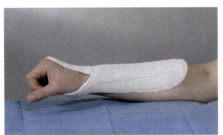

Correct position of the splint on the radial aspect

Klaus Dresing, Jos Engelen

15.8 Palmar short arm splint using plaster of Paris

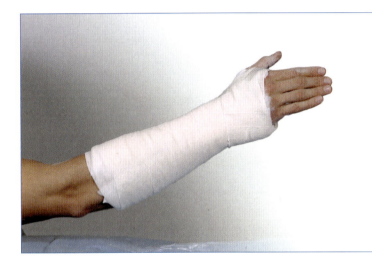

INDICATION

- Stable nondisplaced fractures of the distal radius
- Radial nerve palsy

GOAL

- Stabilization of the distal forearm and wrist

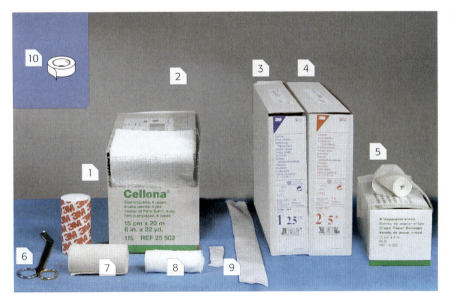

EQUIPMENT

1 Cast padding
2 Plaster of Paris splint 12 cm, 15 cm, or 20 cm
3 Tube bandage 2.5 cm in dispenser box
4 Tube bandage 5 cm in dispenser box
5 Crepe paper bandage
6 Scissors
7 Elastic bandage
8 Gauze bandage
9 Cut tube bandages
10 Surgical tape or bandage clips

PERSONNEL

349

15.8

TECHNIQUES

POSITIONING

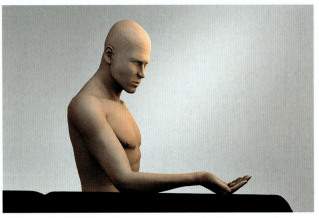

Seat the patient comfortably on a stool.

Place the affected limb on the table in supination during application, and in a functional position during setting.

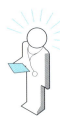

SPECIAL THINGS TO KEEP IN MIND

- The splint extends distally to the distal palmar crease and the metacarpal heads
- The distal palmar crease should remain free
- Metacarpal heads should remain free
- Free flexion of the elbow should be possible
- While the splint is setting, the limb should be positioned halfway between supination and pronation

Klaus Dresing, Jos Engelen

PROCEDURE

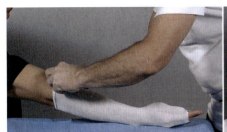

Apply the tube bandage and pull it tight to avoid wrinkles

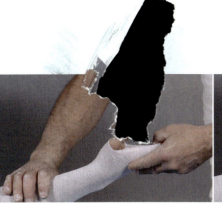

Cut an opening for the thumb

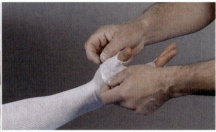

Apply a small tube bandage over the thumb

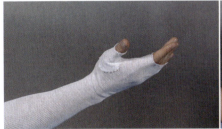

Apply both tube bandages smoothly and free of wrinkles

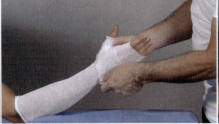

Apply the padding; make an opening for the thumb first

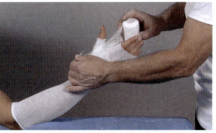

Make a tear in the padding to ensure smooth protection between the thumb and index finger

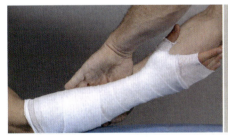

Wrap the forearm using the half-overlapping technique

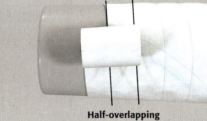

Half-overlapping

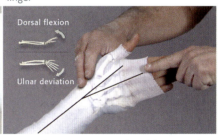

Dorsal flexion

Ulnar deviation

Ensure the wrist is in 20° dorsal flexion and slight ulnar deviation

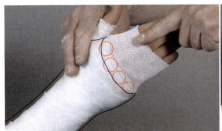

Border of padding and splint at the metacarpal heads

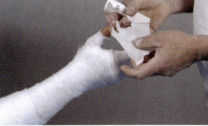

Apply the paper bandage; make a tear to accommodate the thumb. Use the paper bandage to form a barrier between the dry padding and the wet POP

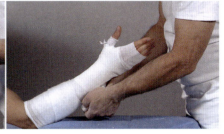

Wrap the forearm using the half-overlapping technique

15.8

TECHNIQUES

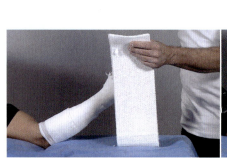

Fold the splint in two to make an 8-layer splint, and trim to the desired shape proximally

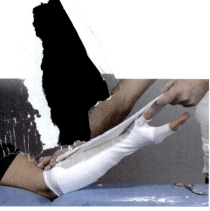

Place the splint two finger's breadth from the elbow crease, and trim to the desired length distally, leaving the MCP joints free

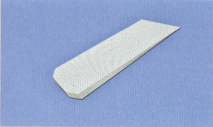

Shape the splint like this

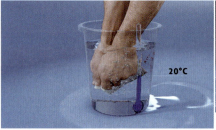

Submerge the splint in water for a few seconds, remove, and squeeze out excess water

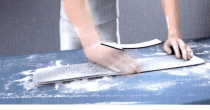

Stretch and smooth out the splint, pressing the layers together, resulting in a compact splint. If this procedure is not done, puff pastry plaster will result, causing an unstable splint

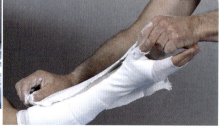

Apply the splint and mold into place

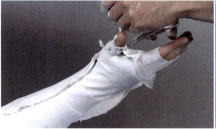

Shape the splint to pass between the thumb and the index finger

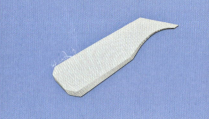

Shape the splint like this

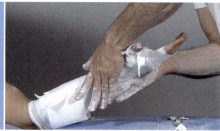

Mold the splint to the hand and forearm

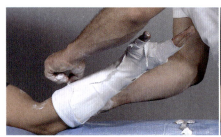

Fold back the tube bandage over the splint, proximally and distally

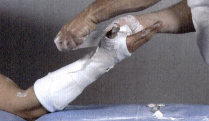

Apply the gauze bandage to hold the splint in position

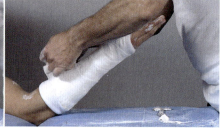

Wrap the forearm using the half-overlapping technique

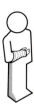

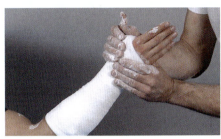

Mold the splint into the desired shape and hold in position until set. Ensure there is 20° dorsal flexion of the wrist

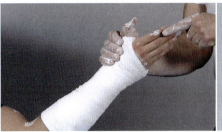

Ensure there is a slight ulnar deviation

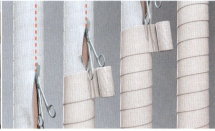

Use the step-by-step splitting and fixing technique to split the splint, and close it with an elastic bandage to avoid loss of reduction

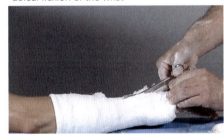

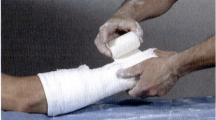

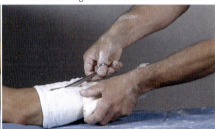

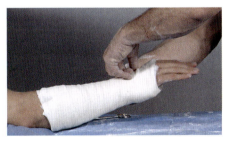

Secure the bandage with surgical tape or bandage clips

15.8

TECHNIQUES

FINAL ASSESSMENT

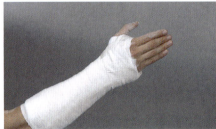

Metacarpal heads remain free

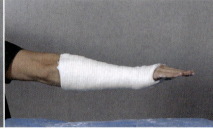

Free flexion and extension of the fingers and thumb

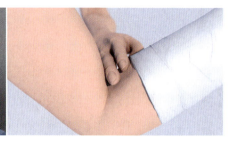

The splint should end two finger's breadth from the elbow crease to allow free motion of the elbow

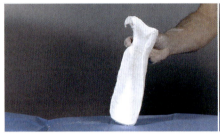

The final shape and contours of the splint show it is molded to the forearm and hand

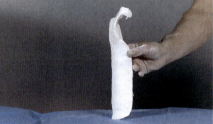

The flap between the thumb and index finger is visible

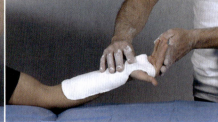

Distal palmar crease is free and the patient is able to make a fist

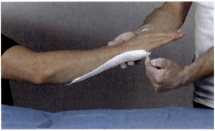

The gutter form of the splint supports the ulna distally

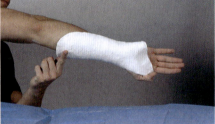

On the palmar side of the wrist, the carpus and the metacarpus are supported

15.9 Palmar short arm splint using synthetic

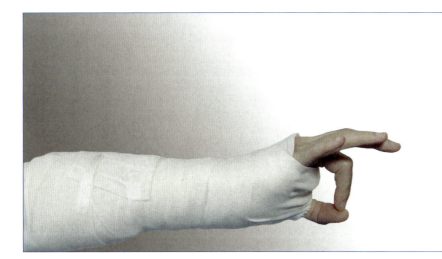

INDICATION

- Stable nondisplaced fractures of the distal radius
- Radial nerve palsy

GOAL

- Stabilization of the distal forearm and wrist

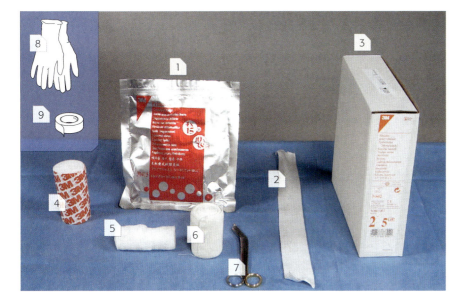

EQUIPMENT

1 Rigid synthetic splint 7.5 cm or 10 cm
2 Cut tube bandage 5 cm
3 Tube bandage 5 cm in dispenser box
4 Cast padding
5 Gauze bandage
6 Elastic bandage
7 Scissors
8 Gloves
9 Surgical tape or bandage clips

PERSONNEL

15.9

TECHNIQUES

POSITIONING

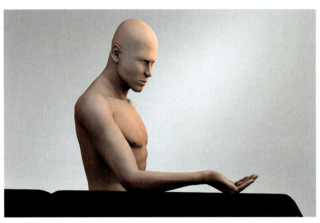

Seat the patient comfortably on a stool.

Place the affected limb on the table in supination during application, and in a functional position during setting.

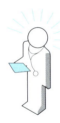

SPECIAL THINGS TO KEEP IN MIND

- The splint extends distally to the distal palmar crease and the metacarpal heads
- The distal palmar crease should remain free
- Metacarpal heads should remain free
- Free flexion of the elbow should be possible
- While the splint is setting, the limb should be positioned halfway between supination and pronation

Klaus Dresing, Jos Engelen

PROCEDURE

15.9

TECHNIQUES

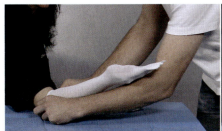

Apply the tube bandage

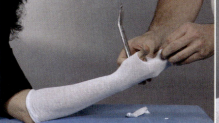

Cut an opening for the thumb

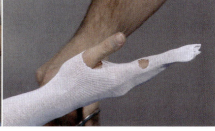

Cut a second opening over the PIP joint of the index finger, to allow the tube bandage to be folded back over the thumb later

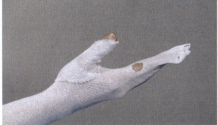

Apply a small tube bandage over the thumb. Apply both tube bandages smoothly and without wrinkles

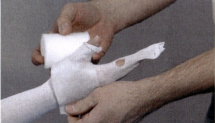

Apply the padding; make an opening for the thumb first

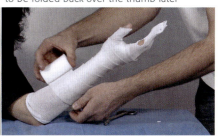

Wrap the forearm using the half-overlapping technique

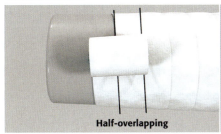

Half-overlapping

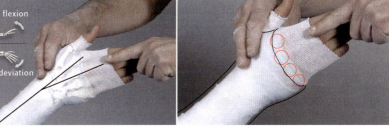

Dorsal flexion

Ulnar deviation

Ensure the wrist is in 20° dorsal flexion and slight ulnar deviation

Border of padding and splint at the metacarpal heads

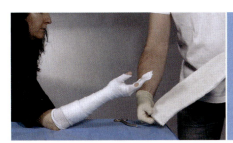

In order to fit the diameter of the forearm, the splint layers must be fanned out proximally; trim the splint to the desired shape

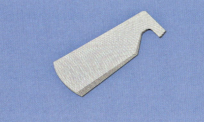

Shape the splint like this

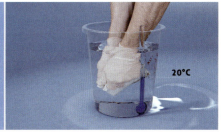

20°C

Submerge the splint in water for a few seconds, remove, and squeeze out excess water

357

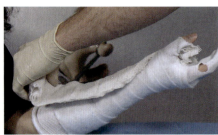

Apply the splint, and trim it two finger's breadth below the elbow crease

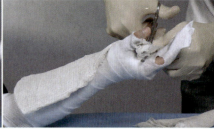

Trim the splint at the distal palmar crease

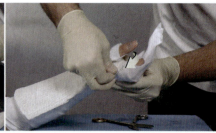

Position the splint flap between the thumb and index finger

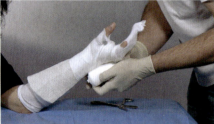

Apply the gauze bandage to hold the splint in position

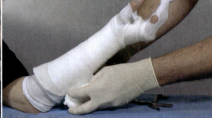

Wrap the forearm using the half-overlapping technique

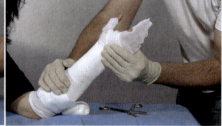

Mold the splint into the desired shape, with the patient's fingers spread, and hold in position until set

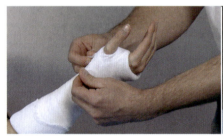

Fold back the tube bandage with the second opening pulled over the thumb

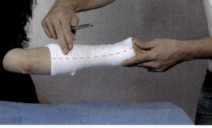

Split the splint completely open, and hold in place with an elastic bandage

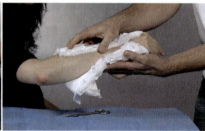

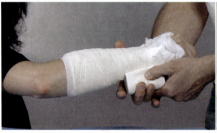

Wrap the forearm using the half-overlapping technique

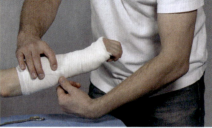

Secure the bandage with surgical tape or bandage clips

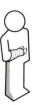

FINAL ASSESSMENT

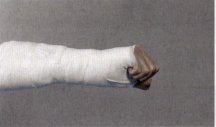

Metacarpal heads remain free

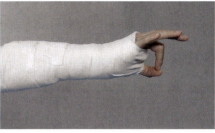

Free flexion and extension of the fingers and thumb

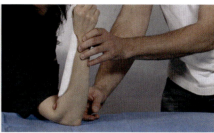

The splint should end two finger's breadth from the elbow crease to allow free flexion of the elbow

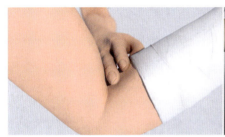

On the palmar side of the wrist, the carpus and the metacarpus are supported

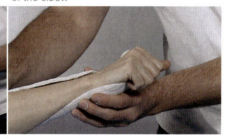

The distal palmar crease is free and the patient is able to make a fist

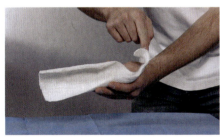

The contours of the hand are clearly visible

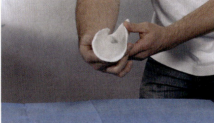

The gutter form of the splint supports the distal forearm and wrist

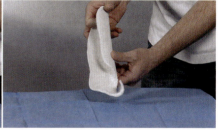

The flap between the thumb and the index finger is visible

Klaus Dresing, Jos Engelen

15.10   Dorsal short arm splint using synthetic

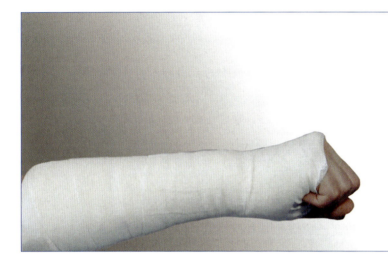

INDICATION

- Stable nondisplaced fractures of the distal radius

GOAL

- Stabilization of the distal forearm and wrist

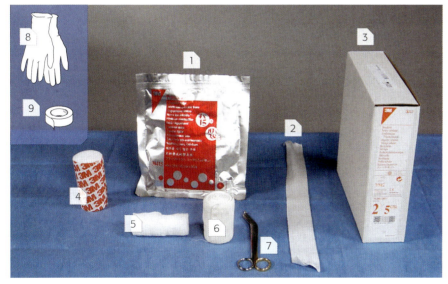

EQUIPMENT

1 Rigid synthetic splint 7.5 cm or 10 cm
2 Cut tube bandage 5 cm
3 Tube bandage 5 cm in dispenser box
4 Cast padding
5 Gauze bandage
6 Elastic bandage
7 Scissors
8 Gloves
9 Surgical tape or bandage clips

PERSONNEL

 (1 surgeon in case of reduction)

POSITIONING

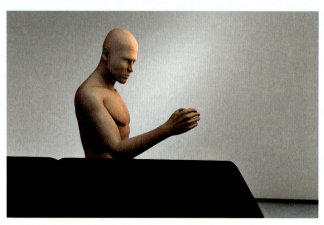

Seat the patient comfortably on a stool.
Place the affected limb on the table, in a functional position.

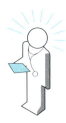

SPECIAL THINGS TO KEEP IN MIND

- The splint extends distally to the metacarpal heads
- The distal palmar crease should remain free
- Metacarpal heads should remain free
- Free flexion of the elbow should be possible

Klaus Dresing, Jos Engelen

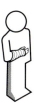

PROCEDURE

15.10

TECHNIQUES

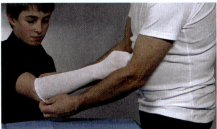

Apply the tube bandage smoothly without wrinkles

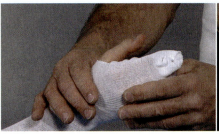

Cut an opening for the thumb

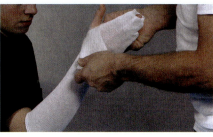

Apply the padding; make an opening for the thumb first

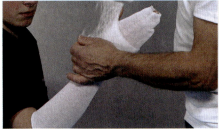

Make a tear in the padding to ensure smooth protection between the thumb and index finger

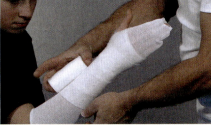

Wrap the forearm using the half-overlapping technique

Half-overlapping

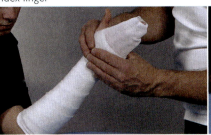

Ensure the metacarpal heads remain free

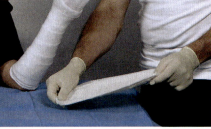

In order to fit the diameter of the forearm, the splint layers must be fanned out proximally

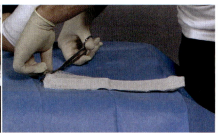

Trim the splint to the desired shape

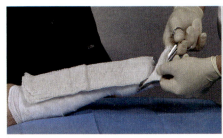

Trim the splint to leave the MCP joints free

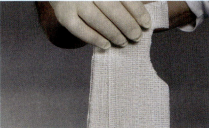

Cut a small section from the splint to allow free movement of the thumb

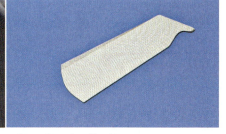

Shape the splint like this

363

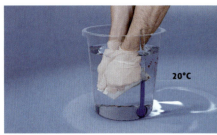

Submerge the splint in water for a few seconds, remove, and squeeze out excess water

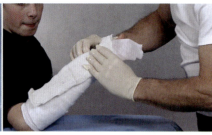

Apply the splint and mold into place

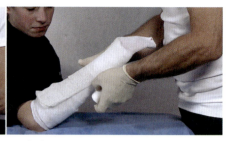

Apply the gauze bandage to hold the splint in place, using the half-overlapping technique

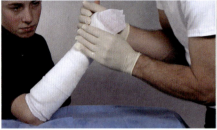

Place the wrist in 20° dorsal flexion using the flat hand technique

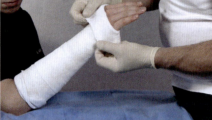

Fold back the tube bandage, proximally and distally

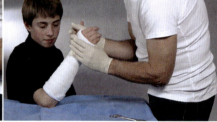

Mold the splint to the desired shape and hold in position until set

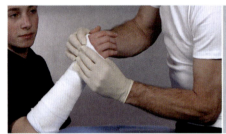

Ensure that the metacarpals are not compressed while molding the splint

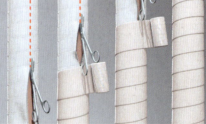

Use the step-by-step splitting and fixing technique to split the splint, and close it with an elastic bandage, to avoid loss of reduction

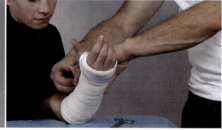

Secure the bandage with surgical tape or bandage clips

Klaus Dresing, Jos Engelen

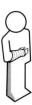

FINAL ASSESSMENT

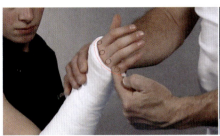

The metacarpal heads remain free

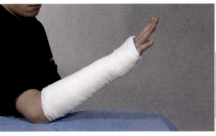

Free flexion and extension of the fingers and thumb

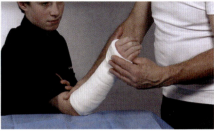

The splint should end two finger's breadth from the elbow crease to allow free flexion of the elbow

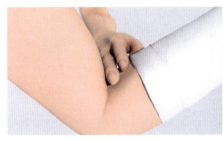

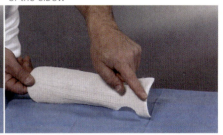

The splint has a gutter form that supports the distal forearm and a flap between the thumb and the index finger

The splint has an oblique edge at the metacarpal heads

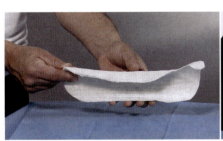

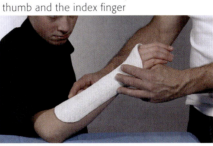

Proximally, the rounded edge allows free movement of the elbow

15.11 Short arm cast using plaster of Paris

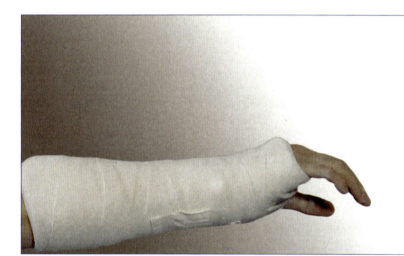

INDICATION

- Fracture of the distal radius

GOAL

- Stabilization of the distal forearm and wrist

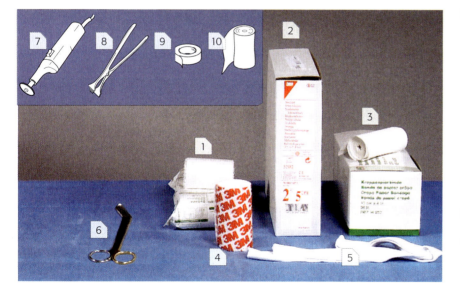

EQUIPMENT

1. Plaster of Paris rolls 8 cm or 10 cm
2. Tube bandage 5 cm in dispenser box
3. Crepe paper bandage
4. Cast padding
5. Cut tube bandage
6. Scissors
7. Oscillating saw
8. Cast spreader
9. Surgical tape or bandage clips
10. Elastic bandage

PERSONNEL

POSITIONING

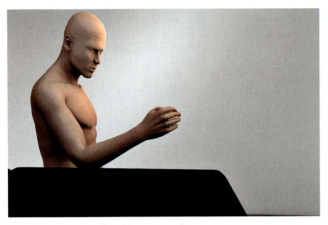

Seat the patient comfortably on a stool.

Place the affected arm on the table, in a functional position.

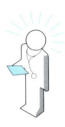

SPECIAL THINGS TO KEEP IN MIND

- Free flexion of the elbow should be possible
- Metacarpal heads should remain free
- The distal palmar crease should remain free
- While the cast is setting, the limb should be positioned halfway between supination and pronation
- In primary fracture care it is necessary to split the cast completely open after setting, or in the case of severe swelling, to remove a small strip

PROCEDURE

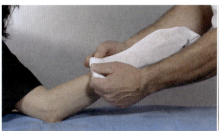

Apply the tube bandage

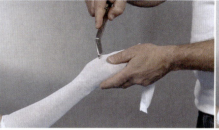

Cut an opening for the thumb

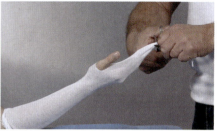

Trim the tube bandage a few centimeters above the fingertips

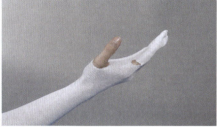

Cut a second opening over the PIP joint of the index finger to fold back over the thumb later

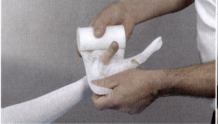

Apply the padding; make a hole for the thumb first

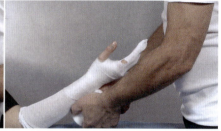

Wrap the forearm using the half-overlapping technique

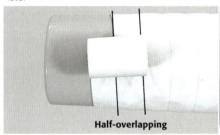

Half-overlapping

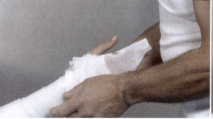

Apply the paper bandage; make a tear to accommodate the thumb

Use the paper bandage to form a barrier between the dry padding and the wet POP

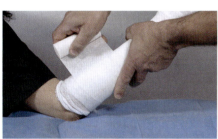

Wrap the forearm using the half-overlapping technique

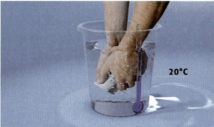

Submerge the roll of POP in water for a few seconds, remove, and squeeze out excess water

20°C

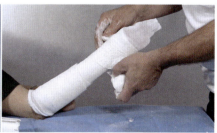

Apply the first roll of POP

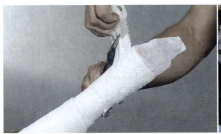

Cut halfway through, from proximal to distal, for easier application between the thumb and index finger

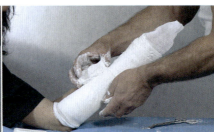

Wrap the forearm using the half-overlapping technique

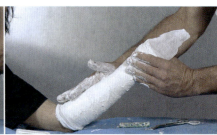

Mold and smooth out the cast

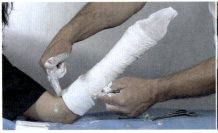

Fold back the tube bandage over the first layer of POP distally

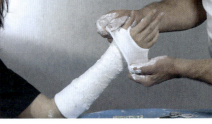

Pass the thumb through the hole in the tube bandage and fold it over the POP

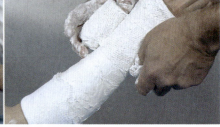

Apply another layer of POP. If extra stability is needed, more splint can be added

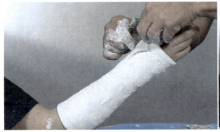

Fold back the end of the POP

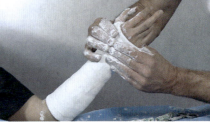

Mold the cast to the required shape

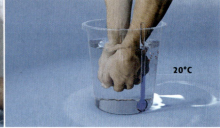

Wet hands make smoothing the cast easier

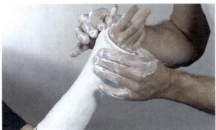

Mold the edges of the cast for a smooth finish

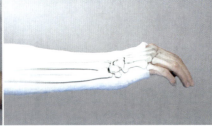

Ensure the metacarpal heads are free to allow movement of the fingers and thumb

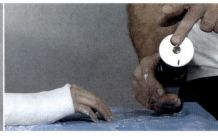

Split the cast with an oscillating saw

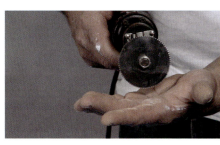

The saw blade oscillates and does not rotate, so there is no direct harm to the skin

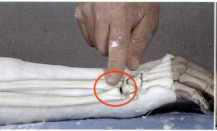

Direct the saw to avoid the bony prominences

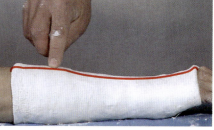

Mark the splitting line

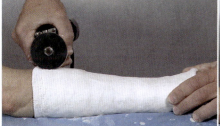

Split the cast from proximal to distal

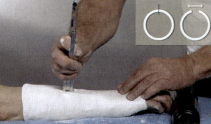

Open the cast with the cast spreaders

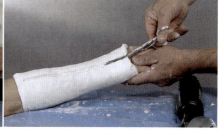

Cut through the padding and the tube bandage with the scissors

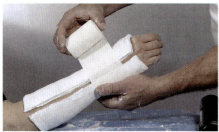

Apply an elastic bandage to fix the cast

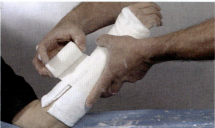

Wrap the forearm using the half-overlapping technique

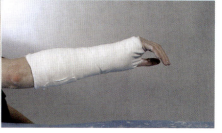

Secure the bandage with surgical tape or bandage clips

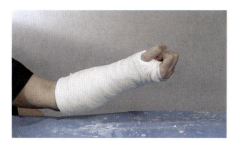

Ensure free movement of the fingers and thumb is possible

SPECIAL PROCEDURE

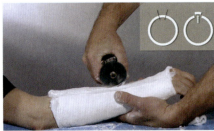

For patients with severe swelling, cut out a strip of the POP cast

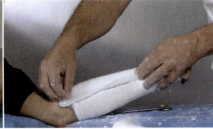

Fill the space with padding to avoid gap edema

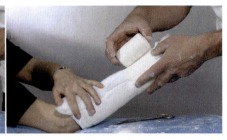

Wrap the cast with an elastic bandage

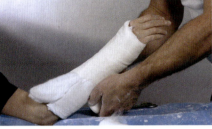

Wrap the forearm using the half-overlapping technique

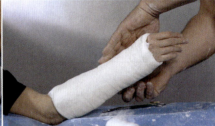

Secure the bandage with surgical tape or bandage clips

FINAL ASSESSMENT

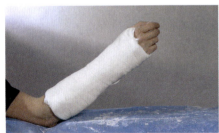

Free flexion of the elbow.

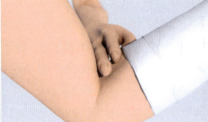

The cast should end two finger's breadth from the elbow crease

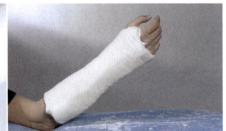

Free movement of the thumb

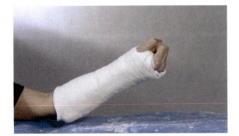

Free flexion of the fingers at the MCP joints

Klaus Dresing, Jos Engelen

15.12 Short arm cast using synthetic, combicast technique

15.12

TECHNIQUES

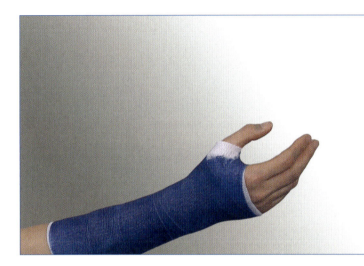

INDICATION

- Fracture of the distal radius

GOAL

- Stabilization of the distal forearm and wrist

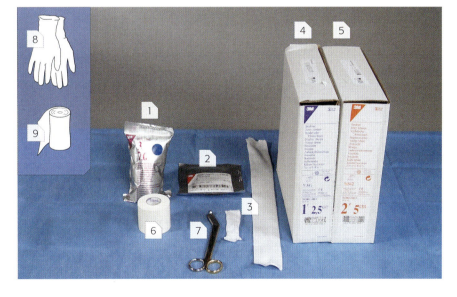

EQUIPMENT

1 Semirigid casting tape 7.5 cm
2 Rigid synthetic splint 7.5 cm x 20 cm
3 Cut tube bandages
4 Tube bandage 2.5 cm in dispenser box
5 Tube bandage 5 cm in dispenser box
6 Elastic foam tape
7 Scissors
8 Gloves
9 Elastic bandage

PERSONNEL

POSITIONING

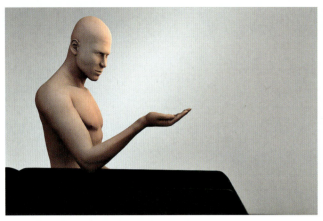

Seat the patient comfortably on a stool.

Place the affected limb on the table, in a functional position.

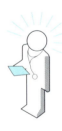

SPECIAL THINGS TO KEEP IN MIND

- Free flexion of the elbow should be possible
- Metacarpal heads should remain free
- The distal palmar crease should remain free
- While the cast is setting, the limb should be positioned halfway between supination and pronation
- In primary fracture care it is necessary to split the cast completely open after setting, or in the case of severe swelling, to remove a small strip

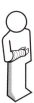

PROCEDURE

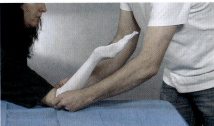

Apply the tube bandage

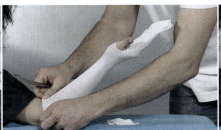

Cut an opening for the thumb

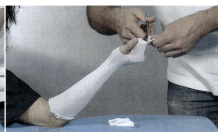

Flex the fingers to allow the excess tube bandage to be cut

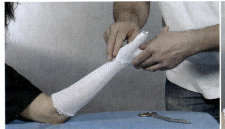

Apply a small tube bandage over the thumb

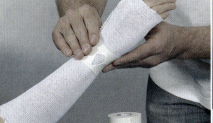

Apply a piece of elastic foam tape, with an opening for the prominent bone, to reduce pressure on the ulnar styloid process

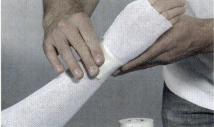

Apply a second piece of elastic foam tape for extra protection

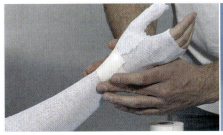

The radial styloid process is also protected with elastic foam tape

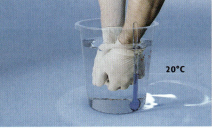

Using wet gloves makes it easier to apply the semirigid casting tape

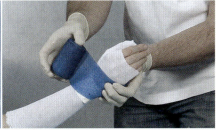

Apply the first layers of semirigid casting tape

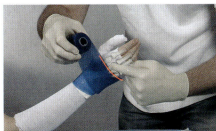

Ensure the metacarpal heads remain free

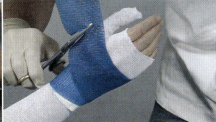

Cut halfway through the casting tape, from proximal to distal, for a smooth application between the thumb and index finger

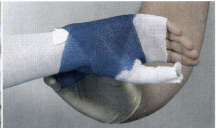

Ensure the distal palmar crease remains free

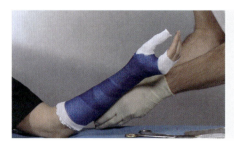

Wrap the forearm using the half-overlapping technique

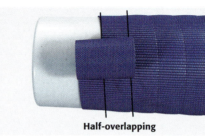

Half-overlapping

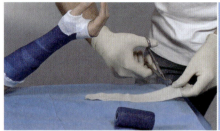

Fold back the tube bandage over the proximal and distal edges of the semirigid casting tape

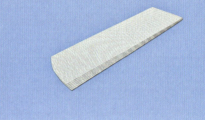

Apply a rigid splint, and if necessary, trim to the desired shape

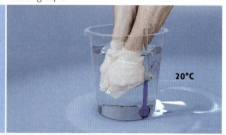

Shape the rigid splint like this; the splint can be used wet or dry

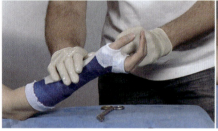

Submerge the rigid splint in water for a few seconds, remove, and squeeze out excess water

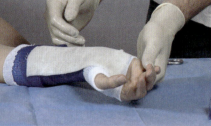

Apply the rigid splint, and mold into place

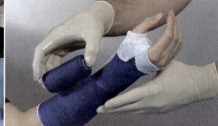

Ensure the distal palmar crease remains free

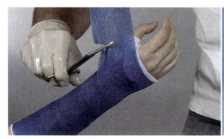

Apply an additional layer of semirigid casting tape using the half-overlapping technique

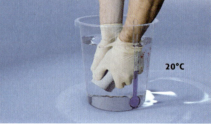

Cut halfway through the casting tape, from proximal to distal, for a smooth application between the thumb and index finger

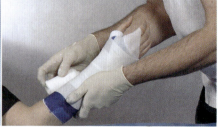

Submerge the elastic bandage in water; using a wet bandage accelerates the setting

Wrap the forearm using the half-overlapping technique

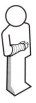

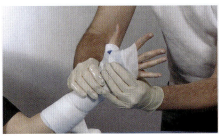

Hold the wrist in 20° dorsal flexion while setting; the fingers should be spread to create enough space in the cast

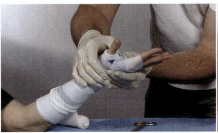

Mold to the palmar crease

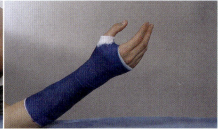

Remove the wet bandage after the cast has set

FINAL ASSESSMENT

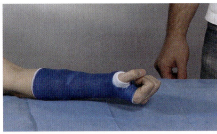

Free flexion of the fingers at the MCP joints

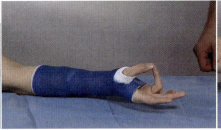

Precise finger movements are possible

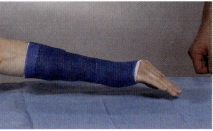

Functional position with 20° dorsal flexion in the wrist

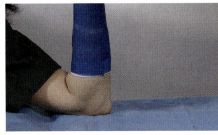
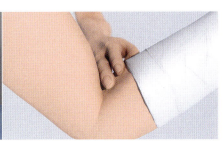

The cast should end two finger's breadth from the elbow crease to allow free flexion of the elbow

377

15.12

TECHNIQUES

CAST REMOVAL

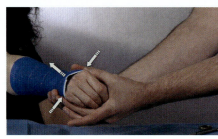

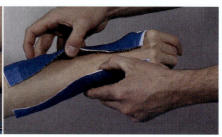

Press on both sides to create a small space for the scissors

Split the cast from distal to proximal, and remove

Klaus Dresing, Jos Engelen

15.13 Thumb spica splint using plaster of Paris

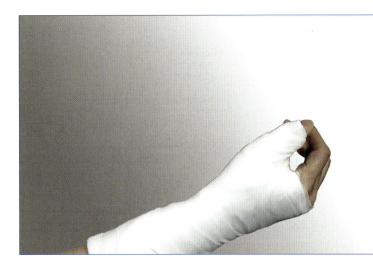

INDICATION

- Fracture of the first metacarpal
- Fracture of the scaphoid

GOAL

- Stabilization of first finger ray

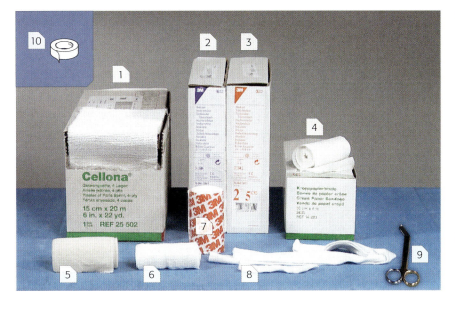

EQUIPMENT

1 Plaster of Paris splint 12 cm or 15 cm
2 Tube bandage 2.5 cm in dispenser box
3 Tube bandage 5 cm in dispenser box
4 Crepe paper bandage
5 Elastic bandage
6 Gauze bandage
7 Cast padding
8 Cut tube bandages
9 Scissors
10 Surgical tape or bandage clips

PERSONNEL

15.13

TECHNIQUES

POSITIONING

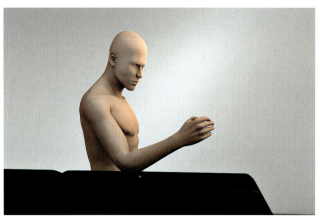

Seat the patient comfortably on a stool.

Place the affected limb on the table, in a functional position.

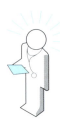

SPECIAL THINGS TO KEEP IN MIND

- The IP joint of the thumb remains free
- Free flexion of the elbow should be possible
- The distal palmar crease should remain free
- While the splint is setting, the limb should be positioned halfway between supination and pronation

Klaus Dresing, Jos Engelen

PROCEDURE

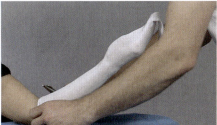

Apply the tube bandage

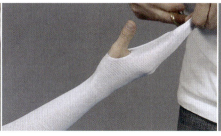

Cut a hole in the tube bandage for the thumb

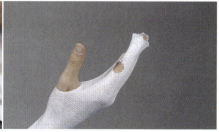

Cut another hole to allow the tube bandage to be pulled back over the thumb later

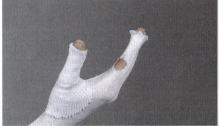

Apply a small tube bandage over the thumb

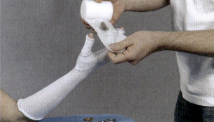

Apply the padding; make a hole for the thumb first

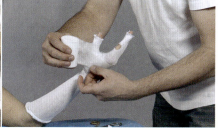

Make a split halfway through the padding, from proximal to distal, to ensure smooth protection between the thumb and index finger

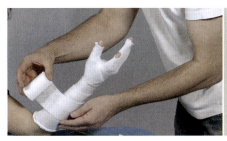

Wrap the forearm using the half-overlapping technique

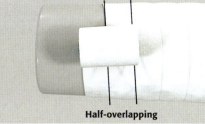

Half-overlapping

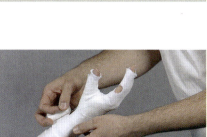

Apply the paper bandage to form a barrier between the dry padding and the wet POP

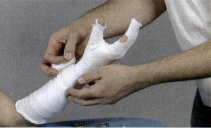

Cut halfway through the bandage, from proximal to distal, for easy application between the thumb and the index finger

Wrap the forearm using the half-overlapping technique

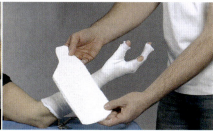

Apply the POP splint, and trim to the required shape

15.13

TECHNIQUES

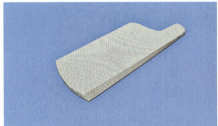

Shape the splint like this

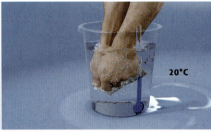

Fold the splint and submerge in water for a few seconds, remove, and squeeze out excess water

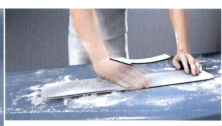

Stretch and smooth out the splint, pressing the layers together, resulting in a compact splint. If this procedure is not done, puff pastry plaster will result, causing an unstable splint

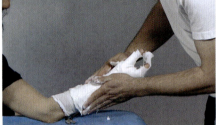

Apply the splint and mold to the arm

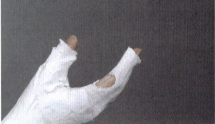

Wrap the splint between the thumb and index finger

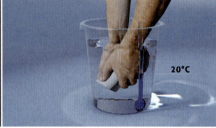

Submerge the gauze bandage in water for a few seconds, remove, and squeeze out excess water

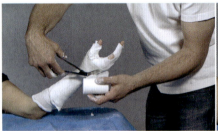

Apply the bandage, cut halfway through, from proximal to distal, for easy application between the thumb and the index finger

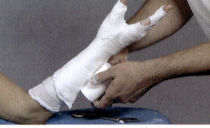

Wrap the forearm using the half-overlapping technique

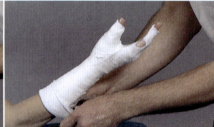

Fold back the tube bandage proximally

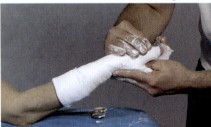

Hold the splint in the desired position during setting, with the thumb and index finger in opposition

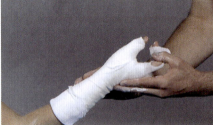

Position the forearm halfway between supination and pronation

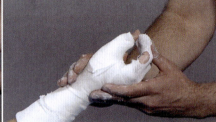

Place the thumb and index finger in opposition, as if holding a baton

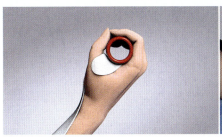

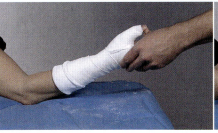

Tap the splint to check it has set

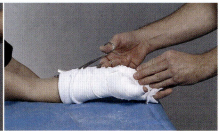

Split the splint completely with scissors

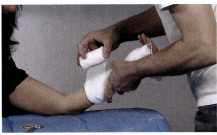

Apply an elastic bandage to close the splint and hold it in position

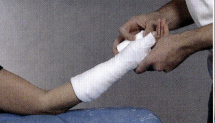

Fold back the tube bandage distally, and hold in place with the elastic bandage

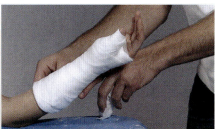

Secure the bandage with surgical tape or bandage clips

FINAL ASSESSMENT

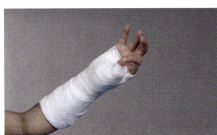

Opposition of the thumb and index finger is possible. Free movement of the IP joint of the thumb is possible

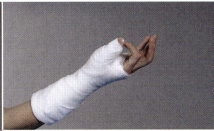

The distal palmar crease is free

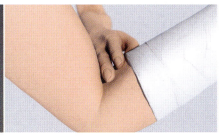

The splint should end two finger's breadth from the elbow

15.13

TECHNIQUES

Klaus Dresing, Jos Engelen

15.14 Thumb spica splint using synthetic

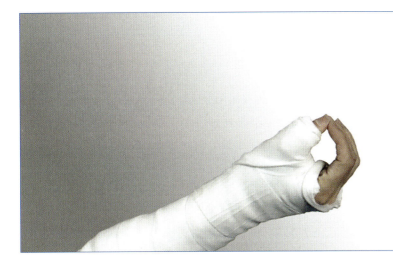

INDICATION

- Fracture of the first metacarpal
- Fracture of the scaphoid

GOAL

- Stabilization of first finger ray

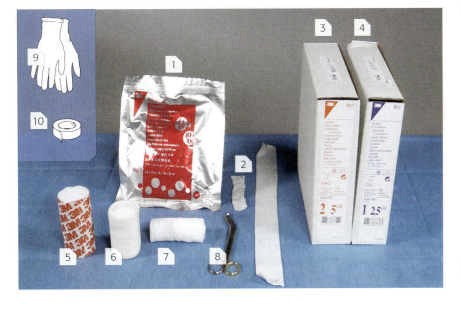

EQUIPMENT

1 Rigid synthetic splint 7.5 cm or 10 cm x 30 cm
2 Cut tube bandages
3 Tube bandage 5 cm in dispenser box
4 Tube bandage 2.5 cm in dispenser box
5 Cast padding
6 Elastic bandage
7 Gauze bandage
8 Scissors
9 Gloves
10 Surgical tape or bandage clips

PERSONNEL

15.14

TECHNIQUES

POSITIONING

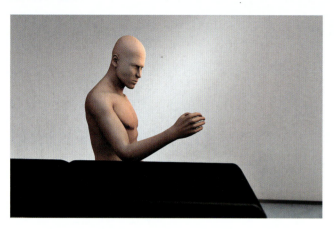

Seat the patient comfortably on a stool.

Place the affected limb on the table, in a functional position.

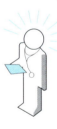

SPECIAL THINGS TO KEEP IN MIND

- The IP joint of the thumb remains free
- Free flexion of the elbow should be possible
- The distal palmar crease should remain free
- While the splint is setting, the limb should be positioned halfway between supination and pronation

Klaus Dresing, Jos Engelen

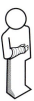

PROCEDURE

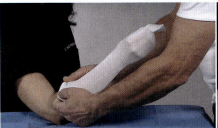

Apply the tube bandage smoothly and without wrinkles

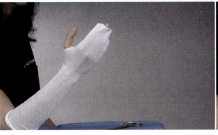

Cut a hole in the tube bandage for the thumb

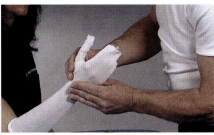

Place a small tube bandage over the thumb

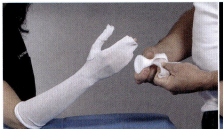

Apply the padding; make a hole for the thumb first

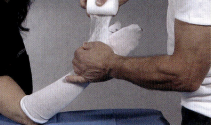

Make a tear in the padding to ensure smooth protection between the thumb and index finger

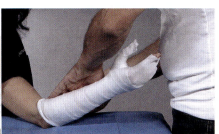

Wrap the forearm using the half-overlapping technique

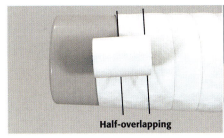

Half-overlapping

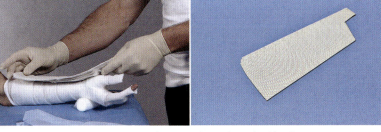

A paper bandage is not needed as synthetic material is used. Check the length of splint, and trim to the desired shape

Shape the splint like this

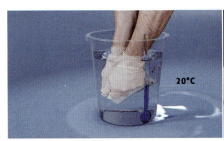

Submerge the splint in water for a few seconds, remove, and squeeze out excess water

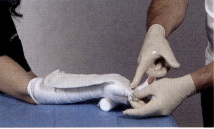

Apply the splint; begin at the distal palmar crease

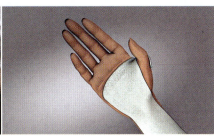

15.14

TECHNIQUES

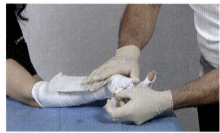

Place the splint around the thumb

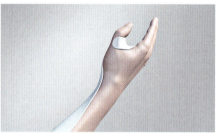

Submerge a gauze bandage in water

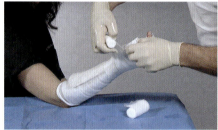

Apply the gauze bandage to hold the splint in place

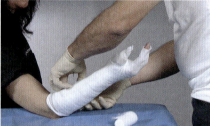

Wrap the forearm using the half-overlapping technique

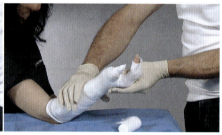

While the splint sets, the limb should be positioned halfway between supination and pronation

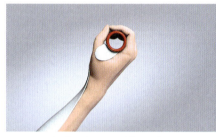

Position the hand as if holding a baton

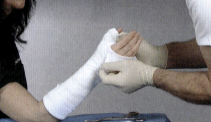

Fold back the tube bandage, proximally and distally

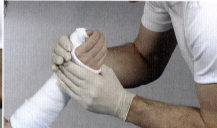

Mold the splint and hold in position until it is set

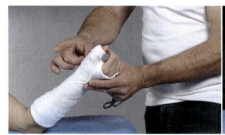

Tap on the splint to check it has set

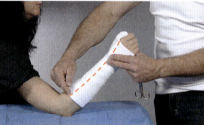

Mark the splitting line

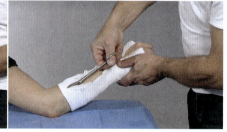

Split the splint completely with scissors, and close with an elastic bandage

Klaus Dresing, Jos Engelen

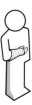

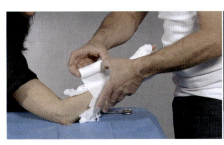

Wrap the forearm using the half-overlapping technique

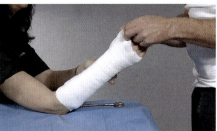

Secure the bandage with surgical tape or bandage clips

FINAL ASSESSMENT

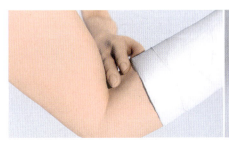

The splint should end two finger's breadth from the elbow

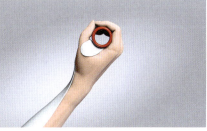

Opposition of the thumb and the index finger is possible

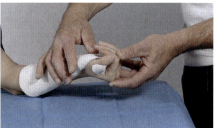

The distal palmar crease is free to allow unrestricted movement of the fingers

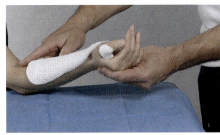

Free movement of the elbow and the IP joint of the thumb are possible

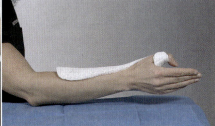

The thumb is protected

Klaus Dresing, Jos Engelen

15.15 Short arm cast using plaster of Paris with traction and reduction

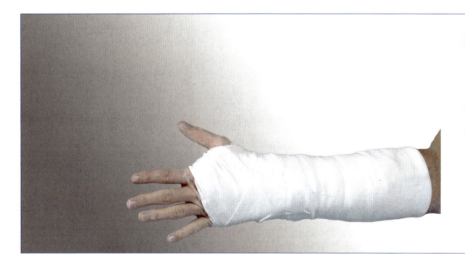

INDICATION

- Displaced fracture of the distal radius

GOAL

- Stabilization of the wrist

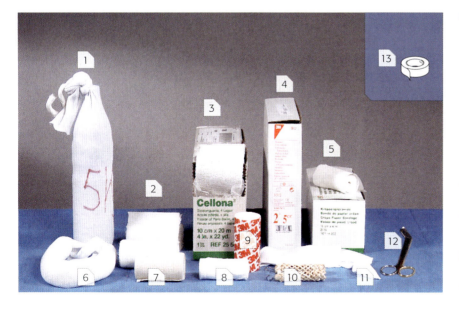

EQUIPMENT

1 A weight
2 Plaster of Paris rolls 10 cm or 12 cm
3 Plaster of Paris splint 12 cm or 15 cm
4 Tube bandage 5 cm in dispenser box
5 Crepe paper bandage
6 Traction sling
7 Elastic bandage
8 Gauze bandage
9 Cast padding
10 Finger traps
11 Cut tube bandage
12 Scissors
13 Surgical tape or bandage clips

PERSONNEL

391

POSITIONING

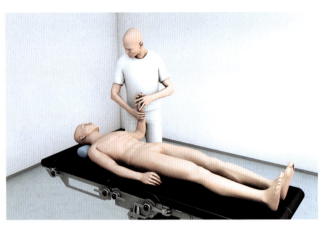

Place the patient supine on a table.

The affected arm is held in abduction by the surgeon, with 90° flexion of the elbow.

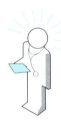

SPECIAL THINGS TO KEEP IN MIND

- The distal palmar crease remains free
- Free flexion of the elbow
- The reduction is performed and held by the surgeon
- X-ray during reduction is advisable, but at the end is mandatory

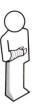

PROCEDURE

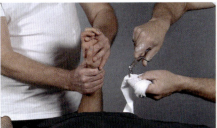

Apply the tube bandage before starting the traction. Cut a hole in the tube bandage for the thumb

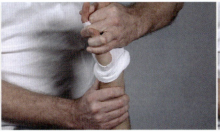

Apply the tube bandage; the wrist needs to be stabilized by the surgeon at all times

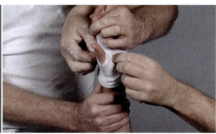

Place a small tube bandage over the thumb

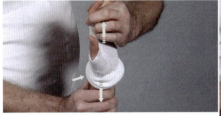

Direction of the traction is over the first and second ray. With the surgeon providing continuous tension and support, apply the finger traps

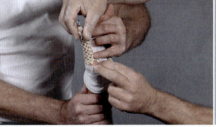

Compress the sleeve to widen it and place over the thumb

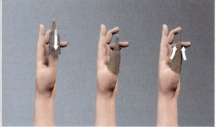

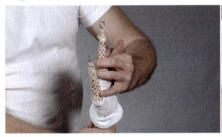

Repeat for the index finger

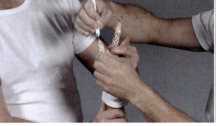

Attach the finger traps to the traction system

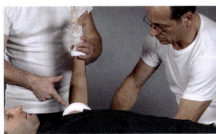

Place a traction sling over the biceps

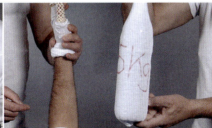

Apply a weight for traction

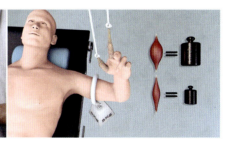

More weight is necessary for more athletic or obese patients, also for patients that are not relaxed

393

15.15

TECHNIQUES

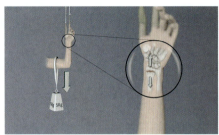

After applying the weight, the traction results in disimpaction of the fracture

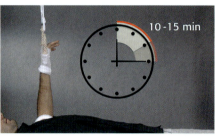

Leave the upper extremity under traction for 10 to 15 minutes

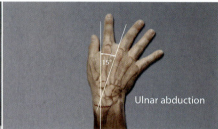

Ulnar abduction of 15° leads to less compression on the fractured radius

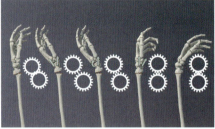

The process involves step-by-step traction and reduction of the fracture (gear-wheel mechanism)

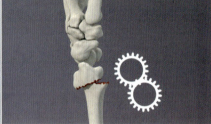

The impacted fracture

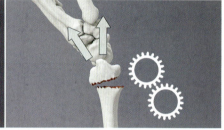

Disimpaction by traction and tension

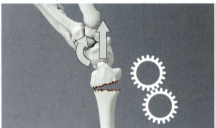

Fragments are reduced dorsally

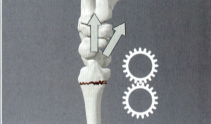

The fragment is rolled over to the palmar side

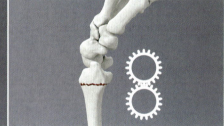

The fracture gap is closed and completely reduced

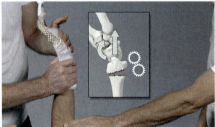

First, move the hand dorsally under extension; the dorsal aspect of the fragments are positioned directly above each other

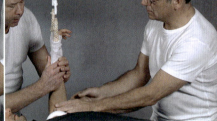

Move the wrist to the functional position under further tension, and then release the extension

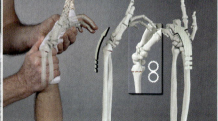

Place the wrist in slight palmar flexion and ulnar abduction to retain the result of the reduction

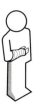

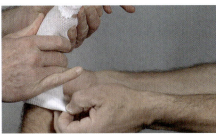

Before fixation, the tube bandage is pulled down over the forearm

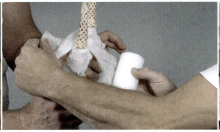

Apply the padding; make a tear from proximal to distal to ensure smooth protection between the thumb and index finger

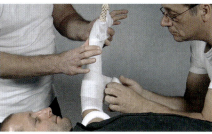

Wrap the forearm using the half-overlapping technique

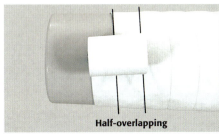

Half-overlapping

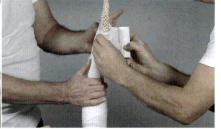

Apply the paper bandage to form a barrier between the dry padding and the wet POP

Cut halfway through the bandage, from proximal to distal, for easy application between the thumb and index finger

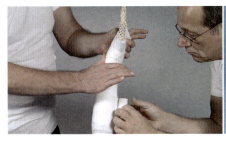

Wrap the forearm using the half-overlapping technique

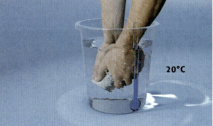

20°C

Submerge a roll of POP in water for a few seconds, remove, and squeeze out excess water

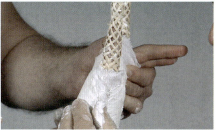

20°C

Apply the roll of POP

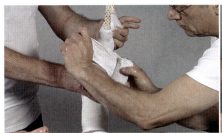

Cut halfway through, from proximal to distal, for easier application between the thumb and the index finger

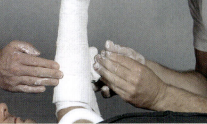

Wrap the forearm using the half-overlapping technique

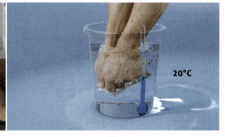

20°C

Submerge the POP splint in water for a few seconds, remove, and squeeze out excess water

395

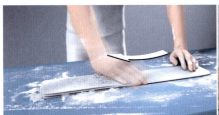

Stretch and smooth out the splint, pressing the layers together, resulting in a compact splint. If this procedure is not done, puff pastry plaster will result, causing an unstable splint

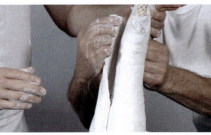

Apply the splint dorsally

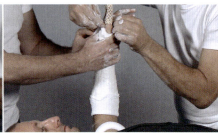

Mold the splint and fold back the tube bandage, proximally and distally

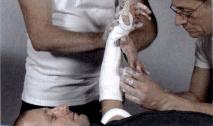

Apply another wet roll of POP. Hold the reduction while the roll of POP is applied

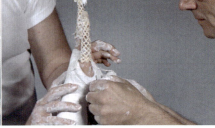

Cut halfway through for easier application between the thumb and index finger

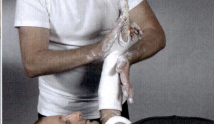

Mold the cast into the final position

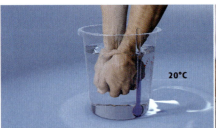

Wet hands make smoothing the cast easier

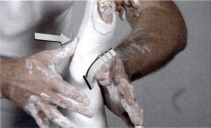

Apply pressure to the distal radius using the thumbs while the cast is molded

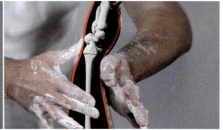

Hold the reduction until the cast is set

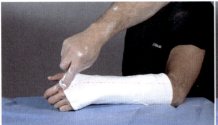

Remove the finger traps after the cast has set. Mark the splitting line

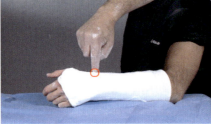

When using the oscillating saw, take care of the prominent bones: the radial and ulnar styloid processes and metacarpal heads

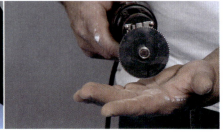

The saw blade oscillates and does not rotate, so there is no direct harm to the skin

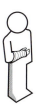

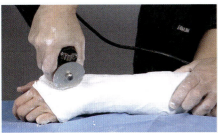

Split the cast from distal to proximal

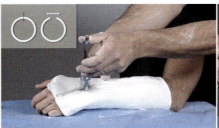

Widen the split with the cast spreader

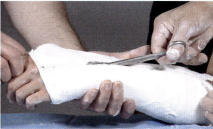

Complete the splitting by cutting the padding and the tube bandage with scissors

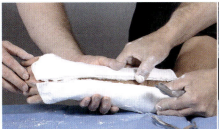

Check that the cast is completely split

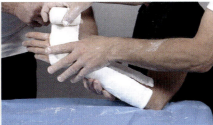

Apply an elastic bandage to secure the cast

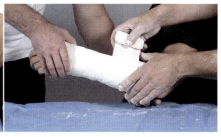

Wrap the forearm using the half-overlapping technique

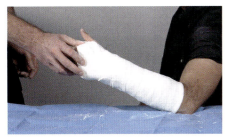

Secure the bandage with surgical tape or bandage clips

15.15

TECHNIQUES

FINAL ASSESSMENT

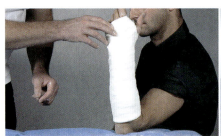

Free flexion of the elbow

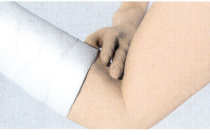

The cast should end two finger's breadth from the elbow crease

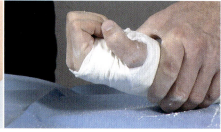

Free flexion of the fingers at the MCP joints

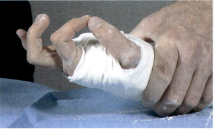

Free movement of the thumb

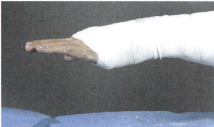

X-ray review is mandatory

Klaus Dresing, Jos Engelen

15.16 Short arm scaphoid cast using synthetic, combicast technique

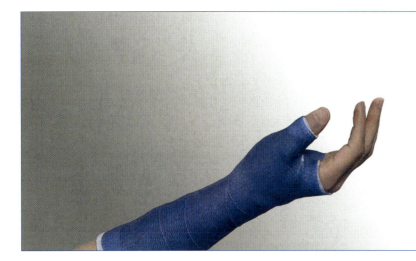

INDICATION

- Fracture of first metacarpal
- Fracture of the scaphoid

GOAL

- Stabilization of the carpal bones and the first finger ray

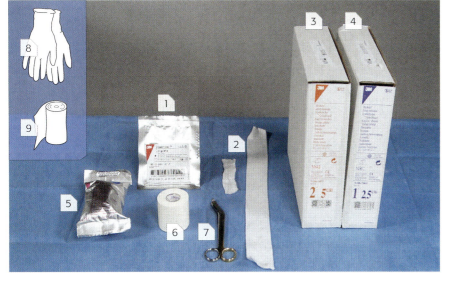

EQUIPMENT

1 Rigid synthetic splint 7.5 cm x 20 cm
2 Cut tube bandages
3 Tube bandage 5 cm in dispenser box
4 Tube bandage 2.5 cm in dispenser box
5 Semirigid casting tape 7.5 cm
6 Elastic foam tape
7 Scissors
8 Gloves
9 Elastic bandage

PERSONNEL

15.16

TECHNIQUES

POSITIONING

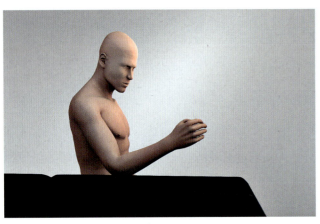

Seat the patient comfortably on a stool.

Place the affected arm on the table, in a functional position.

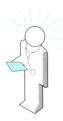

SPECIAL THINGS TO KEEP IN MIND

- The distal palmar crease should remain free
- Metacarpal heads should remain free
- Free flexion of the elbow should be possible
- While the cast is setting, the limb should be positioned halfway between supination and pronation

Klaus Dresing, Jos Engelen

PROCEDURE

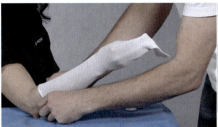

Apply the tube bandage smoothly without wrinkles

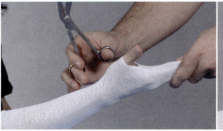

Cut a hole in the tube bandage for the thumb

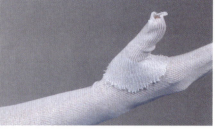

Place a small tube bandage over the thumb

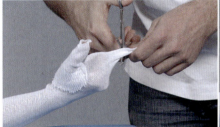

Pull the tube bandage lightly, flex the fingers and trim the bandage to the appropriate length

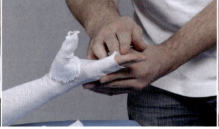

Extend the fingers with the tube bandage now at the correct length

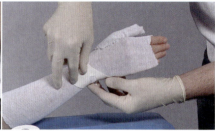

Apply a piece of elastic foam tape over the ulnar styloid process, with an opening for the prominent bone

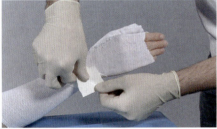

Apply a second piece of elastic foam tape for extra protection

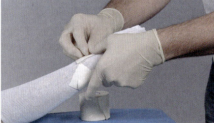

Apply more elastic foam tape to protect the radial styloid process

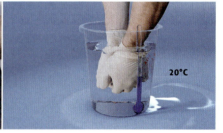

Wet gloves make it easier to apply the semi-rigid casting tape

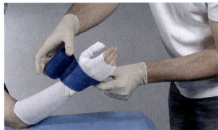

Apply the first layer of semirigid casting tape

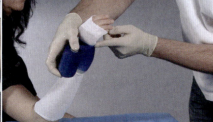

The second wrap should be at the same level as the first

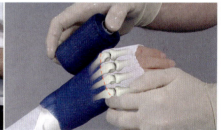

The metacarpal heads should remain free

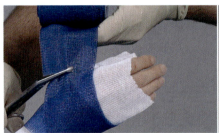

Cut the semirigid casting tape halfway through, from proximal to distal, for smooth application between the thumb and index finger

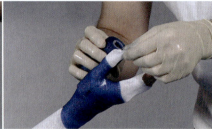

Pull the small tube bandage lightly, and wrap the semirigid casting tape around the thumb, leaving the IP joint free

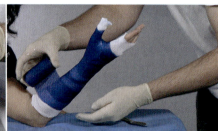

Wrap the forearm using the half-overlapping technique

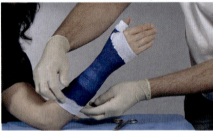

Fold back the tube bandage over the semi-rigid casting tape

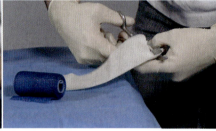

Prepare the rigid splint. Trim the splint to the desired shape

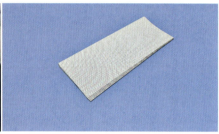

Shape the splint like this

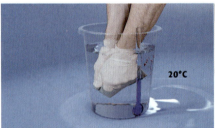

Submerge the splint in water for a few seconds, remove, and squeeze out excess water

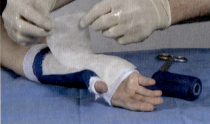

Fold back the outer layer of the splint, from proximal to distal, to give extra stability to the thumb

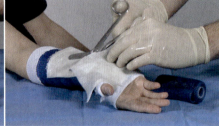

Cut through the fold to avoid pressure from wrinkles and for a smooth surface

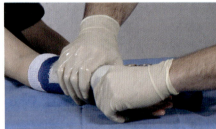

Mold the splint to the hand

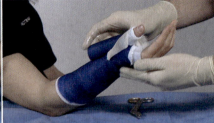

Apply the next layer of semirigid casting tape; use the half-overlapping technique

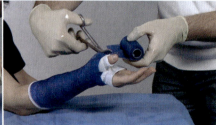

Cut halfway through the semirigid casting tape, from proximal to distal, for smooth application between the thumb and index finger

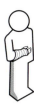

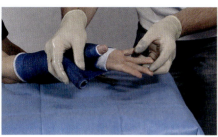

Make sure the fingers can be easily spread to avoid compression across the MCP joints

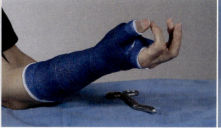

Ensure the thumb and index finger can be placed in opposition

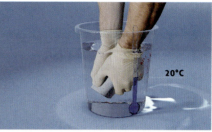

Submerge an elastic bandage in water; using a wet bandage accelerates the setting of the cast

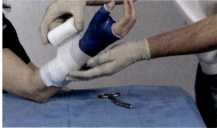

Wrap the forearm using the half-overlapping technique

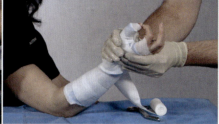

Hold the hand in the desired position until the cast is set

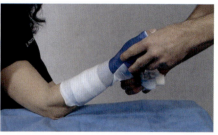

Remove the wet bandage after the cast has set

15.16

TECHNIQUES

FINAL ASSESSMENT

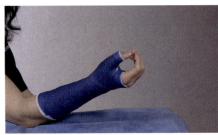

Opposition of the thumb and index finger is possible

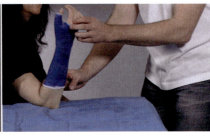

The cast should end two finger's breadth from the elbow crease to allow free flexion of the elbow

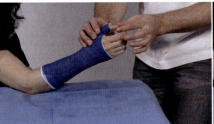

The IP joint of the thumb is free

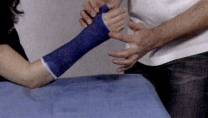

The metacarpal heads remain free

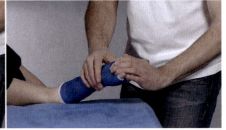

The distal palmar crease remains free to allow a fist to be made

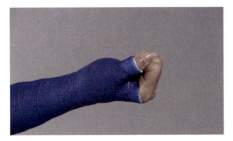

Full motion of the fingers is retained

Klaus Dresing, Jos Engelen

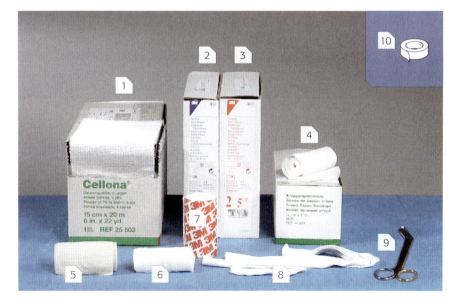

15.17 Dorsopalmar (ulnar gutter) short arm splint including two or more fingers using plaster of Paris

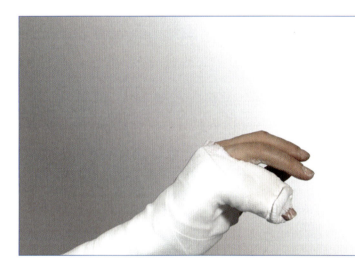

INDICATION

- Fracture of the proximal phalanges II–V
- Fracture of the metacarpals II–V

GOAL

- Stabilization of the fingers and/or metacarpus

EQUIPMENT

1 Plaster of Paris splint 12 cm or 15 cm
2 Tube bandage 2.5 cm in dispenser box
3 Tube bandage 5 cm in dispenser box
4 Crepe paper bandage
5 Elastic bandage
6 Gauze bandage
7 Cast padding
8 Cut tube bandage
9 Scissors
10 Surgical tape or bandage clips

PERSONNEL

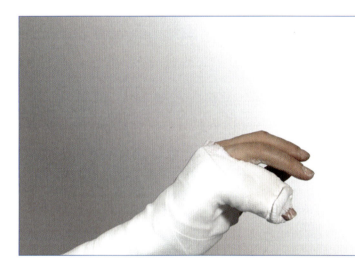

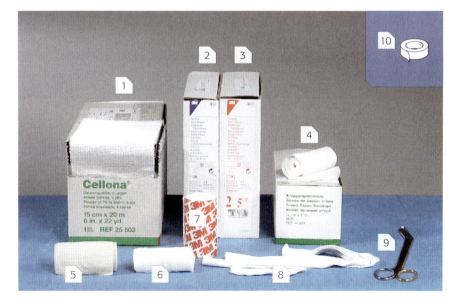

15.17

TECHNIQUES

POSITIONING

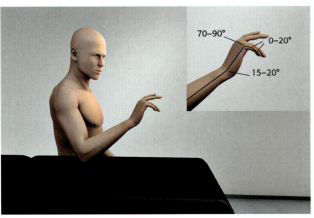

Seat the patient comfortably on a stool.

Place the affected limb on the table during application, with the fingers and MCP joints in the intrinsic-plus position.

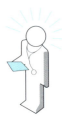

SPECIAL THINGS TO KEEP IN MIND

- Protection of the skin between the fingers to avoid maceration
- The splint should be placed over the dorsopalmar side of the hand and fingers
- While the splint is setting, the limb should be positioned halfway between supination and pronation
- The neighboring finger is included to ensure effective splinting of the fractured finger
- Circulation

PROCEDURE

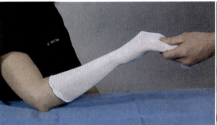

Apply the tube bandage

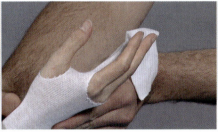

Cut a hole in the tube bandage for the thumb, and another hole for the index and middle finger

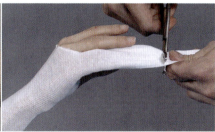

Trim the tube bandage to the required length

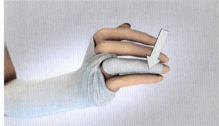

Place a small tube bandage over the ring finger to avoid maceration of the skin

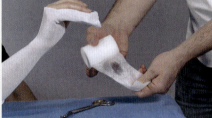

Apply the padding; make a hole for the thumb first

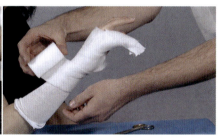

Wrap the forearm using the half-overlapping technique

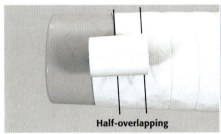

Half-overlapping

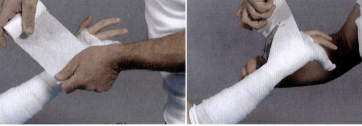

Apply the paper bandage to form a barrier between the dry padding and the wet POP

Cut halfway through the bandage, from proximal to distal, for easy application between the thumb and index finger

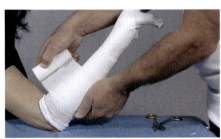

Wrap the forearm using the half-overlapping technique

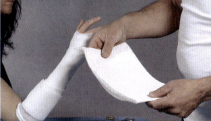

Fold the POP splint in half to give the appropriate length, and trim distally to the width of the hand

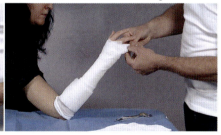

To compensate for the difference in length between the small finger and ring finger, cut out a section of the splint

15.17 Dorsopalmar (ulnar gutter) short arm splint including two or more fingers using plaster of Paris

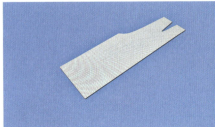

Shape the splint like this

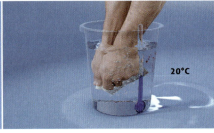

Submerge the POP splint in water for a few seconds, remove, and squeeze out excess water

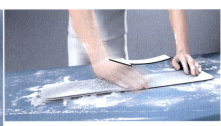

Stretch and smooth out the splint, pressing the layers together, resulting in a compact splint. If this procedure is not done, puff pastry plaster will result, causing an unstable splint

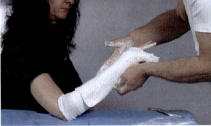

Apply the splint, and if necessary, trim to the desired shape. Mold as an ulnar gutter splint

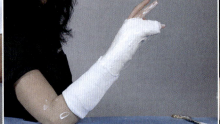

Fold back the tube bandage, distally and proximally, to give smooth edges

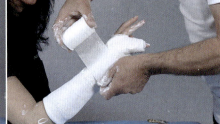

Apply a gauze bandage to hold the splint in place

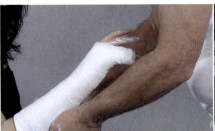

Wrap the forearm using the half-overlapping technique

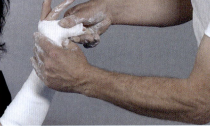

Place the hand in the desired position. Bend the bandaged fingers over the thumb and bring the patient's hand into the intrinsic-plus position

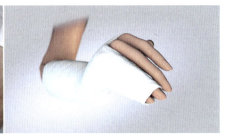

The fingertips should be visible

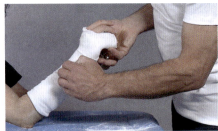

Tap the splint to check it has set

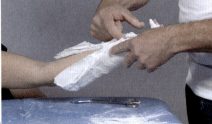

Split the splint completely open with the scissors

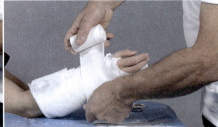

Apply an elastic bandage to close the splint

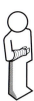

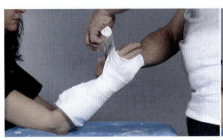

Cut halfway through the bandage, from proximal to distal, for easy application between the thumb and index finger

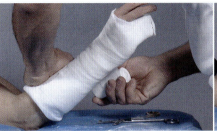

Wrap the forearm using the half-overlapping technique

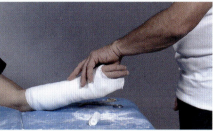

Secure the bandage with surgical tape or bandage clips

FINAL ASSESSMENT

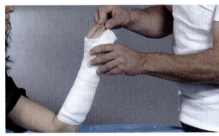

Free flexion of the fingers and thumb

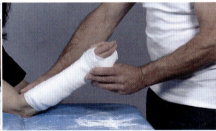

The splint should end two finger's breadth from the elbow crease to allow free flexion of the elbow

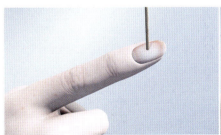

Check for capillary refill

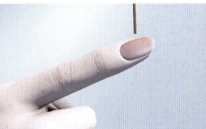

70–90°   0–20°

15–20°

Correct intrinsic-plus position

15.17

Klaus Dresing, Jos Engelen

15.18 Dorsopalmar (ulnar gutter) short arm splint including two or more fingers using synthetic

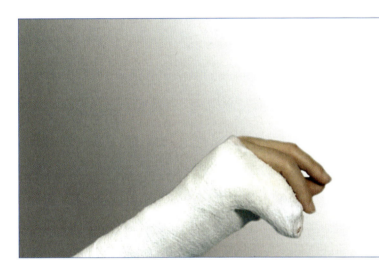

INDICATION

- Fracture of the proximal phalanges II–V
- Fracture of the metacarpals II–V

GOAL

- Stabilization of the fingers and/or metacarpus

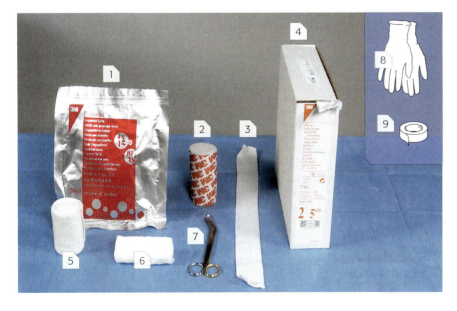

EQUIPMENT

1. Rigid synthetic splint 7.5 cm or 10 cm x 30 cm
2. Cast padding
3. Cut tube bandage
4. Tube bandage 5 cm in dispenser box
5. Elastic bandage
6. Gauze bandage
7. Scissors
8. Gloves
9. Surgical tape or bandage clips

PERSONNEL

15.18 Dorsopalmar (ulnar gutter) short arm splint including two or more fingers using synthetic

15.18

TECHNIQUES

POSITIONING

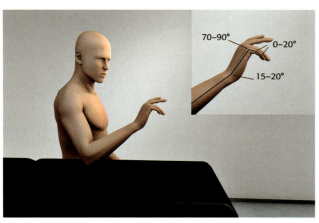

Seat the patient comfortably on a stool.

Place the affected limb on the table during application, with the fingers and MCP joints in the intrinsic-plus position.

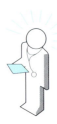

SPECIAL THINGS TO KEEP IN MIND

- Protection of the skin between the fingers to avoid maceration
- The splint should be placed over the dorsopalmar side of the hand and fingers
- While the splint is setting, the limb should be positioned halfway between supination and pronation
- The neighboring finger is included to ensure effective splinting of the fractured finger
- Circulation

Klaus Dresing, Jos Engelen

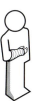

PROCEDURE

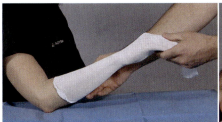

Apply the tube bandage

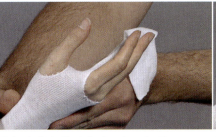

Cut a hole in the tube bandage for the thumb, and another hole for the index and middle finger

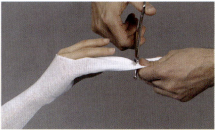

Trim the tube bandage to the required length

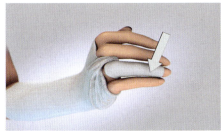

Place a small tube bandage over the ring finger

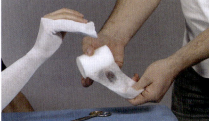

Apply the padding; make a hole for the thumb first

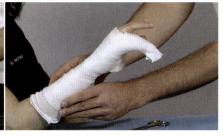

Wrap the forearm using the half-overlapping technique

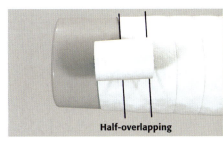

Half-overlapping

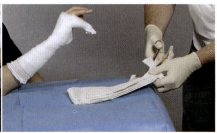

Prepare the rigid synthetic splint. Fan out the layers of the splint to fit to the diameter of the forearm

Trim the splint to the desired shape

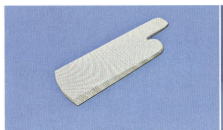

Shape the splint like this

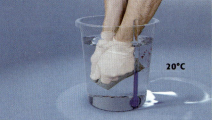

20°C

Submerge the splint in water for a few seconds, remove, and squeeze out excess water

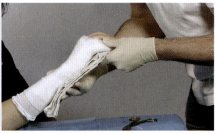

Apply the splint, and trim if necessary

15.18

TECHNIQUES

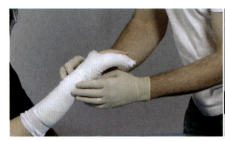

Apply a gauze bandage to hold the splint in place; use the half-overlapping technique

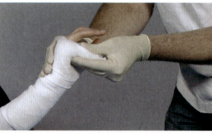

Mold the splint to the required position. The fingers and the MCP joints should be in the intrinsic-plus position. Hold the splint in position until it is set

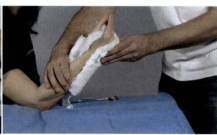

Tap the splint to check it has set, and split the splint completely open with the scissors

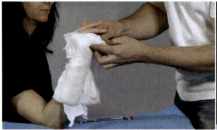

Fold back the tube bandage to free the fingertips

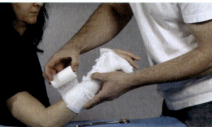

Apply an elastic bandage to hold the splint in position. Secure the bandage with surgical tape or bandage clips

FINAL ASSESSMENT

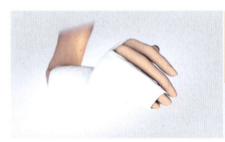

The fingertips are visible

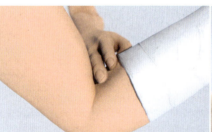

The splint should end two finger's breadth from the elbow crease to allow free flexion of the elbow

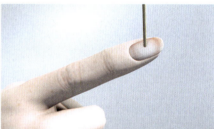

Check for capillary refill

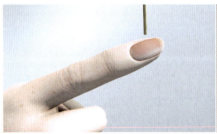

Correct intrinsic-plus position

15.19 Palmar short arm splint including the fingers using plaster of Paris

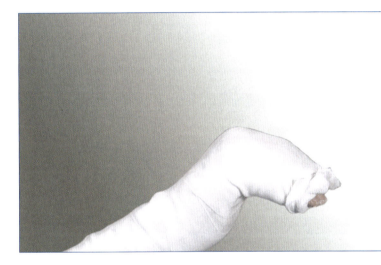

INDICATION

- Fracture of the proximal phalanges II–V
- Fracture of the metacarpals II–V

GOAL

- Stabilization of the fingers and/or metacarpus

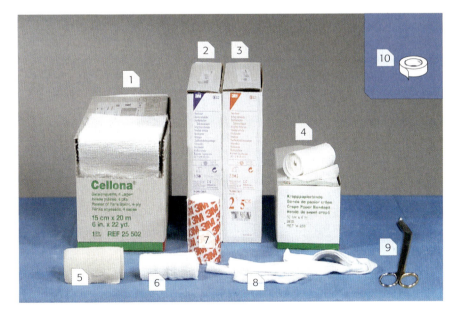

EQUIPMENT

1 Plaster of Paris splint 12 cm or 15 cm
2 Tube bandage 2.5 cm in dispenser box
3 Tube bandage 5 cm in dispenser box
4 Crepe paper bandage
5 Elastic bandage
6 Gauze bandage
7 Cast padding
8 Cut tube bandages
9 Scissors
10 Surgical tape or bandage clips

PERSONNEL

15.19

POSITIONING

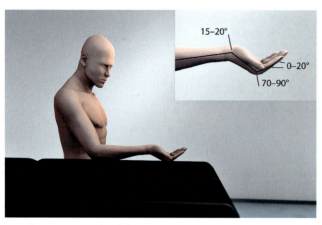

Seat the patient comfortably on a stool.

Place the patient's arm on the table during application, with the fingers and MCP joints in the intrinsic-plus position.

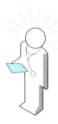

SPECIAL THINGS TO KEEP IN MIND

- Protection of the skin between the fingers to avoid maceration
- The splint should be U-shaped for more stability
- While the splint is setting, the limb should be positioned halfway between supination and pronation
- Circulation

Klaus Dresing, Jos Engelen

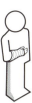

PROCEDURE

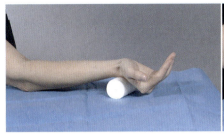

A roll of bandage may be used to support the wrist

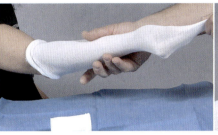

Apply the tube bandage, smoothly and without wrinkles

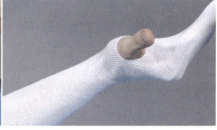

Cut a hole in the tube bandage for the thumb

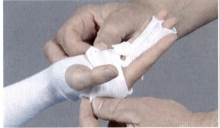

Fold back the tube bandage and apply additional small tube bandages to protect the skin between the fingers

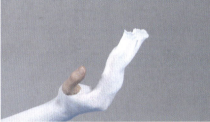

Fold the tube bandage back over the fingers

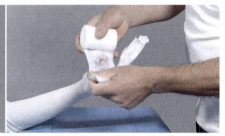

Apply the padding; make a hole for the thumb first

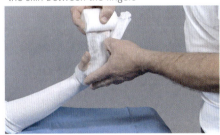

Make a tear in the padding to ensure smooth protection between the thumb and index finger

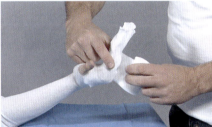

Ensure there is no compression across the fingers

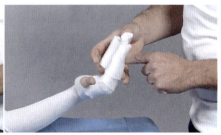

Ensure the padding extends past the fingertips

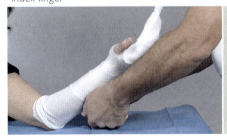

Wrap the forearm using the half-overlapping technique

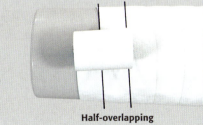

Half-overlapping

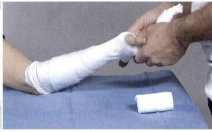

Apply the paper bandage to form a barrier between the dry padding and the wet POP

417

15.19 Palmar short arm splint including the fingers using plaster of Paris

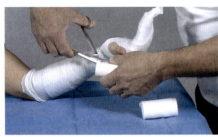

Cut halfway through the bandage, from proximal to distal, for easier application between the thumb and index finger

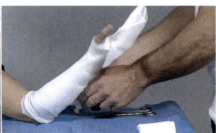

Wrap the forearm using the half-overlapping technique

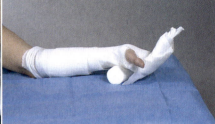

Replace the roll of bandage under the wrist to make positioning of the hand easier

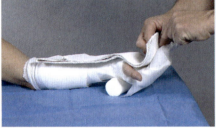

Apply the folded POP splint, starting 2 or 3 cm below the elbow crease. Trim the splint to the desired length and shape

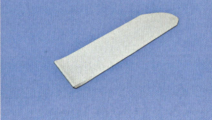

Shape the splint like this

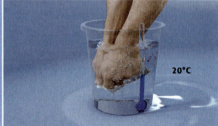

Submerge the POP splint in water for a few seconds, remove, and squeeze out excess water

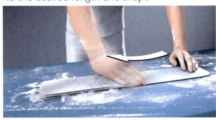

Stretch and smooth out the splint, pressing the layers together, resulting in a compact splint. If this procedure is not done, puff pastry plaster will result, causing an unstable splint

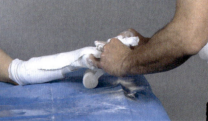

Mold the splint to the hand and the forearm

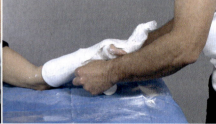

Fold back the tube bandage over the splint, proximally and distally

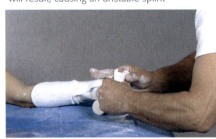

Mold the splint to the desired position. The fingertips should be visible

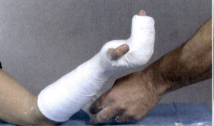

Apply a gauze bandage to hold the splint in position. Wrap the forearm using the half-overlapping technique

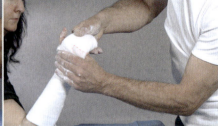

Bend the bandaged fingers over your thumb, while your other hand brings the patient's hand into the intrinsic-plus position. Hold the hand position until the splint is set

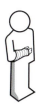

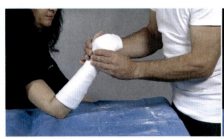
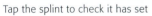

Tap the splint to check it has set

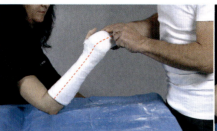

Mark the splitting line

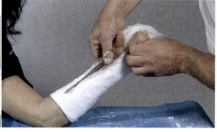

Split the splint completely open with the scissors

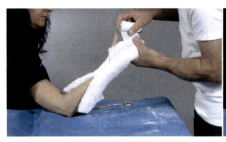

Apply an elastic bandage to hold the splint in position

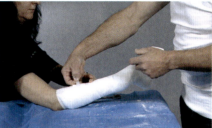

Wrap the forearm using the half-overlapping technique. Secure the bandage with surgical tape or bandage clips

FINAL ASSESSMENT

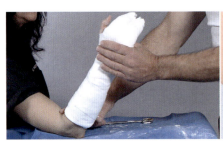

Free flexion of the elbow

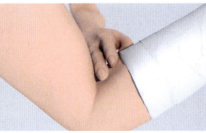

The splint should end two finger's breadth from the elbow crease

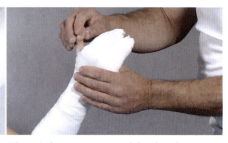

There is free movement of the thumb

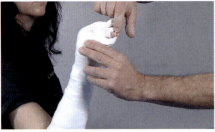

The fingertips are visible

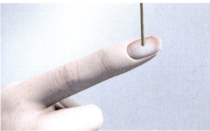

Check for capillary refill

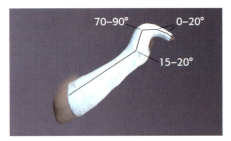

Correct intrinsic-plus position

15.20 Short arm cast including two or more fingers using synthetic, combicast technique

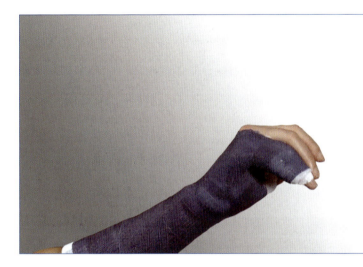

INDICATION

- Fracture of the proximal phalanges II–V
- Fracture of the metacarpals II–V

GOAL

- Stabilization of the fingers and/or the metacarpus

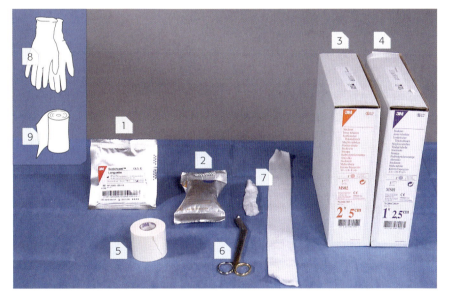

EQUIPMENT

1 Rigid synthetic splint 5 cm or 7.5 cm x 20 cm

2 Semirigid casting tape 5 cm

3 Tube bandage 5 cm in dispenser box

4 Tube bandage 2.5 cm in dispenser box

5 Elastic foam tape

6 Scissors

7 Cut tube bandages

8 Gloves

9 Elastic bandage

PERSONNEL

15.20 Short arm cast including two or more fingers using synthetic, combicast technique

POSITIONING

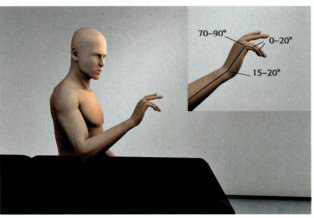

Seat the patient comfortably on a stool.

Place the affected limb on the table during application, with the fingers and MCP joints in the intrinsic-plus position.

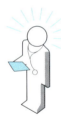

SPECIAL THINGS TO KEEP IN MIND

- Protection of the skin between the fingers to avoid maceration
- While the splint is setting, the limb should be positioned halfway between supination and pronation
- Circulation

Klaus Dresing, Jos Engelen

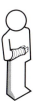
PROCEDURE

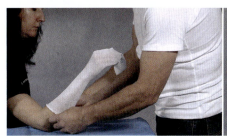

Apply the tube bandage

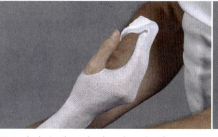

Cut a hole in the tube bandage for the thumb, and pull the bandage tight to remove any wrinkles

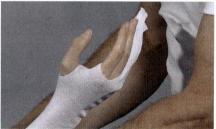

Cut a second hole for the index and middle finger

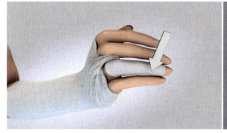

Place a small tube bandage over the ring finger

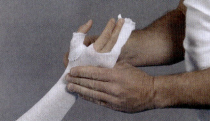

Place an additional small tube bandage to protect the thumb

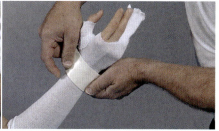

Apply a piece of elastic foam tape to protect the bony prominences; the radial and ulnar styloid processes

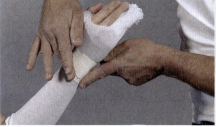

Apply a second piece of elastic foam tape to reduce pressure on the ulnar styloid process

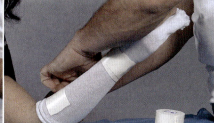

Apply additional elastic foam tape to protect the proximal border of the cast

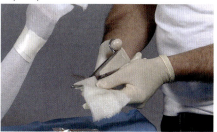

Fold the rigid splint in half, fan out the proximal end to match the shape of the hand, and cut through the distal end

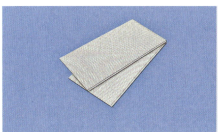

Shape the rigid splint like this

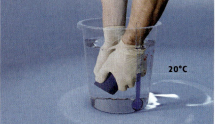

Submerge the semirigid casting tape in water for a few seconds, remove, and squeeze out excess water

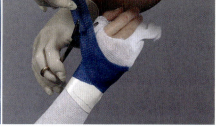

Apply the semirigid casting tape, cut halfway through, from proximal to distal, for easy application between the thumb and index finger

15.20 Short arm cast including two or more fingers using synthetic, combicast technique

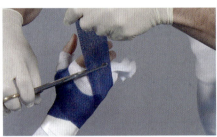

To avoid folds, cut the casting tape halfway through, close to the middle finger, and wrap around the ring and small finger twice

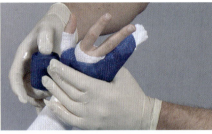

Wrap the semirigid casting tape around the midhand

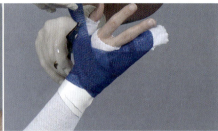

Cut halfway through the semirigid casting tape, and wrap once more between the thumb and index finger

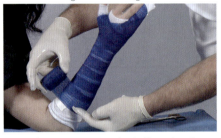

Wrap the forearm using the half-overlapping technique, until half the elastic foam tape is covered

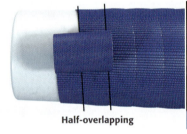

Half-overlapping

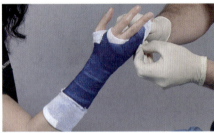

Fold back the tube bandage and the elastic foam tape over the semirigid casting tape proximally

Fold back the tube bandage over the thumb and fingers

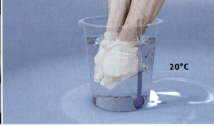

Submerge the rigid splint in water for a few seconds, remove, and squeeze out excess water

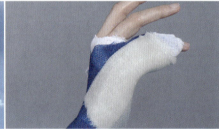

Apply the splint, and if necessary, trim to fit the hand. The fingertips should be visible

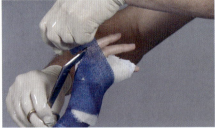

Cut halfway through the semirigid casting tape, from proximal to distal, for easy application between the fingers

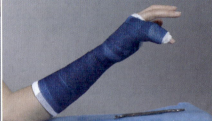

Wrap the forearm using the half-overlapping technique

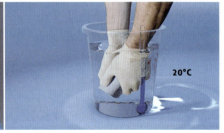

Submerge an elastic bandage in water for a few seconds; using a wet bandage accelerates the setting

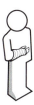

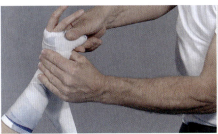

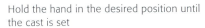

Hold the hand in the desired position until the cast is set

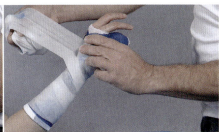

Tap the cast to check it has set and remove the wet bandage

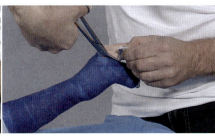

Trim the cast distally to allow free movement of the index and middle finger

15.20 Short arm cast including two or more fingers using synthetic, combicast technique

15.20

TECHNIQUES

FINAL ASSESSMENT

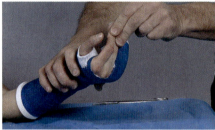

Free movement of the index and middle finger and the thumb

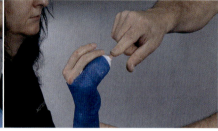

The fingertips of the ring and little finger are visible

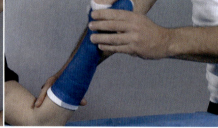

The cast should end two finger's breadth from the elbow crease to allow free flexion of the elbow

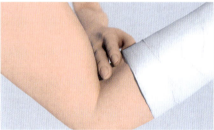

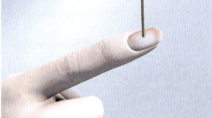

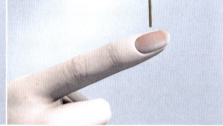

Check for capillary refill

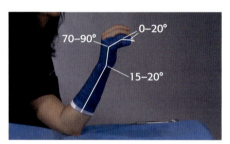

Correct intrinsic-plus position

Casts, Splints, and Support Bandages—Nonoperative Treatment and Perioperative Protection   Klaus Dresing, Peter Trafton

Klaus Dresing, Jos Engelen

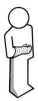

15.21 Kleinert dynamic splint using plaster of Paris

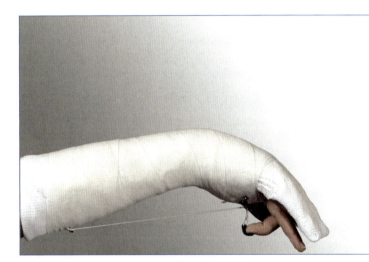

INDICATION

- Lesion of a flexor tendon

GOAL

- Postoperative functional treatment of a flexor tendon lesion

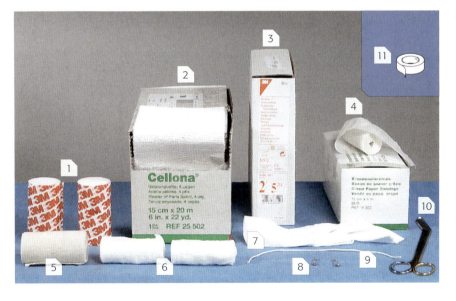

EQUIPMENT

1 Cast padding
2 Plaster of Paris splint 12 cm or 15 cm
3 Tube bandage 5 cm in dispenser box
4 Crepe paper bandage
5 Elastic bandage
6 Two gauze bandages
7 Cut tube bandage
8 Safety pins
9 Piece of elastic
10 Scissors
11 Surgical tape or bandage clips

PERSONNEL

POSITIONING

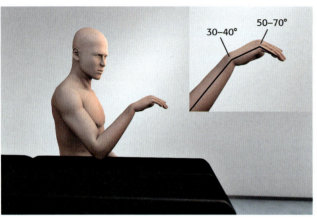

Seat the patient comfortably on a stool.

Place the affected limb on the table, position the wrist at 30–40° and the fingers at 50–70° palmar flexion.

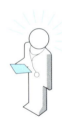

SPECIAL THINGS TO KEEP IN MIND

- For fixation to the nail, a special glue or a suture through the nail can be used
- Metacarpophalangeal joints remain free on the palmar side

PROCEDURE

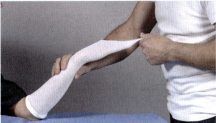

Apply the tube bandage, and stretch it to remove any wrinkles

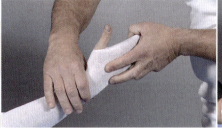

Cut a hole in the tube bandage for the thumb, and trim distally

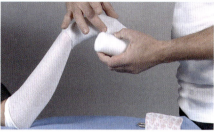

Apply the padding, not too tightly, over the tube bandage. Ensure the fingers are not pressed together, and preserve the angle of the joints

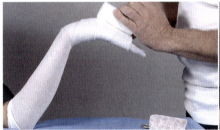

Make a tear in the padding to ensure smooth protection between the thumb and index finger

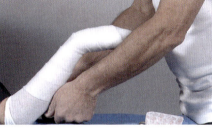

Wrap the forearm using the half-overlapping technique

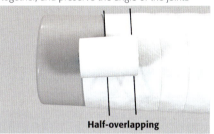

Half-overlapping

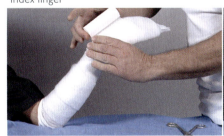

Apply the paper bandage to form a barrier between the dry padding and the wet POP

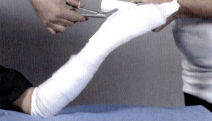

Cut halfway through the bandage for easy application between the thumb and index finger

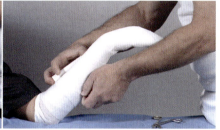

Wrap the forearm using the half-overlapping technique

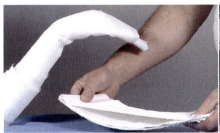

Fold the POP splint in two to make eight layers

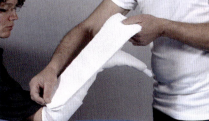

Trim the corners of the splint proximally and place on the forearm

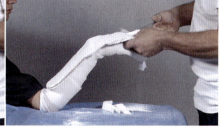

Trim the splint distally to fit the shape of the hand

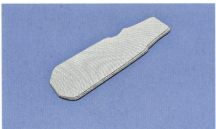

Shape the splint like this

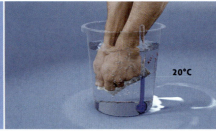

Submerge the POP splint in water for a few seconds, remove, and squeeze out excess water

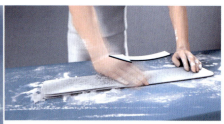

Stretch and smooth out the splint, pressing the layers together, resulting in a compact splint. If this procedure is not done, puff pastry plaster will result, causing an unstable splint

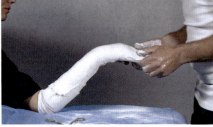

Apply the splint and mold to the hand and forearm

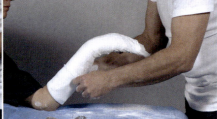

Fold back the tube bandage over the splint proximally

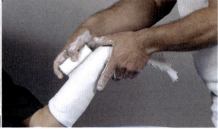

Apply a gauze bandage to hold the splint in position. Wrap the forearm using the half-overlapping technique

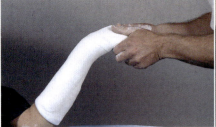

Hold the splint in position while it sets; ensure that no compression is applied across the fingers

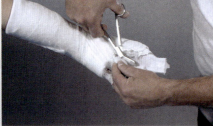

After the splint has set, cut away the gauze bandage and the padding on the distal palmar side

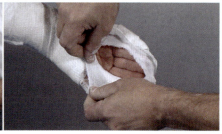

Split the tube bandage and fold it over the splint

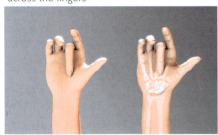

Check the position and direction of the injured finger; in the normal position the finger points to the scaphoid

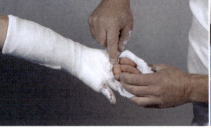

Check that the flexor tendons can fully bend; the fingertip should come as close as possible to the distal palmar crease

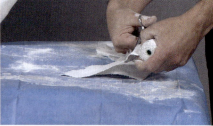

Cut short strips of POP to fix the tube bandage in place; they should be submerged in water one at a time

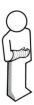

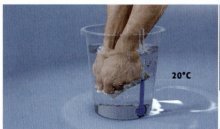

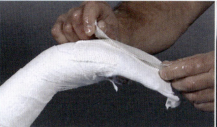

Fold over the tube bandage and hold in place with the POP strips

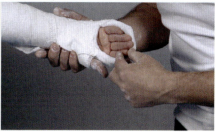

Ensure the distal palmar crease is free to allow movement of the fingers

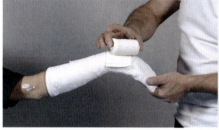

Apply an elastic bandage after the splint has set; it will be used to anchor the safety pins

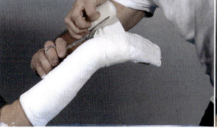

Cut halfway through the bandage, from proximal to distal, for easy application between the thumb and index finger

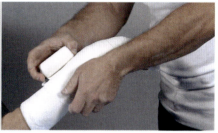

Wrap the forearm using the half-overlapping technique

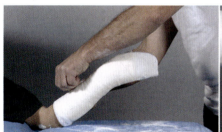

Secure the bandage with surgical tape or bandage clips

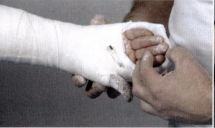

Attach a safety pin to the elastic bandage, distally to the scaphoid, and as close as possible to the distal palmar crease

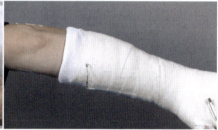

Attach a safety pin proximally

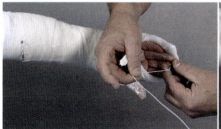

Attach a piece of elastic to the affected finger with glue or a suture through the nail, or as demonstrated here, with a small velcro strip

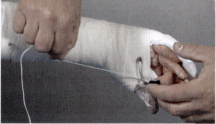

Thread the piece of elastic through both safety pins

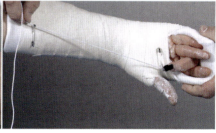

Pull the affected finger into flexion with the elastic

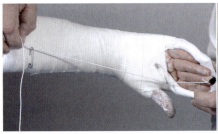

Ensure the patient is able to extend the finger without applying too much force

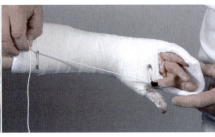

When the patient relaxes, the finger should return to the flexed position

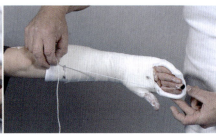

Ensure that complete extension is possible

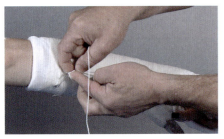

Tie the elastic securely to the proximal safety pin

FINAL ASSESSMENT

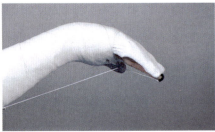

Ensure there is not too much tension on the elastic

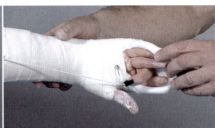

There should be free movement of the unaffected fingers

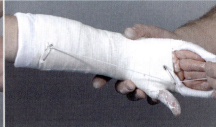

Passive flexion and active extension is possible; this helps to prevent adhesions that limit flexor tendon motion

15.22 Kleinert dynamic splint using synthetic, combicast technique

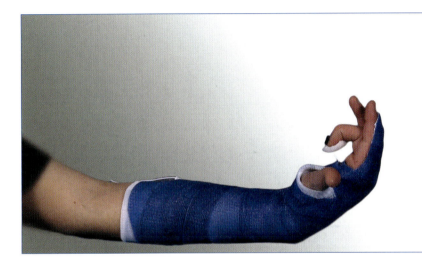

INDICATION

- Lesion of a flexor tendon

GOAL

- Postoperative functional treatment of a flexor tendon lesion

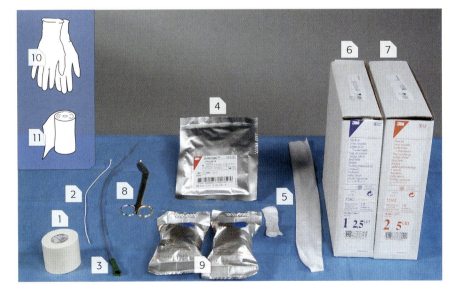

EQUIPMENT

1 Elastic foam tape
2 Piece of elastic
3 Tube, eg, suction tube
4 Rigid synthetic splint 7.5 cm x 45 cm
5 Cut tube bandages
6 Tube bandage 2.5 cm in dispenser box
7 Tube bandage 5 cm in dispenser box
8 Scissors
9 Semirigid casting tape 7.5 cm
10 Gloves
11 Elastic bandage

PERSONNEL

433

POSITIONING

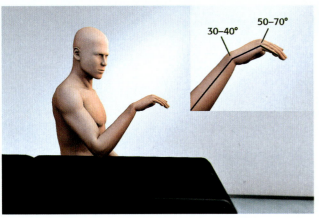

Seat the patient comfortably on a stool.

Place the affected limb on the table, position the wrist at 30–40° and the fingers at 50–70° palmar flexion.

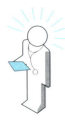

SPECIAL THINGS TO KEEP IN MIND

- For fixation to the nail, special glue or a suture through the nail can be used
- Metacarpophalangeal joints remain free on the palmar side

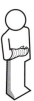

PROCEDURE

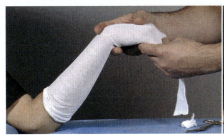

Apply the tube bandage, and stretch it to remove any wrinkles

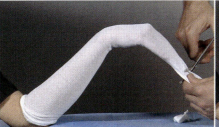

Cut a hole in the tube bandage for the thumb, and trim distally

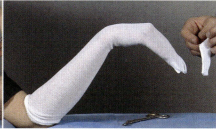

Place a small tube bandage over the thumb

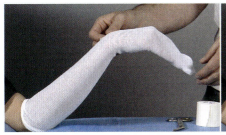

Apply elastic foam tape to protect the bony prominences, starting with the radial styloid process

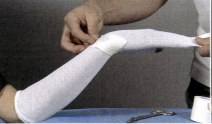

Cut a hole in the first layer of elastic foam tape over the ulnar styloid process, and apply a second layer for extra protection

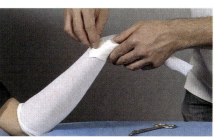

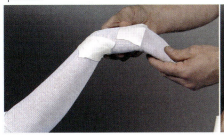

Protect the MCP joints with elastic foam tape

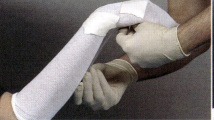

Cut the tubing to the required length

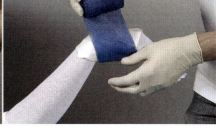

Apply the semirigid casting tape around the hand

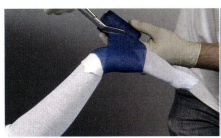

Cut halfway through the semirigid casting tape, from proximal to distal, for easy application between the thumb and index finger

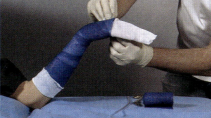

Fold back the tube bandage over the semirigid casting tape proximally, and over the thumb

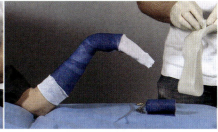

Fold the rigid splint in half, fan out the proximal end to fit the width of the forearm, and cut through the distal end

435

15.22

TECHNIQUES

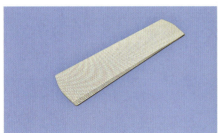

Shape the splint like this

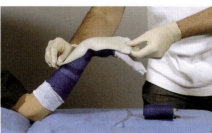

Place the splint on the dorsal side, starting over the PIP joints

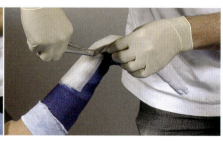

Cut the splint partway through at the wrist to avoid pressure from wrinkles

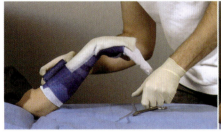

Apply the semirigid casting tape, starting proximally

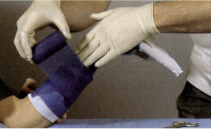

Place the tube at the palmar side; wrap the semirigid casting tape over the tube to hold it in place

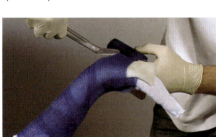

Cut halfway through the semirigid casting tape, from proximal to distal, for easy application between the thumb and index finger

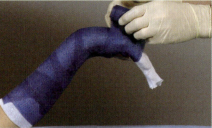

Distally, the semirigid casting tape must be wrapped under the tube

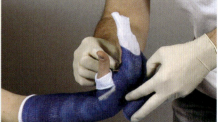

Ensure the desired angle of the wrist and fingers does not change; before continuing, turn the hand 180°

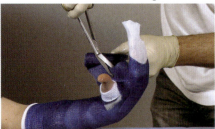

Cut a small hole in the semirigid casting tape and thread the tube through it

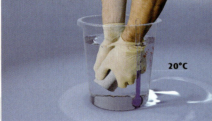

Submerge an elastic bandage in water for a few seconds; using a wet bandage accelerates the setting

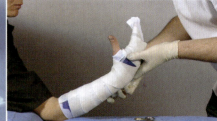

Apply the elastic bandage starting proximally

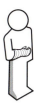

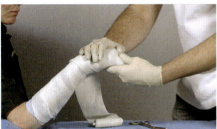

Hold the wrist and fingers in the desired position until the splint is set

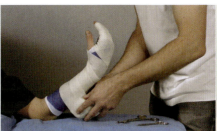

Check that the splint has set and remove the wet bandage

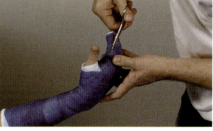

Cut away a section of the splint on the palmar side, down to the distal palmar crease, to free the fingers

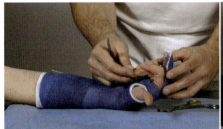

Ensure full flexion of the fingers is possible; the dorsal section prevents overextension

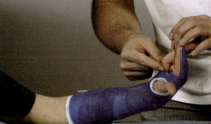

Check that the flexor tendons can fully bend; the fingertip should come as close as possible to the distal palmar crease

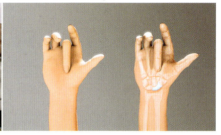

Check the position and direction of the injured finger; in the normal position, the finger points to the scaphoid

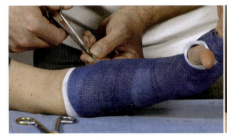

Trim the tube distally, and cut a slit in the proximal end of the tube

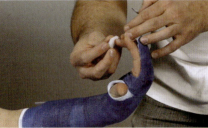

Attach a piece of adhesive foam padding to protect the fingertip of the affected finger

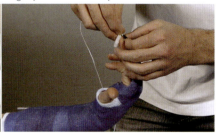

Attach a piece of elastic to the affected finger with glue or a suture through the nail, demonstrated here with a small velcro strip

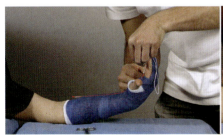

Insert the elastic through the tube

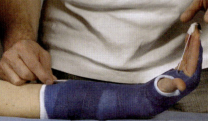

Control the tension of the elastic so that extension of the finger is possible without applying too much force

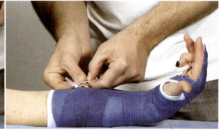

Tie off the elastic proximally with the affected finger in flexion

FINAL ASSESSMENT

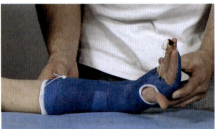

Ensure there is not too much tension on the elastic

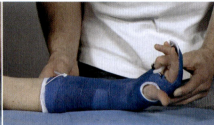

There should be free movement of the unaffected fingers

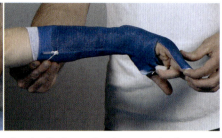

Passive flexion and active extension is possible; this helps to prevent adhesions that limit flexor tendon motion

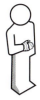

15.23   Metacarpal glove using synthetic, combicast technique

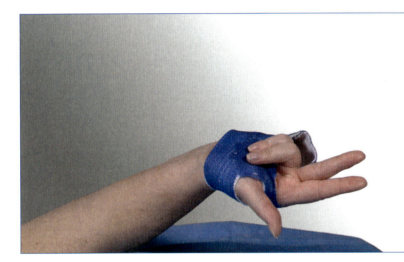

INDICATION

- Nondisplaced or reducible fractures of the fifth metacarpal head
- Also applicable for fractures of the metacarpal heads II–IV in a modified design

GOAL

- Stabilization of the metacarpal heads

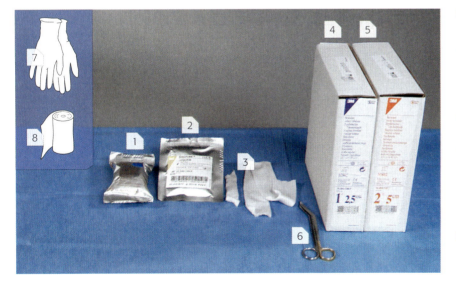

EQUIPMENT

1 Semirigid casting tape 5 cm
2 Rigid synthetic splint 5 cm x 20 cm
3 Cut tube bandages
4 Tube bandage 2.5 cm in dispenser box
5 Tube bandage 5 cm in dispenser box
6 Scissors
7 Gloves
8 Elastic bandage

PERSONNEL

15.23

TECHNIQUES

POSITIONING

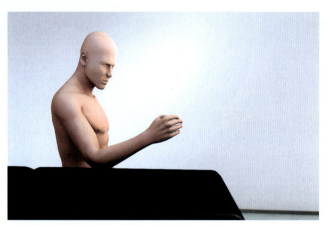

Seat the patient comfortably on a stool.
Place the affected limb on the table.

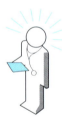

SPECIAL THINGS TO KEEP IN MIND

- Palmar aspect is free, complete flexion of the fingers is possible
- Free movement of the wrist and thumb
- Free interdigital space to avoid friction

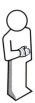

PROCEDURE

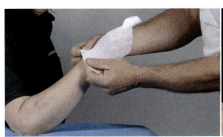

Apply the tube bandage

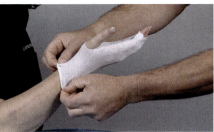

Cut a hole in the tube bandage for the thumb

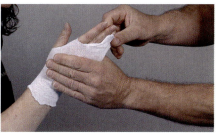

Cut a second hole for the index finger and ring finger

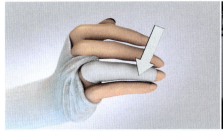

Fold back the tube bandage and place a small tube bandage over the ring finger to protect the skin between the fingers

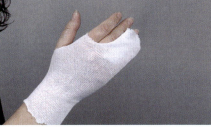

Fold the tube bandage back over the fingers

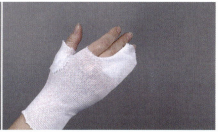

Place a small tube bandage over the thumb

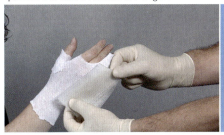

Prepare a rigid splint for the outside of the hand; fan it out, and trim to the desired shape

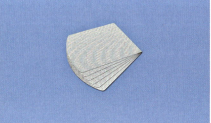

Shape the splint like this

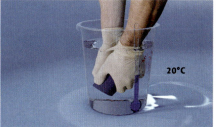

Submerge the semirigid casting tape in water for a few seconds, remove, and squeeze out excess water

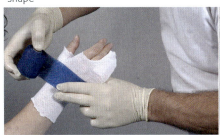

Apply the first layer of semirigid casting tape

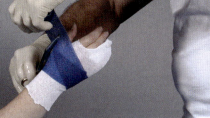

Cut the semirigid casting tape halfway through, from proximal to distal, for easy application between thumb and index finger

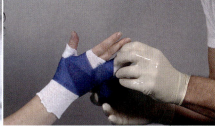

Cut halfway through the semirigid casting tape and wrap between the middle finger and ring finger

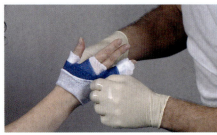

Fold back the tube bandage proximally, and trim

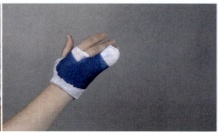

Fold back the small tube bandage from the thumb; leave the rest in place

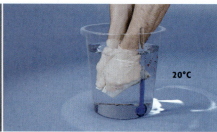

Submerge the splint in water for a few seconds, remove, and squeeze out excess water

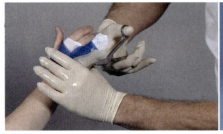

Position the splint and trim to the desired shape

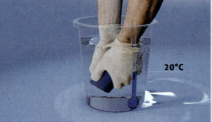

Apply a layer of wet semirigid casting tape to hold the splint in place

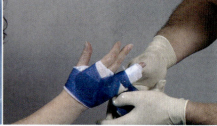

Cut the semirigid casting tape halfway through, from proximal to distal, and wrap around the affected fingers

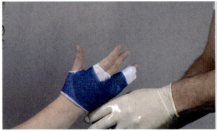

Cut the semirigid casting tape halfway through, from proximal to distal, and wrap between the thumb and index finger

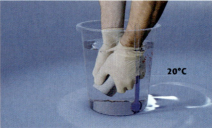

Submerge an elastic bandage in water; using a wet bandage accelerates the setting

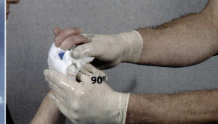

Hold the MCP joints of the affected fingers at 90° while setting

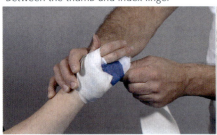

Remove the wet bandage after the glove has set

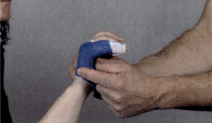

Ensure the MCP joints of the affected fingers are at 90° and the wrist is fully mobile

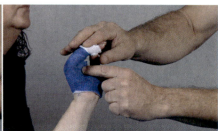

Cut away the material on the palmar side, from over the fingers to the distal palmar crease, to allow free flexion of the MCP joints

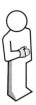

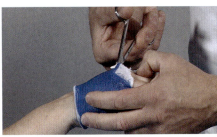

Trimming begins dorsally with small scissors

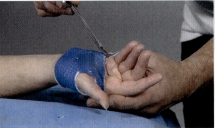

Cut along the MCP joints on the palmar side to allow free flexion of the fingers

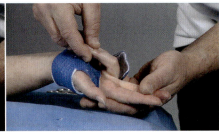

Ensure flexion at the MCP joints is possible

FINAL ASSESSMENT

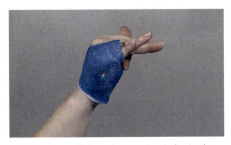

Flexion is possible and extension is limited

Klaus Dresing, Jos Engelen

15.24 Removable thumb orthosis using synthetic

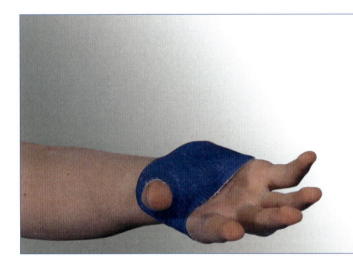

INDICATION

- Ligamentous rupture of the first metacarpophalangeal joint

GOAL

- Stabilization of the first metacarpophalangeal joint

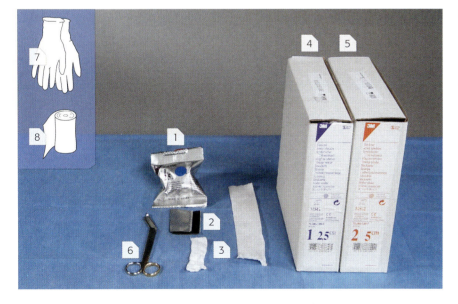

EQUIPMENT

1. Semirigid casting tape 2.5 cm
2. Adapted adhesive velcro strips (hook and loop)
3. Cut tube bandages
4. Tube bandage 2.5 cm in dispenser box
5. Tube bandage 5 cm in dispenser box
6. Scissors
7. Gloves
8. Elastic bandage

PERSONNEL

POSITIONING

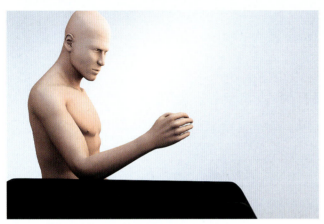

Seat the patient comfortably on a stool.

Place the affected limb on the table with the thumb in opposition.

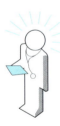

SPECIAL THINGS TO KEEP IN MIND

- Wrist should remain free
- Interphalangeal joint of the thumb should remain free

PROCEDURE

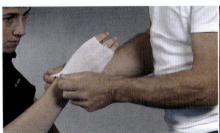

Apply the tube bandage

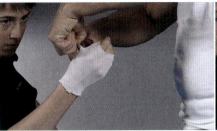

Cut a hole in the tube bandage over the MCP joint of the thumb, and slide the thumb through the hole

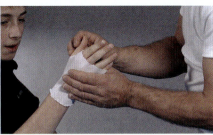

Place the fingers in extension and the thumb in the desired position

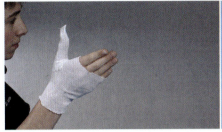

Place a small tube bandage over the thumb

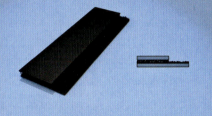

Prepare two adhesive velcro strips of different widths, one hook and one loop, and place together, overlapping on one side

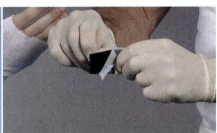

Remove the adhesive protection layers

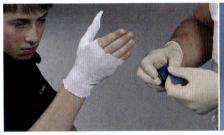

As a ligament injury does not usually need rigid splint support, only semirigid casting tape is applied

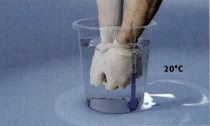

Using wet gloves makes application of the semirigid casting tape easier

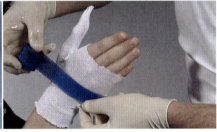

Apply the semirigid casting tape, beginning below the thumb

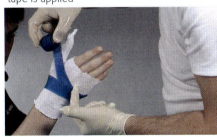

Follow the MCP joints and pass the semirigid casting tape between the thumb and index finger and across the distal palmar crease

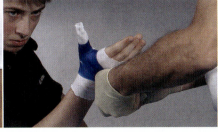

Wrap the semirigid casting tape twice around the thumb

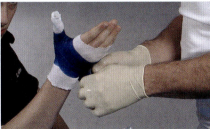

Continue wrapping until all gaps are covered

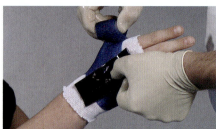

Place the combined velcro strips on the semirigid casting tape and wrap with another layer of semirigid casting tape

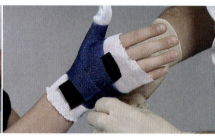

Important: while fixing the velcro strips with another layer of semirigid casting tape, keep the same borders as the first layer

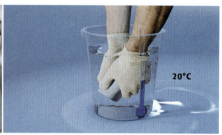

Submerge an elastic bandage in water for a few seconds; using a wet bandage accelerates the setting

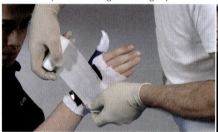

Apply the wet elastic bandage

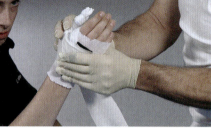

Place the thumb in opposition while the orthosis sets

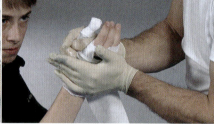

Support the thumb on the ulnar side to reduce stress on the ulnar collateral ligament

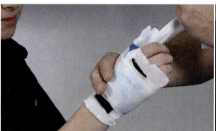

Tap on the orthosis to check it has set, and remove the wet bandage

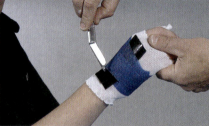

Remove the orthosis before trimming it to the desired shape. The first step is to open the velcro

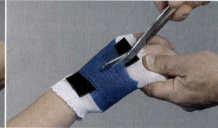

Place the scissors underneath the outer layers of semirigid casting tape where the velcro overlaps, and cut through the tape

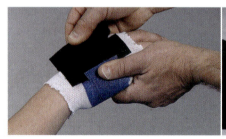

Open and fold back the velcro; the lower layer of semirigid casting tape can be seen

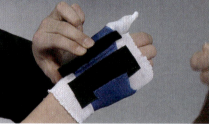

The patient holds the velcro in place

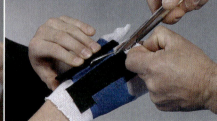

Place the scissors under the tube bandage, and cut through the lower layer of semirigid casting tape and tube bandage

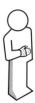

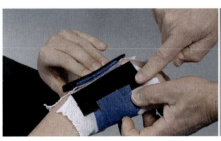

The velcro strips are on either side of the orthosis, which can now be opened and closed easily

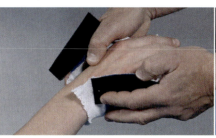

Remove the orthosis

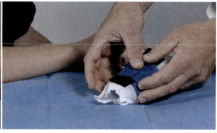

Close the orthosis and trim to the desired shape

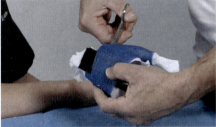

Trim the proximal edge of the orthosis to allow free movement of the wrist

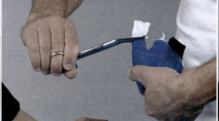

Trim the orthosis to allow free movement of the IP joint of the thumb

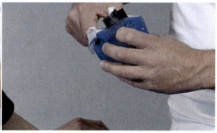

Trim the distal edges to allow free movement of the MCP joints

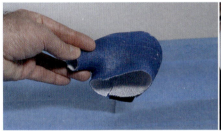

The contours of the hand can be clearly seen in the orthosis

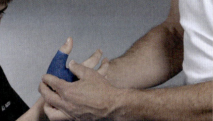

Open the velcro and slide the orthosis over the thumb

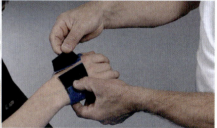

To give support to the injury, pull on the upper velcro strip to close the orthosis

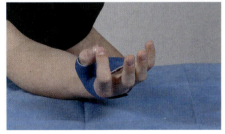

There should be enough freedom of movement to bring the thumb and index finger into opposition

449

FINAL ASSESSMENT

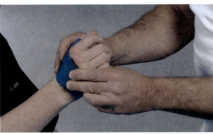 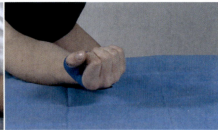

Free movement of the wrist and fingers   Free flexion of the fingers

Klaus Dresing, Jos Engelen

15.25 Removable finger splint using synthetic

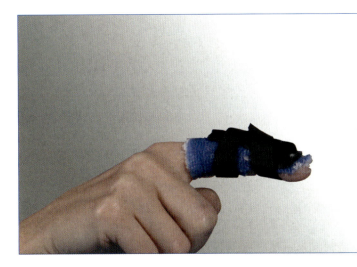

INDICATION

- Fracture of the intermediate phalanx or ligamentous rupture of the proximal interphalangeal joint

GOAL

- Stabilization of the proximal interphalangeal joint

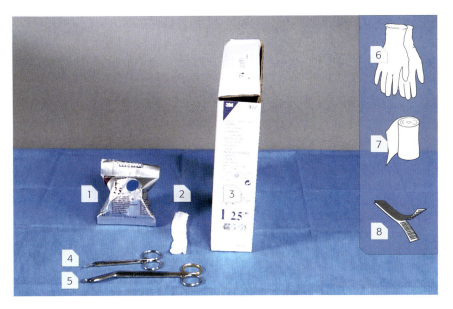

EQUIPMENT

1. Semirigid casting tape 2.5 cm
2. Cut tube bandage 2.5 cm
3. Tube bandage 2.5 cm in dispenser box
4. Small scissors
5. Scissors
6. Gloves
7. Elastic bandage
8. Adhesive and nonadhesive velcro

PERSONNEL

POSITIONING

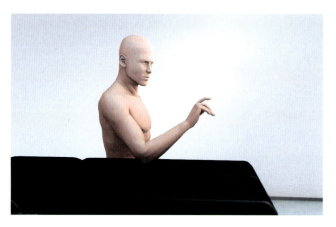

Seat the patient comfortably on a stool.
Place the affected limb on the table.

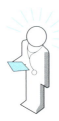

SPECIAL THINGS TO KEEP IN MIND

- The splint should cover as much of the proximal phalanx as possible
- Free movement of the metacarpophalangeal joint
- Space is made for the nail

Klaus Dresing, Jos Engelen

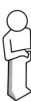

PROCEDURE

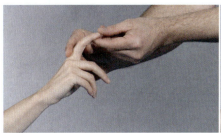

Place the finger in the functional position

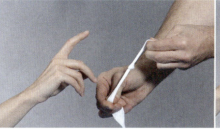

Make a knot at one end of the tube bandage, and trim the excess

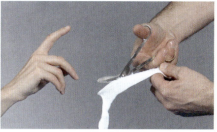

Cut along the length of the tube bandage, leave enough material uncut to cover the finger

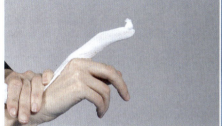

Place the tube bandage over the finger and position the knot over the fingernail

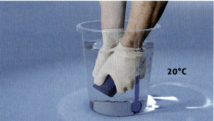

Submerge the semirigid casting tape in water for a few seconds, remove, and squeeze out excess water

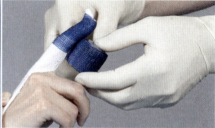

Wrap the finger with three layers of semirigid casting tape, using the half-overlapping technique

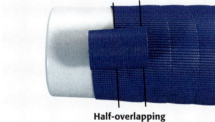

Half-overlapping

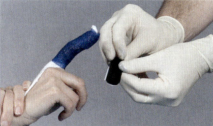

Place an adhesive strip of velcro (with loops) on the dorsal side

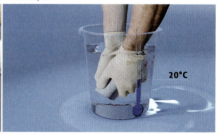

Submerge an elastic bandage in water; using a wet bandage accelerates the setting

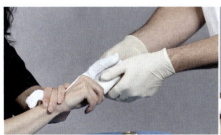

Apply the bandage with the finger placed in a functional position with slight flexion of the PIP and DIP joints

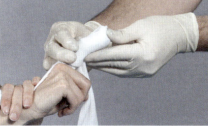

Ensure the knot is still on the fingernail

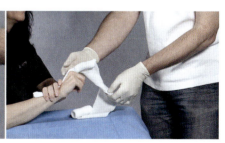

Remove the wet bandage when the splint has set

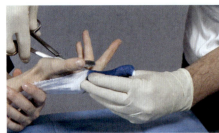

Cut a slit in the splint with the scissors to make removal easier

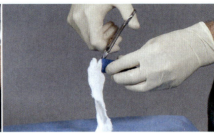

Trim the proximal end of the splint

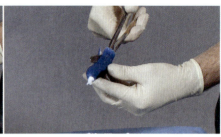

Cut a slit in the splint up to the DIP joint on the palmar side

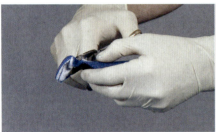

Remove the section of the splint that covers the palmar distal phalanx, along with the knot

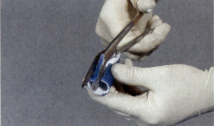

Widen the split in the splint

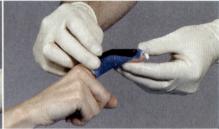

Place the splint back on the finger; ensure there is free movement of the distal phalanx

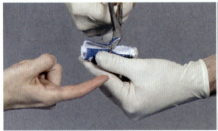

Make any final adjustments that are necessary

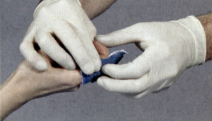

Make a final check to ensure free movement of the DIP joint

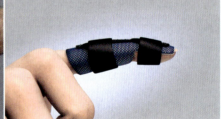

Apply velcro strips (with hooks) or adhesive tape to close the splint

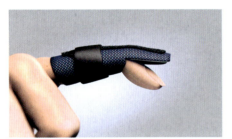

If functional treatment is allowed, the distal velcro strip can be removed to allow free flexion and extension

FINAL ASSESSMENT

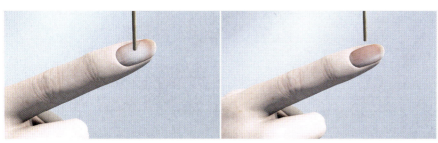

Check for capillary refill

Klaus Dresing, Jos Engelen

15.26 Mallet finger splint using synthetic

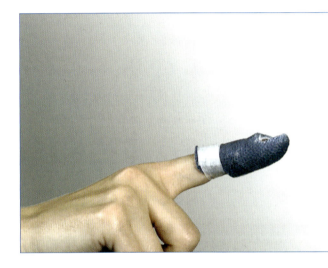

INDICATION

- Extensor tendon injury at the distal interphalangeal joint (mallet or baseball finger)

GOAL

- Full extension of the distal interphalangeal joint

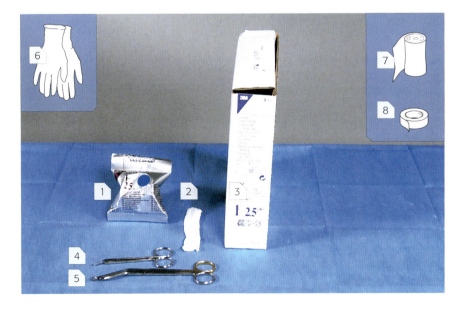

EQUIPMENT

1 Semirigid casting tape 2.5 cm
2 Cut tube bandage 2.5 cm
3 Tube bandage 2.5 cm in dispenser box
4 Small scissors
5 Scissors
6 Gloves
7 Elastic bandage
8 Surgical tape

PERSONNEL

POSITIONING

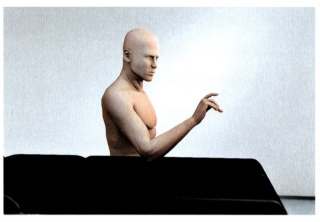

Seat the patient comfortably on a stool.
Place the affected limb on the table.

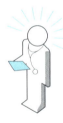

SPECIAL THINGS TO KEEP IN MIND

- Avoid hyperextension of the distal interphalangeal joint
- Nail bed should be free
- Flexion of the proximal interphalangeal joint should be possible

Klaus Dresing, Jos Engelen

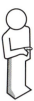

PROCEDURE

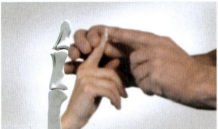

Place the affected finger in full extension

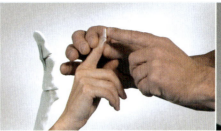

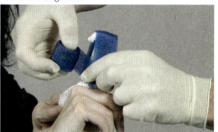

Make a knot at one end of the tube bandage and place it over the finger. Position the knot over the fingernail

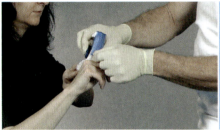

Measure enough semirigid casting tape to reach from PIP joint to PIP joint, sagittally

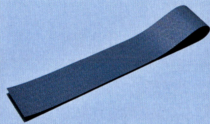

Fold over the semirigid casting tape to make a two-layer splint and trim like this

Place the splint over the finger, and wrap the finger with three layers of semirigid casting tape, using the half-overlapping technique

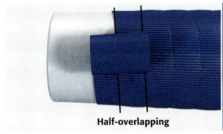

Half-overlapping

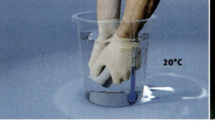

20°C

Submerge an elastic bandage in water; using a wet bandage accelerates the setting

Apply the wet bandage with the finger in full extension

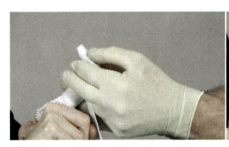

Mold the end of the splint during setting. Ensure the knot is still on the fingernail

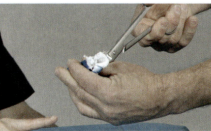

Remove the splint after it has set, and trim to the desired shape

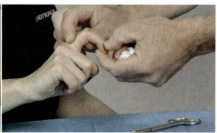

Free movement of the PIP joint is necessary

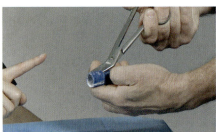

Remove a palmar section of the splint to allow movement of the PIP joint

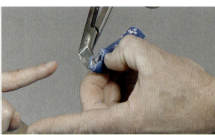

Make an opening for the fingernail

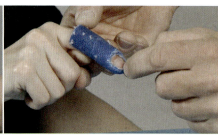

Place the prepared splint over the finger. Ensure the complete fingernail is free

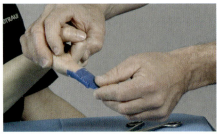

Ensure free flexion and extension of the PIP joint is possible

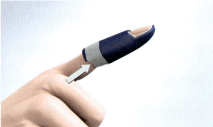

Hold the splint in place with surgical tape

FINAL ASSESSMENT

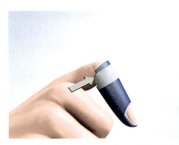

Free flexion and extension of the PIP joint

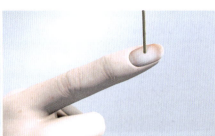

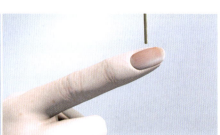

Control of the capillary refill

TECHNIQUES

16 Lower extremity

16 Lower extremity

Klaus Dresing, Jos Engelen

16.1 One-and-a-half leg hip spica cast using plaster of Paris

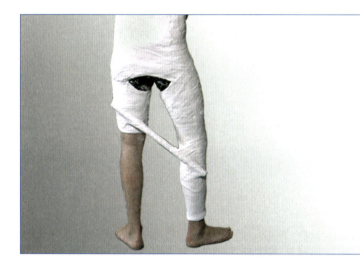

INDICATION

- Pediatric fracture of the femur

GOAL

- Stabilization of the leg and hip

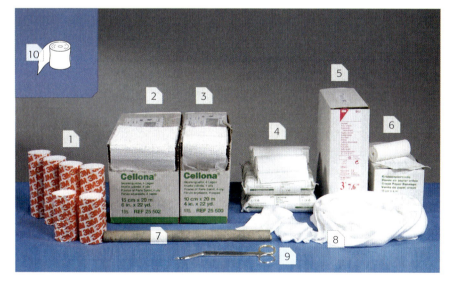

EQUIPMENT

1 Cast padding
2 Plaster of Paris splint 12 cm or 15 cm
3 Plaster of Paris splint 10 cm or 12 cm
4 Plaster of Paris rolls 12 cm or 15 cm
5 Tube bandage 7.5 cm in dispenser box
6 Crepe paper bandage
7 Broomstick
8 Cut tube bandages
9 Scissors
10 Adhesive tape

PERSONNEL

3 (1 surgeon if needed)

16.1

TECHNIQUES

POSITIONING

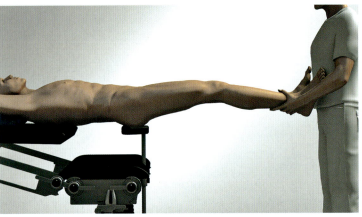

Patient is lying with the sacrum on a support.

Place the legs in a foot support, or held by an assistant, ensure slight flexion of the hip and knee.

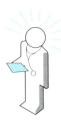

SPECIAL THINGS TO KEEP IN MIND

- Free movement of the knee on the contralateral side
- Protection of the bony prominences
- Slight flexion of the hip and knee joint is necessary
- Two or three people are needed for this procedure

Klaus Dresing, Jos Engelen

PROCEDURE

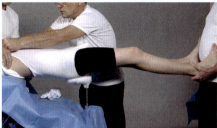

Apply a tube bandage or cast trousers

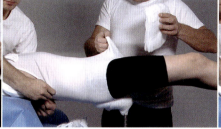

Apply padding over the stomach to provide space for breathing and eating

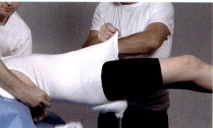

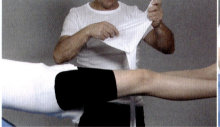

Make a slit in the proximal end of a long tube bandage, roll it up and apply over the affected leg up to the hip

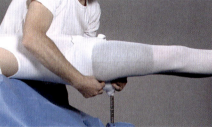

Pull the bandage tight to remove any wrinkles

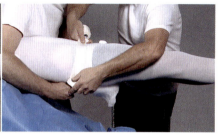

Apply strips of adhesive tape to hold the tube bandage in place

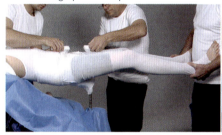

Apply a tube bandage over the other leg, and hold it in place with strips of adhesive tape

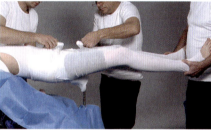

Apply rolls of padding over both tube bandages using the half-overlapping technique

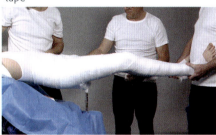

Apply the padding down to the ankle of the affected leg, and down to the knee of the other leg

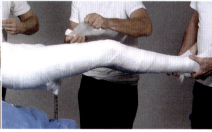

Apply a layer of paper bandage to cover all the padding to form a barrier between the dry padding and the wet POP

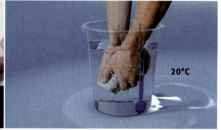

Submerge the rolls of POP in water for a few seconds, remove, and squeeze out excess water

465

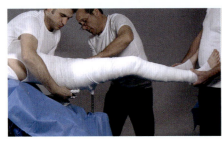

Apply the rolls of POP using the half-overlapping technique

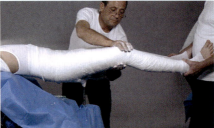

Smooth the POP with wet hands

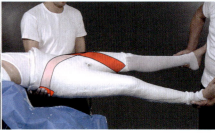

Apply the first POP splint from the left knee to the right hip

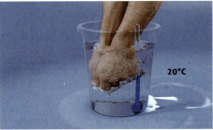

Submerge the POP splint in water for a few seconds, remove, and squeeze out excess water

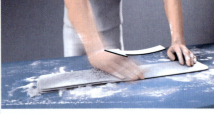

Stretch and smooth out the splint, pressing the layers together, resulting in a compact splint. If this procedure is not done, puff pastry plaster will result, causing an unstable splint

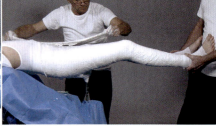

POP splints are used to reinforce the POP cast at specific locations

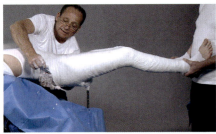

Start at the knee, pass under the body, ending above the pelvis on the contralateral side; do not pass the splint over the stomach

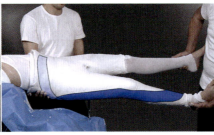

Apply a longer, second POP splint to the right leg

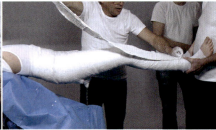

Apply the splint starting at the ankle, and follow the lateral tibia

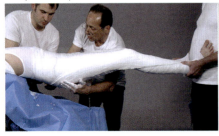

Continue over the femur to the top of the pelvis, and pass the splint under the body to the contralateral side

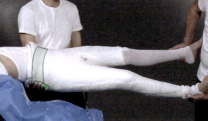

Apply a third splint around the posterior pelvis; this splint provides extra stability

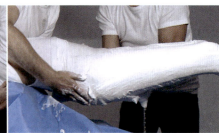

Klaus Dresing, Jos Engelen

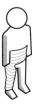

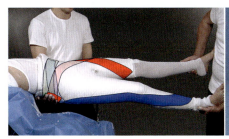

Position of the three reinforcement POP splints

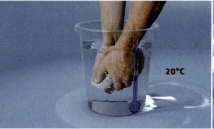

Submerge the rolls of POP in water for a few seconds, remove, and squeeze out excess water

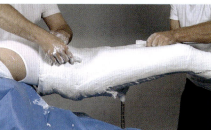

Apply the rolls of POP using the half-overlapping technique, to hold the POP splints in place

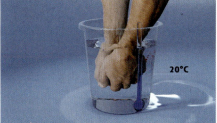

Wet hands make smoothing the POP easier

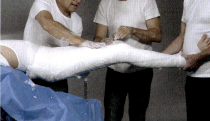

Smooth the complete cast and mold where needed

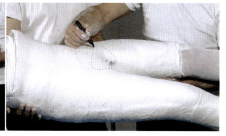

After the cast has set, it is marked for removal and trimming

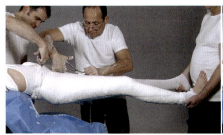

Cut out the marked area and trim the edges

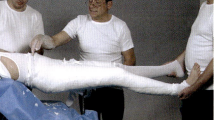

The tube bandage must be folded over the edges of the cast

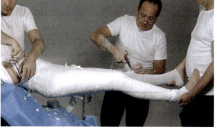

Trim the tube bandage above and below the cast

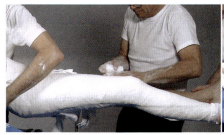

Apply extra padding to areas where it is needed

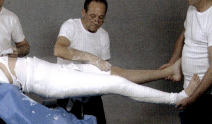

Push the edge of the padding under the cast and fold back the tube bandage

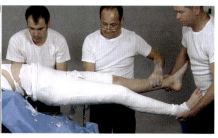

The unaffected knee has complete freedom of motion

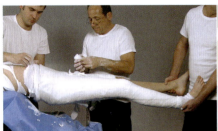

Fold back the tube bandage over the proximal edge of the cast

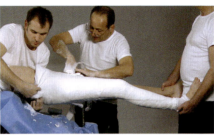

Add padding where the section of the cast was removed, and fold back the tube bandage

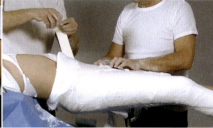

Apply strips of adhesive tape to hold the edges of the tube bandage in place

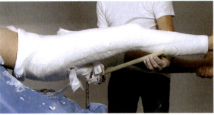

Place a piece of broomstick on the dorsal aspect of the legs to give added stability. Place the broomstick at an angle, from the healthy to the injured leg

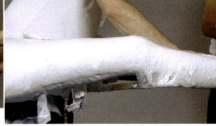

Secure the broomstick to the cast with several layers of POP, using the figure-of-eight technique

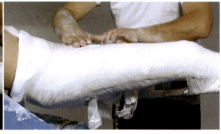

Apply a short strip of POP to attach the folded-over tube bandage to the cast

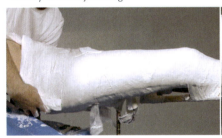

Secure the tube bandage in place with a roll of POP

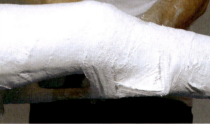

Reinforce the attachment of the broomstick to the cast with a roll of POP

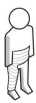

FINAL ASSESSMENT

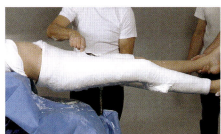

Carrying out personal hygiene is possible

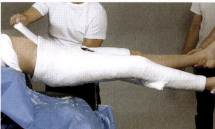

Remove the padding from the stomach to allow enough space for free breathing and eating

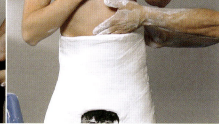

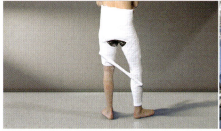

Dorsal view of the cast

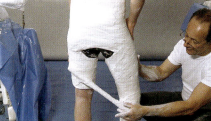

The broomstick reinforces the structure of the cast

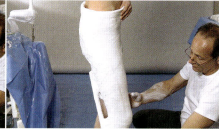

Slight flexion of the hip and knee is visible

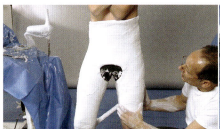

Bodily functions are possible

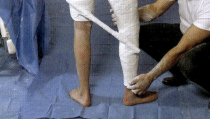

Pressure sores are prevented by the soft smooth edges of the cast

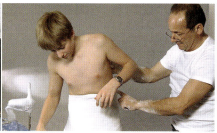

Smooth edges also allow free movement of the upper body

Casts, Splints, and Support Bandages—Nonoperative Treatment and Perioperative Protection   Klaus Dresing, Peter Trafton

Klaus Dresing, Jos Engelen

16.2   Single leg hip spica cast using synthetic, combicast technique

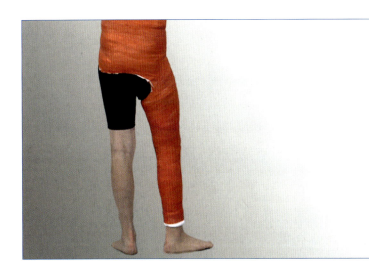

INDICATION

- Pediatric fracture of the femur

GOAL

- Stabilization of the leg and hip

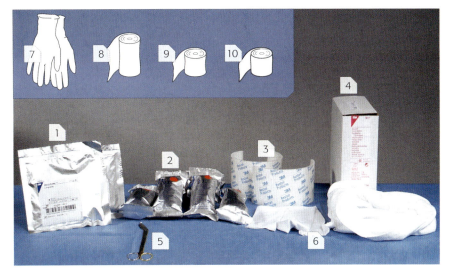

EQUIPMENT

1 Rigid synthetic splint 7.5 cm x 70 cm or 10 cm x 76 cm

2 Semirigid casting tape 7.5 cm or 10 cm

3 Adhesive foam padding

4 Tube bandage 7.5 cm in dispenser box

5 Scissors

6 Cut tube bandages

7 Gloves

8 Elastic bandage

9 Adhesive tape

10 Elastic foam tape

PERSONNEL

3 (1 surgeon if needed)

16.2

TECHNIQUES

POSITIONING

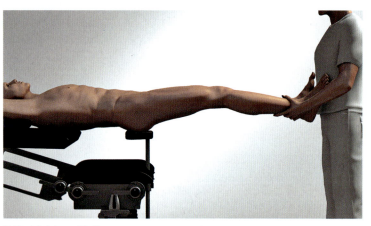

Patient is lying with the sacrum on a support.

Place the legs in a foot support, or held by an assistant, ensure slight flexion of the hip and knee.

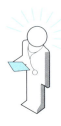

SPECIAL THINGS TO KEEP IN MIND

- Free movement of the hip on the contralateral side
- Protection of the bony prominences
- Slight flexion of the hip and knee joint is necessary
- Two or three people are needed for this procedure
- The greater stability of synthetic material allows minimizing the hip spica cast—contralateral leg is not included

Klaus Dresing, Jos Engelen

PROCEDURE

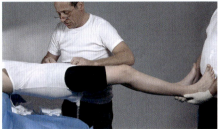

Apply a tube bandage or cast trousers

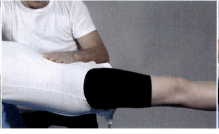

Apply additional padding for the stomach to provide space for breathing and eating

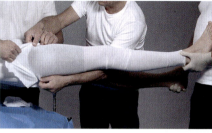

Make a slit in the proximal end of a long tube bandage, roll it up and apply over the affected leg up to the hip

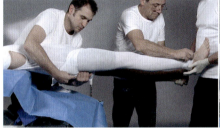

Pull the bandage tight to remove any wrinkles

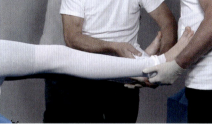

Apply a shorter tube bandage over the other leg, from the knee to the hip

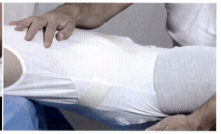

Apply strips of adhesive tape to hold the tube bandages in place

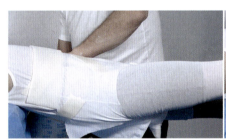

Apply strips of adhesive foam padding for added protection

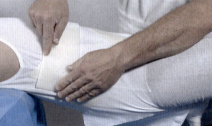

Place the padding just under the costal arches to provide a smooth edge when it is folded back over the cast

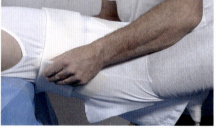

Apply a second strip of padding on the patient's back, at the same level as the first

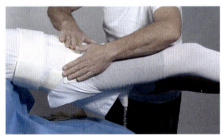

Add strips of elastic foam tape to protect the prominent areas of the pelvis

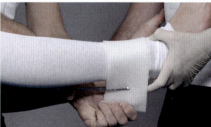

Apply adhesive foam padding over the distal bony prominences, ensure it does not completely encircle the leg

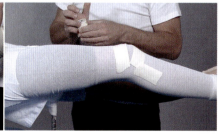

Protect all the prominent bones around the knee with elastic foam tape

16.2 Single leg hip spica cast using synthetic, combicast technique

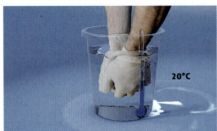

Using wet gloves makes it easier to apply the semirigid casting tape

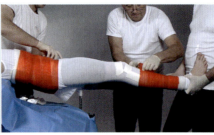

Apply the semirigid casting tape, from proximal and distal, using the half-overlapping technique

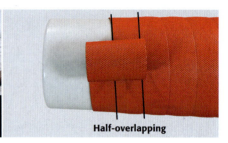

Half-overlapping

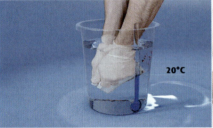

Submerge the rigid splint in water for a few seconds, remove, and squeeze out excess water

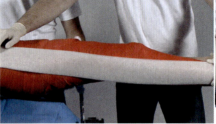

Apply the first splint along the axis of the affected leg

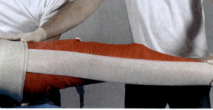

Place the second splint around the pelvis; leave the contralateral ventral aspect of the hip joint free. Position the splint over the sacrum but avoid the perineal area

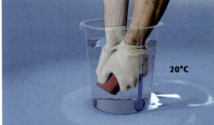

Submerge the semirigid casting tape in water for a few seconds, remove, and squeeze out excess water

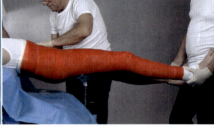

Apply the semirigid casting tape to hold the splints in place

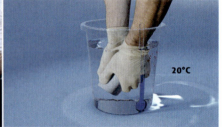

Submerge an elastic bandage in water; using a wet bandage accelerates the setting

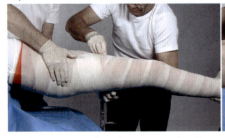

Apply the wet bandage from proximal and distal, to cover the semirigid casting tape

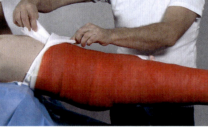

Tap on the cast to make sure it is set, and remove the wet bandage and the extra stomach padding

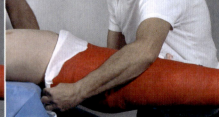

Fold the foam padding and the tube bandage over the cast

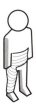
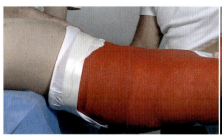

Apply strips of adhesive tape to hold the tube bandage in place

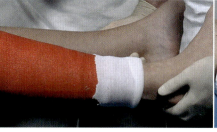

Fold over the tube bandage and foam padding distally and trim

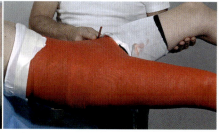

Trim the cast in the inguinal and perineal region; ensure that the hip joint of the unaffected leg has full range of motion

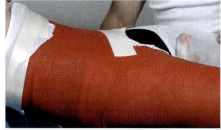

Cut through the tube bandage, fold it back over the cast and secure with strips of adhesive tape

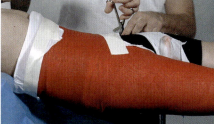

Remove any cast that may hinder free movement of the hip

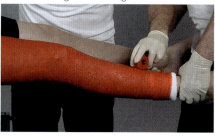

Wet semirigid casting tape is used to wrap all the edges of the cast

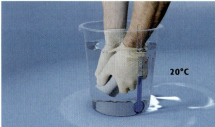

Submerge an elastic bandage in water

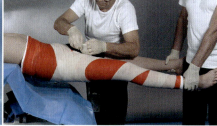

Applying a wet bandage accelerates the setting

FINAL ASSESSMENT

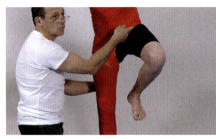

Free movement of the contralateral leg

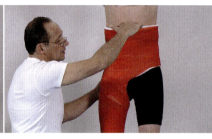

There is enough space for free breathing and eating

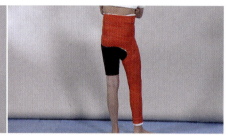

Dorsal view of the cast

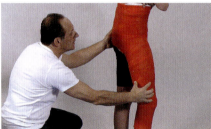

Slight flexion of the hip and knee is visible

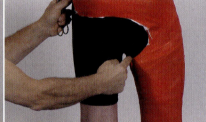

Bodily functions are possible

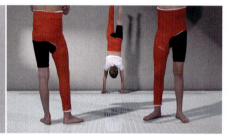

Combicast technique still allows a wide range of activities

Klaus Dresing, Jos Engelen

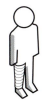

16.3 Cylinder long leg cast using synthetic, combicast technique

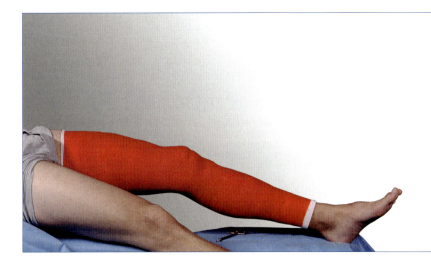

INDICATION

- Fracture of the distal femur
- Fracture of the proximal tibia
- Fracture of the patella
- Ligamentous rupture of the knee

GOAL

- Stabilization of the knee joint

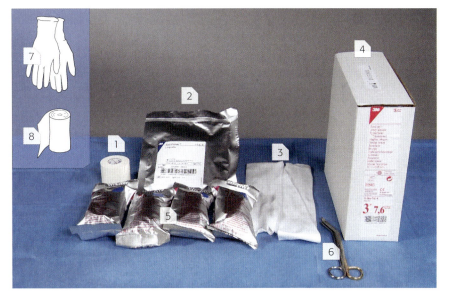

EQUIPMENT

1 Elastic foam tape
2 Rigid synthetic splint 10 cm or 12.5 cm x 90 cm
3 Cut tube bandage
4 Tube bandage 7.5 cm in dispenser box
5 Semirigid casting tape 7.5 cm or 10 cm
6 Scissors
7 Gloves
8 Elastic bandage

PERSONNEL

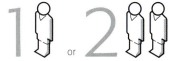

477

16.3

TECHNIQUES

POSITIONING

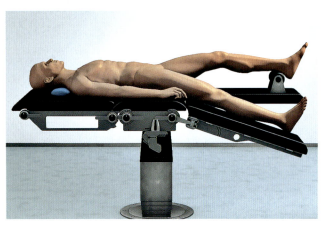

Place the patient supine on a table.

Place the ankle on a foot rest with 10-20° flexion at the knee.

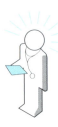

SPECIAL THINGS TO KEEP IN MIND

- Proximal extension: lesser trochanter–greater trochanter
- Distal extension: two fingers proximal of the malleoli, to allow free movement of the ankle
- Molding to the femoral condyles, to avoid the cast slipping down the patient's leg
- Pressure sore on the Achilles tendon
- In some indications, an assistant is needed to support the knee/leg

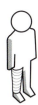

PROCEDURE

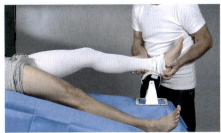

Apply a tube bandage up to the hip. Pull the tube bandage tight to avoid wrinkles

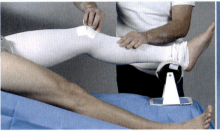

Apply elastic foam tape to protect the bony prominences around the knee

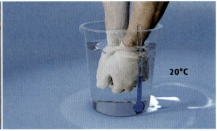

Wet gloves make application of the semirigid casting tape easier

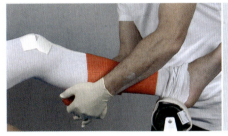

Apply the first layer of semirigid casting tape, from distal to proximal, using the half-overlapping technique

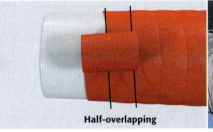

Half-overlapping

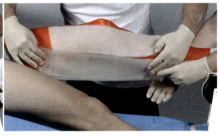

Ensure the semirigid casting tape covers the lesser trochanter and greater trochanter

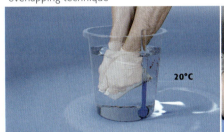

Submerge the rigid synthetic splint in water for a few seconds, remove, and squeeze out excess water

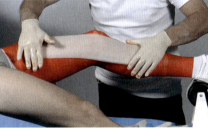

Cut the splint in half; apply the first splint medially and fix in place proximally with semirigid casting tape

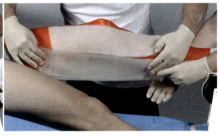

Apply the second splint dorsally; fix both splints in place with semirigid casting tape, using the half-overlapping technique

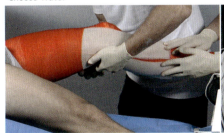

An assistant may be needed to hold the splints in place distally

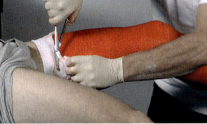

Fold back the tube bandage over the semirigid casting tape, proximally and distally, and trim the excess

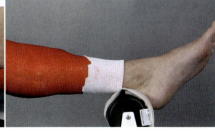

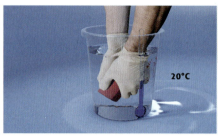

Apply a second layer of wet semirigid casting tape, from distal to proximal, using the half-overlapping technique

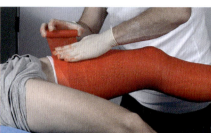

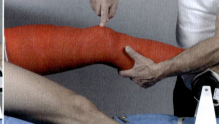

Submerge an elastic bandage in water

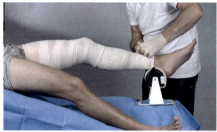

Applying a wet bandage accelerates the setting

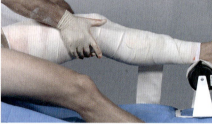

Mold the cast to the femoral condyles, the patella, and the popliteal fossa

Remove the wet bandage after the cast has set. Ensure there is no pressure on the patella, as there is no splint in this position

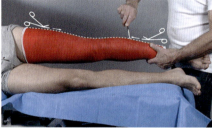

Mark the splitting line; split the cast from distal to the knee, then from proximal to the knee

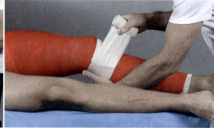

Wrap the split cast with an elastic bandage; start at the knee using the half-overlapping technique

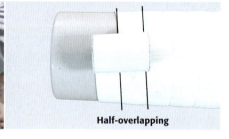

Half-overlapping

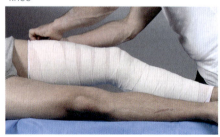

Secure the bandage with surgical tape or bandage clips

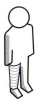

Klaus Dresing, Jos Engelen

FINAL ASSESSMENT

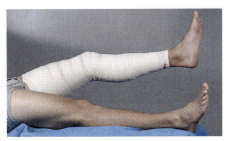

Hip joint and ankle joint have free range of
motion

16.3

TECHNIQUES

16.3

TECHNIQUES

16.4 Hinged knee brace

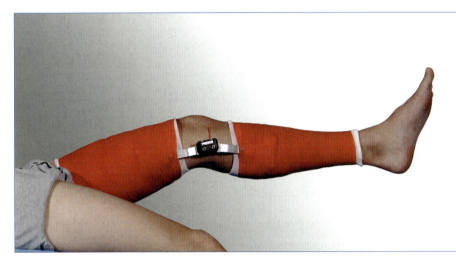

INDICATION

- Fracture of the diaphyseal and distal femur
- Fracture of the proximal tibia
- Knee dislocations and ligamentous lesions
- As an alternative to a prefabricated orthosis
- This hinged brace is not for primary care

GOAL

- Stabilization of the knee allowing limited motion of knee joint
- Functional treatment of the knee

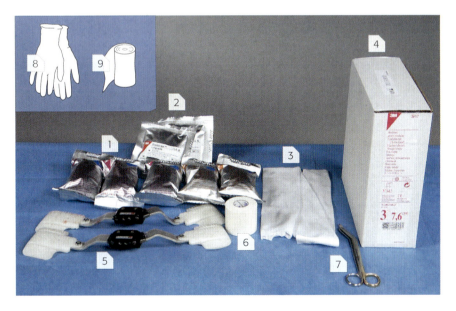

EQUIPMENT

1. Semirigid casting tape 7.5 cm or 10 cm
2. Rigid synthetic splint 7.5 cm x 70 cm
3. Cut tube bandages
4. Tube bandage 7.5 cm in dispenser box
5. Hinges
6. Elastic foam tape
7. Scissors
8. Gloves
9. Elastic bandage

PERSONNEL

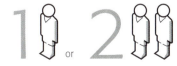

16.4

TECHNIQUES

POSITIONING

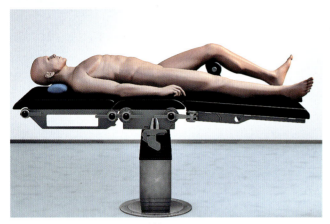

Place the patient supine on a table.
Place the knee on a knee support in approximately 30° flexion.

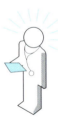

SPECIAL THINGS TO KEEP IN MIND

- Positioning of the hinges (axis)
- Perfect fit of the proximal and distal cast cylinders

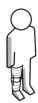

PROCEDURE

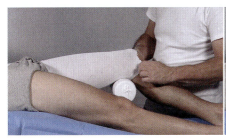

Apply a tube bandage from the knee to the hip. Pull the bandage tight to avoid any wrinkles

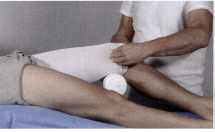

Ensure the proximal cast will leave the femoral condyles free, and will end as high as possible

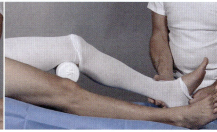

Apply a second tube bandage from the foot to the knee

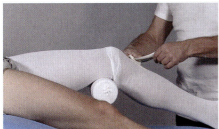

Apply elastic foam tape over the tibial tuberosity and the fibular head to protect the bony prominences

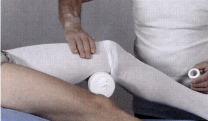

Proximally, no additional padding is needed because of the soft tissue covering

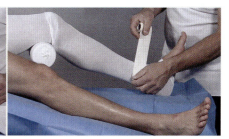

Apply elastic foam tape to the distal tibia to stop the cast sliding; ensure the tape does not encircle the bone

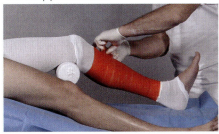

Apply the first layer of semirigid casting tape, using the half-overlapping technique, but leave the knee joint free

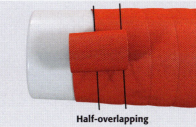

Half-overlapping

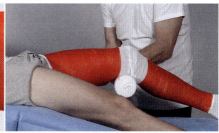

Apply a wider roll of semirigid casting tape to wrap the upper leg, using the half-overlapping technique

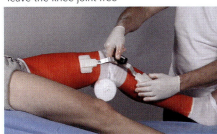

Position the hinges at their fixation points, the distal femur and the proximal tibia; two rigid splints will be placed here

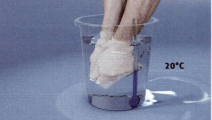

20°C

Submerge the rigid splints in water for a few seconds, remove, and squeeze out excess water

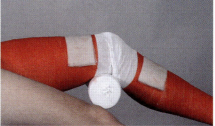

Apply the rigid splints only halfway around the leg

16.4

TECHNIQUES

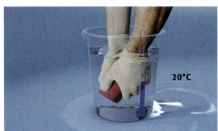

Apply a layer of wet semirigid casting tape to fix the rigid splint on the lower leg using the half-overlapping technique

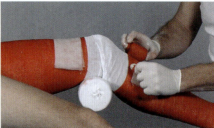

Fold back the tube bandage, trim and hold in place with semirigid casting tape

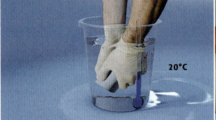

Submerge an elastic bandage in water

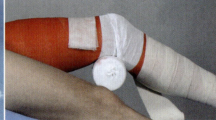

Applying a wet bandage accelerates the setting

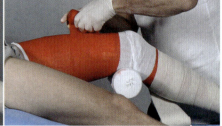

Apply a layer of wet semirigid casting tape to the upper leg to fix the rigid splint in place

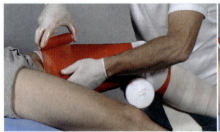

Fold back the tube bandage and hold it in place with semirigid casting tape

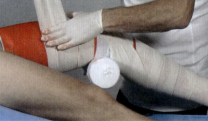

Wrap the wet bandage around the upper leg

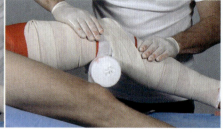

Mold the material over the femoral condyles and the tibial condyles while it sets

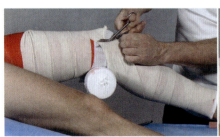

Clear the knee of elastic bandage and tube bandage

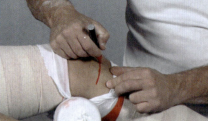

Identify and mark the level of the knee joint

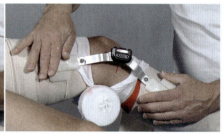

Position a hinge centered over the joint and if needed contour to the leg. Repeat the procedure with the second hinge

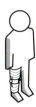

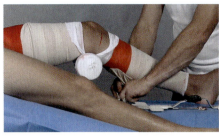

Remove the wet bandage after the casts have set

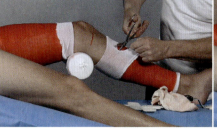

Fold back the ends of the tube bandage over the casts and trim

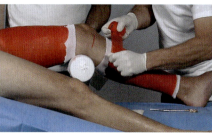

Prepare a roll of semirigid casting tape and apply to the lower leg

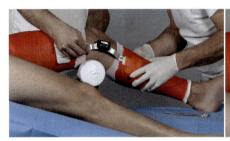

Mount both hinges and wrap the distal ends with semirigid casting tape to hold them in place

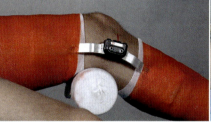

Wrap the proximal ends of the hinges with semirigid casting tape

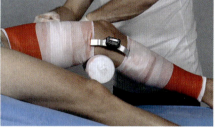

Wrap a wet elastic bandage around the new layer of semirigid casting tape to accelerate the setting

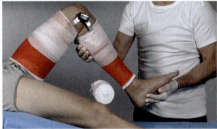

Ensure the hinges allow full extension and flexion of the knee

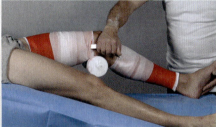

After the casts have set, ensure the hinges are solidly set in place, and remove the wet bandage

FINAL ASSESSMENT

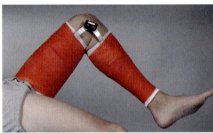

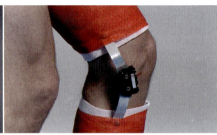

Free flexion and extension of the knee with unblocked hinges

Depending on the injury, flexion and extension of the knee can be limited by blocking the hinges

Klaus Dresing, Jos Engelen

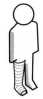

16.5 Dorsal long leg splint using plaster of Paris

16.5

TECHNIQUES

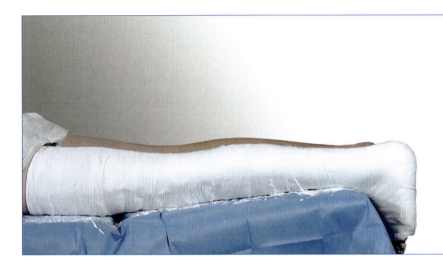

INDICATION

- Fracture of the tibia
- Fractures around the knee

GOAL

- Stabilization of the knee and lower leg

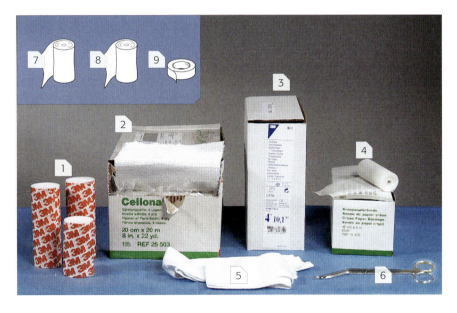

EQUIPMENT

1 Cast padding
2 Plaster of Paris splint 20 cm
3 Tube bandage 10 cm in dispenser box
4 Crepe paper bandage
5 Cut tube bandage
6 Scissors
7 Elastic bandage
8 Gauze bandage
9 Surgical tape or bandage clips

PERSONNEL

2

489

16.5

TECHNIQUES

POSITIONING

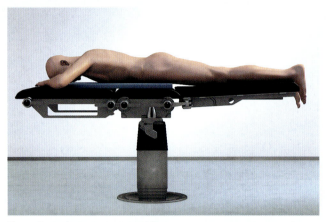

Place the patient prone on a table.

Place the ankle joint in 90° flexion and the knee in 10° flexion.

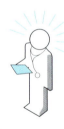

SPECIAL THINGS TO KEEP IN MIND

- An assistant is necessary to support positioning of the affected limb
- Attention should be paid to keep the ankle joint in a functional position (90°)
- When possible, free movement of the toes
- Proximal extension: lesser trochanter–greater trochanter

PROCEDURE

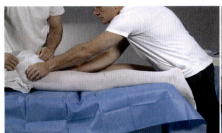

Apply a tube bandage up to the hip.
Pull the bandage tight to avoid any wrinkles

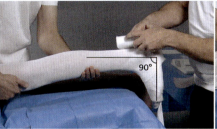

Apply padding over the tube bandage, starting at the foot. Support the knee during application; ensure that the ankle joint is at 90° flexion

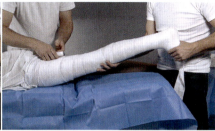

Wrap the leg using the half-overlapping technique

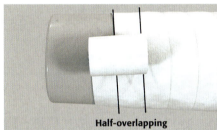

Half-overlapping

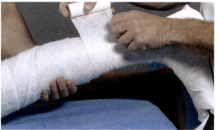

Apply a paper bandage to form a barrier between the dry padding and the wet POP

Wrap the leg using the half-overlapping technique

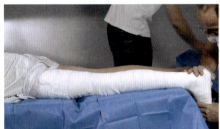

Lay the leg back on the table

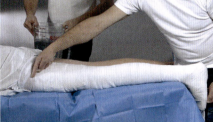

Measure the length of POP splint needed, from the toes to the lesser trochanter – greater trochanter

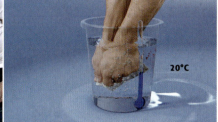

Submerge the POP splint in water for a few seconds, remove, and squeeze out excess water

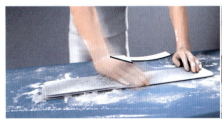

Stretch and smooth out the splint, pressing the layers together, resulting in a compact splint. If this procedure is not done, puff pastry plaster will result, causing an unstable splint

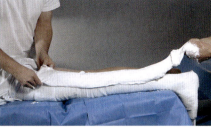

An assistant fans out and molds the proximal end of the splint

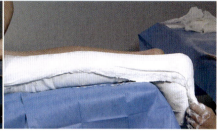

Mold the distal end of the splint to the underside of the foot and trim to the desired shape

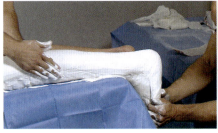

Mold the splint to the desired shape along the complete length

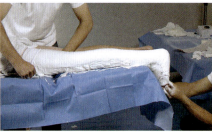

Trim the tube bandage distally and proximally, and fold back over the splint

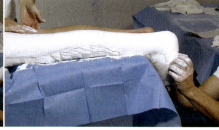

Apply a gauze bandage to the lower leg, from distal to proximal, to hold the splint in place

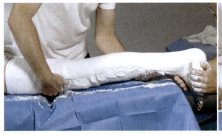

The assistant lifts the leg during application of the gauze bandage

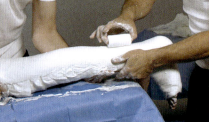

Wrap the lower leg using the half-overlapping technique

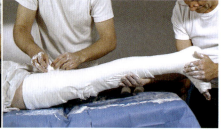

Wrap the upper leg with a gauze bandage

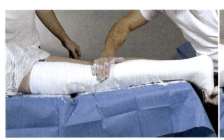

Ensure the knee is at 10° flexion and the ankle joint at 90° flexion

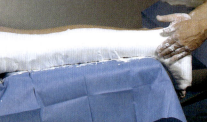

Ensure the splint is molded over the Achilles tendon, both malleoli, the condyles, and there is support for the thigh muscles

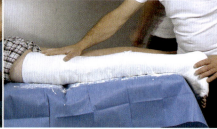

Tap on the splint to check it has set

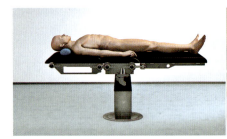

Place the patient in the supine position before splitting the splint

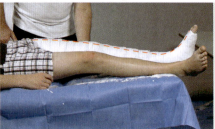

Mark the splitting line, and split all layers on the ventral side

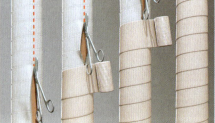

Use the step-by-step splitting and fixing technique to avoid loss of reduction

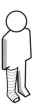

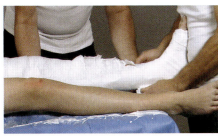

Apply an elastic bandage distally to close the splint

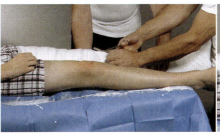

Continue splitting proximally and close with the elastic bandage

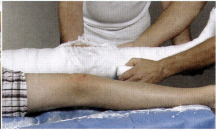

Ensure the knee is supported during the splitting and wrapping

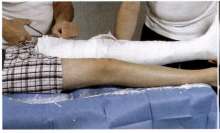

Finish the splitting from proximal and close with the elastic bandage

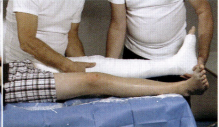

Secure the bandage with surgical tape or bandage clips. Continue supporting the knee for a short time after the splint is closed

FINAL ASSESSMENT

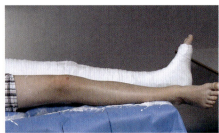

Free movement of the toes

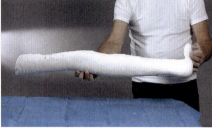

The splint is formed around the contours of the leg and foot

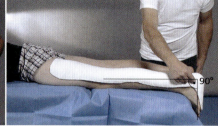

The knee is in 10° flexion and the ankle joint is in 90° flexion

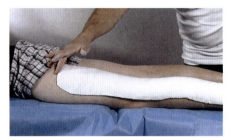

There is sufficient support of the thigh muscles on the dorsal side

Klaus Dresing, Jos Engelen

16.6

TECHNIQUES

16.6 Long leg cast using plaster of Paris

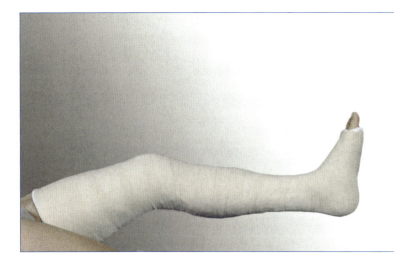

INDICATION

- Fracture of the distal femur
- Fracture of the proximal tibia
- Fracture of the tibial shaft

GOAL

- Stabilization of the distal upper leg and the lower leg

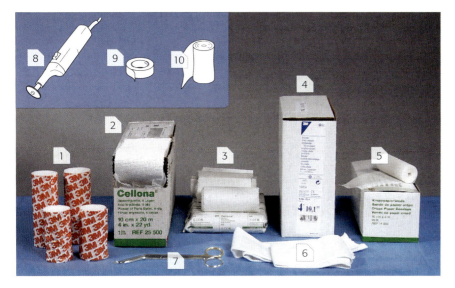

EQUIPMENT

1 Cast padding
2 Plaster of Paris splint 10 cm or 12 cm
3 Plaster of Paris rolls 12 cm or 15 cm
4 Tube bandage 10 cm in dispenser box
5 Crepe paper bandage
6 Cut tube bandage
7 Scissors
8 Oscillating saw
9 Surgical tape or bandage clips
10 Elastic bandage

PERSONNEL

2

495

16.6

TECHNIQUES

POSITIONING

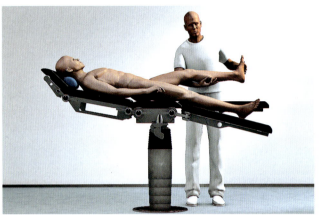

Place the patient supine or seated on a table.

An assistant supports the affected leg; the ankle joint in 90° flexion and the knee in 10–20° flexion.

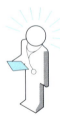

SPECIAL THINGS TO KEEP IN MIND

- An assistant is necessary to support positioning of the affected limb
- Attention should be paid to keep the ankle joint in a functional position (90°)
- When possible, free movement of the toes
- Proximal extension: lesser trochanter–greater trochanter

PROCEDURE

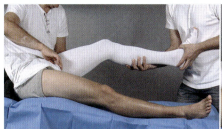

Apply a tube bandage from the foot to the hip. Pull the bandage tight to avoid any wrinkles

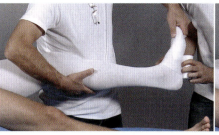

Apply padding over the tube bandage, starting at the foot

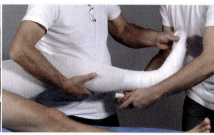

Wrap the leg using the half-overlapping technique

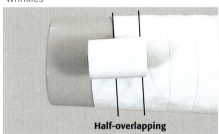

Half-overlapping

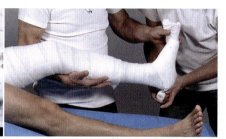

Use a wider roll of padding for the upper leg to make application easier

Apply a paper bandage to form a barrier between the dry padding and the wet POP

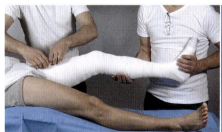

Wrap the leg using the half-overlapping technique

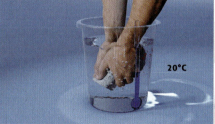

Submerge the roll of POP in water for a few seconds, remove, and squeeze out excess water

20°C

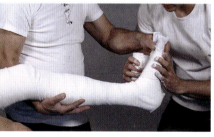

Apply the roll of POP starting distally

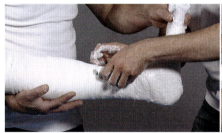

Wrap the leg using the half-overlapping technique

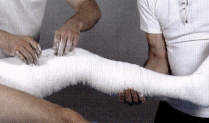

Use a wider roll of POP for the upper leg to make application easier

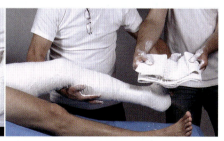

Measure out an 8-layer POP splint and fold it up

497

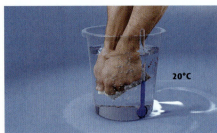

Submerge the POP splint in water for a few seconds, remove, and squeeze out excess water

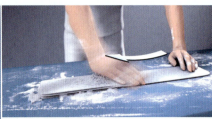

Stretch and smooth out the splint, pressing the layers together, resulting in a compact splint. If this procedure is not done, puff pastry plaster will result, causing an unstable splint

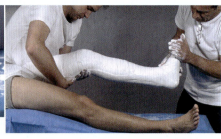

Apply the POP splint and mold to the underside of the foot and the back of the leg

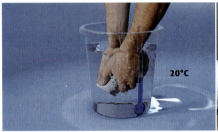

Submerge a roll of POP in water for a few seconds, remove, and squeeze out excess water

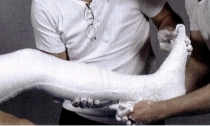

Apply the roll of POP, from distal to proximal, using the half-overlapping technique

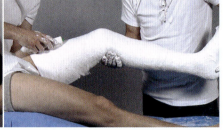

Fold back the tube bandage over the cast proximally, and wrap with POP to hold it in place

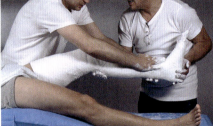

Smooth the complete cast around the leg

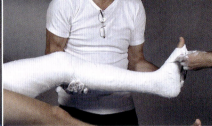

Fold back the tube bandage over the cast distally

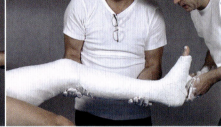

Apply a roll of POP to hold the tube bandage in place

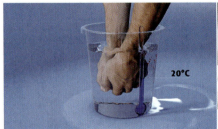

Wet hands make smoothing the cast easier

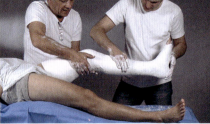

Smooth the complete cast, and mold to the femoral condyles, the patella, and the tibial crest

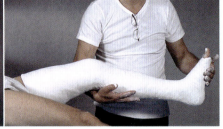

Hold the cast in the desired position while setting

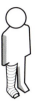

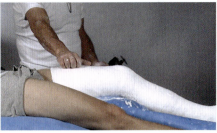

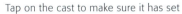

Tap on the cast to make sure it has set

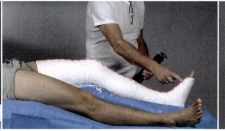

Mark the splitting line on the ventral side

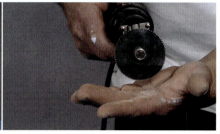

The saw blade oscillates and does not rotate, so there is no direct harm to the skin

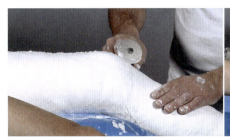

Split the cast; pass laterally to the patella

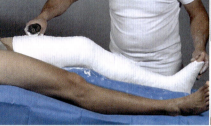

Make a second split, approximately 1 cm laterally to the first, to ensure there is enough space for any swelling

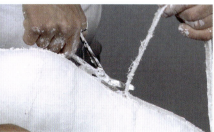

Cut through the padding and the tube bandage completely with the scissors, and remove the strip of cast

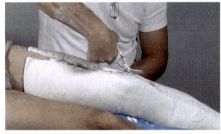

Cut through any remaining material to create a gap in the cast

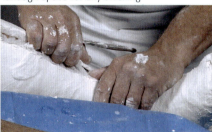

Pull apart the cast slightly to ensure it is completely separated

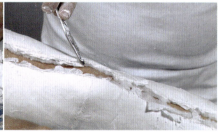

Ensure the split passes laterally to the patella and is on the lateral side of the foot

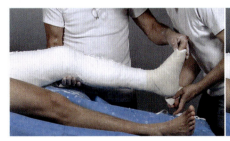

Wrap the complete cast with an elastic bandage

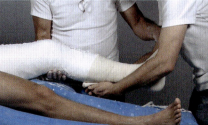

Wrap the leg using the half-overlapping technique

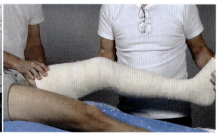

Secure the bandage with surgical tape or bandage clips

FINAL ASSESSMENT

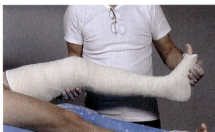
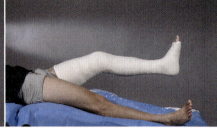

Free movement of the toes and capillary refill

Proximal and distal ends of the cast are smooth to avoid irritation. The ankle joint is in 90° flexion and the knee in 10–20° flexion

Klaus Dresing, Jos Engelen

16.7 Long leg cast using synthetic, combicast technique

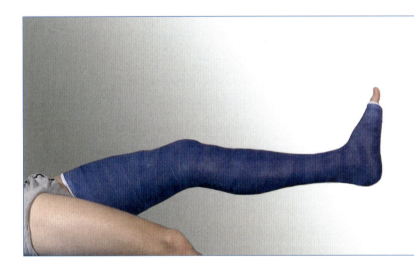

INDICATION

- Fracture of the distal femur
- Fracture of the proximal tibia
- Fracture of the tibial shaft

GOAL

- Stabilization of the distal upper leg and the lower leg

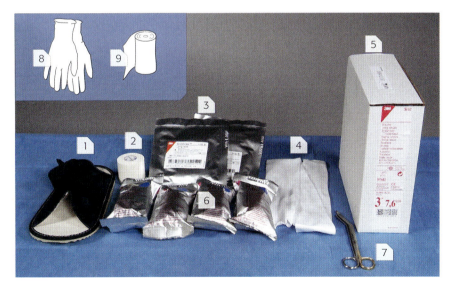

EQUIPMENT

1 Cast shoe
2 Elastic foam tape
3 Rigid synthetic splint 7.5 cm x 70 cm
4 Cut tube bandage
5 Tube bandage 7.5 cm in dispenser box
6 Semirigid casting tape 7.5 cm or 10 cm
7 Scissors
8 Gloves
9 Elastic bandage

PERSONNEL

POSITIONING

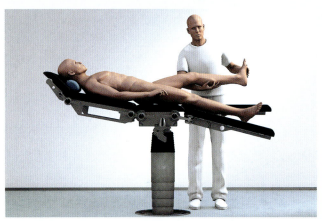

Place the patient supine or seated on a table.

An assistant supports the affected leg; the ankle joint in 90° flexion and the knee in 10–20° flexion

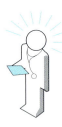

SPECIAL THINGS TO KEEP IN MIND

- An assistant is necessary to support positioning of the affected limb
- Attention should be paid to keep the ankle joint in a functional position (90°)
- When possible, free movement of the toes
- Proximal extension: lesser trochanter–greater trochanter

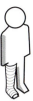

PROCEDURE

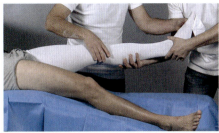

Apply a tube bandage from the foot to the hip. Pull the tube bandage tight to avoid any wrinkles

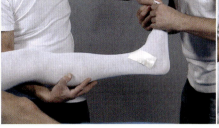

Apply elastic foam tape to protect the bony prominences of the ankle. Ensure there are no wrinkles in the tube bandage

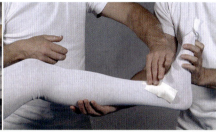

Ensure the extensor tendons are also protected

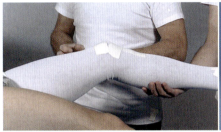

Protect the tibial tuberosity and the patella

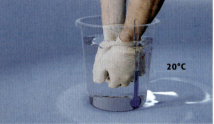

Wet gloves make application of the semirigid casting tape easier

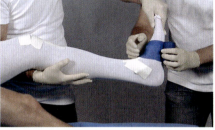

Wrap the semirigid casting tape around the forefoot

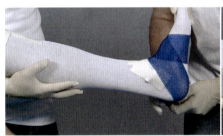

Pass diagonally over the heal and around the forefoot distally

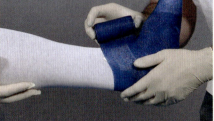

Pass diagonally beneath the foot and over the Achilles tendon

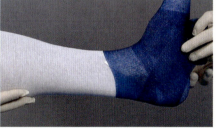

Pass over the heal and diagonally beneath the foot

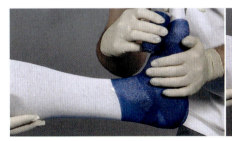

Ensure the ankle joint is in 90° flexion

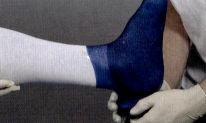

Pass around the forefoot and diagonally down to wrap the ankle

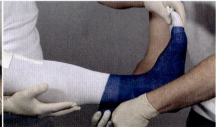

Wrap the leg using the half-overlapping technique

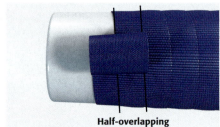

Half-overlapping

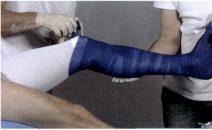

Ensure there are no wrinkles over the knee

Wrap at an angle from the greater trochanter to the lesser trochanter

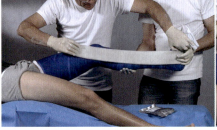

Place the first rigid splint medially, extending just past the knee; an assistant holds it in place distally

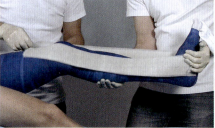

Place a second rigid splint laterally; ensure the ventral and dorsal sides remain open

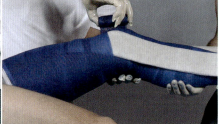

Apply another layer of semirigid casting tape from proximal, to hold the splints in place, using the half-overlapping technique

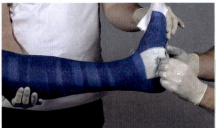

Ensure the splints lie flat over the sole of the foot

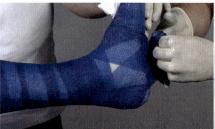

Wrap the ankle using the figure-of-eight technique

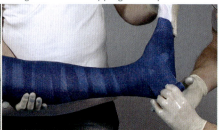

Avoid too many forward wraps, and ensure enough support and stability at the sole of the foot

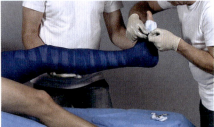

Trim the tube bandage distally, and fold it back over the semirigid casting tape

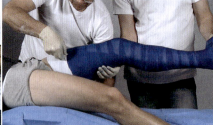

Fold back the tube bandage over the semirigid casting tape proximally

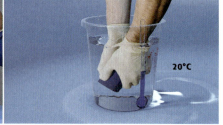

20°C

Submerge the semirigid casting tape in water for a few seconds, remove, and squeeze out excess water

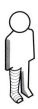

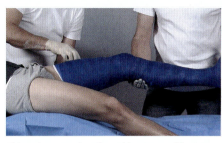

Wrap the complete leg with a second layer of semirigid casting tape, from distal to proximal

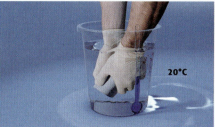

Submerge an elastic bandage in water; using a wet bandage accelerates the setting

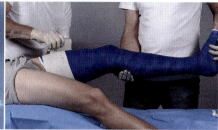

Apply the wet bandage from proximal to distal

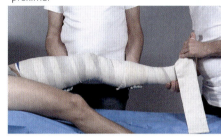

Ensure the ankle joint is in 90° flexion; mold the cast to the arch of the foot

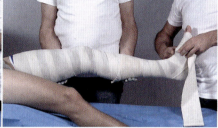

Ensure there are no wrinkles in the cast from dorsal over-flexion of the ankle

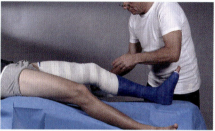

Tap the cast to make sure it has set, and remove the wet bandage

FINAL ASSESSMENT

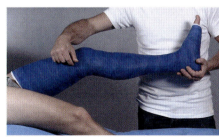

Knee in 10-20° flexion and the ankle joint in 90° flexion

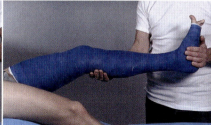

Free movement of the toes, and capillary refill

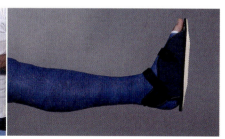

A cast shoe can easily be worn

CAST REMOVAL

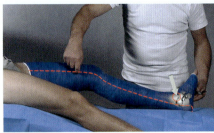

Ensure the splitting line passes dorsally to the medial malleolus

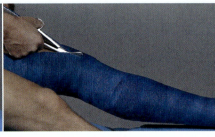

Use the scissors to cut completely through the cast, from proximal to distal

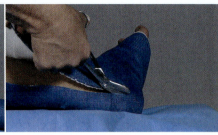

Guide the scissors dorsally to the medial malleolus

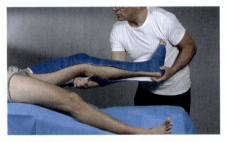

Fold back the cut section and gently remove the cast

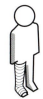

16.8 Sarmiento (patella tendon bearing) cast using plaster of Paris

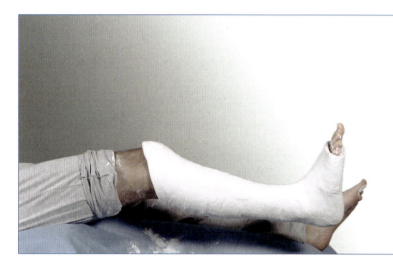

INDICATION

- Stable diaphyseal fractures of the tibia limited to the distal two-thirds of the tibial shaft
- Primary unstable tibial fractures at the hard callus formation stage

GOAL

- Stabilization of the lower leg

EQUIPMENT

1. Cast padding
2. Plaster of Paris splint 12 cm or 15 cm
3. Plaster of Paris rolls 12 cm or 15 cm
4. Tube bandage 7.5 cm in dispenser box
5. Crepe paper bandage
6. Cut tube bandage
7. Scissors

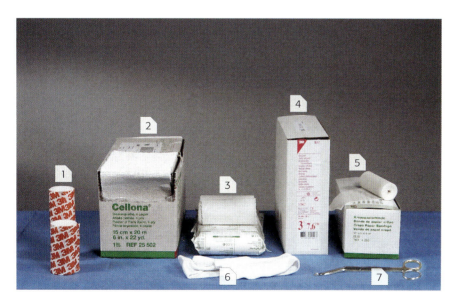

PERSONNEL

507

16.8 Sarmiento (patella tendon bearing) cast using plaster of Paris

16.8

TECHNIQUES

POSITIONING

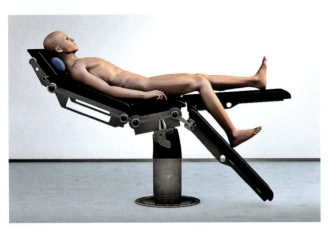

Place the patient supine or seated on a table.
Place the knee in approximately 60° flexion and the ankle joint in 90° flexion.

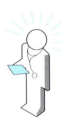

SPECIAL THINGS TO KEEP IN MIND

- Support at the patella tendon and the tibial condyles
- Free movement of the knee joint
- Free movement of the toes

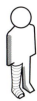
PROCEDURE

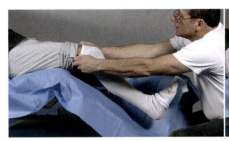

Apply a tube bandage from the foot to over the knee

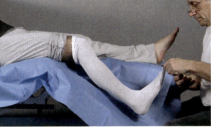

Pull the tube bandage tight to avoid any wrinkles, and trim distally

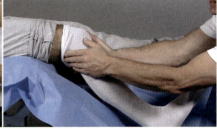

Ensure the tube bandage extends past the femoral condyles

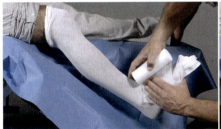

Apply the padding over the tube bandage

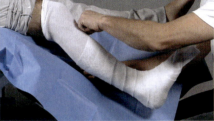

Wrap the leg using the half-overlapping technique

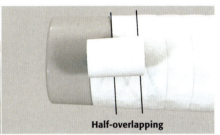

Half-overlapping

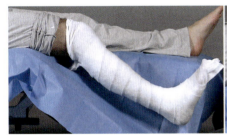

Ensure the padding covers the entire patella

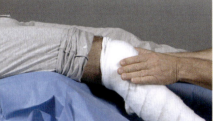

Apply a thick layer of padding over the patella, and a thin layer over the tibial tuberosity, to provide the correct support

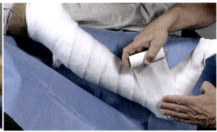

Apply a paper bandage to form a barrier between the dry padding and the wet POP

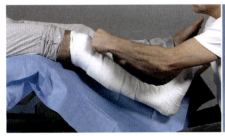

Wrap the leg using the half-overlapping technique

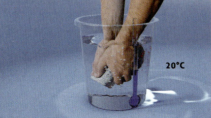

Submerge a roll of POP in water for a few seconds, remove, and squeeze out excess water

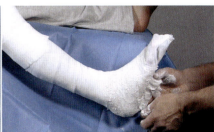

Apply the roll of POP starting distally

16.8 Sarmiento (patella tendon bearing) cast using plaster of Paris

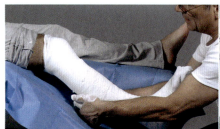

Wrap the leg using the half-overlapping technique

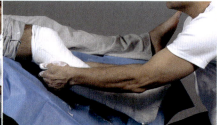

Apply extra layers of POP over the patella

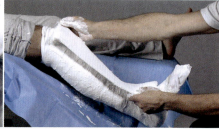

Prepare a POP splint to be applied ventrally, and over the patella

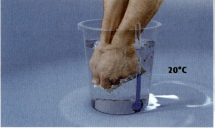

Submerge the POP splint in water for a few seconds, remove, and squeeze out excess water

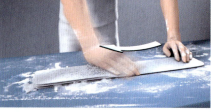

Stretch and smooth out the splint, pressing the layers together, resulting in a compact splint. If this procedure is not done, puff pastry plaster will result, causing an unstable splint

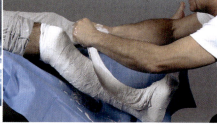

Apply the POP splint ventrally

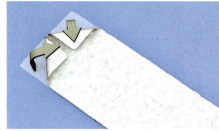

Fold over the proximal corners

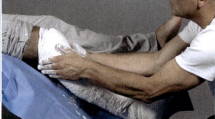

Mold the splint to the knee

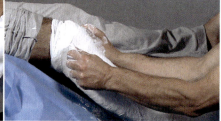

Apply a short POP splint across the tibial condyles for extra support

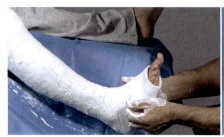

Fold back the tube bandage over the cast distally

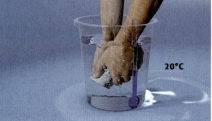

Submerge a roll of POP in water for a few seconds, remove, and squeeze out excess water

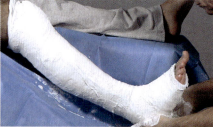

Apply the roll of POP, from distal to proximal, to fix the tube bandage and the POP splint in place

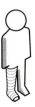

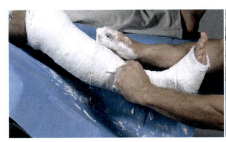

Wrap the leg using the half-overlapping technique

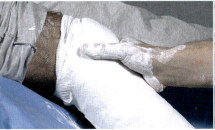

As the POP begins to set, it must be perfectly molded to the patella tendon and the tibial condyles

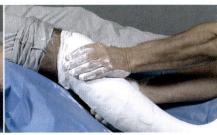

Mold the POP splint to form two dents at the tibial condyles, medial and lateral of the tibial tuberosity

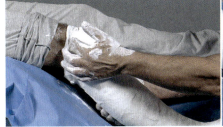

After the cast has set, trim it to allow free movement of the knee

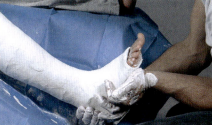

Ensure the ankle joint is in 90° flexion

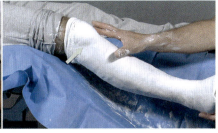

Lateral dent is visible on the cast

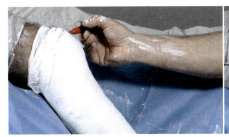

Mark the cast where it should be trimmed proximally

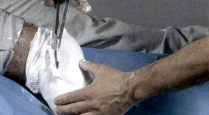

Trim the cast with cast scissors or an oscillating saw

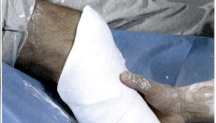

Fold back the tube bandage and the padding over the cast to form a smooth edge

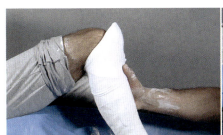

Ensure free movement of the knee is possible

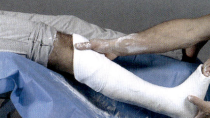

In extension, the support lies over the patella and the patella tendon

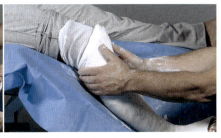

Fold back the tube bandage to reveal the padding

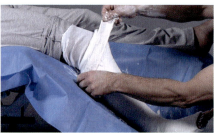

Apply wet strips of POP to fix the padding to the cast

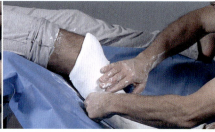

Fold back the tube bandage over the cast

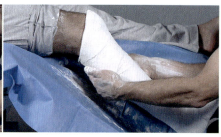

Apply a wet roll of POP to fix the tube bandage to the cast

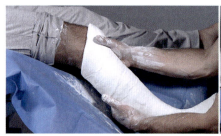

Mold the cast to give a smooth finish proximally

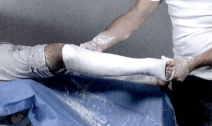

Ensure perfect molding of the cast to the patella tendon and the tibial condyles has occurred

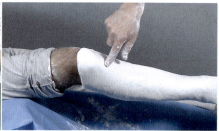

The triangular shape allows control of rotation

FINAL ASSESSMENT

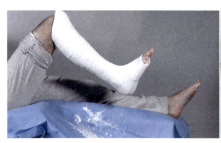

There is flexion and extension of the knee and toes

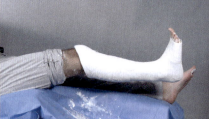

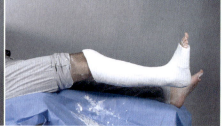

During weight bearing, the force is transmitted from the condyles to the cast to protect the fracture region from weight bearing

16.9 Sarmiento tibial brace using synthetic, combicast technique

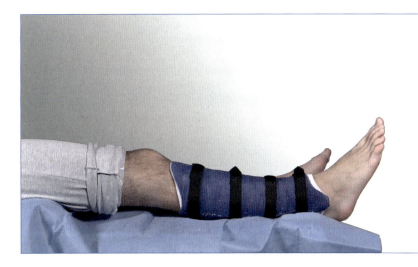

INDICATION

- Some diaphyseal fractures of the tibia
- Not recommended for primary fracture care

GOAL

- Stabilization of the tibia

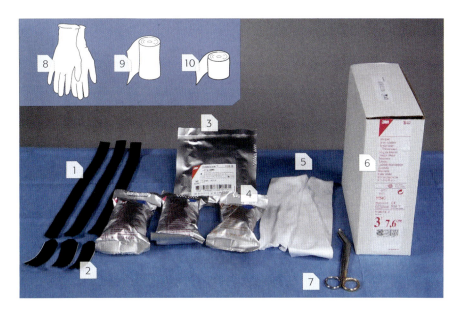

EQUIPMENT

1 Velcro strips nonadhesive (hook)
2 Velcro strips adhesive (loop)
3 Rigid synthetic splint 7.5 cm x 45 cm
4 Semirigid casting tape 7.5 cm
5 Cut tube bandage
6 Tube bandage 7.5 cm in dispenser box
7 Scissors
8 Gloves
9 Elastic bandage
10 Elastic foam tape

PERSONNEL

POSITIONING

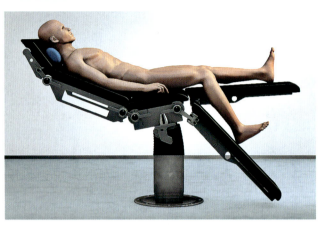

Place the patient supine or seated on a table.

Place the knee in approximately 60° flexion and the ankle joint in 90° flexion.

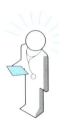

SPECIAL THINGS TO KEEP IN MIND

- The casting material is applied circularly; after it is split it will be reapplied and used as a brace fixed with velcro straps
- The brace must be tight enough to obtain the compression effect
- Free movement of the knee and ankle joint
- Functional treatment

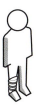

Klaus Dresing, Jos Engelen

PROCEDURE

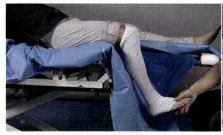

Apply a tube bandage from the foot to over the knee

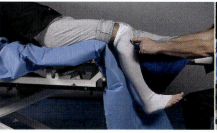

On the ventral side, a rigid splint will be applied to give support; elsewhere, semirigid material will be used

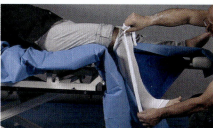

Insert a second tube bandage under the first on the dorsal side; it will be used later to make splitting the brace easier

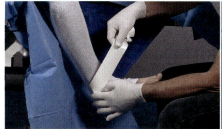

Apply elastic foam tape to protect the bony prominences

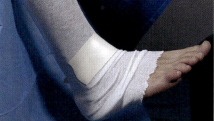

Place the first strip of elastic foam tape from the lateral malleolus to the medial malleolus

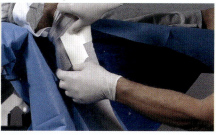

Apply elastic foam tape over the tibial tuberosity and the fibular head

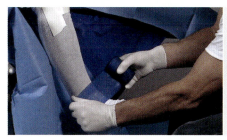

Apply semirigid casting tape from distal to proximal; begin with circular wraps, then use the half-overlapping technique

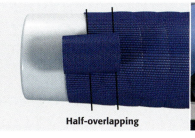

Half-overlapping

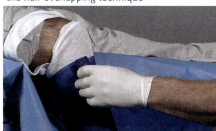

The leg hangs free during this procedure

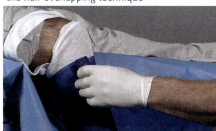

Apply the semirigid casting tape over the elastic foam tape; it will be trimmed later

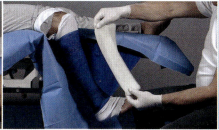

Apply a rigid splint on the ventral side for extra support. Fold the rigid splint in half and fan out the proximal end

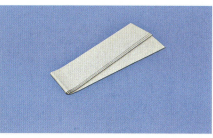

515

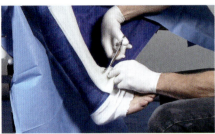

Trim the rigid splint distally to avoid pressure on the extensor tendons

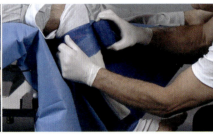

Apply a second layer of semirigid casting tape proximally

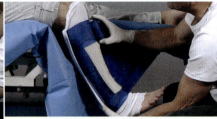

Fold the inner tube bandage back, from proximal to distal, and wrap with semirigid casting tape. This procedure will allow the brace to be closed with an overlapping edge

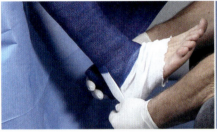

Apply the semirigid casting tape distally to cover the rigid splint, and mold it to the malleoli

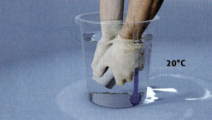

Submerge the elastic bandage in water; using a wet bandage accelerates the setting

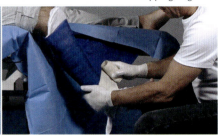

Apply the wet bandage, from distal to proximal, using the half-overlapping technique

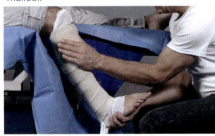

Hold the ankle in dorsiflexion, and mold the brace to the tibia

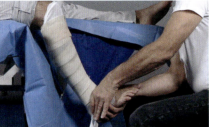

Hold the brace in the desired position until it is set

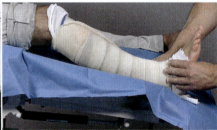

When the brace has set, place the leg in the horizontal position, and remove the wet bandage

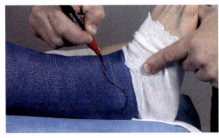

Prepare the brace for trimming; mark the distal tibia, the lateral malleolus, and the medial malleolus. Connect these points to mark the distal trimming line

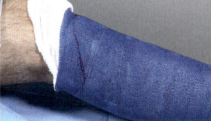

The proximal border of the brace is from the tibial tuberosity to 2 cm below the fibular head, to allow free movement of the knee

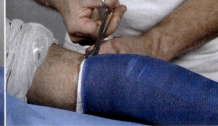

Cut through the folded-over tube bandage proximally

Klaus Dresing, Jos Engelen

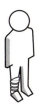

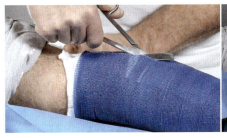

Slide one blade of the scissors into the outer tube bandage and split open the outer layer of semirigid casting tape

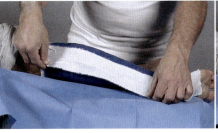

Trim the tube bandage distally, fold back the split layer, and remove the outer section of the tube bandage

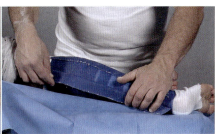

This flap will be used as an overlap when the brace is closed

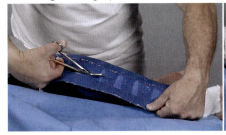

The flap is opened and the tube bandage and the lower layer are cut through, contralaterally to the first cut

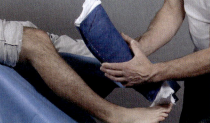

Lower the leg and remove the brace

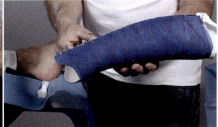

Trim the brace along the marked edges with the scissors

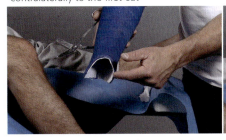

The shape of the lateral malleolus and the medial malleolus are visible in the brace

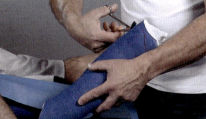

Trim the proximal edge of the brace

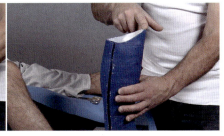

The elastic foam tape is cut through; the ventral and dorsal height difference is clear

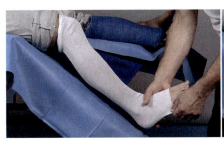

Apply a new tube bandage, or a long sock, to prevent any irritation of the skin

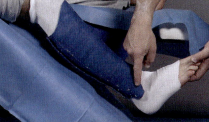

Reapply the brace. Distally, the support lies directly over the lateral malleolus and the medial malleolus

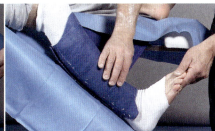

Ensure free movement of the ankle joint is possible

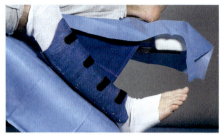

Apply four short strips of adhesive velcro (with hooks) to the brace

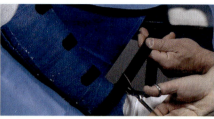

Attach a long strip of velcro (with loops) to the short velcro, pass around the leg, tighten, and close the brace. Trim any excess velcro by making two 45° cuts

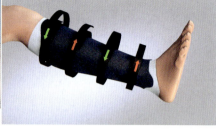

Alternate the direction of the velcro strips to avoid any rotation of the brace

FINAL ASSESSMENT

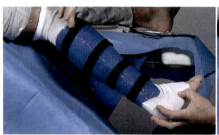

The brace is closed on the dorsal side

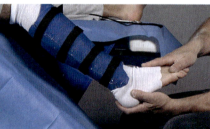

Free flexion and extension of the ankle joint

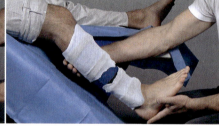

Fold over the tube bandage, distally and proximally, to protect the skin

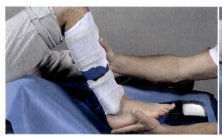

Free movement of the knee

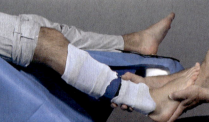

Due to closure with velcro, the brace does not slip

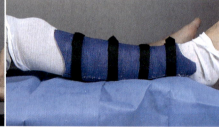

If the brace becomes loose, the velcro strips allow easy retightening

16.10 Dorsal short leg splint using plaster of Paris

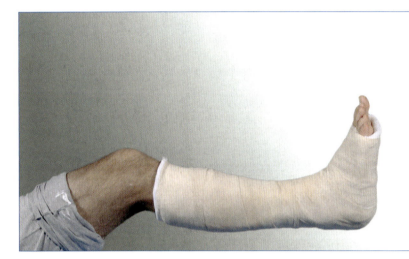

INDICATION

- Fracture of the ankle
- Fracture of the tarsal bones
- Ligamentous ruptures

GOAL

- Stabilization of the ankle joint and foot

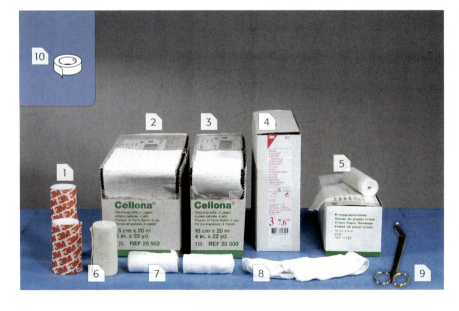

EQUIPMENT

1 Cast padding
2 Plaster of Paris splint 15 cm or 20 cm
3 Plaster of Paris splint 10 cm
4 Tube bandage 7.5 cm in dispenser box
5 Crepe paper bandage
6 Elastic bandage
7 Gauze bandage
8 Cut tube bandage
9 Scissors
10 Surgical tape or bandage clips

PERSONNEL

POSITIONING

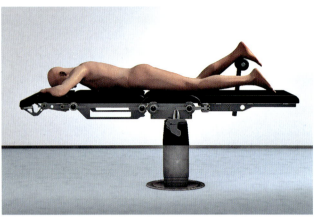

Place the patient prone (whenever possible) or supine on a table.
Place the affected leg on a support, with the ankle joint in 90° flexion.

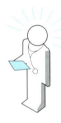

SPECIAL THINGS TO KEEP IN MIND

- Ensure the fibula head remains free a minimum of 2 cm to avoid pressure on the peroneal nerve
- Free flexion of the knee
- When possible, free movement of the toes

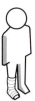

PROCEDURE

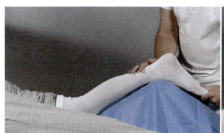

Apply a tube bandage from the foot to over the knee

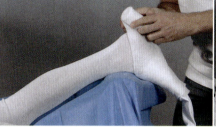

Apply the padding over the tube bandage, from distal to proximal

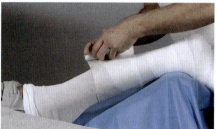

Wrap the leg using the half-overlapping technique

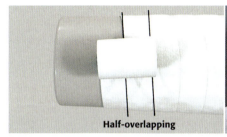

Half-overlapping

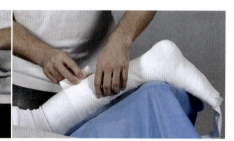

Apply a paper bandage to form a barrier between the dry padding and the wet POP

Wrap the leg using the half-overlapping technique

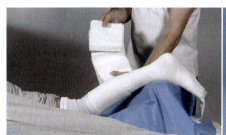

Prepare the posterior POP splint

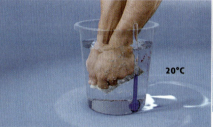

20°C

Submerge the POP splint in water for a few seconds, remove, and squeeze out excess water

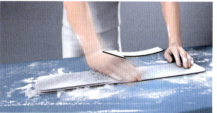

Stretch and smooth out the splint, pressing the layers together, resulting in a compact splint. If this procedure is not done, puff pastry plaster will result, causing an unstable splint

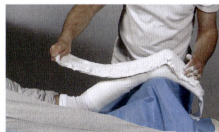

Apply the L-shaped POP splint, starting at the foot

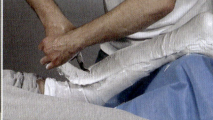

Trim the splint proximally, and mold it to the leg

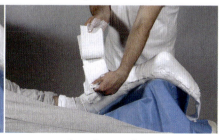

Prepare a U-shaped POP splint

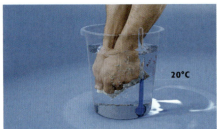

Submerge the POP splint in water for a few seconds, remove, and squeeze out excess water

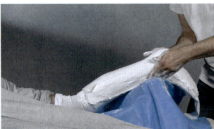

Apply the U-shaped POP splint under the heel, and medially and laterally along the lower leg. Mold the splint from distal to proximal

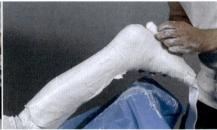

Wrap the splint with a gauze bandage, beginning distally

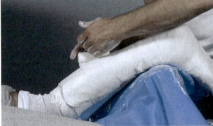

Wrap the leg using the half-overlapping technique

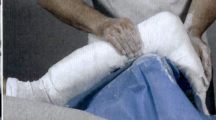

Mold the complete splint to the desired shape

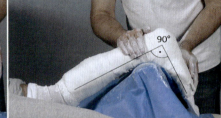

Hold the ankle joint in 90° flexion while setting

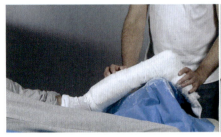

Tap on the splint to check it has set

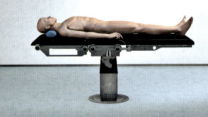

After the splint has set, turn the patient from the prone to the supine position

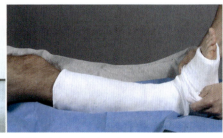

Fold back the tube bandage over the splint, proximally and distally

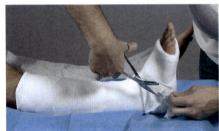

Trim the excess tube bandage

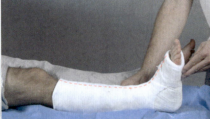

Mark the splitting line

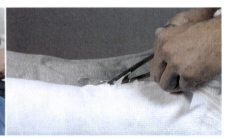

Split the complete splint, including the tube bandage, with the scissors

Klaus Dresing, Jos Engelen

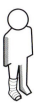

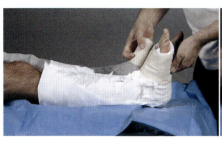

Wrap the splint with an elastic bandage, from distal to proximal

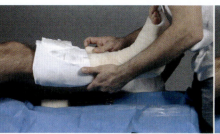

Wrap the leg using the half-overlapping technique

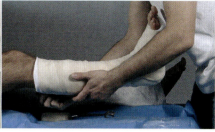

Secure the bandage with surgical tape or bandage clips

FINAL ASSESSMENT

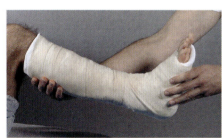

Free flexion of the knee

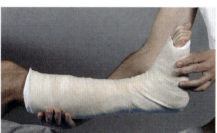

Free movement of the toes

16.10

TECHNIQUES

Klaus Dresing, Jos Engelen

16.11 Dorsal short leg splint using synthetic

16.11

TECHNIQUES

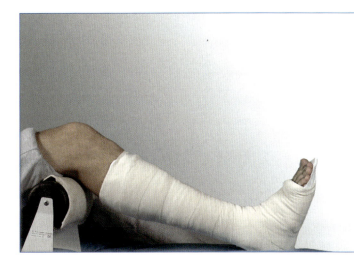

INDICATION

- Fracture of the ankle
- Fracture of the tarsal bones
- Ligamentous ruptures

GOAL

- Stabilization of the ankle joint and foot

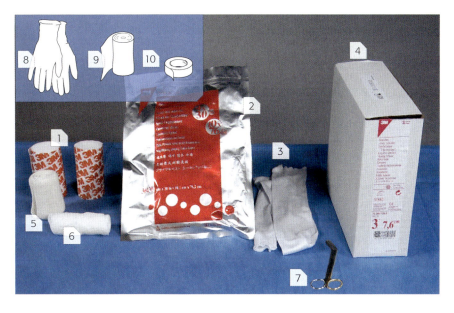

EQUIPMENT

1 Cast padding
2 Rigid synthetic splint 10 cm or 12.5 cm x 76 cm
3 Cut tube bandage
4 Tube bandage 7.5 cm in dispenser box
5 Elastic bandage
6 Gauze bandage
7 Scissors
8 Gloves
9 Elastic bandage
10 Surgical tape or bandage clips

PERSONNEL

525

16.11

TECHNIQUES

POSITIONING

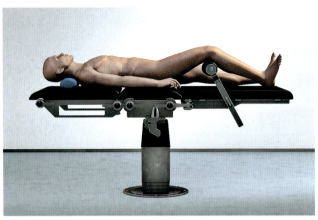

Place the patient supine or prone on a table.

Place the affected leg on a support, with the ankle joint in 90° flexion.

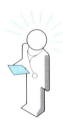

SPECIAL THINGS TO KEEP IN MIND

- Ensure the fibula head remains free a minimum of 2 cm to avoid pressure on the peroneal nerve
- Free flexion of the knee
- When possible, free movement of the toes

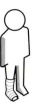

PROCEDURE

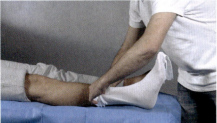

Apply a tube bandage over the foot and ankle

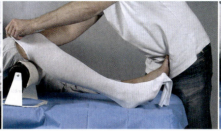

Place the knee on a support; pull the tube bandage over the knee and pull it tight to avoid any wrinkles

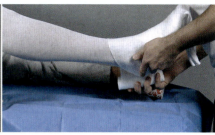

Apply the padding, from distal to proximal

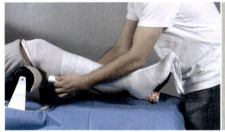

Wrap the leg using the half-overlapping technique

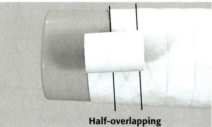

Half-overlapping

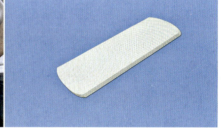

Prepare two U-shaped splints and a footplate splint

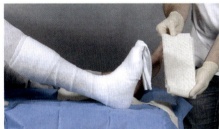

Remove one layer of splint and fold in three to make the footplate splint

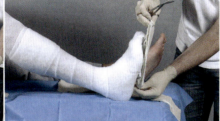

Trim the splint to fit the foot

Shape the splint like this

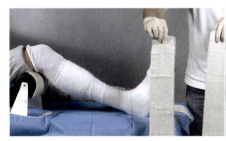

Separate the remaining splint layers in two to make the U-shaped splints

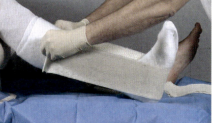

Place the first splint beneath the foot, and at equal length along both sides of the leg

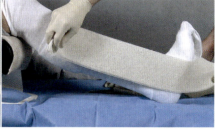

For patients with longer legs, place more of the splint on one side of the leg than the other

527

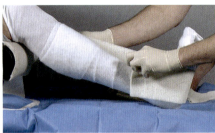

Place a second splint on the other side of the leg

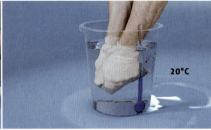

Submerge the rigid splint in water for a few seconds, remove, and squeeze out excess water

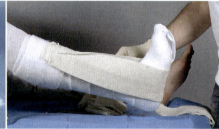

If you are working alone, apply the first U-shaped splint and fold the ends over each other

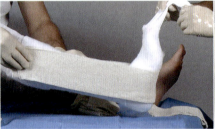

If an assistant is available, they hold the first U-shaped splint in place while the footplate splint is applied

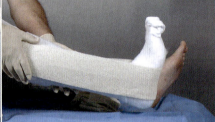

Fold up the distal end of the tube bandage

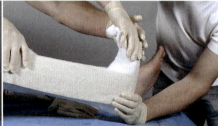

Apply the wet footplate splint; fan out the splint over the heel to prevent a thick edge forming, and mold to the sole of the foot

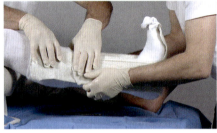

Apply the second U-shaped splint over the first

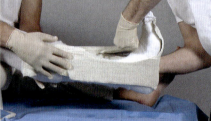

Remove a section of the splints over the dorsal distal tibia with the scissors

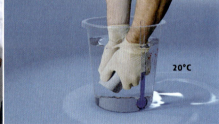

Submerge a gauze bandage in water for a few seconds, remove, and squeeze out excess water

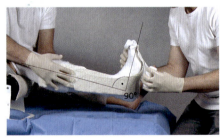

Ensure the ankle joint is in 90° flexion; apply the gauze bandage starting distally

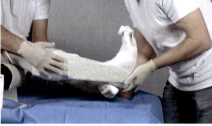

As the gauze bandage is applied, mold the splint to the foot and leg

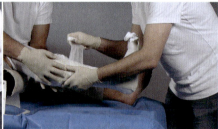

Wrap the leg using the half-overlapping technique

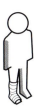

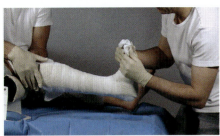

Mold the complete splint to the desired shape

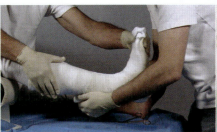

Apply a second layer of wet gauze bandage, beginning proximally

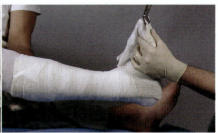

Trim the footplate splint to match the shape of the toes

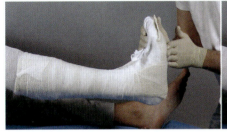

Mold the footplate splint to match the contours of the foot

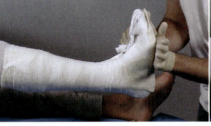

When working on the right leg, apply the ball of the left thumb to the arch of the foot to mold the splint

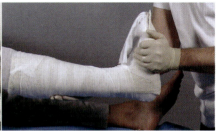

Hold the foot in the desired position until the splint is set

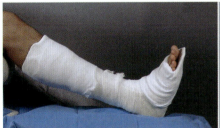

Tap on the splint to check it has set. Fold back the tube bandage over the splint, distally and proximally

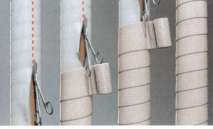

Split the splint completely, using the step-by-step splitting and fixing technique

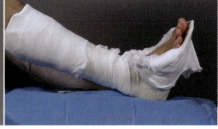

Begin the splitting distally, cutting through all layers

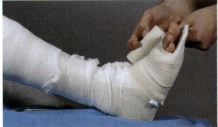

Fix the cut section with an elastic bandage

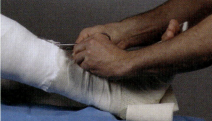

Cut through another section of the splint

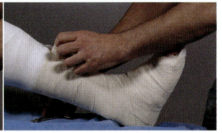

Wrap the leg using the half-overlapping technique

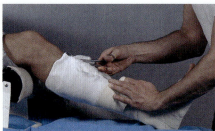

Split and fix the rest of the splint; using the splitting and fixing technique avoids loss of reduction

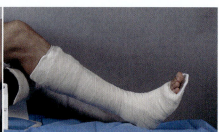

Secure the bandage with surgical tape or bandage clips

FINAL ASSESSMENT

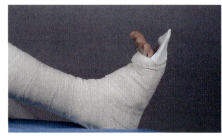

Extension and flexion of the toes is possible

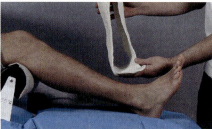

In the frontal aspect, the splint is U-shaped

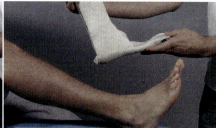

In the lateral aspect, the ankle joint is at 90°

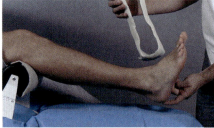

In the dorsal aspect, the splint is U-shaped and molded to the sole of the foot and covers the toes

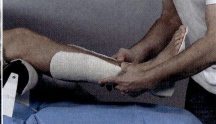

The splint stops two finger's breadth below the fibula head

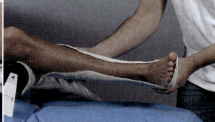

The splint is formed to the sole of the foot and the leg

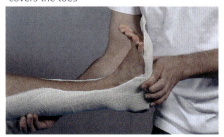

The splint allows free movement of the toes

Klaus Dresing, Jos Engelen

16.12 Short leg cast using rigid synthetic

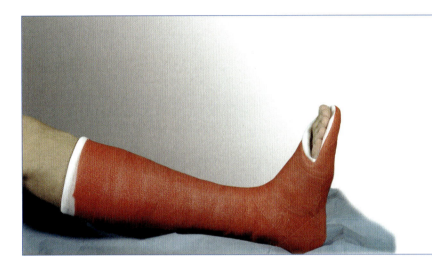

INDICATION

Secondary treatment of:
- Fracture of the distal tibia
- Fracture of the ankle
- Fracture of the foot

GOAL

- Stabilization of the distal tibia, the ankle, and the foot

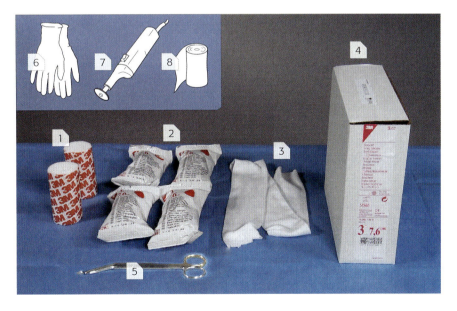

EQUIPMENT

1 Cast padding
2 Rigid casting tape 7.5 cm or 10 cm
3 Cut tube bandage
4 Tube bandage 7.5 cm in dispenser box
5 Scissors
6 Gloves
7 Oscillating saw
8 Elastic bandage

PERSONNEL

16.12

TECHNIQUES

POSITIONING

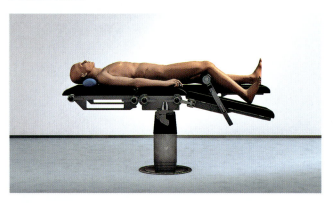

Place the patient supine on a table.

Place the knee on a support in 45-60° flexion and the ankle joint in 90° flexion.

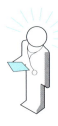

SPECIAL THINGS TO KEEP IN MIND

- Ensure the fibula head remains free a minimum of 2 cm to avoid pressure on the peroneal nerve
- Free flexion of the knee
- Free extension, and if possible, flexion of the toes
- Pressure sores

Klaus Dresing, Jos Engelen

PROCEDURE

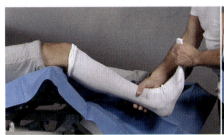

Apply a tube bandage from the foot to the knee

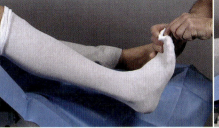

Tie a knot in the tube bandage and place the knot between the first and second toes to avoid excess compression across the toes

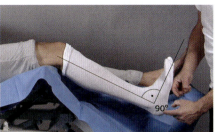

Position the ankle joint in 90° flexion

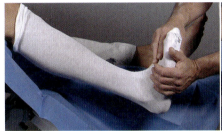

Ensure the foot is positioned halfway between supination and pronation

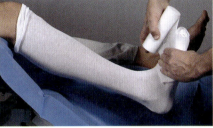

Apply the padding; wrap the padding past the end of the toes to provide extra protection

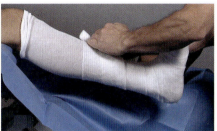

Wrap the leg using the half-overlapping technique

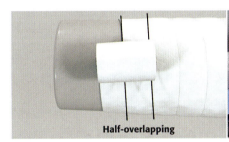

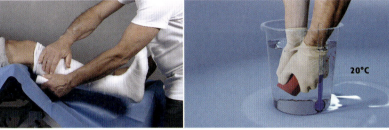

Extend the padding higher than the final height of the cast; when it is folded over, there is a soft edge to the cast

Submerge a roll of rigid casting tape in water for a few seconds, remove, and squeeze out excess water

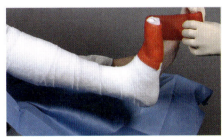

Apply the rigid casting tape; wrap the ends of the toes three times, without applying any compression

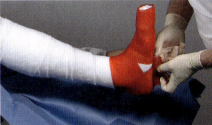

Wrap the ankle using the figure-of-eight technique

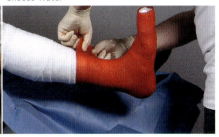

Wrap the leg using the half-overlapping technique

533

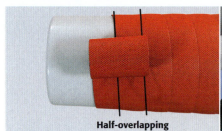

Half-overlapping

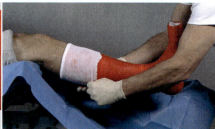

Fold back the tube bandage and the padding over the rigid casting tape proximally

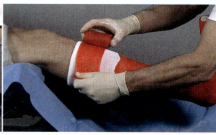

Apply another layer of wet rigid casting tape, starting proximally

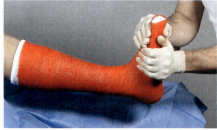

Mold the cast to the contours of the foot

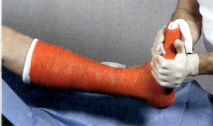

Pull out the tube bandage from between the toes to release pressure and allow movement of the toes

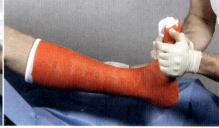

Hold the foot and ankle in the desired position until the cast is set

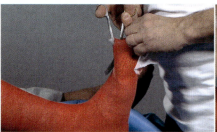

Remove part of the cast over the toes, cut down to the base of the big toe

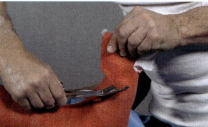

Cut across to the base of the little toe

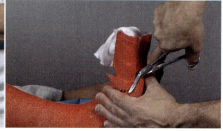

Cut below the level of the little toe to ensure it is completely free at the dorsal aspect to allow free movement

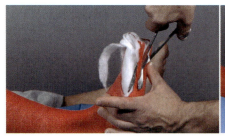

Trim the base of the cast to match the shape of the foot

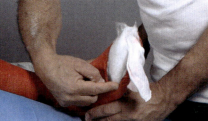

Ensure the cast is open from the base of the big toe to the base of the little toe

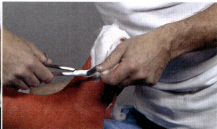

Remove the padding from over the toes

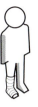

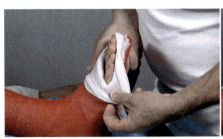

Fold back the tube bandage to check that all the toes are free

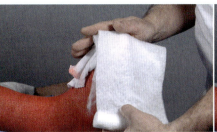

Apply additional layers of padding beneath the toes for extra protection and comfort

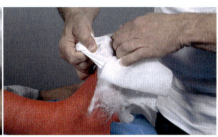

Tuck the padding under the tube bandage and cut off the excess

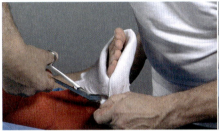

Fold back the tube bandage over the cast, and trim

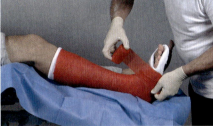

Apply another layer of wet rigid casting tape over the tube bandage

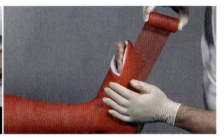

Apply longitudinal plantar fixation of the forefoot to finish the cast

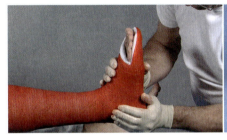

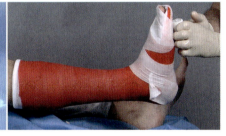

Submerge an elastic bandage in water; using a wet bandage accelerates the setting

Apply the wet elastic bandage around the foot

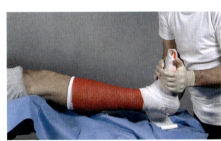

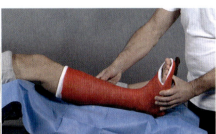

Hold the foot and ankle in the desired position during setting

After the cast has set, remove the wet bandage

FINAL ASSESSMENT

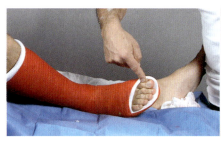 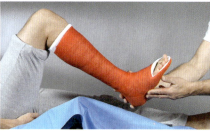 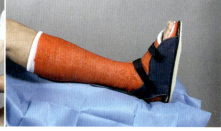

All toes are free and have a full extension

Flexion and extension of the knee is possible and the ankle joint is in 90° flexion

If weight bearing is allowed, the use of a cast shoe is mandatory

CAST REMOVAL

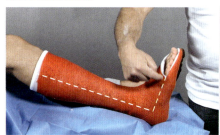 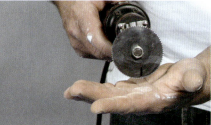 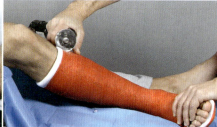

Mark the splitting lines; avoid the lateral and the medial malleolus

The saw blade oscillates and does not rotate, so there is no direct harm to the skin

Split the cast with the oscillating saw; begin on the medial side

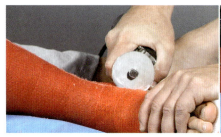 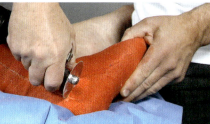 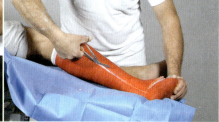

To remove the anterior section of the cast, cut just above the medial malleolus and just below the lateral malleolus

Turn the leg and split the lateral side of the cast

Cut through the padding and the tube bandage on both sides of the cast using scissors

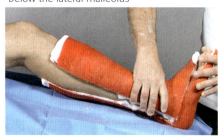

Remove both sections of the cast

Klaus Dresing, Jos Engelen

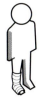

16.13 Short leg cast using synthetic, combicast technique

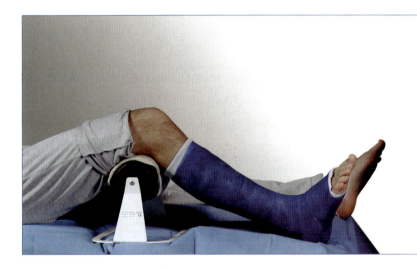

INDICATION

Secondary treatment of:
- Fracture of the distal tibia
- Fracture of the ankle
- Fracture of the foot

GOAL

- Stabilization of the distal tibia, the ankle, and the foot

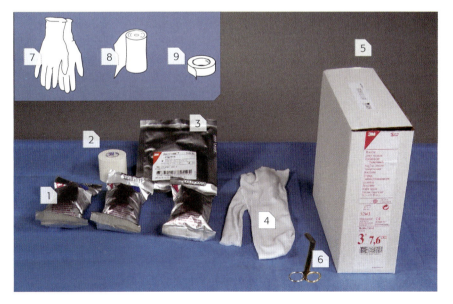

EQUIPMENT

1 Semirigid casting tape 7.5 cm
2 Elastic foam tape
3 Rigid synthetic splint 7.5 cm x 70 cm
4 Cut tube bandage
5 Tube bandage 7.5 cm in dispenser box
6 Scissors
7 Gloves
8 Elastic bandage
9 Surgical tape or bandage clips

PERSONNEL

POSITIONING

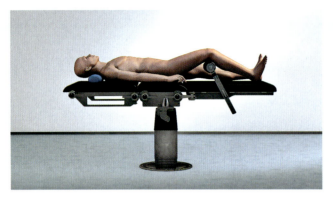

Place the patient supine on a table.

Place the knee on a support in 45–60° flexion and the ankle joint in 90° flexion.

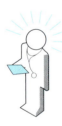

SPECIAL THINGS TO KEEP IN MIND

- Ensure the fibula head remains free a minimum of 2 cm to avoid pressure on the peroneal nerve
- Free flexion of the knee
- Free extension, and if possible, flexion of the toes
- Pressure sores

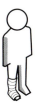

PROCEDURE

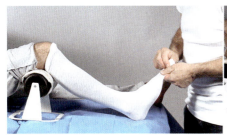

Apply a tube bandage from the foot to the knee. Pull the tube bandage tight to avoid any wrinkles

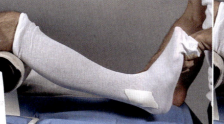

Apply elastic foam tape to protect the bony prominences: the lateral malleolus and the medial malleolus

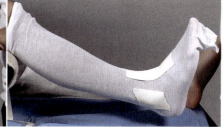

The extensor tendons should also be protected

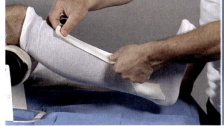

The tibial crest should also be protected

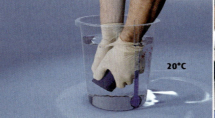

Submerge the semirigid casting tape in water for a few seconds, remove, and squeeze out excess water

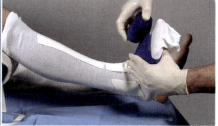

Apply the semirigid casting tape around the forefoot, leaving the toes free

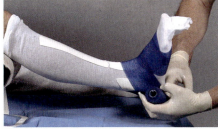

Wrap diagonally over the ankle, to the medial malleolus, and across the Achilles tendon

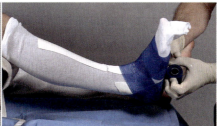

Pass diagonally beneath the foot

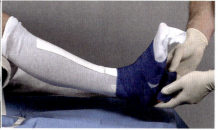

Pass over the lateral malleolus, the ankle joint, the Achilles tendon, and diagonally beneath the foot

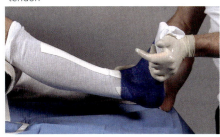

Support the lateral side of the foot

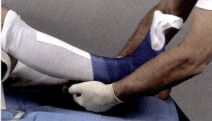

Wrap the leg using the half-overlapping technique

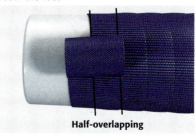

Half-overlapping

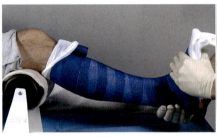

Fold back the tube bandage proximally to hold the roll of semirigid casting tape in place

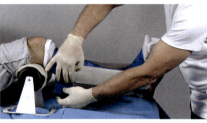

Apply a U-shaped rigid splint beneath the foot, and medially and laterally along the lower leg. Hold the rigid splint in place with semirigid casting tape

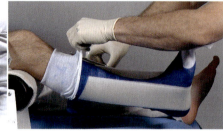

Fold back the tube bandage over the semirigid casting tape, proximally and distally, and trim it

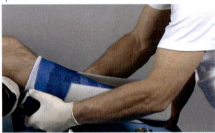

Apply another layer of wet semirigid casting tape over the rigid splint

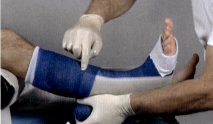

Ensure the rigid splint does not cover the ventral side of the leg

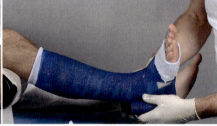

Wrap the ankle using the figure-of-eight technique

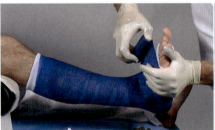

Wrap the distal edge of the cast, lateral to medial, to avoid supination

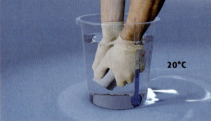

Submerge an elastic bandage in water; using a wet bandage accelerates the setting

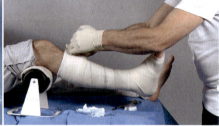

Wrap the complete cast with the elastic bandage

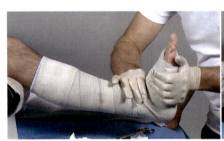

Mold the cast to the desired position

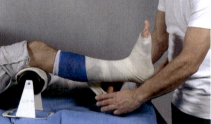

Tap on the cast to check it has set, and remove the wet bandage

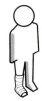

Klaus Dresing, Jos Engelen

16.14 Antirotation short leg cast using synthetic, combicast technique

16.14

TECHNIQUES

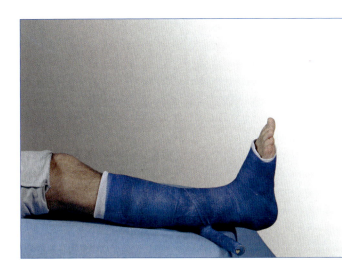

INDICATION

- Traumatic hip dislocation
- Hip dislocation after arthroplasty

GOAL

- To prevent rotation of the leg

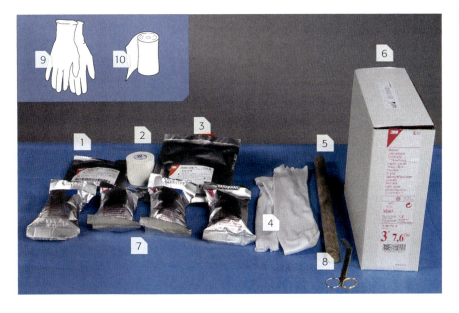

EQUIPMENT

1 Rigid synthetic splint 7.5 cm x 20 cm
2 Elastic foam tape
3 Rigid synthetic splint 7.5 cm x 70 cm
4 Cut tube bandage
5 Broomstick
6 Tube bandage 7.5 cm in dispenser box
7 Semirigid casting tape 7.5 cm
8 Scissors
9 Gloves
10 Elastic bandage

PERSONNEL

543

POSITIONING

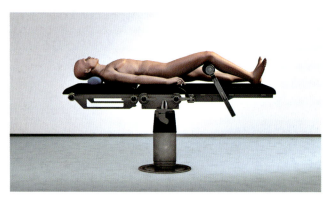

Place the patient supine on a table.

Place the knee on a support in 45–60° flexion, and the ankle joint in 90° flexion.

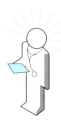

SPECIAL THINGS TO KEEP IN MIND

- Ensure the fibula head remains free a minimum of 2 cm to avoid pressure on the peroneal nerve
- Free flexion of the knee
- Free flexion and extension of the toes
- Pressure sores
- No disturbance of the contralateral leg

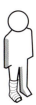

PROCEDURE

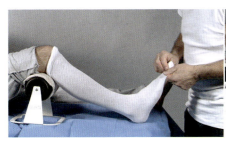

Apply a tube bandage from the foot to the knee. Pull the tube bandage tight to avoid any wrinkles

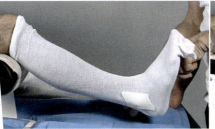

Apply elastic foam tape to protect the bony prominences: the lateral malleolus and the medial malleolus

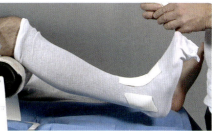

The extensor tendons are also protected

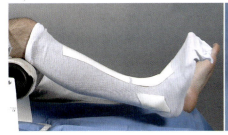

The tibial crest should be protected

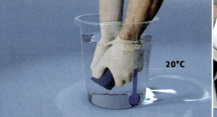

Submerge the semirigid casting tape in water for a few seconds, remove, and squeeze out excess water

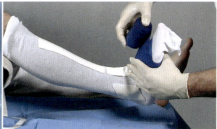

Apply the semirigid casting tape around the forefoot, leaving the toes free

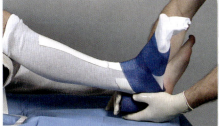

Wrap diagonally over the ankle, to the medial malleolus, and across the Achilles tendon

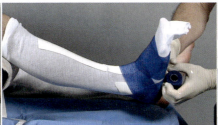

Pass diagonally beneath the foot

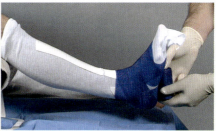

Pass over the lateral malleolus, the ankle joint, the Achilles tendon, and diagonally beneath the foot

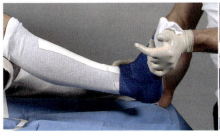

Support the lateral side of the foot

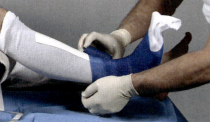

Wrap the leg using the half-overlapping technique

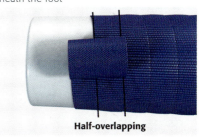

Half-overlapping

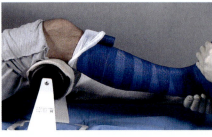

Fold back the tube bandage proximally to hold the roll of semirigid casting tape in place

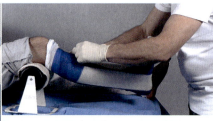

Apply a U-shaped rigid splint beneath the foot, and medially and laterally along the lower leg. Hold the rigid splint in place with semirigid casting tape

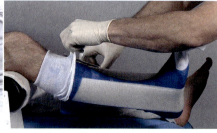

Fold back the tube bandage over the semirigid casting tape, proximally and distally, and trim it

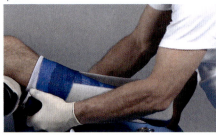

Apply another layer of wet semirigid casting tape over the rigid splint

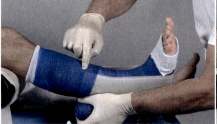

Ensure the rigid splint does not cover the ventral side of the leg

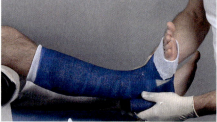

Wrap the ankle using the figure-of-eight technique

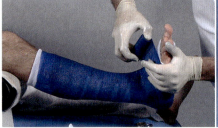

Wrap the distal edge of the cast, lateral to medial, to avoid supination

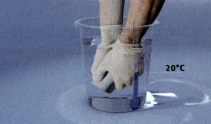

Submerge an elastic bandage in water; using a wet bandage accelerates the setting

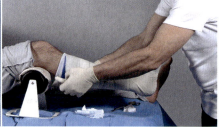

Wrap the complete cast with the elastic bandage

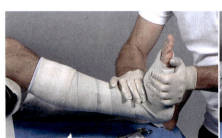

Mold the cast to the desired position

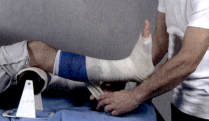

Tap on the cast to check it has set, and remove the wet bandage

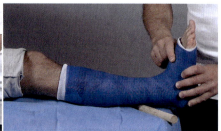

Place a broomstick or wooden rod beneath the leg to prevent any exorotation or endorotation

Klaus Dresing, Jos Engelen

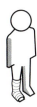

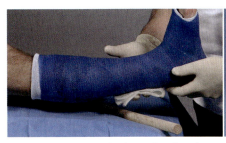

Prepare the short rigid splint to be placed between the cast and the broomstick

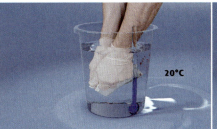

Submerge the rigid splint in water for a few seconds, remove, and squeeze out excess water

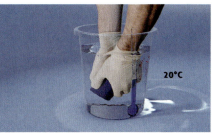

Submerge a roll of semirigid casting tape in water for a few seconds, remove, and squeeze out excess water

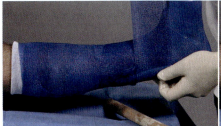

Place the rigid splint on the cast over the Achilles tendon, and wrap with semirigid casting tape

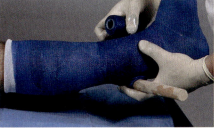

Place the broomstick over the rigid splint, and attach to the leg with semirigid casting tape using the figure-of-eight technique

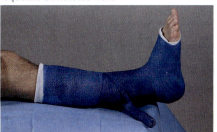

Completely wrap the broomstick with semirigid casting tape

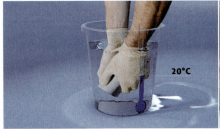

Submerge an elastic bandage in water; using a wet bandage accelerates the setting

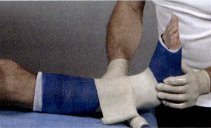

Wrap the wet bandage around the wet semirigid casting tape and the broomstick

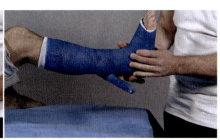

Remove the wet bandage after the cast has set

FINAL ASSESSMENT

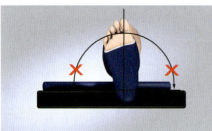 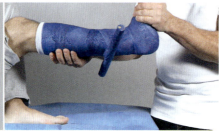

No rotation of the leg is possible

Free movement of the contralateral leg is possible

16.15   Removable ankle splint using synthetic, combicast technique

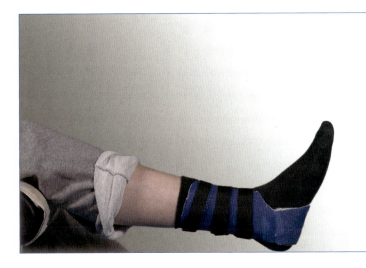

INDICATION

- Postoperative protection after ankle osteosynthesis
- Nondisplaced ankle fractures
- Ligamentous ruptures
- Ankle sprain
- Fracture of the proximal fifth metatarsal

GOAL

- Stabilization of the ankle joint

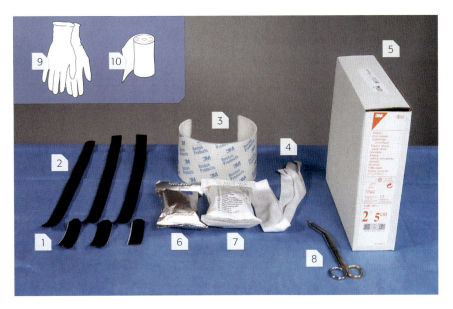

EQUIPMENT

1 Velcro strips adhesive (loop)
2 Velcro strips nonadhesive (hook)
3 Adhesive foam padding
4 Cut tube bandage
5 Tube bandage 5 cm in dispenser box
6 Semirigid casting tape 5 cm
7 Rigid casting tape 5 cm
8 Scissors
9 Gloves
10 Elastic bandage

PERSONNEL

POSITIONING

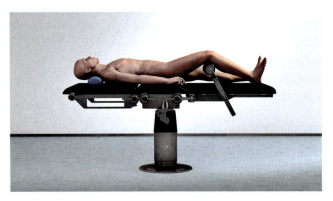

Place the patient supine or seated on a table.

Place the knee on a support, and the ankle joint in 90° flexion.

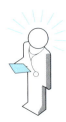

SPECIAL THINGS TO KEEP IN MIND

- Bony prominences
- Ensure soft edges of the splint

Klaus Dresing, Jos Engelen

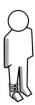

PROCEDURE

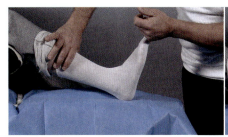

Apply a tube bandage over the foot and ankle. Pull the tube bandage tight to avoid any wrinkles

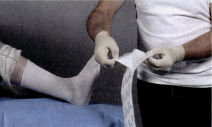

Cut the required length of adhesive foam padding and remove the protective paper layer

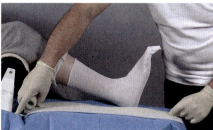

Place three layers of rigid casting tape on the adhesive surface of the foam padding

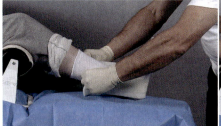

Apply the foam padding around the base of the foot and over the ankle; ensure the rigid casting tape faces outward

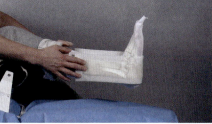

The patient holds the foam padding in place; ensure the rigid casting tape lies over the lateral malleolus and the medial malleolus

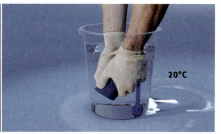

Submerge the semirigid casting tape in water for a few seconds, remove, and squeeze out excess water

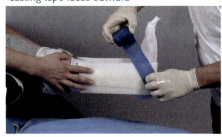

Apply the semirigid casting tape around the ankle and the base of the foot

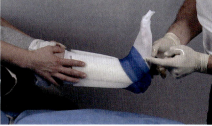

Ensure the semirigid casting tape is not wrapped too far distally

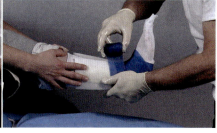

Wrap the leg using the half-overlapping technique

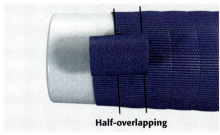

Half-overlapping

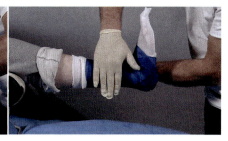

Ensure the ankle joint is in 90° flexion

Extend the semirigid casting tape a minimum of a handbreadth above the malleoli

16.15

TECHNIQUES

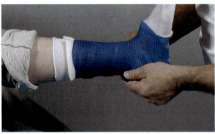

Attach three short strips of adhesive velcro (with loops) to the dorsal surface of the splint

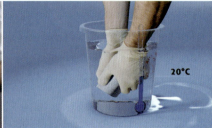

Submerge an elastic bandage in water; using a wet bandage accelerates the setting

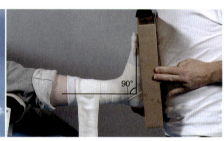

Ensure the ankle joint is in 90° flexion during setting

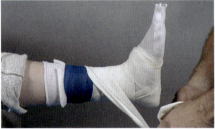

After the splint has set, remove the wet bandage

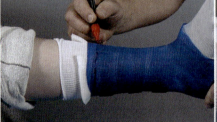

Mark the splint for trimming

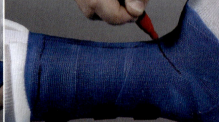

Split the splint on the ventral side; ensure free movement of the ankle joint

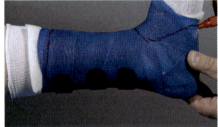

Leave enough of the splint to support the foot

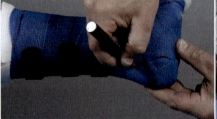

Ensure the calcaneus is free up to the insertion of the Achilles tendon

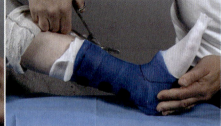

Split the splint on the ventral side, from proximal to distal, using the scissors

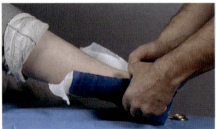

Open the splint and remove it

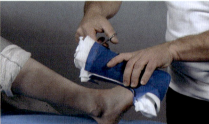

Trim the splint to the desired shape

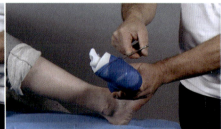

Ensure that enough splint is removed on the medial side to allow free movement

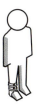

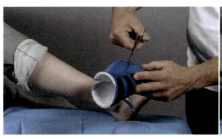

The splint supports the lateral side of the foot to prevent supination

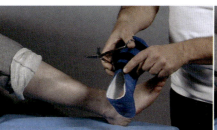

The heel must be completely free

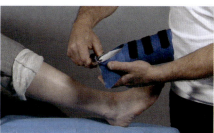

Ensure there is no pressure over the Achilles tendon

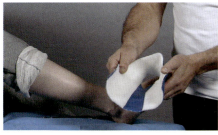

The padding gives more comfort for the patient

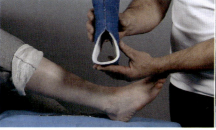

The shape of the lateral side of the foot can be seen in the splint

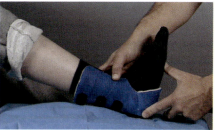

The splint can be worn over a sock

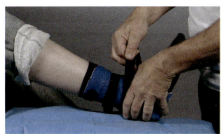

Attach three strips of velcro (with hooks) to close the splint

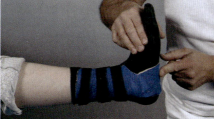

The splint supports the lateral edge of the foot against supination

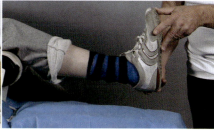

The patient can wear a normal shoe, preferably a lace-up or velcro shoe

16.15

TECHNIQUES

FINAL ASSESSMENT

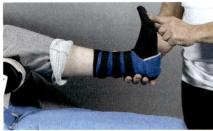 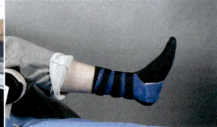

Free flexion and extension of the ankle joint   The splint has no sharp edges

16.16 Fifth metatarsal cast using synthetic, combicast technique

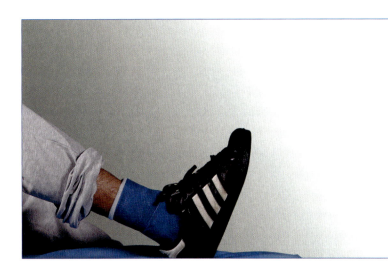

INDICATION

- Fracture of the proximal fifth metatarsal
- Fracture of the ankle, type Weber A
- Avulsion fracture of the medial malleolus

GOAL

- Stabilization of the ankle joint and the tarsus

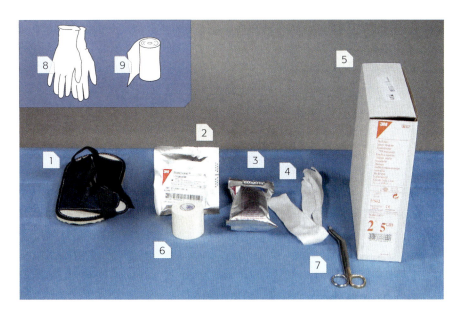

EQUIPMENT

1 Cast shoe
2 Rigid synthetic splint 7.5 cm x 45 cm
3 Semirigid casting tape 7.5 cm
4 Cut tube bandage
5 Tube bandage 5 cm in dispenser box
6 Elastic foam tape
7 Scissors
8 Gloves
9 Elastic bandage

PERSONNEL

16.16

TECHNIQUES

POSITIONING

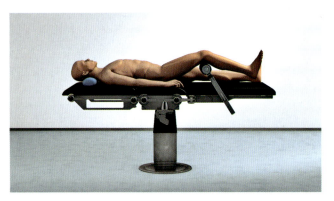

Place the patient supine or seated on a table.

Place the knee on a support, and the ankle joint in 90° flexion.

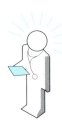

SPECIAL THINGS TO KEEP IN MIND

- Padding of the malleoli
- Functional position of the ankle (90°)
- Halfway between supination and pronation
- In case of severe swelling the cast should be split

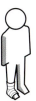

PROCEDURE

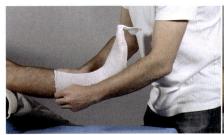

Apply a tube bandage over the foot and ankle. Pull the tube bandage tight to avoid any wrinkles

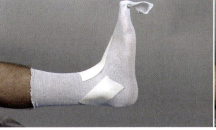

Apply elastic foam tape to protect the lateral malleolus, the medial malleolus, and the instep of the foot

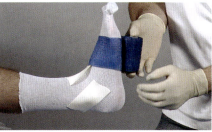

Apply the first layer of semirigid casting tape, beginning at the level of the small toe, with a circular wrap

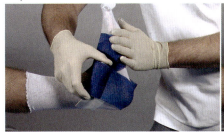

Pass the semirigid casting tape over the heel; ensure the ankle joint is in 90° flexion

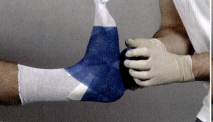

Continue by using the figure-of-eight technique over the Achilles tendon and diagonally beneath the foot

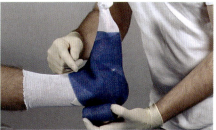

Pass once more over the Achilles tendon and diagonally beneath the foot

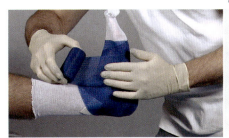

Pass diagonally over the foot and wrap the distal tibia using the half-overlapping technique

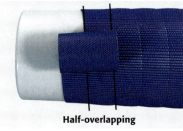

Half-overlapping

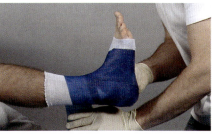

Trim the tube bandage distally, and fold back over the semirigid casting tape

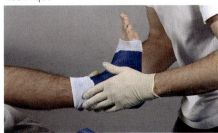

Cut the semirigid casting tape proximally, and fold back the tube bandage

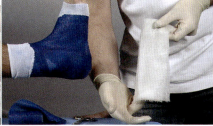

Fan out the layers of the rigid splint at one end

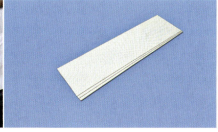

Shape the splint like this

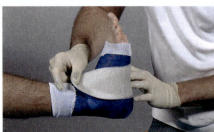

The splint should be applied over the fifth metatarsal and laterally over the foot

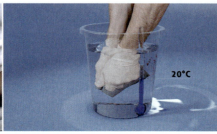

Submerge the splint in water for a few seconds, remove, and squeeze out excess water

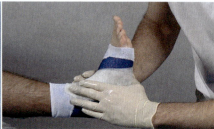

Apply the wet splint; the layers of the splint should be fanned out

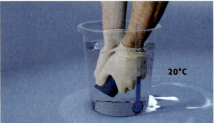

Submerge the semirigid casting tape in water for a few seconds, remove, and squeeze out excess water

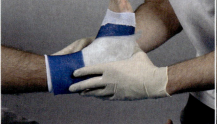

Apply the semirigid casting tape; begin proximally with a circular wrap

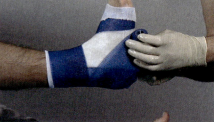

Pass over the Achilles tendon, and wrap diagonally beneath the foot

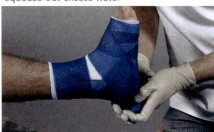

Apply a circular wrap distally, and pass diagonally over the heel

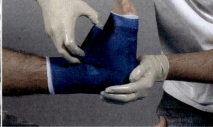

Ensure the ankle joint is in dorsiflexion while applying the last wraps

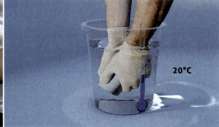

Submerge an elastic bandage in water; using a wet bandage accelerates the setting

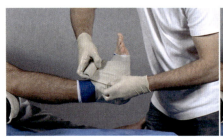

Apply the wet bandage using the same technique as with the semirigid casting tape

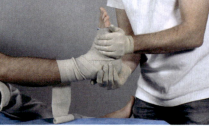

Mold the cast and hold in position until it is set

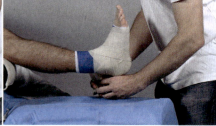

After the cast has set, remove the wet bandage

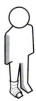

FINAL ASSESSMENT

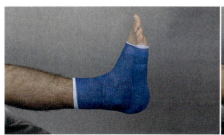
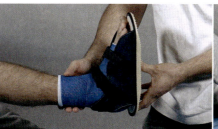
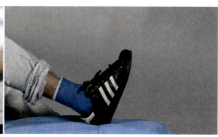

The ankle joint is in 90° flexion. The cast has smooth edges, and there is free movement of the toes

A cast shoe can be worn during weight bearing

The patient can also wear a normal shoe, preferably a lace-up or velcro shoe

Casts, Splints, and Support Bandages—Nonoperative Treatment and Perioperative Protection   Klaus Dresing, Peter Trafton

Klaus Dresing, Jos Engelen

16.17 Removable fifth metatarsal cast using synthetic, combicast technique

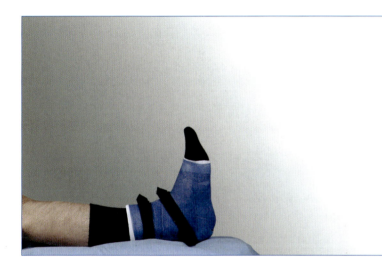

INDICATION

- Fracture of the proximal fifth metatarsal
- Fracture of the ankle, type Weber A
- Avulsion fracture of the medial malleolus

GOAL

- Stabilization of the ankle joint and the tarsus

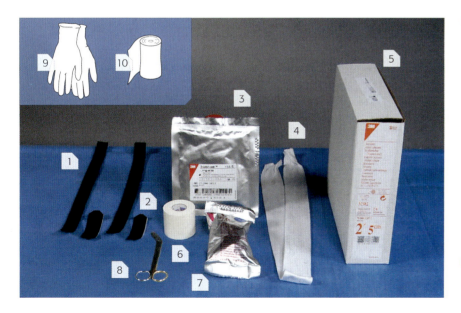

EQUIPMENT

1. Velcro strips nonadhesive (hook)
2. Velcro strips adhesive (loop)
3. Rigid synthetic splint 7.5 cm x 45 cm
4. Cut tube bandage
5. Tube bandage 5 cm in dispenser box
6. Elastic foam tape
7. Semirigid casting tape 7.5 cm
8. Scissors
9. Gloves
10. Elastic bandage

PERSONNEL

16.17

TECHNIQUES

POSITIONING

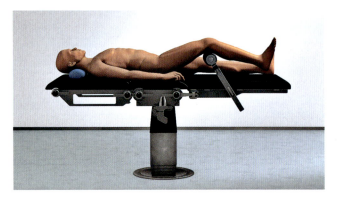

Place the patient supine or seated on a table.

Place the knee on a support, and the ankle joint in 90° flexion.

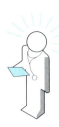

SPECIAL THINGS TO KEEP IN MIND

- Padding of the malleoli
- Functional position of the ankle (90°)
- Halfway between supination and pronation
- In case of severe swelling the cast should be split
- The patient can wear their own sock under the cast

Klaus Dresing, Jos Engelen

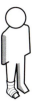

PROCEDURE

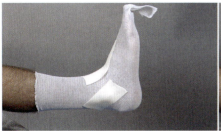

Apply a tube bandage over the foot and ankle. Pull the tube bandage tight to avoid any wrinkles

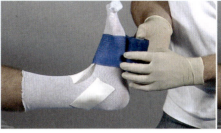

Apply elastic foam tape to protect the lateral malleolus, the medial malleolus, and the instep of the foot

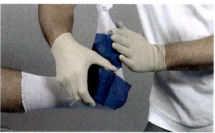

Apply the first layer of semirigid casting tape, beginning at the level of the small toe, with a circular wrap

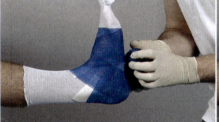

Pass the semirigid casting tape over the heel; ensure the ankle joint is in 90° flexion

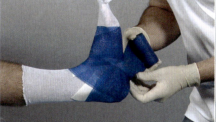

Continue by using the figure-of-eight technique over the Achilles tendon and diagonally beneath the foot

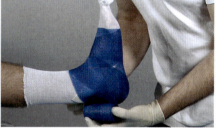

Pass once more over the Achilles tendon and diagonally beneath the foot

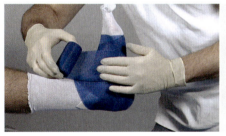

Pass diagonally over the foot and wrap the distal tibia using the half-overlapping technique

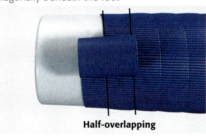

Half-overlapping

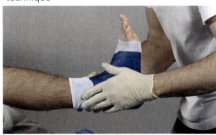

Trim the tube bandage distally, and fold back over the semirigid casting tape

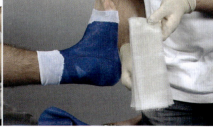

Cut the semirigid casting tape proximally, and fold back the tube bandage

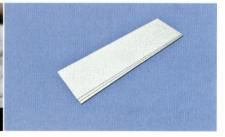

Fan out the layers of the rigid splint at one end

Shape the splint like this

563

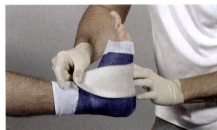

The splint should be applied over the fifth metatarsal and laterally over the foot

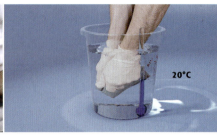

Submerge the splint in water for a few seconds, remove, and squeeze out excess water

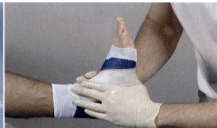

Apply the wet splint; the layers of the splint should be fanned out

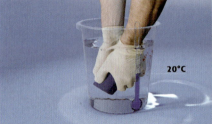

Submerge the semirigid casting tape in water for a few seconds, remove, and squeeze out excess water

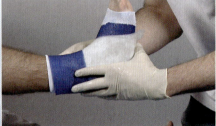

Apply the semirigid casting tape; begin proximally with a circular wrap

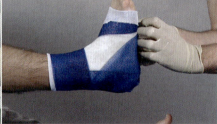

Pass over the Achilles tendon, and wrap diagonally beneath the foot

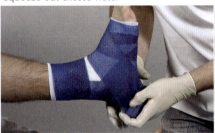

Apply a circular wrap distally, and pass diagonally over the heel

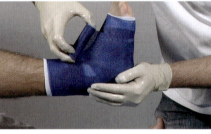

Ensure the ankle joint is in dorsiflexion while applying the last wraps

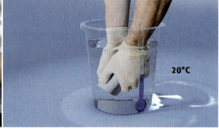

Submerge an elastic bandage in water; using a wet bandage accelerates the setting

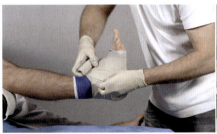

Apply the wet bandage using the same technique as with the semirigid casting tape

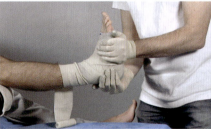

Mold the cast and hold in position until it is set

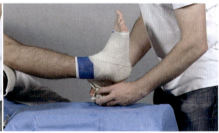

After the cast has set, remove the wet bandage

Klaus Dresing, Jos Engelen

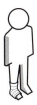
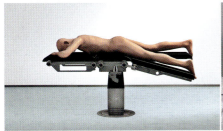

Place the patient in the prone position before splitting the cast

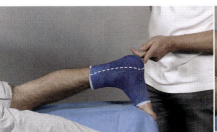

Mark the splitting line along the Achilles tendon and over the hindfoot

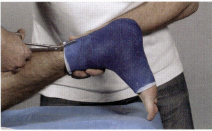

Squeeze the cast together before splitting to create more space to insert the scissors

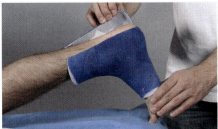

Split the cast, open the flap, and remove the cast

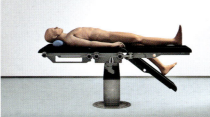

Place the patient in the supine position to reapply the cast

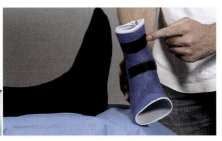

Attach two adhesive velcro strips (with loops) to the ventral aspect of the cast

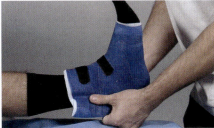

Reapply the cast; patients should wear their own sock

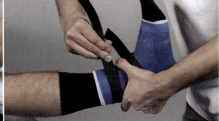

Attach two long velcro strips (with hooks) to close the cast. A cast shoe or a normal lace-up shoe can be worn

FINAL ASSESSMENT

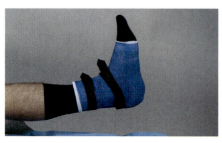

The ankle joint is in 90° flexion. The cast has smooth edges, and there is free movement of the toes. A cast shoe or a lace-up or velcro shoe can be worn

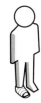

16.18 Foot cast using synthetic, combicast technique

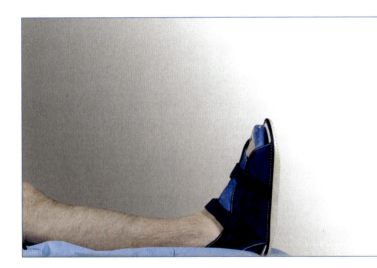

INDICATION

- Fracture of the metatarsals
- Fracture of tarsals
- Postoperative treatment after osteosynthesis of tarsals and metatarsals

GOAL

- Stabilization of hindfoot, midfoot and forefoot

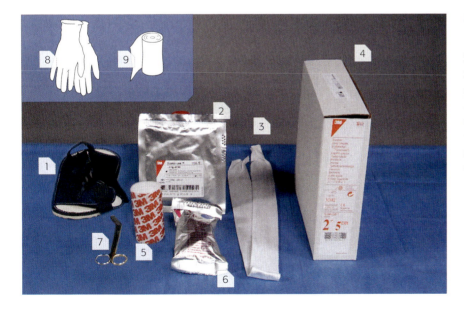

EQUIPMENT

1 Cast shoe
2 Rigid synthetic splint 7.5 cm x 45 cm
3 Cut tube bandages
4 Tube bandage 5 cm in dispenser box
5 Cast padding
6 Semirigid casting tape 7.5 cm
7 Scissors
8 Gloves
9 Elastic bandage

PERSONNEL

POSITIONING

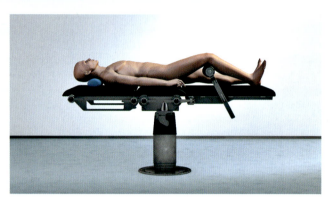

Place the patient supine on a table.

Place the knee on a support, and ensure free movement of the toes.

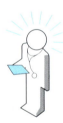

SPECIAL THINGS TO KEEP IN MIND

- Free movement of the ankle joint
- Ensure free movement of the toes by opening the dorsal aspect of the cast

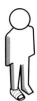
PROCEDURE

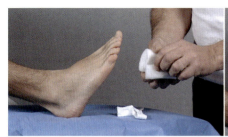

Apply a small folded piece of padding between each toe

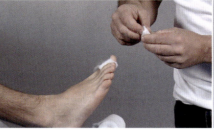

Padding ensures there is enough space in the foot cast to allow the patient to walk without discomfort

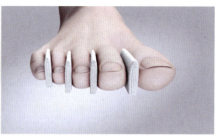

Padding holds the toes apart

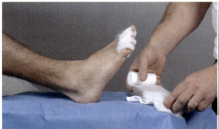

Fold five or six layers of additional padding and apply over the end of the toes

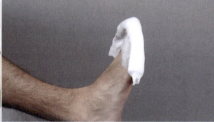

Insert the padding into a tube bandage to create a roll of padding for the toes

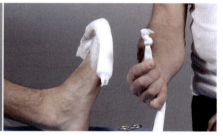

Make a knot at one end of a second tube bandage; the knot will be placed over the first and second toe

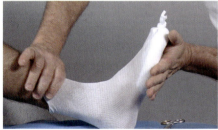

Apply the tube bandage to above the ankle; ensure the padding remains in the desired position

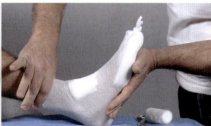

Apply additional padding to protect the extensor tendons

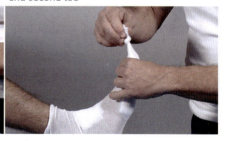

Apply tension to the knot and place it between the first and second toe

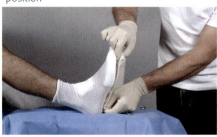

Prepare the footplate using a 3-layer rigid splint. Fold the splint to make a 6-layer splint to match the length and width of the foot

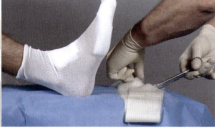

Fan out the splint and trim both ends

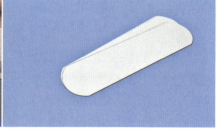

Shape the splint like this

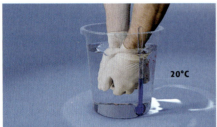

Using wet gloves makes it easier to apply the semirigid casting tape

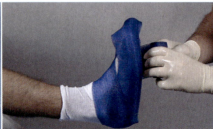

Apply two layers of semirigid casting tape longitudinally; hold it in place with circular wraps

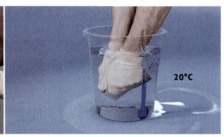

Submerge the rigid splint in water for a few seconds, remove, and squeeze out excess water

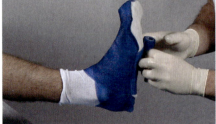

Apply the footplate splint; hold in place with a layer of semirigid casting tape

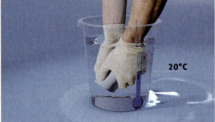

Submerge an elastic bandage in water; using a wet bandage accelerates the setting

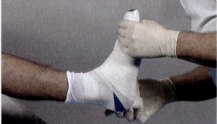

Apply the wet bandage using the same technique as with the semirigid casting tape

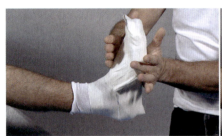

Mold the arch of the foot using the ball of the thumb; do not dorsiflex the toes

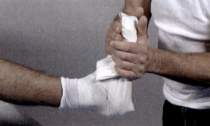

Provide plantar support under the toes and metatarsal heads

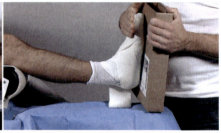

If a flat sole is needed for the cast, hold a flat surface against it

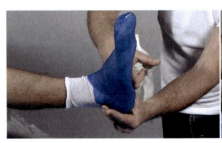

Remove the wet bandage after the cast has set. Ensure the cast has been molded to the arch of the foot

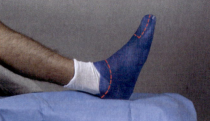

Trim the cast to allow free movement of the toes and ankle

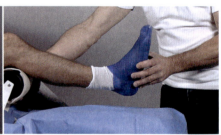

Remove the knee support before trimming the cast

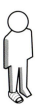

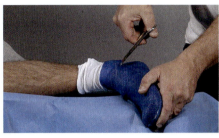

Trim the cast below the medial malleolus and the lateral malleolus

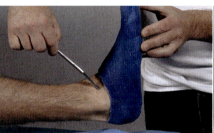

Ensure free movement of the ankle joint is possible

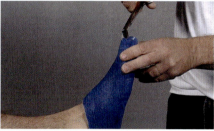

Remove the dorsal distal section of the cast to free the toes; begin by making a small hole over the padding

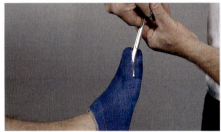

Insert the scissors and split the cast laterally to the base of the fifth metatarsal

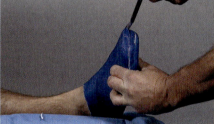

Split the cast down to the base of the first metatarsal and remove the padding tube

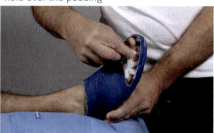

Remove the padding between the toes

16.18

TECHNIQUES

FINAL ASSESSMENT

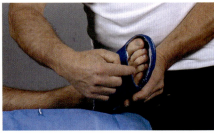 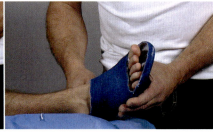 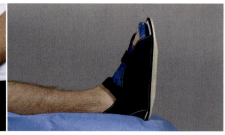

Free movement of the ankle and the toes during weight bearing

Ensure the base of the toes are supported during any movement

Use a cast shoe if weight bearing is allowed

Klaus Dresing, Jos Engelen

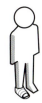

16.19 Removable foot cast using synthetic, combicast technique

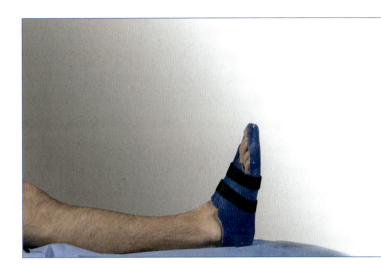

INDICATION

- Fracture of the metatarsals
- Fracture of tarsals
- Postoperative treatment after osteosynthesis of tarsals and metatarsals

GOAL

- Stabilization of hindfoot, midfoot and forefoot

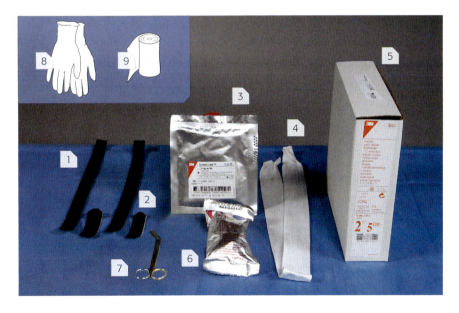

EQUIPMENT

1. Velcro strips nonadhesive (hook)
2. Velcro strips adhesive (loop)
3. Rigid synthetic splint 7.5 cm x 45 cm
4. Cut tube bandages
5. Tube bandage 5 cm in dispenser box
6. Semirigid casting tape 7.5 cm
7. Scissors
8. Gloves
9. Elastic bandage

PERSONNEL

POSITIONING

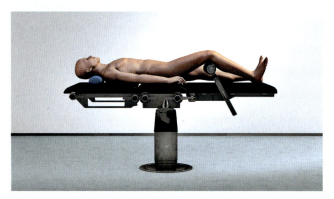

Place the patient supine on a table.

Place the knee on a support, and ensure free movement of the toes.

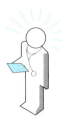

SPECIAL THINGS TO KEEP IN MIND

- Free movement of the ankle joint
- Ensure free movement of the toes by opening the dorsal aspect of the cast

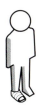

PROCEDURE

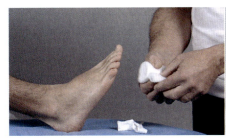

Apply a small folded piece of padding between each toe

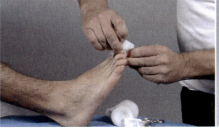

Padding ensures there is enough space in the foot cast to allow the patient to walk without discomfort

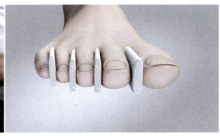

Padding holds the toes apart

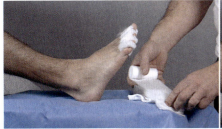

Fold five or six layers of additional padding and apply over the end of the toes

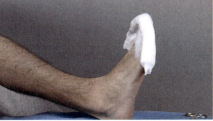

Insert the padding into a tube bandage to create a roll of padding for the toes

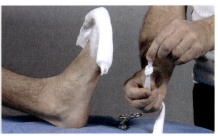

Make a knot at one end of a second tube bandage; the knot will be placed over the first and second toe

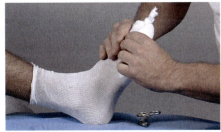

Apply the tube bandage to above the ankle; ensure the padding remains in the desired position

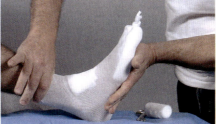

Apply additional padding to protect the extensor tendons

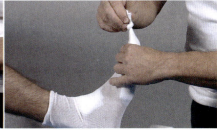

Apply tension to the knot and place it between the first and second toe

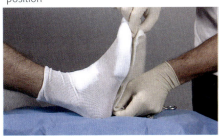

Prepare the footplate using a 3-layer rigid splint. Fold the splint to make a 6-layer splint to match the length and width of the foot

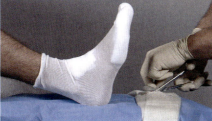

Fan out the splint and trim both ends

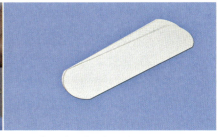

Shape the splint like this

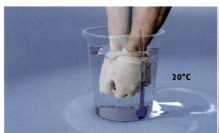

Using wet gloves makes it easier to apply the semirigid casting tape

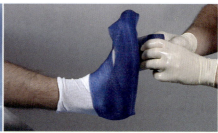

Apply two layers of semirigid casting tape longitudinally; hold in place with circular wraps

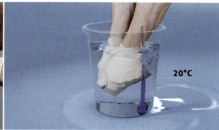

Submerge the rigid splint in water for a few seconds, remove, and squeeze out excess water

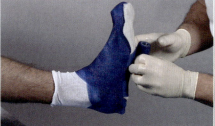

Apply the footplate splint; hold it in place with a layer of semirigid casting tape

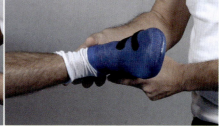

Apply two adhesive velcro strips (with loops) to the dorsomedial side of the cast

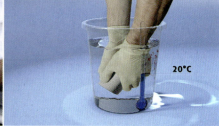

Submerge an elastic bandage in water; using a wet bandage accelerates the setting

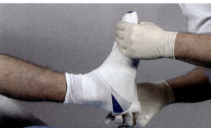

Apply the wet bandage using the same technique as with the semirigid casting tape

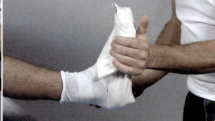

Mold the arch of the foot using the ball of the thumb; do not dorsiflex the toes

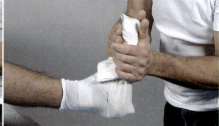

Provide plantar support under the toes and metatarsal heads

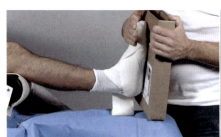

If a flat sole is needed for the cast, hold a flat surface against it

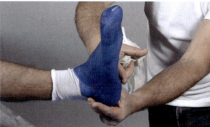

Remove the wet bandage after the cast has set. Ensure the cast has been molded to the arch of the foot

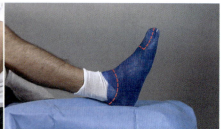

Trim the cast to allow free movement of the toes and ankle

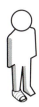

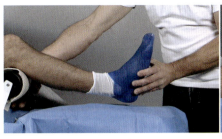

Remove the knee support before trimming the cast

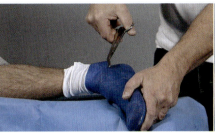

Trim the cast below the medial malleolus and the lateral malleolus

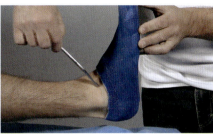

Ensure free movement of the ankle joint is possible

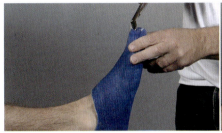

Remove the dorsal distal section of the cast to free the toes; begin by making a small hole over the padding

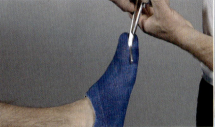

Insert the scissors and split the cast laterally to the base of the fifth metatarsal

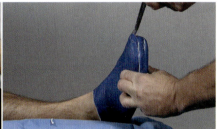

Split the cast down to the base of the first metatarsal and remove the padding tube

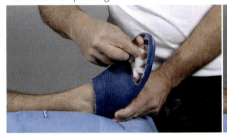

Remove the padding between the toes

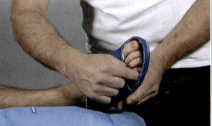

Be aware that during weight bearing the toes need more space

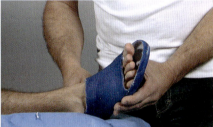

Ensure the base of the toes are supported during any movement

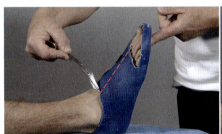

Mark the splitting line on the dorsal side of the cast

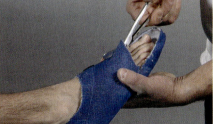

The cast is split from the base of the second toe, directed toward the lateral malleolus

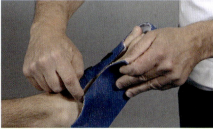

The split should be oblique, and should lie over the extensor muscles

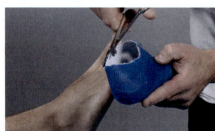

Remove the cast and trim the edges

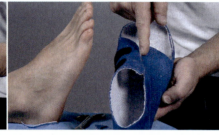

Round off the sharp edges and remove
2–3 mm to leave a gap between the edges

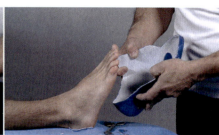

Reapply the cast

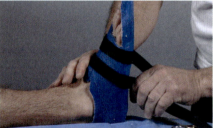

Attach two long velcro strips (with hooks)
and wrap them around the foot under
tension to close the cast

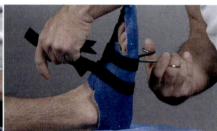

Trim the velcro strips to the required length
with two 45° cuts

FINAL ASSESSMENT

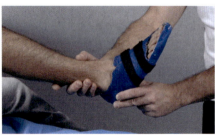

Free movement of the ankle joint is possible

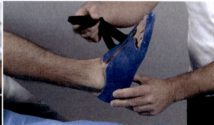

The velcro strips allow easy removal and
reapplication of the cast

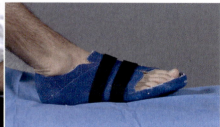

The rounded edges of the cast avoid irritation
of the instep. There is enough space for
movement of the toes

Klaus Dresing, Jos Engelen

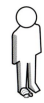

16.20 First toe orthosis using synthetic, combicast technique

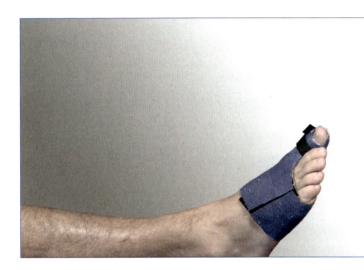

INDICATION

- Fracture of the first toe
- Perioperative protection after hallux valgus surgery

GOAL

- Stabilization of the first toe and first ray

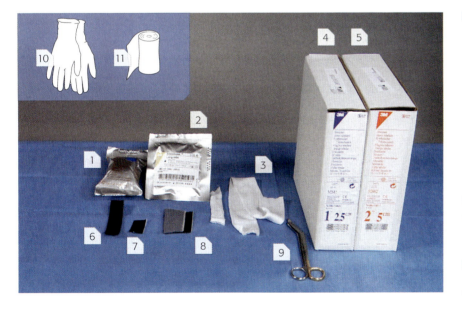

EQUIPMENT

1 Semirigid casting tape 5 cm
2 Rigid synthetic splint 7.5 cm x 45 cm
3 Cut tube bandages
4 Tube bandage 2.5 cm in dispenser box
5 Tube bandage 5 cm in dispenser box
6 Velcro strip nonadhesive (hook)
7 Velcro strip adhesive (loop)
8 Combined adapted velcro strips adhesive (loop and hook)
9 Scissors
10 Gloves
11 Elastic bandage

PERSONNEL

579

16.20

TECHNIQUES

POSITIONING

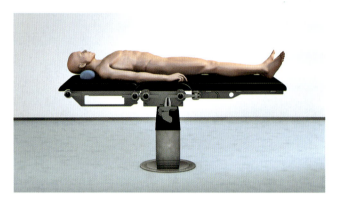

Place the patient supine or seated on a table.

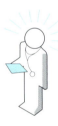

SPECIAL THINGS TO KEEP IN MIND

- First toe in functional position
- Enough interdigital space to avoid friction and skin irritation

PROCEDURE

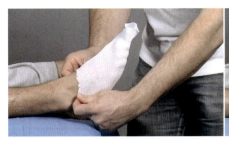

Apply a short tube bandage over the toes and part of the foot

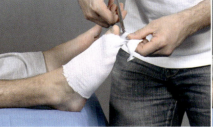

Cut an opening in the tube bandage for toes I-III and trim the excess

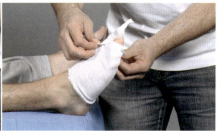

Apply a small tube bandage, with a slit at one end, over the first toe

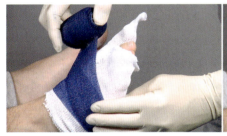

Apply the semirigid casting tape from lateral, around the forefoot, and then diagonally to the base of the first toe

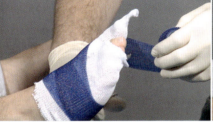

Cut halfway through the casting tape, from proximal to distal, for easier application between the first and second toe

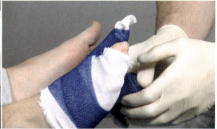

Cut again, and wrap once more around the first toe

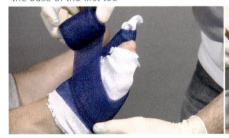

Wrap below the fifth toe and across the forefoot, and trim

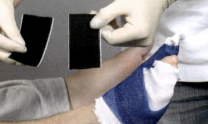

Use two strips of adhesive velcro (one with loops and one with hooks) to open and close the orthosis

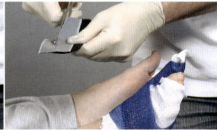

Attach the velcro strips half-overlapping, and trim to the required width

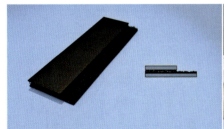

Ensure the velcro with loops is below and the velcro with hooks is above

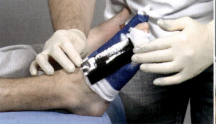

Remove the backing and attach the adhesive velcro (with loops) to the semirigid casting tape

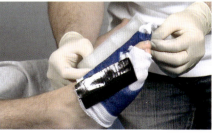

Trim a rigid splint to fit the first toe and the medial side of the forefoot

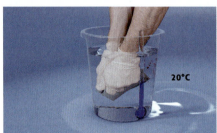

Submerge the rigid splint in water for a few seconds, remove, and squeeze out excess water

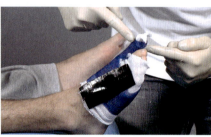

Apply the rigid splint under the first toe and along the medial side of the forefoot

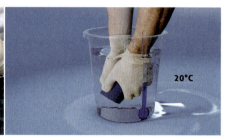

Submerge the semirigid casting tape in water for a few seconds, remove, and squeeze out excess water

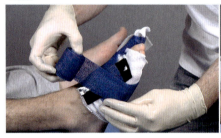

Apply the semirigid casting tape over the velcro, using the same technique as with the first layer

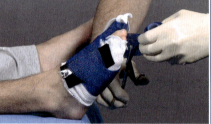

Cut halfway through the casting tape, from proximal to distal, for easier application between the first and second toe

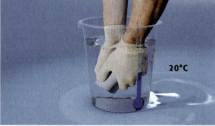

Submerge an elastic bandage in water; using a wet bandage accelerates the setting

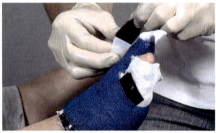

Attach a small strip of adhesive velcro (with loops) to the medial side of the cast over the first toe

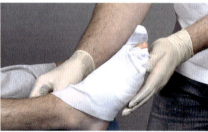

Apply the wet bandage over the complete orthosis

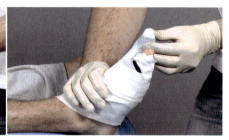

Mold the orthosis to the desired position while it sets

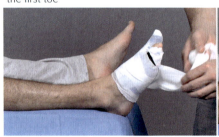

Remove the wet bandage after the orthosis has set

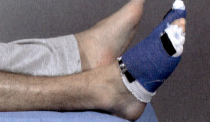

Before trimming the orthosis to the desired shape, it is removed. The first step is to open the velcro

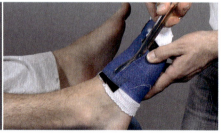

Slide the scissors beneath the outer layer of the orthosis where the velcro overlaps, and cut through the orthosis

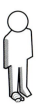

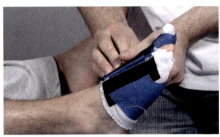

Open and fold back the velcro; the lower layer of the orthosis can be seen

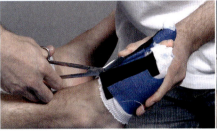

Slide the scissors beneath the tube bandage, and cut through the lower layer of the orthosis

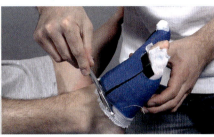

Close the velcro; the orthosis must be trimmed to free the ankle joint and toes II-V

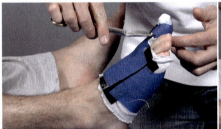

The material between the first and second toe must be removed to avoid friction and skin irritation by the orthosis

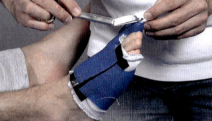

Make a cut along the inside of the first toe to allow the orthosis to be adjusted around the toe

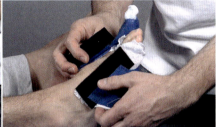

Open the orthosis and remove it

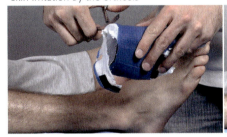

Trim the orthosis to the desired shape, proximally and distally, to free the hindfoot and the toes II-V

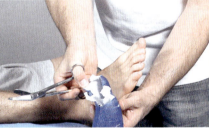

The section over the first toe is also split

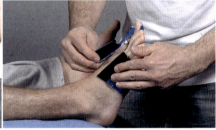

Open the velcro, slide the orthosis over the first toe, and close with the velcro

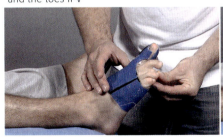

Ensure the orthosis has been trimmed correctly and does not interfere with free movement of the toes

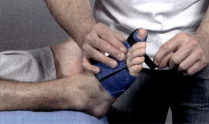

Attach a narrow strip of velcro (with hooks) to close the orthosis around the first toe

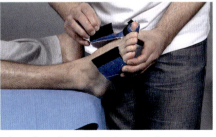

The velcro allows the patient to adjust the orthosis if there is too much pressure on the first toe

FINAL ASSESSMENT

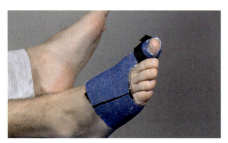

Free movement of the ankle joint and the
toes, except the first toe

TECHNIQUES

17 Spine

17 Spine

Klaus Dresing, Jos Engelen

17.1 Corset using plaster of Paris

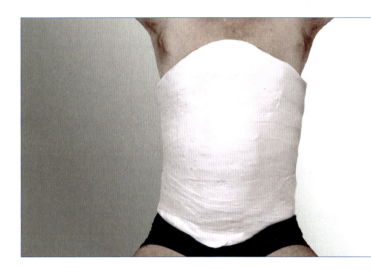

INDICATION

- Fracture of the lower thoracic spine
- Fracture of the lumbar spine

GOAL

- Stabilization of the spine

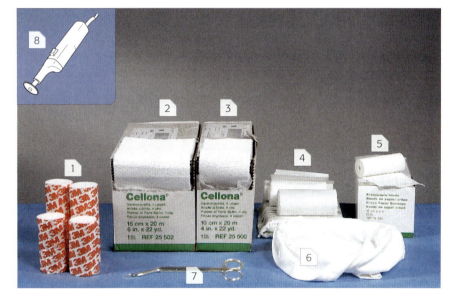

EQUIPMENT

1 Cast padding
2 Plaster of Paris splint 12 cm or 15 cm
3 Plaster of Paris splint 10 cm
4 Plaster of Paris rolls 15 cm or 20 cm
5 Crepe paper bandage
6 Cut tube bandage or cast shirt
7 Scissors
8 Oscillating saw

PERSONNEL

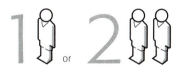

1 or 2

POSITIONING

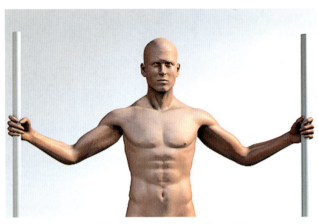

Stand the patient upright between supports if possible.

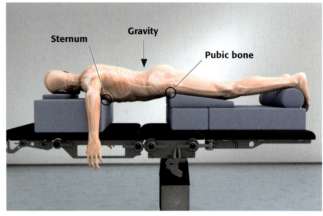

If the patient requires anesthesia, place the patient in lordosis using the three-point principle.

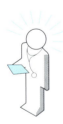

SPECIAL THINGS TO KEEP IN MIND

- Ensure the axillary fossa is free
- Free movement of the hips
- Three-point support: sternum, pubic bone, lumbar spine
- Be aware of the edges: padding of the edges
- Ventral window to allow normal food intake might be necessary in slim patients

Klaus Dresing, Jos Engelen

PROCEDURE

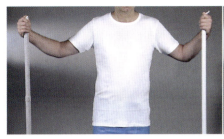

Apply a large tube bandage or cast shirt

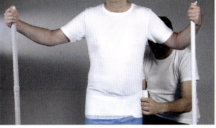

Apply the padding over the cast shirt, from distal to proximal; be aware of bony prominences at the superior anterior iliac spine

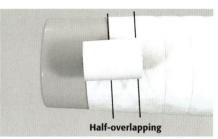

Half-overlapping

Use the half-overlapping technique

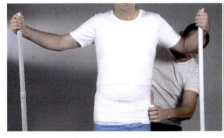

Apply a paper bandage as a barrier between the dry padding and the wet POP. Use the half-overlapping technique

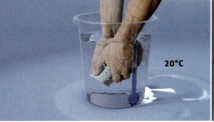

20°C

Submerge the roll of POP in water for a few seconds, remove, and squeeze out excess water

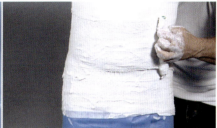

Apply the roll of POP using the half-overlapping technique

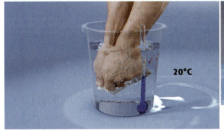

20°C

Reinforce the corset with a ventral POP splint, either in one or two sections

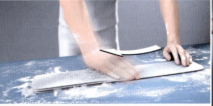

Stretch and smooth out the splint, pressing the layers together, resulting in a compact splint. If this procedure is not done, puff pastry plaster will result, causing an unstable splint

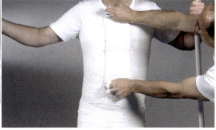

Apply the first POP splint to the front of the corset

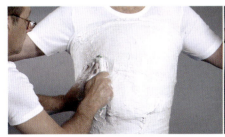

Apply wet rolls of POP over the POP splint, using the half-overlapping technique

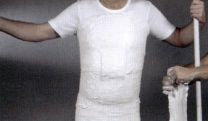

Apply a long POP splint to the back of the corset

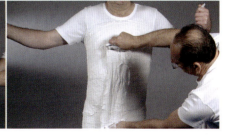

Apply a second POP splint to the front of the corset and trim the excess

589

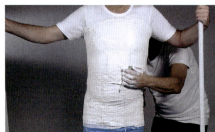

Apply another layer of POP to cover the splints, using the half-overlapping technique

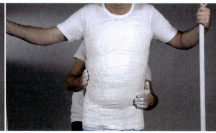

Smooth out the corset

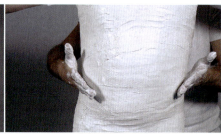

Mold the corset to the iliac crests

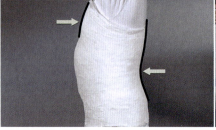

Mold the corset while it is setting, to provide support for the sternum and the lumbar spine

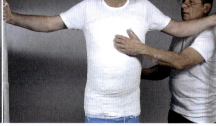

Tap on the corset to check it has set and mark the edges of the cast for trimming

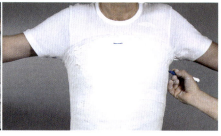

Ensure the axillae are free to provide unhindered movement of the shoulders

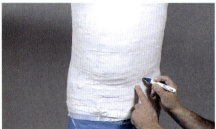

Mark the pubic bone and the iliac crests; they must be free of material

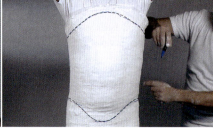

Mark the complete splitting line on the corset

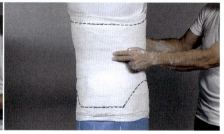

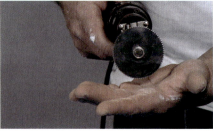

The saw blade oscillates and does not rotate, so there is no direct harm to the skin

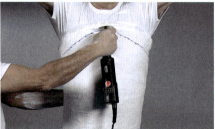

Remove the excess material with the oscillating saw or a plaster knife

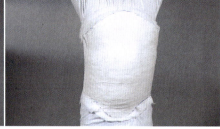

The final shape of the corset after trimming

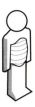

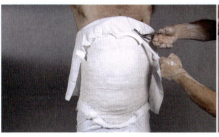

Remove the excess cast shirt; leave enough to fold over the corset

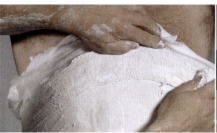

Apply wet rolls of POP to the edges of the trimmed corset

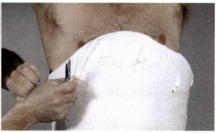

Fold back the cast shirt over the corset and press onto the wet POP

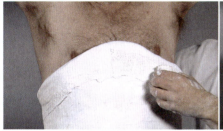

Apply wet rolls of POP to give a smooth finish to the edges of the corset

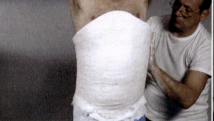

Smooth out the POP to give an even finish

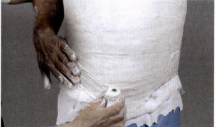

Repeat the procedure at the distal border of the corset

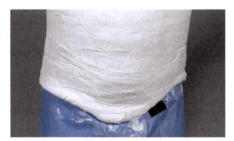

Apply wet rolls of POP to give a smooth finish to the edges of the corset

FINAL ASSESSMENT

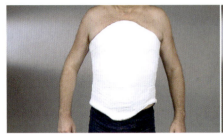

The edges of the corset are smooth

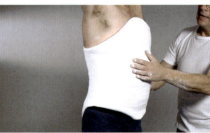

The axillae are completely free

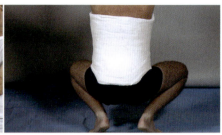

Free movement of the shoulders, hips and lower body is possible

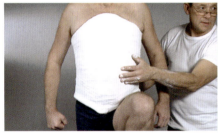

Hip flexion of at least 90° is possible to allow comfortable sitting

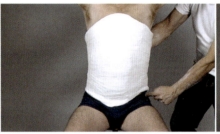

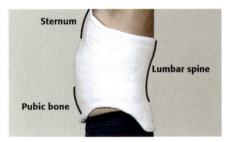

There are two or three finger's breadth between the distal border of the corset and the seating area

The corset supports the sternum, lumbar spine, and pubic bone: the three-point principle

CORSET REMOVAL

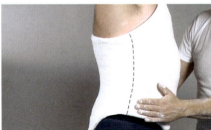

Mark the splitting line

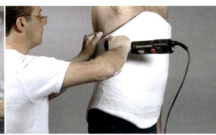

Split the corset with the oscillating saw

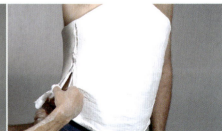

Cut through the padding and the cast shirt with scissors, and remove the corset

Klaus Dresing, Jos Engelen

17.2 Corset using synthetic, combicast technique

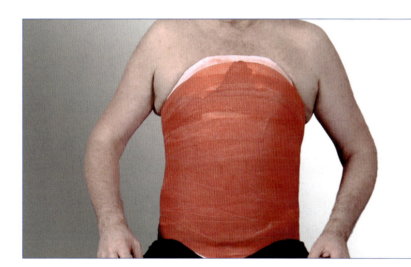

INDICATION

- Fracture of the lower thoracic spine
- Fracture of the lumbar spine

GOAL

- Stabilization of the spine

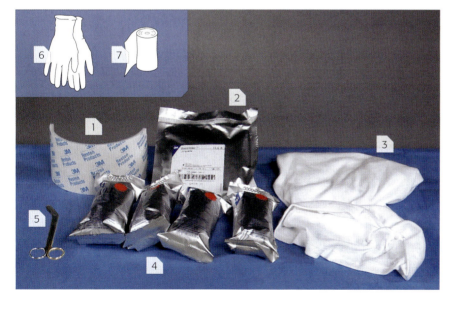

EQUIPMENT

1 Adhesive foam padding
2 Rigid synthetic splint 10 cm or 12.5 cm x 90 cm
3 Cut tube bandage or cast shirt
4 Semirigid casting tape 10 cm or 12.5 cm
5 Scissors
6 Gloves
7 Elastic bandage

PERSONNEL

1 or 2

POSITIONING

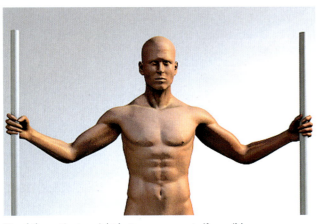

Stand the patient upright between supports if possible.

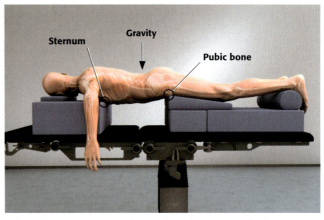

If the patient requires anesthesia, place the patient in lordosis using the three-point principle .

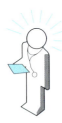

SPECIAL THINGS TO KEEP IN MIND

- Ensure the axillary fossa is free
- Free movement of the hips
- Three-point support: sternum, pubic bone, lumbar spine
- Be aware of the edges: padding of the edges
- Ventral window to allow normal food intake might be necessary in slim patients

Klaus Dresing, Jos Engelen

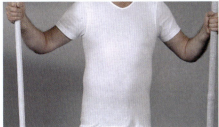

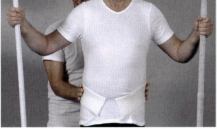

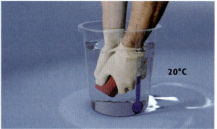

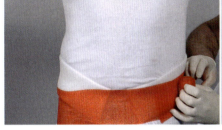

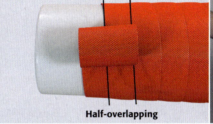

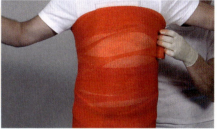

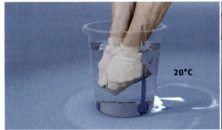

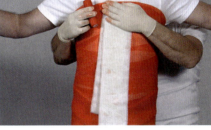

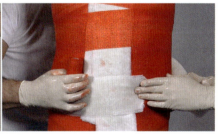

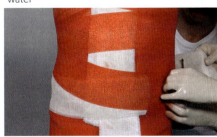

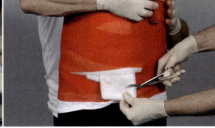

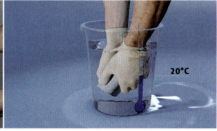

PROCEDURE

Apply a large tube bandage or cast shirt

Apply adhesive foam padding to protect the iliac crests and the sternum

Submerge the semirigid casting tape in water for a few seconds, remove, and squeeze out excess water

Apply the semirigid casting tape; start by covering the foam padding over the iliac crests

Continue the application, using the half-overlapping technique

Half-overlapping

Extend the semirigid casting tape to cover the foam padding protecting the sternum

Submerge the rigid splint in water for a few seconds, remove, and squeeze out excess water

Apply the first rigid splint anteriorly, and hold it in place with another layer of semirigid casting tape

Apply a second rigid splint at the level of the iliac crest, and hold it in place with semirigid casting tape

Trim the rigid splint; ensure that it does not completely encircle the body

Trim the first rigid splint to the desired length

Submerge an elastic bandage in water; using a wet bandage accelerates the setting

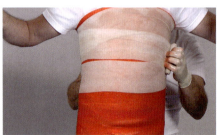

Apply the wet elastic bandage over the semirigid casting tape

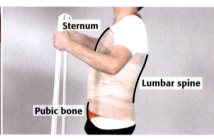

Ensure there is support of the sternum, lumbar spine, and pubic bone to create the required lordosis

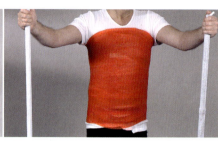

Remove the wet bandage after the corset has set

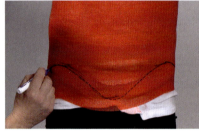

Mark the edges of the corset for trimming

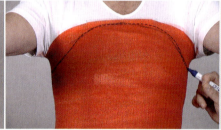

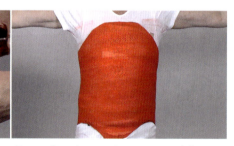

Ensure the axillae and the hips are free of material

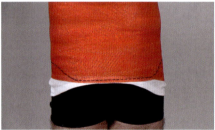

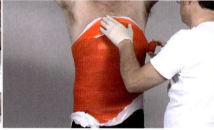

Trim the corset along the marked lines with the scissors

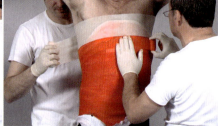

Ensure there is enough space around the axillae to allow free movement of the shoulders

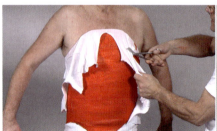

Cut the cast shirt free and fold it back over the corset

Apply another layer of wet semirigid casting tape to hold the edges of the cast shirt in place

Apply a wet elastic bandage to accelerate the final setting

Klaus Dresing, Jos Engelen

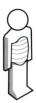

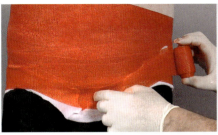

Repeat the procedure at the distal border of the corset

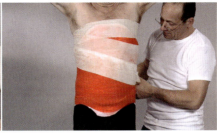

Remove the wet bandage after the corset has set

FINAL ASSESSMENT

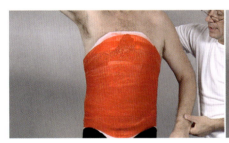

The axillae are completely free

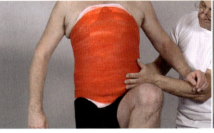

Free movement of the shoulders, hips and lower body is possible

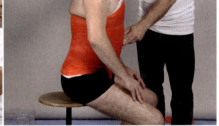

Hip flexion of at least 90° is possible to allow comfortable sitting

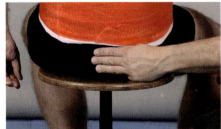

There are two or three finger's breadth between the distal border of the corset and the seating area

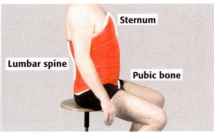

The corset supports the sternum, lumbar spine, and pubic bone: the three-point principle

598

Casts, Splints, and Support Bandages—Nonoperative Treatment and Perioperative Protection   Klaus Dresing, Peter Trafton

17.3   Removable corset using synthetic, combicast technique

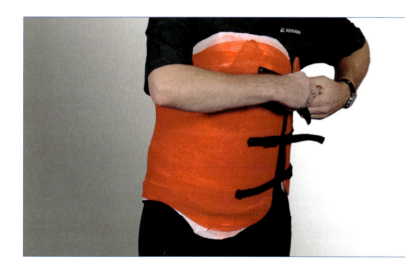

INDICATION

- Fracture of the lower thoracic spine
- Fracture of the lumbar spine

GOAL

- Stabilization of the spine

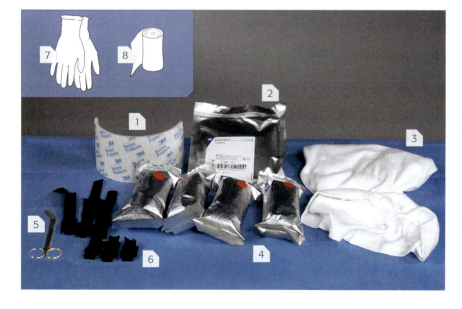

EQUIPMENT

1. Adhesive foam padding
2. Rigid synthetic splint 10 cm or 12.5 cm x 90 cm
3. Cut tube bandage or cast shirt
4. Semirigid casting tape 10 cm or 12.5 cm
5. Scissors
6. Velcro straps or rivet straps
7. Gloves
8. Elastic bandage

PERSONNEL

 or

17.3

TECHNIQUES

POSITIONING

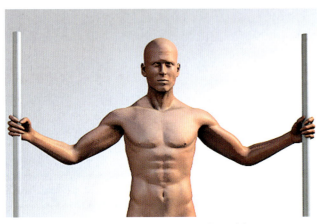

Stand the patient upright between supports if possible

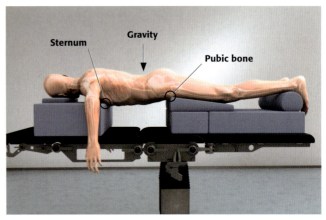

Sternum   Gravity   Pubic bone

If the patient requires anesthesia, place the patient in lordosis using the three-point principle

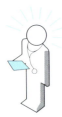

SPECIAL THINGS TO KEEP IN MIND

- Ensure the axillary fossa is free
- Free movement of the hips
- Three-point support: sternum, pubic bone, lumbar spine
- Be aware of the edges: padding of the edges
- Ventral window to allow normal food intake might be necessary in slim patients
- The caregiver should explain how best to remove and reapply the corset

Klaus Dresing, Jos Engelen

PROCEDURE

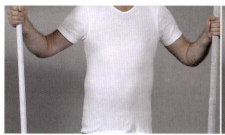

Apply a large tube bandage or cast shirt

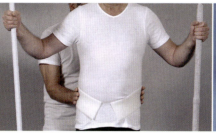

Apply adhesive foam padding to protect the iliac crests and the sternum

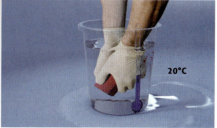

Submerge the semirigid casting tape in water for a few seconds, remove, and squeeze out excess water

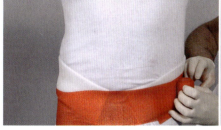

Apply the semirigid casting tape; start by covering the foam padding over the iliac crests

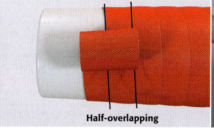

Half-overlapping

Continue the application, using the half-overlapping technique

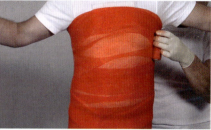

Extend the semirigid casting tape to cover the foam padding protecting the sternum

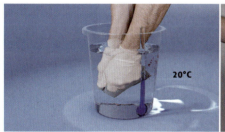

Submerge the rigid splint in water for a few seconds, remove, and squeeze out excess water

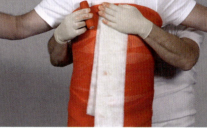

Apply the first rigid splint anteriorly, and hold it in place with another layer of semirigid casting tape

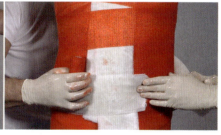

Apply a second rigid splint at the level of the iliac crest, and hold it in place with semirigid casting tape

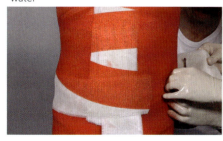

Trim the rigid splint; ensure that it does not completely encircle the body

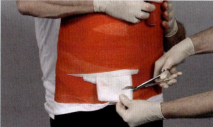

Trim the first rigid splint to the desired length

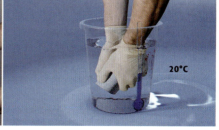

Submerge an elastic bandage in water; using a wet bandage accelerates the setting

17.3

TECHNIQUES

601

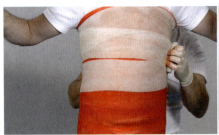

Apply the wet elastic bandage over the semirigid casting tape

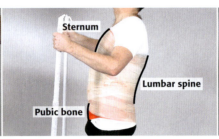

Ensure there is support of the sternum, lumbar spine, and pubic bone to create the required lordosis

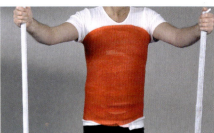

Remove the wet bandage after the corset has set

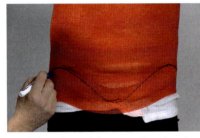

Mark the edges of the corset for trimming

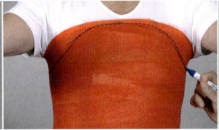

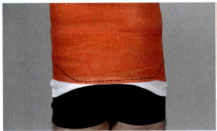

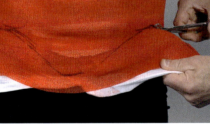

Ensure the axillae and the hips are free of material

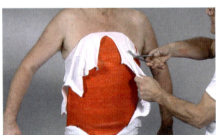

Trim the corset along the marked lines with the scissors

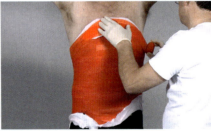

Ensure there is enough space around the axillae to allow free movement of the shoulders

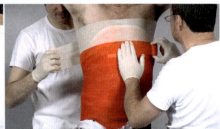

Cut the cast shirt free and fold it back over the corset

Apply another layer of wet semirigid casting tape to hold the edges of the cast shirt in place

Apply a wet elastic bandage to accelerate the final setting

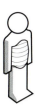

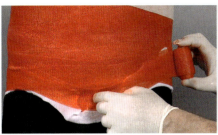

Repeat the procedure at the distal border of the corset

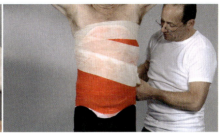

Remove the wet bandage after the corset has set

FINAL ASSESSMENT

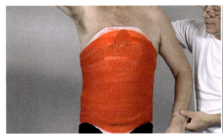

The axillae are completely free

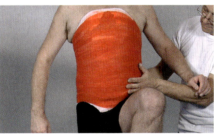

Free movement of the shoulders, hips and lower body is possible

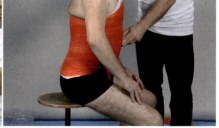

Hip flexion of at least 90° is possible to allow comfortable sitting

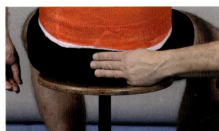

There are two or three finger's breadth between the distal border of the corset and the seating area

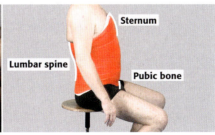

The corset supports the sternum, lumbar spine, and pubic bone: the three-point principle

SPLITTING AND REAPPLYING

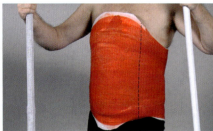

Mark the splitting line on the lateral side of the corset

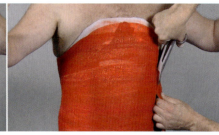

Split the corset using the cast scissors

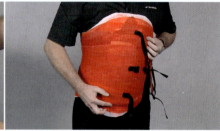

Velcro straps or rivet straps are applied to make opening and closing easier

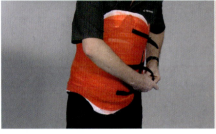

The patient can put on, or take off, the corset without any help

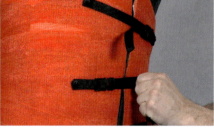

Adjustments can be made with the straps. The straps should be fully tightened to keep the corset in the correct position

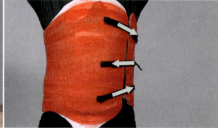

The alternate direction of the straps avoids any rotation of the corset

TECHNIQUES

18 Support bandages

18 Support bandages

Klaus Dresing, Jos Engelen

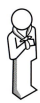

18.1   Collar and cuff bandage

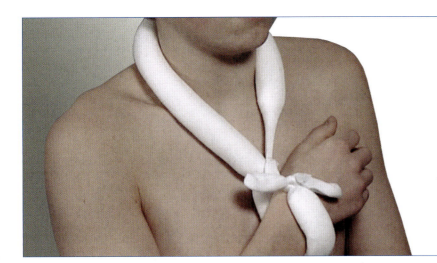

INDICATION

- Fracture of the supracondylar humerus in children
- Temporary immobilization in proximal diaphyseal humeral fractures and shoulder injuries in adults

GOAL

- Elbow in flexion to maintain position, depending on the extent of swelling

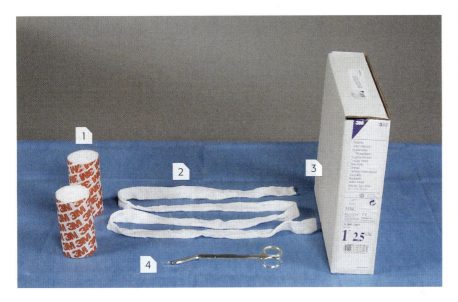

EQUIPMENT

1 Cast padding
2 Cut tube bandage
3 Tube bandage 2.5 cm in dispenser box
4 Scissors

PERSONNEL

POSITIONING

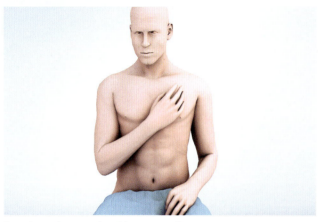

Seat the patient comfortably on a stool.

In children: elbow in greater than 90° flexion.

In adults: elbow in functional position (90° flexion).

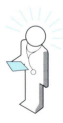

SPECIAL THINGS TO KEEP IN MIND

- Swelling
- Circulation
- Skin irritation under the axilla
- In adults: temporary immobilization only

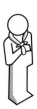

Klaus Dresing, Jos Engelen

PROCEDURE

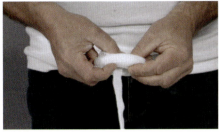

To make the collar and cuff, a tube bandage is rolled inside out

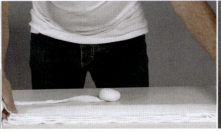

Eight layers of padding are laid out

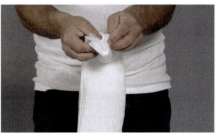

Fold the padding in half lengthways

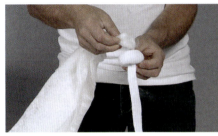

Insert the folded padding into the tube bandage

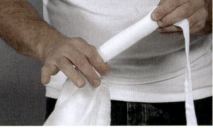

Roll out the tube bandage over the padding to make a padded roll

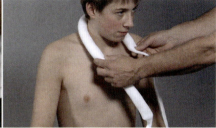

Place the padded roll around the neck of the patient

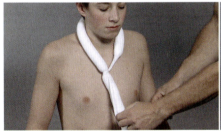

Make a knot in the padded roll to fix the sling

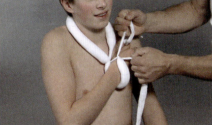

Bend the elbow and pass the padded roll around the wrist. Make a knot to fix the wrist in place

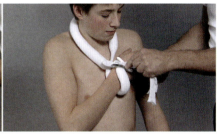

Trim the excess tube bandage with the scissors

FINAL ASSESSMENT

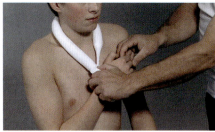

Check that the bandage is not too tight by taking the pulse

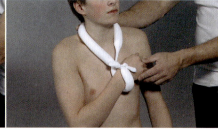

Check there is sufficient padding around the neck

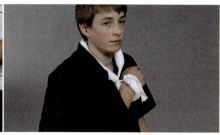

Important: As the material loses tension, it is necessary to adjust the collar and cuff after a few days

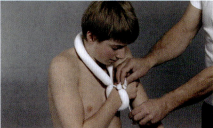

Adapt the flexion of the elbow to the amount of swelling. Loosen the knot and slide it up the padded roll

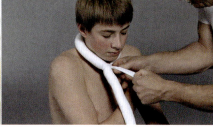

Retighten the knot at the desired position

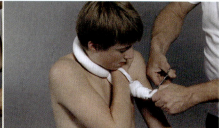

Roll back the tube bandage and trim the excess padding

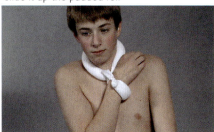

Retie the knot to hold the wrist at the desired position

Klaus Dresing, Jos Engelen

18.2   Clavicle bandage

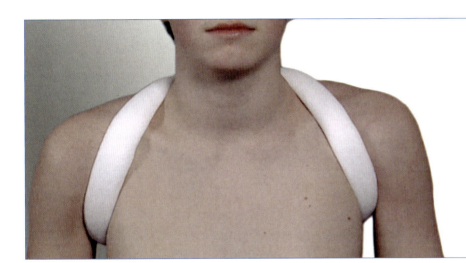

INDICATION

- Fracture of the clavicle

GOAL

- Retraction of both shoulders to prevent overlapping of the ends of the clavicular fracture

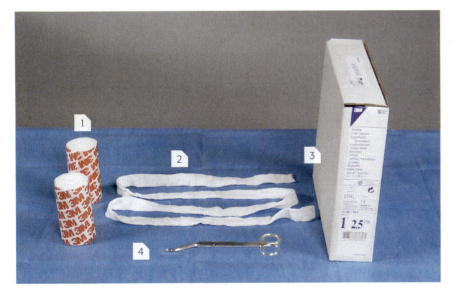

EQUIPMENT

1 Cast padding
2 Cut tube bandage
3 Tube bandage 2.5 cm in dispenser box
4 Scissors

PERSONNEL

18.2

TECHNIQUES

POSITIONING

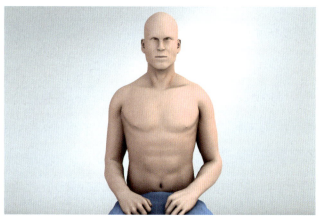

Seat the patient comfortably on a stool.
Place the affected limb hanging in the functional position.

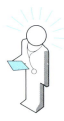

SPECIAL THINGS TO KEEP IN MIND

- Circulation
- Irritation of the brachial plexus
- Skin irritation under the axillae
- Beware of arm swelling due to reduced venous drainage

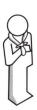

PROCEDURE

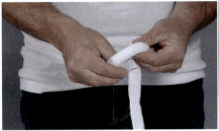

To make a clavicle bandage, a tube bandage is rolled inside out

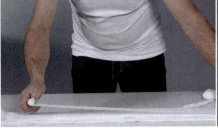

Eight layers of padding are laid out

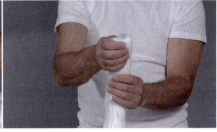

Fold the padding in half lengthways

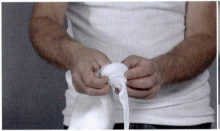

Insert the folded padding into the tube bandage

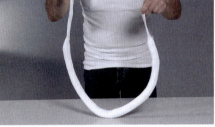

Roll out the tube bandage over the padding to make a padded roll

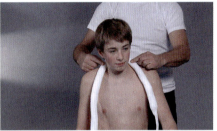

Place the padded roll around the back of the patient's neck and under both axillae. Extend the shoulders under slight tension

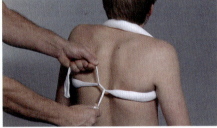

Tie the ends of the bandage together

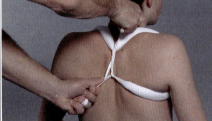

Pull together the sections behind the neck and the back to create more tension

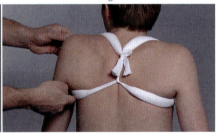

Tie together both sections between the shoulder blades

18.2

TECHNIQUES

FINAL ASSESSMENT

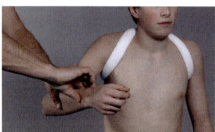

Check that the bandage is not too tight by taking the pulse

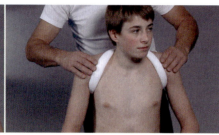

Check sensation in the upper extremities and skin irritation under the bandage

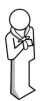
18.3   Gilchrist bandage

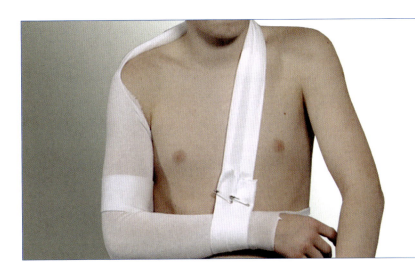

INDICATION

- Fracture of the proximal humerus
- Shoulder injuries

GOAL

- Stabilization of the proximal humerus and the shoulder

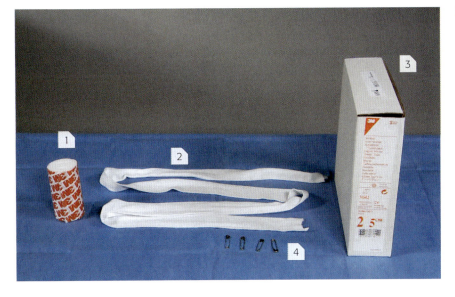

EQUIPMENT

1   Cast padding
2   Cut tube bandage
3   Tube bandage 5 cm in dispenser box
4   Safety pins

PERSONNEL

18.3

TECHNIQUES

POSITIONING

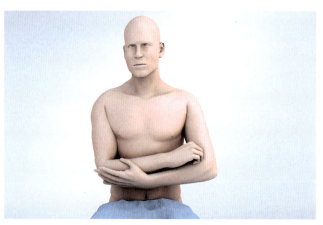

Seat the patient comfortably on a stool.
Place the affected limb hanging with 90° flexion in the elbow.

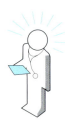

SPECIAL THINGS TO KEEP IN MIND

- Skin irritation under the axilla
- Circulation

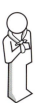

PROCEDURE

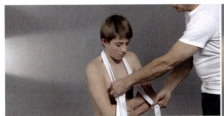

Select a tube bandage 3 to 4 times the length of the patient's arm. The length of the tube bandage may vary depending on the size of the patient's waist

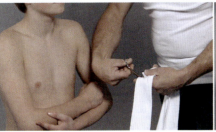

Make an opening in the middle of the tube bandage for the affected arm

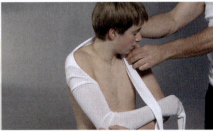

Slide the tube bandage over the affected arm and around the neck

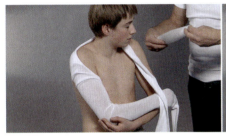

Fold the padding lengthways and insert into the tube bandage to prevent excessive pressure on the neck

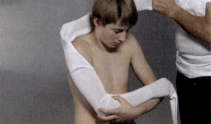

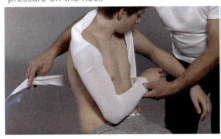

Make an opening in the tube bandage distally, to free the hand and allow movement of the fingers

The distal section of the tube bandage will be passed around the patient's back

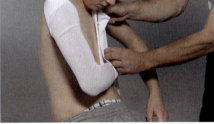

The proximal section of the tube bandage is made into a sling to support the forearm, and fixed with safety pins or clips

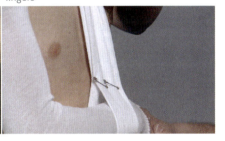

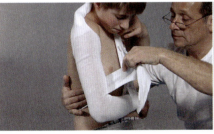

Wrap the distal section of the tube bandage around the body; it should pass between the body and the affected arm

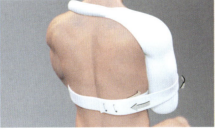

Wrap the tube bandage around the upper arm and fix in place dorsally with safety pins or clips

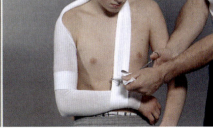

Trim the excess tube bandage with scissors

18.3

TECHNIQUES

FINAL ASSESSMENT

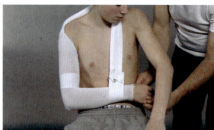

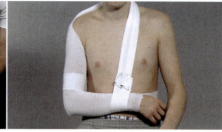

Ensure the forearm is supported.
Ensure there is free movement of the wrist

Check that the bandage is not too tight by taking the pulse. Check sensation in the upper extremities and skin irritation under the bandage

18.4   Wrist bandage

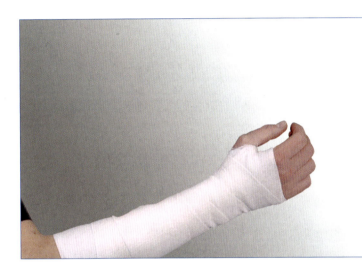

INDICATION

- Strain
- Sprain

GOAL

- Stabilization and pain relief

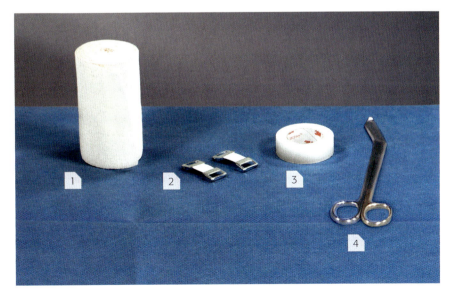

EQUIPMENT

1   Elastic bandage
2   Bandage clips
3   Surgical tape
4   Scissors

PERSONNEL

18.4

TECHNIQUES

POSITIONING

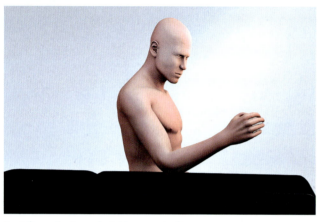

Seat the patient comfortably on a stool.
Place the affected limb on the table in a functional position.

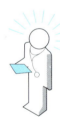

SPECIAL THINGS TO KEEP IN MIND

- A bandage of appropriate size is applied with the bandage roll always facing outward
- Bandages are normally applied in a pronated direction from distal to proximal
- The extremity should not be pulled in an extreme pronate or supinate position by the bandage
- Each diagonal turn needs to be fixed with a straight circular turn
- Be aware of an undiagnosed scaphoid fracture

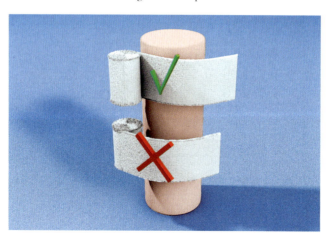

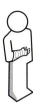

PROCEDURE

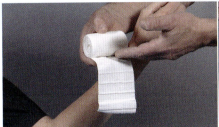

Ensure the bandage roll always faces outward

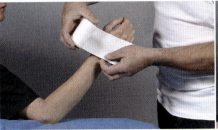

Begin laterally; the first wrap is diagonal towards the base of the thumb

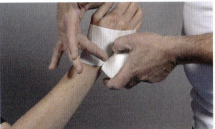

Wrap from the ulnar styloid process, over the hand and between the thumb and index finger

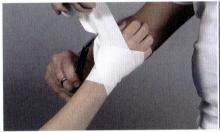

Cut halfway through the bandage, from proximal to distal, to avoid excessive folds between the thumb and index finger

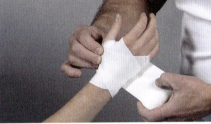

The next wrap follows the metacarpal heads, then after another cut, passes between the thumb and index finger

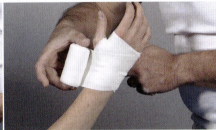

Wrap from lateral to the base of the thumb

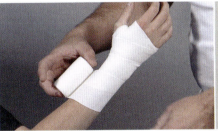

If the forearm is of uniform width, wrap from distal to proximal, using the half-overlapping technique

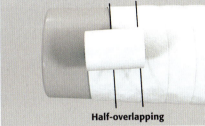

Half-overlapping

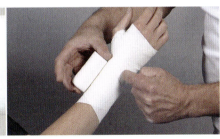

If the forearm is tapered, use the criss-cross technique up to the elbow

Criss-cross

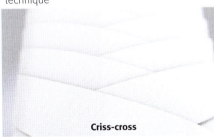

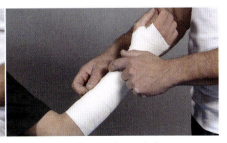

Keep the bandage close to the arm at all times

Secure the bandage with surgical tape or bandage clips at a place that does not irritate the patient

18.4

TECHNIQUES

FINAL ASSESSMENT

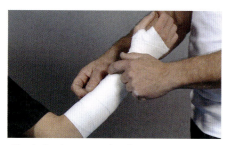

Circulation is not restricted

18.5 Elbow bandage

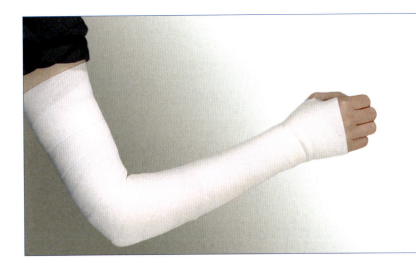

INDICATION

- Strain
- Sprain

GOAL

- Stabilization and pain relief

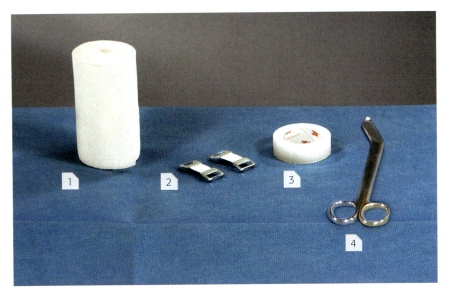

EQUIPMENT

1 Elastic bandage
2 Bandage clips
3 Surgical tape
4 Scissors

PERSONNEL

18.5

TECHNIQUES

POSITIONING

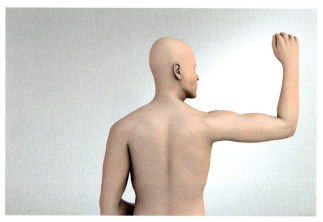

Seat the patient comfortably on a stool.
Place the elbow in 90° flexion.

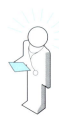

SPECIAL THINGS TO KEEP IN MIND

- A bandage of appropriate size is applied with the bandage roll always facing outward
- Bandages are normally applied in a pronated direction from distal to proximal
- The extremity should not be pulled in an extreme pronate or supinate position by the bandage
- Each diagonal turn needs to be fixed with a straight circular turn

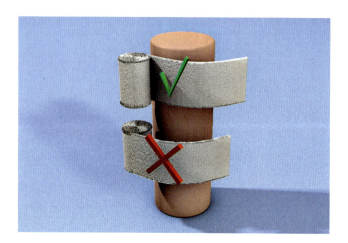

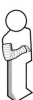

PROCEDURE

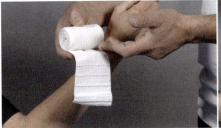

Ensure the bandage roll always faces outward

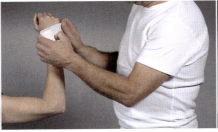

Begin laterally; the first wrap is diagonal towards the base of the thumb

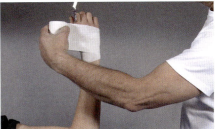

Wrap from the ulnar styloid process, over the hand and between the thumb and index finger

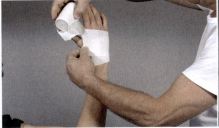

Cut halfway through the bandage, from proximal to distal, to avoid excessive folds between the thumb and index finger

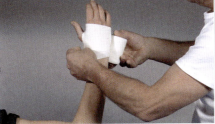

The next wrap follows the metacarpal heads, then after another cut, passes between the thumb and index finger

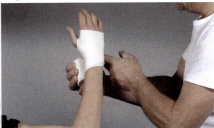

Wrap from lateral to the base of the thumb

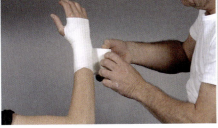

If the forearm is of uniform width, wrap from distal to proximal, using the half-overlapping technique

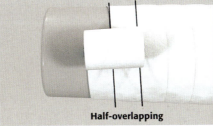

Half-overlapping

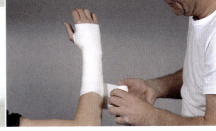

If the forearm is tapered, use the criss-cross technique

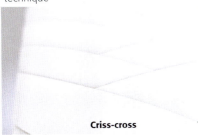

Criss-cross

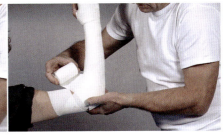

Use the figure-of-eight technique at the elbow to avoid an excessive amount of layers

Fix the figure-of-eight in place with circular wraps

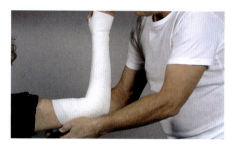

Secure the bandage with surgical tape or
bandage clips at the upper arm

FINAL ASSESSMENT

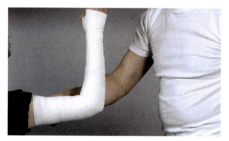

The elbow is in 90° flexion and circulation is
not restricted

Klaus Dresing, Jos Engelen

18.6 Ankle and foot bandage

18.6

TECHNIQUES

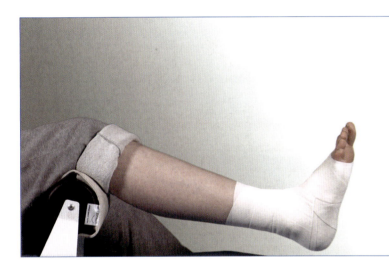

INDICATION

- Ankle sprain
- Instability of the ankle joint

GOAL

- Stabilization of the ankle joint

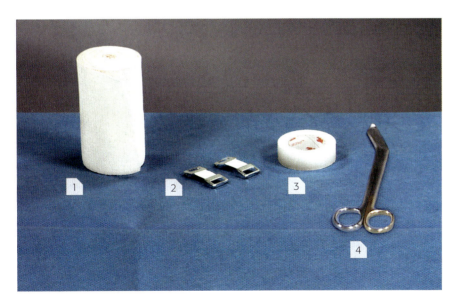

EQUIPMENT

1. Elastic bandage
2. Bandage clips
3. Surgical tape
4. Scissors

PERSONNEL

627

POSITIONING

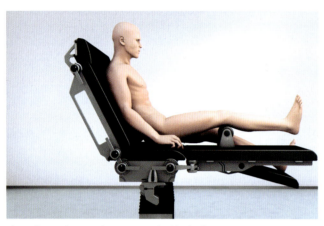

Place the patient supine or seated with the knee on a support.
Place the ankle in 90° flexion.

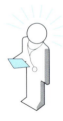

SPECIAL THINGS TO KEEP IN MIND

- A bandage of appropriate size is applied with the bandage roll always facing outward
- Bandages are normally applied in a pronated direction from distal to proximal
- The extremity should not be pulled in an extreme pronate or supinate position by the bandage
- Each diagonal turn needs to be fixed with a straight circular turn

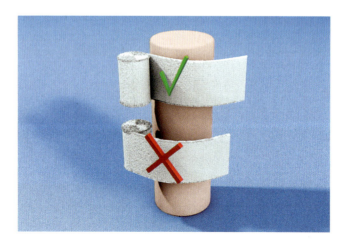

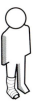

PROCEDURE

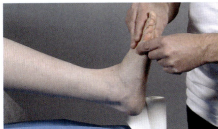

Avoid supination by wrapping the foot in pronation

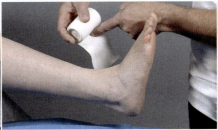

Ensure that the roll of bandage faces outward not inward

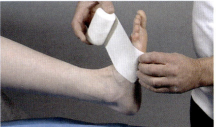

Start laterally and wrap once around the forefoot

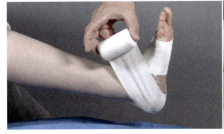

Pass the bandage diagonally over the heel and across the subtalar joint

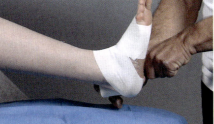

Pass the bandage over the medial malleolus

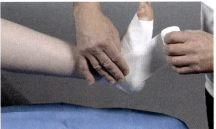

Pass the bandage over the Achilles tendon and diagonally beneath the foot

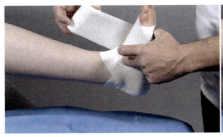

Secure the bandage on the lateral side with a finger and pass the bandage over the medial arch

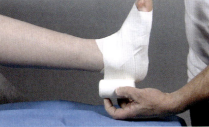

Pass the bandage across the lateral malleolus and the Achilles tendon

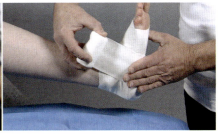

Pass the bandage beneath the foot to the lateral side; pull the lateral side of the foot up slightly

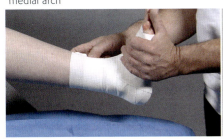

Wrap the lower leg, from distal to proximal, using the half-overlapping technique

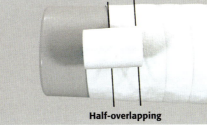

Half-overlapping

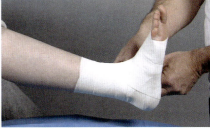

Now wrap the bandage from proximal to distal; wrap from lateral to medial across the medial malleolus

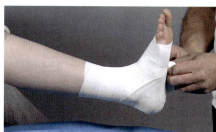

Pass the bandage over the Achilles tendon and diagonally beneath the foot

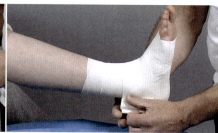

Pass the bandage across the foot and over the lateral malleolus and the Achilles tendon

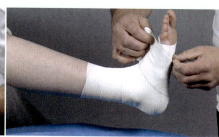

Pass the bandage beneath the foot and apply a circular wrap around the foot

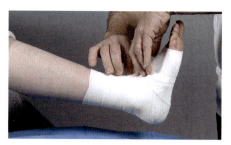

Wrap the remaining bandage over the Achilles tendon and secure with surgical tape or bandage clips

FINAL ASSESSMENT

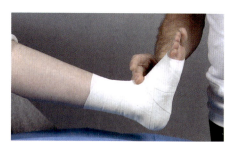

The circulation must not be restricted. The ankle joint is in 90° flexion

Casts, Splints, and Support Bandages—Nonoperative Treatment and Perioperative Protection   Klaus Dresing, Peter Trafton

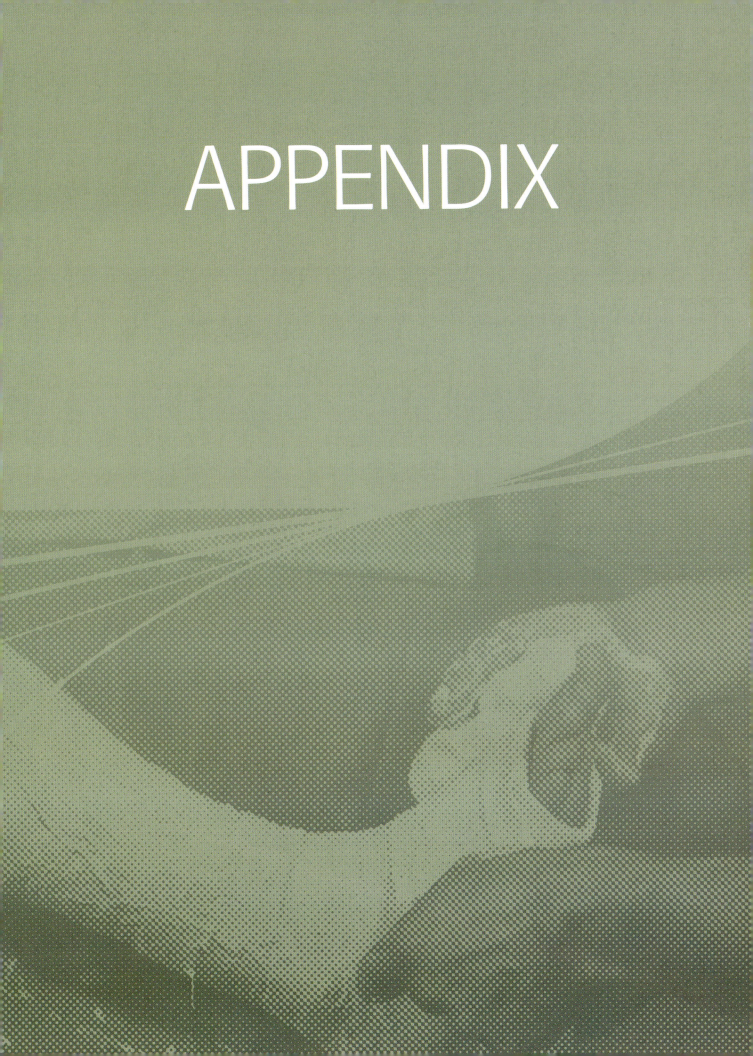

APPENDIX

Appendix

This document is available from AOTrauma and the Thieme Media Center website

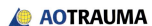 **AOTRAUMA**

Casts and Splints— Instructions for Patients

What is a cast?

A cast is a hard bandage wrapped around your arm or leg to support and protect an injury such as a broken bone, a sprain, or the site of an operation. The cast holds the injured area still and straight, protecting it during healing, and helps to relieve pain. A splint is a firm support, like a cast, but the hard part does not wrap all the way around your injured limb, allowing some room for swelling.

Casts and splints usually include padding or cushioning to protect the skin, the bones, and any nerves that are close to the surface. You must leave this padding where it is so the cast continues to protect you. Casts and splints should only ever be taken off or changed when advised by your doctor.

Your doctor has recommended a cast or splint as part of your treatment. But since each person and their medical problems are unique, the following information provides general instructions only on how best to look after your injury and your cast. However, if at any time you develop any of the warning signs described, or have any questions or worries, contact your doctor immediately.

Warning signs

You should contact your doctor immediately if you develop any of the following warning signs:

- Cast/splint is too tight
- Fingers or toes are swollen (a little is normal; a lot is bad)
- Numbness (loss of feeling) in fingers or toes
- Can't move fingers or toes
- Pain keeps getting worse
- "Hot spot" (burning and/or rubbing) under the cast.

Don't leave without written follow-up instructions from your doctor, including telephone number, address, and next appointment date.

How to prevent swelling

Your limbs usually swell following a serious injury. To reduce the swelling, rest and elevate the injured area above the level of your heart. An injured foot or ankle should be up on pillows while you are lying or sitting partially upright. Once elevated, gentle finger or toe motion is alright, but vigorous use may irritate the injured area, increasing swelling and pain.

Apply ice to the injured area using a waterproof bag. This helps relieve pain and swelling, even through the cast or bandage.

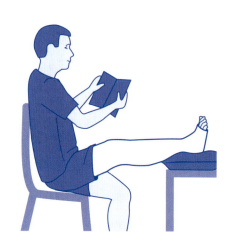

How to prevent stiffness

As soon as you can, completely bend and straighten the fingers/toes of your injured limb for a few seconds every hour while you are awake. Gentle stretching of the joints above the cast (elbow, shoulder, knee, hip) is also a good idea in most cases. Even if not injured, your shoulder especially can become stiff and uncomfortable if not used normally for long periods of time. If needed, use your other hand to help move limbs and joints through a full range of motion.

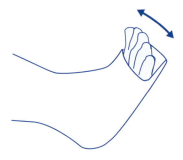

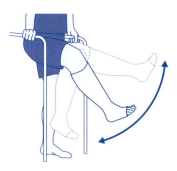

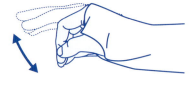

2

Casts and Splints—Instructions for Patients

634   Casts, Splints, and Support Bandages—Nonoperative Treatment and Perioperative Protection   Klaus Dresing, Peter Trafton

Walking on your cast

Some leg casts allow the patient to put weight on their leg or even to walk while wearing the cast (once it has completely dried). Walking casts may have an attached heel for this purpose, or be provided with a removable cast shoe. If your cast is not intended for walking you must obtain crutches or a walking frame, and learn how to use these safely. Check with your doctor for specific instructions.

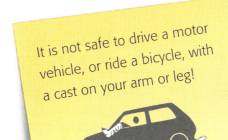

It is not safe to drive a motor vehicle, or ride a bicycle, with a cast on your arm or leg!

Taking care of your cast

While casts are made of strong material they can still be easily damaged, reducing their effectiveness. Follow these simple guidelines to keep your cast working properly.

- Keep your cast dry: Plaster casts "melt" if they get wet, and your skin can be harmed from wet padding. Always use a waterproof cover or heavy plastic bag when showering (no swimming or baths), and use a hair dryer set to a low temperature if it becomes damp. Contact your doctor if the cast becomes significantly wet.

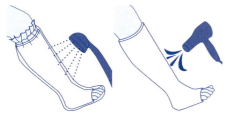

- Keep your cast clean: Avoid dirty or dusty places, beaches, fields, etc, and avoid activities that might soil your cast.
- Don't overheat your cast: If your cast is near a heater or fireplace it can become overheated and burn you.
- Don't put anything inside your cast: Sometimes your skin itches inside the cast. This can be relieved by applying an ice pack, or placing a hair dryer or vacuum cleaner against one of the ends of the cast to draw air through it and across your skin.

- Is my cast too tight? Casts should feel snug, but not too tight. Tightness develops from swelling inside the cast. Elevate and rest the limb. Eventually, the swelling decreases. If tightness does not improve, call your doctor promptly.
- Is my cast too loose? Sometimes, as healing progresses, the cast begins to feel loose. This can usually be checked by your doctor during a routine follow-up, but if the cast slides significantly up or down your limb it should be checked promptly.
- What if my cast gets soft or breaks? This can happen with any type of cast resulting in a cast that does not protect your injury well, or that irritates your skin, perhaps causing blisters or sores. Visit your doctor to get the cast repaired or replaced. If it's on your leg, stop walking on the cast and use crutches.
- How about jewelry and nail polish? Immediately after an injury, remove any rings, bracelets, and body piercings. Because of swelling, they can become too tight. Your doctor may ask you to remove nail polish or artificial nails.

3

Cast removal and recovery

Your cast will be removed with either scissors or a special cast saw that vibrates its way through the cast. Even though your injury has started to heal, the joints inside will become stiff, and muscles have become weaker. Skin and hair growth may change under the cast, but these usually resolve after cast removal. However, muscles and joints require several months of exercise and use before they have fully recovered.

Never remove your cast by yourself. You may injure yourself or disturb the healing process.

These instructions have been provided by orthopedic specialists with many years' experience treating patients with casts and splints. Following these simple instructions will help you to achieve the best possible result for your injury, and will help you get back to work and play as quickly and as safely as possible.

Since every patient and every injury is unique, you must obtain and follow your own doctor's advice.

The AO Foundation is a medically guided nonprofit organization led by an international group of surgeons specialized in the treatment of trauma and disorders of the musculoskeletal system.